The Interaction of Cancer and Host

The Interaction of Cancer and Host
Its Therapeutic Significance

MICHAEL F. A. WOODRUFF

M.D., D.Sc., M.S. (Melb.), F.R.C.S. (Engl. and Edinb.),
F.R.A.C.S., F.A.C.S. (Hon.), F.R.S.

EMERITUS PROFESSOR OF SURGERY
UNIVERSITY OF EDINBURGH, SCOTLAND

Grune & Stratton
A Subsidiary of Harcourt Brace Jovanovich, Publishers
New York   London   Toronto   Sydney   San Francisco

Library of Congress Cataloging in Publication Data

Woodruff, Michael F   A   Sir.
   The interaction of cancer and host.

   Bibliography:
   Includes index.
   1. Cancer—Immunological aspects. 2. Immunotherapy.
3. Carcinogenesis.   I. Title. [DNLM: 1. Neoplasm
invasiveness. 2. Neoplasm metastasis. 3. Neoplasms—
Immunology. 4. Neoplasms—Therapy. QZ200 W894i]
RC268.3.W66   616.99'4079   80-23645
ISBN 0-8089-1265-8

Grune & Stratton, Inc.
111 Fifth Avenue
New York, New York 10003

Distributed in the United Kingdom by
Academic Press, Inc. (London) Ltd.
24/28 Oval Road, London NW 1

Library of Congress Catalog Number 80-23645
International Standard Book Number 0-8089-1265-8

Printed in the United States of America

DEDICATED TO PROFESSOR H. J. EVANS

Director, Medical Research Council
Clinical Population and Cytogenetics Unit
Edinburgh, Scotland

*WITHOUT WHOSE "RESCUE OPERATION" MY RESEARCH
WOULD HAVE ENDED IN 1977 AND THIS BOOK
WOULD NOT HAVE BEEN WRITTEN*

CONTENTS

ACKNOWLEDGMENTS   xv

PREFACE   xvii

CHAPTER 1. METHODS OF INVESTIGATION

1.1 **The study of cancer in man**   1
    1.11   Methods   1
        1.111   Epidemiological investigations   1
        1.112   Study of patients treated by standard procedures   2
        1.113   Clinical therapeutic trials   4
    1.12   Ethical and other limitations   6
1.2 **The study of animal tumors** *in vivo*   7
    1.21   Autochthonous tumors   8
        1.211   Spontaneous tumors   8
        1.212   Experimentally induced tumors   9
    1.22   Transplanted tumors   10
    1.23   Choice of animal model   12
1.3 **The growth of human tumors in animals**   12
1.4 *In vitro* **methods**   13

CHAPTER 2. ORIGIN AND NATURE OF THE CANCER CELL

2.1 **Mechanisms of carcinogenesis**   15
    2.11   Carcinogenesis by chemicals   19
    2.12   Carcinogenesis by radiation   21
    2.13   Effect of trauma, and contact with films of plastic, metal, or glass   23

2.14   Viral carcinogenesis   24
    2.141   Experimental observations   24
    2.142   The role of oncogenic viruses in man   28
2.15   The effect of hormonal imbalance   31
2.16   Immunologically induced carcinogenesis   32
2.17   Genetic factors   33
2.2   Experimental inhibition of carcinogenesis   34
**2.3   Homeostatic mechanisms to prevent
the emergence of cancer cells**   37

CHAPTER 3.   STRUCTURE, GROWTH, AND FUNCTIONAL ACTIVITY OF TUMORS

3.1   Structure of tumors   40
    3.11   Tumor cells   42
        3.111   Chromosomal abnormalities   42
        3.112   Changes in intracellular and surface antigens   43
        3.113   Cell hybridization and the analysis
of malignancy   43
        3.114   Evidence of monoclonality   45
    3.12   Leukocytes and macrophages   47
    3.13   Supporting tissue. Angioneogenesis   49
3.2   Progression and regression of primary tumors   50
3.3   Invasion and metastasis   52
    3.31   Metastasis by lymphatics   52
    3.32   Metastasis by the bloodstream   54
    3.33   Metastasis by surface implantation   57
    3.34   Dormancy and regression of metastases   58
3.4   Growth curves   62
3.5   Cell population kinetics   66
3.6   Functional activity of tumors   70

CHAPTER 4.   THE RELATIONSHIP OF TUMOR AND HOST

4.1   The concept of antagonistic symbiosis   73
4.2   Response of tumors to normal controls   73
    4.21   Contact with neighboring structures and cells   74
    4.22   Chalones   74
    4.23   Antigen deletion   75
    4.24   Hormone-dependent tumors   75
4.3   Homeostatic mechanisms   78
4.4   The deleterious effect of cancer on the host   79
    4.41   General effects   79
    4.42   Effect on immunological and
para-immunological responsiveness   80

CHAPTER 5. IMMUNOLOGICAL AND PARA-IMMUNOLOGICAL MECHANISIMS AFFECTING TUMOR GROWTH

5.1 General Considerations   86

5.2 Tumor-associated antigens   86

    5.21   Tumor-associated transplantation antigens   88

       5.211   Chemically induced tumors   90

       5.212   Tumors of viral origin   91

       5.213   Plasmacytomas   93

       5.214   Other induced tumors   93

       5.215   Spontaneous tumors   94

    5.22   Antigens of primary autochthonous tumors   95

       5.221   Histological evidence of an immunological reaction to human tumors   95

       5.222   Tumor-bound immunoglobulin   96

       5.223   Xenogeneic immunization   97

       5.224   *In vitro* tests for humoral immunity   98

       5.225   *In vitro* tests for antibody-dependent cell-mediated cytotoxicity   99

       5.226   *In vitro* tests for lymphocyte-mediated cytotoxicity   100

       5.227   Migration and leukocyte adherence inhibition assays   102

       5.228   Mixed lymphocyte–tumor cell cultures (MLTC)   103

       5.229   Skin hypersensitivity reactions   104

    5.23   Oncofetal antigens (OFA)   105

       5.231 α-Fetoprotein (AFP)   106

       5.232   Carcinoembryonic antigen (CEA)   106

       5.233   Other human OFA detected with xenogeneic or allogeneic sera   107

       5.234   OFA immunogenic in isogeneic and autochthonous hosts   107

    5.24   Antigens of recurrent and metastatic tumors   110

    5.25   Further characterization of TAA   111

    5.26   Release of antigen by tumor cells   112

5.3 Regulation of the immune response to cancer   113

    5.31   Cytotoxic mechanisms   114

       5.311   Role of antiviral and cytotoxic antibody   114

       5.312   Antibody-dependent cell-mediated cytotoxicity (ADCC)   115

       5.313   Cell-mediated cytotoxicity not dependent on antibody   116

    5.32   Helper mechanisms   117

       5.321   Subclasses of T cells   117

       5.322   Cell cooperation   118

       5.323   MHC restriction   120

5.4 Para-immunological mechanisms   121

    5.41   Allogeneic inhibition   121

    5.42   Other forms of radioresistant inhibition   122

    5.43   Macrophage-mediated cytotoxicity   123

        5.431   Cytotoxic effect of macrophages
                    on tumor cells *in vitro*   123

        5.432   Macrophage-mediated cytotoxicity *in vivo*   125

    5.44   Cytotoxicity mediated by NK cells   127

        5.441   NK-cell activity in mice   128

        5.442   NK-cell activity in other species   131

        5.443   Role of NK cells in resistance to
                    tumors *in vivo*   132

5.5 Surveillance   133

    5.51   The hypothesis of Thomas and Burnet   133

    5.52   Criticism and countercriticism   134

        5.521   Escape from surveillance   134

        5.522   Immunostimulation   138

        5.523   Tumors arising in immunodeficient hosts   139

        5.524   Non-immunogenic tumors   144

        5.525   Monoclonality and immunoselection   145

    5.53   A more general hypothesis   146

CHAPTER 6.   THERAPEUTIC IMPLICATIONS OF THE HOST REACTION

6.1 Introduction   148

6.2 Therapeutic objectives   148

6.3 Limitations of current methods of treatment   149

    6.31   Surgical treatment and radiotherapy   150

    6.32   Chemotherapy   156

        6.321   Chemotherapy as the primary
                    or sole procedure   156

        6.322   Adjuvant chemotherapy   158

    6.33   Endocrinological procedures   161

6.4 New approaches to prophylaxis and treatment   162

CHAPTER 7.   THE EXPERIMENTAL BASIS OF IMMUNOTHERAPY

7.1 Introduction   164

7.2 Passive immunization with serum, plasma, or immunoglobulin   165

    7.21   Mechanisms of tumor inhibition and stimulation   165

        7.211   Inhibition of tumor growth   165

        7.212   Stimulation of tumor growth   166

    7.22   Isogeneic and allogeneic donors   166

    7.23   Xenogeneic donors   167

    7.24   Reasons for failure. Attempts to overcome them.   169

7.3   Immunochemotherapy   172

7.4   Passive immunization with cells and cell products   173

     7.41   Isogeneic and autochthonous cells   175
          7.411   Non-immune unstimulated cells   175
          7.412   Cells from immunized or
                  tumor-bearing donors   176
          7.413   Cells immunized or armed *in vitro*   176
          7.414   Non-specifically stimulated cells   178
     7.42   Allogeneic, semiallogeneic, and xenogeneic cells   179
          7.421   Recipients subjected to radiotherapy
                  or chemotherapy   179
          7.422   Semiallogeneic (P to Fl) cells without
                  immunosuppression   183
          7.423   Allogeneic or xenogeneic cells without
                  radiotherapy or chemotherapy   184
     7.43   Immune RNA   185

7.5   Non-specific immunopotentiation   187

     7.51   BCG and derivatives   188
          7.511   General immunological properties   190
          7.512   Systemic treatment of tumors with live BCG   192
          7.513   Live BCG mixed with tumor cell inoculum   193
          7.514   Intralesional injection of BCG   194
          7.515   Killed BCG and BCG derivatives   195
     7.52   *"Corynebacterium Parvum"* (CP)   197
          7.521   General immunological properties   197
          7.522   Systemic treatment of tumors with CP   205
          7.523   CP mixed with tumor cell inoculum   210
          7.524   Local injection of CP   210
          7.525   Mechanisms underlying the therapeutic
                  effect of CP   211
          7.526   CP derivatives   212
     7.53   Other bacterial preparations   213
     7.54   Viral infection   214
     7.55   Polynucleotides   215
          7.551   Immunopotentiation and macrophage
                  activation   215
          7.552   Interferon induction   218
          7.553   Cytotoxicity for tumor cells   219
          7.554   Effect on tumor growth *in vivo*   219
     7.56   Levamisole   220
     7.57   Anticoagulants and fibrinolytic agents   221
     7.58   Interferon   221
     7.59   Other agents   222

7.6   Specific active immunization   223

     7.61   Unmodified and irradiated cells. Cell extracts   223
     7.62   Neuraminidase-treated tumor cells   224
     7.63   Modified tumor cells and cross-reacting antigen   227
     7.64   Selected subpopulations of tumor cells   228

7.7 Combined immunotherapeutic procedures 229
7.71 Combined active specific and
non-specific immunotherapy 229
7.711 Immunopotentiating agents mixed
with tumor cells or antigen 231
7.712 Separate administration of specific and
non-specific agents 231
7.72 Combined passive and active immunotherapy 231
7.8 Procedures to eliminate blocking factors and suppressor cells 231
7.81 Thoracic duct drainage and plasmapheresis 232
7.82 Administration of antibody 232
7.821 Unblocking serum 232
7.822 Anti-plasma-cell and anti-immunoglobulin sera 233
7.823 Anti-I-J alloserum 233
7.824 Anti-idiotype antibody 233
7.83 Other procedures 233

CHAPTER 8. IMMUNOTHERAPY OF HUMAN CANCER

8.1 Introduction 234
8.2 Clinical trials 235
8.21 Passive immunotherapy with serum, plasma,
or immunoglobulin 237
8.211 Allogeneic serum or plasma 237
8.212 Xenogeneic serum 238
8.22 Immunochemotherapy 240
8.23 Passive immunization with cells and cell products 240
8.231 Bone marrow 241
8.232 Non-immune unstimulated lymphoid cells 242
8.233 Immune and non-specifically stimulated
lymphoid cells 244
8.234 Transfer factor 247
8.235 Immune RNA 249
8.24 Non-specific immunopotentiation 249
8.241 Coley's bacterial toxins 250
8.242 BCG and derivatives 251
8.243 "C. Parvum" (CP) 259
8.244 Other bacterial preparations 263
8.245 Viral infection 264
8.246 Polynucleotides 265
8.247 Levamisole 266
8.248 Anticoagulants and fibrinolytic agents 268
8.249 Phytohemagglutinin, polysaccharides, thymosin 269
8.24(10) Substances to evoke a local
hypersensitivity reaction 269
8.24(11) Hyperthermia 270
8.25 Active specific immunization 271
8.251 Early investigations 271

		8.252	Unmodified or irradiated tumor cells with or without adjuvants	272
		8.253	Enzyme-treated tumor cells	273
		8.254	Antigenic tumor extracts	273
		8.255	Xenogenized tumor cells	274
		8.256	Paternal cells or tissue in chorioncarcinoma	275

8.26   Combined non-specific and active specific immunotherapy   275

8.27   Plasmapheresis   280

8.3   Present position and future prospects   280

8.31   The present position   280

8.32   The way ahead   282

     8.321   Passive immunization   282

     8.322   Active immunotherapy   283

     8.323   Administration of interferon   284

     8.324   Other procedures   284

     8.325   Combined immunotherapy   284

References   287

Postscript   421

Index   423

ACKNOWLEDGMENTS

Ars longa, vita brevis The university surgeon becomes painfully aware of the truth of this maxim. There are so many exciting questions he wants to investigate, but the overriding demands of patients, coupled with teaching and administrative responsibilities, leave insufficient time for research, and it becomes increasingly difficult to keep abreast of scientific developments relevant to his clinical fields.

Encouraged by the example of senior colleagues in various parts of the world, I decided that after I retired from the practice of surgery I would, for a few years, devote myself to study and research—and, incidentally, write this book. The problem of finding a place in which to work was solved when Professor H. J. Evans, the director of the Medical Research Council's *Clinical and Population Cytogenetics Research Unit* at the Western General Hospital in Edinburgh, Scotland, offered to accommodate me in his unit. I am deeply grateful to Professor Evans and his colleagues for their warm welcome and for the privilege of working in this stimulating environment. The other problem—that of obtaining financial support—proved to be more difficult because the organizations that provide most of the money for cancer research in the United Kingdom did not seem to share my belief that a retired clinician can contribute significantly to biomedical research. I was, however, able to carry on for nearly two years with the help of the Nuffield Foundation, which agreed to support the immunological aspects of my work; the Wellcome Foundation, which supported a clinical trial; the Melville Trust; and a fund established in my old department by gifts from patients, until I was awarded a project grant by the Medical Research Council. I express my grateful thanks to these organizations and to former patients and their relatives who established the Woodruff Fund.

I am deeply indebted to Mrs. Margaret Doe, who has typed successive drafts of the manuscript of the book with unfailing patience and accuracy; to Dr. Felix Rapaport for many helpful suggestions; to S. Karger and Dr. Helen C. Nawts and to the *Lancet* and Dr. Lise Davignon, for permission to include the data presented in Table 1 and Tables 2 and 3 respectively; to various colleagues for permission to cite unpublished works; and to the staff of Grune & Stratton for their patience during the book's long gestation and for their excellent production. Last, but not least, I thank my wife, who has maintained my collection of several thousand reprints, checked references, read and criticized the manuscript, helped to correct the proofs, and provided much needed encouragement when it looked as if the book would never be finished.

PREFACE

Not so long ago it was widely believed and taught that malignant tumors are, as Ewing (1940) expressed it, autonomous new growths of tissue. The precise meaning which different people attach to *"autonomous"* is not always entirely clear, but in general the term seems to imply, firstly, that tumors are not influenced by any of the factors that control the growth and equilibrium of normal tissues, and, secondly, that no special homeostatic mechanisms, even of the most rudimentary kind, have evolved for controlling carcinogenesis and tumor growth.

Today the dogma of autonomy in its extreme form seems untenable in the light of evidence (to be reviewed in detail later) that malignant tumors occasionally regress or reappear suddenly after a long period of latency; that some tumors at some stage in their life history are influenced by hormonal stimulation or lack of stimulation or other factors that influence the growth of normal tissues; and that some tumor cells carry antigenic determinants or other surface markers that can trigger homeostatic mechanisms. It may, however, pertinently be asked whether, except perhaps in a few rare special cases, the host reaction has any decisive effect on the development of a tumor and what, if any, are the therapeutic implications of the interaction of tumor and host.

Neither the tumor biologist, who often knows little of the clinical features of human cancer, nor the clinician, who has often for one reason or another abandoned the struggle to familiarize himself with modern developments in tumor biology, is well placed to answer these questions single-handedly. What is required is a concerted effort by people in each camp and by those with a foothold, however precarious, in both, based on free communication and mutual understanding. It is hoped that this book, addressed to people of all disciplines who are concerned with the problem of cancer, will help to promote such understanding.

In any book about cancer, questions of terminology arise. Faced with the alternatives of accepting some redundancy or attempting to translate the publications cited into the terminology which I myself prefer, I have opted for the former. Throughout the book, therefore, the words tumor and neoplasm are used synonomously. They refer to both benign and malignant lesions, but since we shall be concerned primarily with malignant conditions the term tumor will often be used in this restricted sense when it seems clear from the context what is intended. When this is not clear the appropriate qualification will be added; alternatively, malignant neoplasms, whatever their origin, will be referred to collectively as cancer.

Among clinicians it is quite common, and indeed etymologically correct, to restrict the term "tumor" to neoplasms in which a localized swelling exists or is in process of developing, but many biologists do not follow this practice; where such a qualification seems necessary, therefore, the term "solid tumor" will be used. The terms "malignant lymphoma" and "lymphatic leukemia" are sometimes used interchangeably by tumor biologists; in clinical practice, however, malignant lymphoma includes, but is not synonymous with, lymphatic leukemia, and this usage will be adhered to throughout the book.

The meaning attached to terms like "carcinoma" and "sarcoma", which specify the type of tissue in which a tumor originated, conform to generally accepted usage. Agents that induce malignant tumors, which in the writer's view should be termed "oncogens," are so often referred to as carcinogens that we shall use these terms synonymously.

The Interaction of Cancer and Host

1
Methods of Investigation

Tumor biology can be studied as, for example, number theory can be studied, for its own sake, without thought of possible practical applications; cancer engenders such fear, however, and causes so much misery to so many people that for most investigators the ultimate objective in cancer research is to discover more effective ways of preventing and treating human cancer. To suggest that this can be achieved solely by laboratory experiments is to suggest that one can have Hamlet without the Prince: the etiology and natural history of human cancer can be established only be observing human populations and individual patients; the comparative value of different forms of treatment only by clinical trial. Moreover, what McQuarrie (1944) has aptly called *the experiments of nature,* which daily confront clinicians, have provided key clues leading to many important fundamental discoveries, not least in the field of tumor biology (Haddow, 1971). On the other hand, the difficulties inherent in clinical research, and the ethical and other limitations to which it is subject, are such that it can never be completely self-sufficient but must be based on controlled laboratory experiments in animals and *in vitro.* These permit the study in depth of phenomena revealed by clinical observation and provide a rational basis for planning new clinical investigations.

1.1   THE STUDY OF CANCER IN MAN

1.11   Methods

The methods available for the study of cancer in man include:

1. Epidemiological investigations.
2. Studies of cancer patients treated by standard procedures.
3. Clinical trials of new methods of treatment.

1.111   EPIDEMIOLOGICAL INVESTIGATIONS

Epidemiological investigations are concerned with the incidence and clinical behavior of tumors of various kinds, and the death rate associated with them, in relation

1

to such factors as the patient's age, sex, family history, ethnic group, associated genetic markers, geographical location, occupation, diet, smoking and other addictions, and contact with other people who have, or have had, similar tumors and also with animals.

Many epidemiological studies involve comparisons among patients in different regions or countries; others are concerned with groups of patients collected at different times in the same region, or even the same hospital.

Caution is required in interpreting epidemiological data, particularly when such data are drawn from diverse sources, because they are greatly influenced by such variables as the availability and quality of primary medical care, and of the hospital and laboratory services, and the proportion of patients certified as dying from cancer in whom the diagnosis is confirmed, or established for the first time, at autopsy. Despite this, epidemiological investigations have provided important information concerning the etiology of some human tumors (2.1) and are beginning to throw some light on the question of whether homeostatic mechanisms (4.3) play any significant role in relation to cancer in man.

1.112   STUDY OF PATIENTS TREATED BY STANDARD PROCEDURES

Studies of patients presenting for, and receiving, standard forms of treatment are based on clinical examination; radiological examination including computerized axial tomography, lymphangiography, and radioisotope scans; thermography or more elaborate procedures for measuring the amount of heat produced by an accessible tumor (Gautherie, Armand, and Gros, 1975); biochemical hematological, and immunological investigations; and histological examination of specimens of the tumor and related lymph nodes obtained by biopsy, at operation, or at autopsy.

It would seem particularly important to compare the results of such investigations in patients who respond well to treatment and those who do not. At present, apart from attempts to correlate histological findings with clinical behavior, this is a rather neglected area of cancer research.

In interpreting the findings, due weight must be given to the resolving power of the methods used. Thus, for example, the proportion of patients with breast cancer who are reported as presenting with evidence of skeletal metastases will be much higher in hospitals which routinely perform bone scans than in those which rely solely on routine radiography (Galasko, 1969, 1975; Citrin et al., 1976; El-Domeiri and Shroff, 1976); computerized tomography is a more sensitive way of detecting pulmonary metastases than conventional chest radiography and whole lung tomography (Muhm, Brown, and Crowe, 1977); lymphangiography may demonstrate metastases in lymph nodes (Fuchs, Davidson, and Fisher, 1969; Ariel, 1974); and detailed studies of the cellular content of tumors (3.1), and of cell population kinetics (3.5), will yield information which is unobtainable by routine histological examination.

Immunological investigations are of particular interest in relation to the study of the interaction of tumor and host, and the extent to which this may be modified by treatment. The results will be discussed later (4.42; Chapter 5), but the main methods used are listed below:

1.   Investigation of the patient's general level of immunological and para-immunological responsiveness (4.42).

(1) Determination of serum levels of immunoglobulin (Ig) classes and sub-
     classes.
(2) Study of the primary and secondary responses to a variety of antigens.
(3) Study of cutaneous delayed-type hypersensitivity to recall antigens (i.e.,
     antigens which many patients are likely to have encountered previously)
     and new antigens.
(4) Determination of the number of T, B, and null lymphocytes in blood and
     tissues, and also the proportion of different categories of T lymphocytes,
     by means of their surface markers.
(5) Study of the response of the patient's lymphocytes *in vitro* to phytohem-
     agglutinin (PHA) and other mitogens.
(6) Study of the capacity of the patient's lymphocytes to mount a graft-ver-
     sus-host (GVH) reaction in animals.
(7) Studies of macrophage function, including phagocytic activity, response
     of macrophages to chemotactic stimuli *in vitro,* accumulation of macro-
     phages at inflammatory sites, and serum levels of lysozyme.
(8) Studies of polymorphonuclear leukocytes.

2. Investigation of tumor-associated antigens and of the patient's capacity to react
    immunologically or para-immunologically against his tumor (5.2).

(1) Assay of antibody in the patient's serum which reacts with autochthon-
     ous tumor cells, or established tumor cell lines, as shown by cytotoxicity,
     immunofluorescence, complement fixation, or immune adherence (5.21;
     5.224).
(2) Tests for antibody-dependent cell-mediated cytotoxicity (ADCC), using
     the patient's serum, autochthonous tumor cells, or allogeneic cell lines as
     targets, and various kinds of effector cells (5.225).
(3) Assay of immune complexes in the patient's serum (5.521).
(4) Detection and characterization of cell-bound Ig (5.222).
(5) Study of cutaneous delayed-type hypersensitivity to antigenic tumor ex-
     tracts (5.229).
(6) Study of mixed cultures of tumor cells and the patient's lymphocytes
     (5.228).
(7) Study of the effect of tumor extracts on leukocyte and macrophage mi-
     gration *in vitro* (5.227)
(8) Study of cell-mediated immunity *in vitro,* using the patient's lymphocytes
     as effector cells and autochthonous tumor cells or allogeneic tumor cell
     lines as targets (5.226).
(9) Study of *in vitro* cytotoxicity for tumor cells mediated by macrophages
     (5.431) and NK cells (5.442).
(10) Assay of carcinoembryonic antigen (CEA), α-feto protein, and other sub-
      stances which occur also in fetal tissues, in the patient's serum (5.23).

There have in addition been some studies of autotransplants (Grace and Kondo,
1958; Southam and Brunschwig, 1961; J. M. Howard, 1963) and allotransplants
(Southam, Moore, and Rhoads, 1957; Itoh and Southam, 1963; Levin *et al.,* 1964;
Southam, 1968) of human tumors. It was considered at the time by those who performed these experiments that, with careful monitoring, there would be little danger
to the volunteers who participated, but the report of one case in which a melanoma allo-

transplant proliferated and disseminated in the recipient with resulting death (Scanlon, Hawkins, Fox, and Smith, 1965) shows that this is not necessarily the case, and it would be difficult to justify further experiments of this kind. The situation is of course quite different when non-viable (for example, heavily irradiated) tumor cells are transplanted for therapeutic purposes (8.25).

It has been suggested that in assessing the response to treatment a distinction should be drawn between the response of the tumor and the response of the patient, and some standard criteria for assessing the response of the tumor in patients with cancer of the breast have been proposed (British Breast Group, 1974). Insofar as this facilitates valid comparison of data from different centers it is to be welcomed, but it is important to be clear about the precise connotation of the word tumor in this context. If it denotes a particular palpable lump, which may or may not have been biopsied, or a particular shadow in a radiograph, then the proposed criteria can be applied provided due allowance is made for observer error (Yorkshire Breast Cancer Group, 1977), but such lumps and shadows always contain a component of non-neoplastic cells, and sometimes we do not know whether a palpable lump in relation to a tumor—for example, a palpable axillary lymph node in a patient with breast cancer—contains any neoplastic cells at all. It would seem wise, therefore, to avoid trying to draw a rigid distinction between the response of the patient and the response of the tumor, but to distinguish rather between objective criteria and those which are, to a greater or lesser extent, subjective.

One parameter which is absolutely clear cut is the length of survival from the start of treatment. This will of course vary greatly with the stage of the disease when treatment was begun, so that there is no escaping the difficult task of trying to develop standard staging criteria. Survival data are often expressed in terms of the proportion of patients alive after some given time, often five years, from the start of treatment. Metcalf (1974) has usefully drawn attention to the fact that since the proportion of survivors can often be expressed as an exponential function of the time since the start of treatment, or as the sum of two exponential functions, it is possible, and more informative, to use the half time $t_{1/2} = 0.693 /k$, derived from the regression of survival on time expressed by the equation

$$\ln Y = a - bX$$

where Y is the number (or percentage) of survivors, X the time in years, a, b are constants ($a = \ln Y_0, b = k$), Y_t the value of Y when $X = t$, and

$$k = \frac{1}{t} \ln \frac{Y_0}{Y_t} = \frac{2.303}{t} \log \frac{Y_0}{Y_t}$$

Other statistical methods applicable to survival time studies are discussed by Kaplan and Meier (1958) and Gehan (1965, 1975), and one particular method, termed the log rank test, is described in detail by Peto et al. (1976, 1977).

1.113 CLINICAL THERAPEUTIC TRIALS

The clinical trial of new methods of treatment, without which therapeutics would not advance, imposes a heavy burden of responsibility on those who undertake it. In the first place, patients may be exposed to unforeseen risks. Secondly, erroneous conclusions, if published, may result in serious harm to other people suffering from the same disease as those in the trial, either because useless or harmful treatment is prescribed or because treatment which might have been effective is withheld. It is therefore extremely important to design clinical trials in such a way that these dangers are minimized (London Hospital Clinical Trials Unit, 1977).

It is customary to distinguish three stages in the clinical assessment of a new form of treatment, and to designate trials appropriate to these stages as Phase I, Phase II, and Phase III trials, respectively (Staquet, 1973; Union Internationale Contre le Cancer, 1974; Forbes, 1977a, 1977b).

A Phase I trial is a pilot study to assess the feasibility of a new method of treatment suggested by laboratory and animal studies, and to provide information about dosage and toxicity. It is normally conducted in patients with advanced disease for whom standard treatment has little to offer. If the new treatment appears feasible, and free from unacceptable complications, a further pilot study (Phase II) may be undertaken in a small number (e.g., 15–30) of patients, to decide whether or not the therapeutic effect is sufficient to warrant setting up a large scale (Phase III) trial. Phase II trials are often undertaken in patients with advanced disease, but if the disease is so advanced as to virtually preclude the possibility of any demonstrable therapeutic effect the trial will be useless. It is a moot question whether or not to use randomized controls (*vide infra*) in Phase II trials (see Staquet and Sylvester, 1977).

A Phase III trial should be designed, in the light of all available evidence from animal experiments and earlier clinical trials, to answer a specific question concerning the efficacy of one particular agent, or of a group of agents combined in a rational way on the basis of data concerning their mode of action and efficacy when used alone. Empirical attempts to win a therapeutic jackpot are unlikely to pay off.

In Phase III trials properly randomized controls and efficient methods of statistical analysis should be used whenever possible because it is then much easier to draw reliable conclusions than it is when survival and other data from patients receiving a new form of treatment are compared with data from patients previously treated in other ways (so-called historical controls), or from a non-random sample of patients treated simultaneously in the same or another hospital (Wood, Gillis, and Blumgart, 1976; Pocock, 1977). The value of randomized trials was established by the British Medical Research Council's (1948) trial of streptomycin in tuberculosis, and this has served as a model for many subsequent trials (Hill, 1963); more recently, statistical guidelines for the design and conduct of such trials have been put forward by Peto *et al.* (1976, 1977), with particular reference to the use of life tables and the log rank test. If these procedures are used, the most usual, and as a rule the most useful, end point is length of survival from the day of randomization, but other end points, such as length of remission after a course of chemotherapy, or the period of freedom from local recurrence and manifest metastasis after surgical excision of a primary tumor or radiotherapy, may be used instead. Of course, as Powles (1976) has emphasized, the fact that a patient is alive when the results are analyzed does not exclude the possibility of his dying later as a direct result of his tumor, and the chances of this happening are clearly greater the earlier the analysis is made.

Every attempt should be made to admit all the patients likely to be needed in as short a time as possible to avoid the situation which may otherwise arise in which a difference between treated and control patients, or between two treatment groups, is sufficient to make one reluctant to continue with one particular regimen but insufficient to carry conviction throughout the world if the trial is terminated at this stage and the results are subsequently published (Woodruff, 1963). This is likely to necessitate multi-center trials, and the logistic and psychological problems which this entails must be overcome (Woodruff, 1977a, 1977b).

To avoid unconscious bias by doctor or patient an attempt is sometimes made to devise control treatments, sometimes referred to as *placebos,* which resemble in form the treatment being tested, so that neither doctor nor patient knows who is getting what. Such double blind trials are often hard to arrange because in many cases the treatment involves procedures such as repeated intravenous injection, or causes side effects, which it seems unreasonable to inflict on control patients, but in practice it should not, and usually does not, matter much if both a patient and the doctor responsible for his care know that he is receiving special treatment, provided that some independent person who does not know this is responsible for assessing the patient's condition at follow-up examinations. The results of the trial should be monitored by sequential analysis so that large differences do not pass unnoticed, but, as a further precaution against bias, should not be communicated to participants until the end of the trial unless such differences are detected.

1.12 Ethical and Other Limitations

The study of cancer in man is limited by the number of patients with particular kinds of tumor available for study, by the heterogeneity of different populations in respect of their genetic constitution and the environment in which they live, and, most importantly, by ethical constraints (Woodruff, 1970).

Some procedures are clearly so dangerous that their trial in man is never justifiable. It would, for example, be unthinkable to study carcinogenesis by deliberately exposing people to agents which are known to be highly carcinogenic in animals or in people who have been exposed to them accidentally. Conversely, there are procedures which have already proved so efficacious that it would be unjustifiable to withhold them from particular groups of patients in order to obtain further evidence for statistical analysis unless there was insufficient material to treat more than a small number of patients, as was the case in the Medical Research Council trial of streptomycin mentioned in the previous section.

These extreme situations are far from typical, and much more commonly the questions to be faced are whether it is justifiable to withhold one form of treatment which is moderately effective in order to assess another which might turn out to be either better or worse, and whether the difference in response to two forms of treatment, reported by others or revealed by a trial in progress, is sufficient to make a further trial, or continuation of a trial in progress, unjustified. Such dilemmas are sometimes unavoidable, and each case must then be decided on its merits in relation to some accepted ethical standard, as, for example, that embodied in the Code of Ethics of the World Medical Association (1964, 1975). Often, however, the problem would not have arisen if a properly designed trial had been undertaken in the first instance (British Medical Journal, 1977a).

A more difficult problem is what to say to patients when they are invited to participate in a trial. Consider, for example, a trial of some form of adjuvant therapy (6.321) following operation for an apparently localized tumor. There are four possibilities to consider (Woodruff, 1976):

1. Undertake a properly randomized trial but do not tell patients that this is being done. This is surely ethically wrong, and has the practical disadvantage that many patients in the group (or groups) given adjuvant therapy are likely to drop out.

2. Assign patients by randomization to control and adjuvant therapy groups *before* obtaining their agreement to participate in the trial. This is often done, but is statistically invalid because some of the patients assigned to the adjuvant therapy groups will almost certainly decline to participate if they do not like the option they have drawn, and the remainder cannot therefore be regarded as a truly random sample of the population.

3. Inform patients in advance that a randomized trial is being undertaken and explain what this means. Describe the various forms of treatment being tested and their possible side effects. The disadvantage is that inviting a patient to participate in a trial of adjuvant therapy implies that the doctor considers that there is a risk of recurrence after operation, and, if adjuvant therapy is liable to cause unpleasant symptoms or serious inconvenience to the patient (e.g., admission to hospital every few weeks for an intravenous infusion), that he regards this risk as appreciable. Some patients may not realize that their tumor may recur or, what is more likely, will not want to be reminded of this possibility; others, with greater insight, may feel frustrated if, after agreeing to participate in the trial, they find themselves assigned to an "operation only" group. To meet this last objection one can prescribe a placebo (1.113). In some types of trial this may be a useful maneuvre, for example, when one is comparing the effect of different routes of administration of the same drug, since some patients can be given the drug by the first route and the placebo by the second, and others *vice versa*. When, however, one wants to compare the effect of a particular drug or combination of drugs with no treatment it is often difficult to conceal from both doctors and patients which patients are receiving the supposedly active drug and which the placebo (Hill, Nunn, and Fox, 1976; Lancet, 1976), and in this event administration of a placebo seems pointless.

4. Undertake a non-randomized trial. This, despite its disadvantages from the point of view of statistical analysis, is at least better than a phoney trial which purports to be randomized but, in fact, is not.

Of these possibilities only the last two seem to merit serious consideration. If the third is chosen it is important to restrict the choice of patients invited to participate to those whom it is considered will not suffer psychologically as a result of the invitation. This selection, provided it is carried out before random assignment to the various treatment groups, does not invalidate the trial as regards statistical analysis. It does impose a restriction on the conclusion to be drawn if there is a significant difference in survival between two or more of the treatment groups in that instead of being able to say that this difference holds good for all patients presenting for treatment one must add the qualification that it has been demonstrated only in respect of patients who were considered to have sufficient insight to be invited to participate in the trial and who accepted this invitation. In practice, however, this limitation is unlikely to be of much consequence.

1.2 THE STUDY OF ANIMAL TUMORS *IN VIVO*

The study of tumors in animals is not subject to the ethical restrictions which limit the study of cancer in man. This is not to say that no ethical problems arise. They are, however, of a different order, and many procedures which would be totally unacceptable in people are rightly regarded as reasonable in experimental animals. For those who demur the case has been argued elsewhere (Woodruff, 1970). But to what extent can animal tumors be regarded as valid models of human cancer, and what weight can be attached to the data they provide when planning new clinical investigations? To attempt to answer these questions we must examine critically various experimental systems and the extent to which they conform to the clinical situation.

1.21   Autochthonous Tumors

An *autochthonous tumor* is a tumor growing in the animal (or patient) in which it originated, and this animal is termed the *autochthonous host.* Such tumors may have developed undisturbed, but the term autochthonous is still used even if the tumor has been removed and replaced in the autochthonous host, either immediately or after being maintained in tissue culture or stored at low temperature.

A distinction is usually drawn between autochthonous tumors which have arisen spontaneously and those induced experimentally with radiation, chemical carcinogens, oncogenic viruses, or other means. This distinction, however, is essentially an operational one and does not necessarily reflect important biological differences, since exposure to carcinogenic agents can occur "accidentally," i.e., without any deliberate effort on the part of the experimenter.

1.211   SPONTANEOUS TUMORS

It is convenient to distinguish three categories of operationally spontaneous tumors, since the spectrum of immunological and other properties which they exhibit may be somewhat different:

1. Tumors arising in domestic and farm animals and in non-inbred laboratory animals.
2. Tumors arising in inbred strains of laboratory animals in which there is a high incidence of tumors of the kind in question.
3. Tumors arising in inbred strains of laboratory animals in which the incidence of tumors of the kind in question, or of all tumors, is low.

Spontaneous tumors occur in many species of domestic and farm animal (Lancet, 1968; Cotchin, 1976; Owen, 1977); examples include mammary and skin carcinomas, melanomas, and sarcomas of various kinds in dogs; leukemia in cats; leukoses and sarcomas in birds; squamous cell carcinomas in cattle; and melanomas in horses. There have been numerous epidemiological studies with tumors of this kind (Cotchin, 1976), and these have yielded important information concerning, *inter alia,* the role of oncogenic viruses in avian leukoses and sarcomas (Ellerman and Bang, 1908; Rous, 1910b, 1911; Payne, 1977) and feline leukemia (Jarrett *et al.,* 1973); exposure to solar ultraviolet light in bovine squamous cell carcinoma of the eyelid (Anderson and Skinner, 1961); hormonal factors in canine mammary cancer (Hamilton, 1975; Evans and Pierrepoint, 1976); and genetic factors in equine melanoma and other tumors. It has been suggested (Priester, 1975) that it would be of interest to compare the geographical incidence of human and animal tumors originating in similar tissues or organs. Little work of this kind appears to have been done, though Priester refers briefly to a correlation between the incidence of cancer of the pharynx and esophagus in poultry and in people in different regions, and the level of nitrosamines in food and water. While visiting the Cancer Research Institute in Canton the writer learned that nasopharyngeal carcinoma occurs also in pigs in some parts of China, but the geographical distribution differs from that of human nasopharyngeal carcinoma, and the pig tumor does not appear to be associated with the Epstein-Barr (EB) virus (2.142).

In addition to being the subject of epidemiological studies, domestic animals bearing spontaneous tumors have also been used in therapeutic trials, e.g., that of Owen (1964) relating to osteosarcoma in dogs, but these have been on a small scale.

Comparative studies of human and animal tumors, like that of Misdorp and den Herder (1966) relating to bone metastases from human and canine mammary cancer, can be illuminating, but it is unsafe to extrapolate from animals to man simply because some similarities in tumor behavior have been observed. It is important also to note that restrictions similar to those which limit the study of human tumors may arise, partly because the number of cases with a particular kind of tumor available for study may be inadequate and partly because animals brought to a veterinary surgeon for treatment are rightly regarded by both owner and veterinarian as patients. The second of these limitations is, however, less absolute than it is with human patients; it does not arise in the case of laboratory animals, and the status of a veterinary patient may be changed with the owner's consent to that of experimental animal.

Spontaneous tumors in inbred strains of mice (Hoag, 1963; Fraser, 1971; Wrathmell, 1976), rats (Dunning and Curtis, 1946; Olcott, 1950; Crain, 1958; Hard and Grasso, 1976), and other small laboratory animals have the advantage that variation due to differences in genetic background is eliminated. Breeding programs can usually be arranged to provide a modest but useful number of new tumors for study, and these can be freely transplanted within the strain of origin (1.22). The highly inbred animals is, however, a laboratory artefact, and the incidence and behavior of tumors in members of an inbred strain depend on the rules which governed the selection of animals for breeding when the strain was first established (see Woodruff, 1977a, 1977b). A noteworthy feature of spontaneous tumors in strains with a low tumor incidence, to which we shall return later (5.215), is that they are often weakly immunogenic, or even apparently non-immunogenic, in the strain of origin.

1.212   EXPERIMENTALLY INDUCED TUMORS

Exposure of animals to chemical carcinogens, oncogenic viruses, and other agents able to induce tumors, and transplantation of embryonic or normal tissue mixed or pretreated with such agents, are important techniques for the study of carcinogenesis (2.1). Useful statistical guidelines for the analysis of tumor incidence and death rates have been published by Peto (1974). These techniques are also important in the search for evidence of surveillance (5.5), because material for histological study can be obtained, and experimental procedures which potentiate or inhibit postulated surveillance mechanisms can be applied, at any desired time in relation to initial exposure to the carcinogen. Plasma cell tumors, which can be induced readily in some strains of mice by injection of mineral oil, have the special feature that each tumor secretes one particular immunoglobulin, from which it is concluded that they are monoclonal in origin (3.114).

Induced tumors also provide a convenient source of material for experimental therapeutic studies, both in the autochthonous host and also, with the limitations discussed below (1.22), after transplantation to another animal.

Tumors induced with chemical carcinogens and oncogenic viruses are typically highly immunogenic in the animal of origin and after isogeneic transplantation (1.22), but the extent to which different tumors induced by the same carcinogen share common antigens is markedly different in the two cases (5.211, 5.212).

1.22 Transplanted Tumors

It was shown many years ago by Hanau (1889) and Jensen (1903) that cancer could sometimes be transmitted from one animal to another by transplantation of tumor tissue. Soon after Jensen's paper appeared Paul Ehrlich (1906, 1907) reported that reinoculation of tumor cells to mice with an established tumor often failed to produce a further tumor, but the true nature of this phenomenon was not realized until many years later, when the immunological basis of allograft rejection was established (see Woodruff, 1960). In consequence, as Woglom (1929) trenchantly argued in a review that has become a classic, much of the early work with transplanted tumors was misinterpreted and has contributed little to our understanding of cancer. It would be absurd to denigrate the remarkable achievements of pioneers like Ehrlich himself in Germany, Bashford, Haaland, and Murray at the laboratories of the Imperial Cancer Research Fund in London, and Peyton Rous (1910a) in New York, because they failed to anticipate advances which were made possible only when, as a result of the work of Strong and Lyttle at the Jackson Laboratories, inbred strains of animals became generally available (see Bittner, 1935; Barrett, 1940, 1955; Gorer, 1948; Snell, 1948, 1952; Kaliss, 1961), though it is noteworthy that as early as 1909 Leo Loeb had initiated the study of tumors in animals of known ancestry. What is astonishing and regrettable is that the errors inherent in drawing conclusions about the host reaction to cancer, and the comparative value of different methods of treatment, from studies with tumor allografts, are still far from being universally recognised.

This is not to say that tumor allografts should never be used. It is of biological interest that some tumors, like the Ehrlich ascites tumor of mice (see, e.g., Wheatley and Easty, 1964; Lala, 1974b), the Walker rat carcinoma, and the venereal sarcoma of dogs (Novinsky, 1876; Wade, 1908; Karlson and Mann, 1952; Alexander, Braunstein, and Altemeier, 1964), can be transplanted allogeneically and sometimes even xenogeneically, though the mechanism underlying this phenomenon has not yet been fully elucidated. It is also of interest to compare the local and general reactions evoked by tumor allografts and isografts, and a case can perhaps be made for continuing to use the Ehrlich and similar tumors in the preliminary screening of new therapeutic agents.

Xenografts are normally rejected even more rapidly than allografts, but may survive and grow in immunologically privileged sites and in immunodeficient hosts. The main value of these procedures is that they make it possible to grow some human tumors in laboratory animals (1.3).

Transplants between members of a strain which has been maintained by brother–sister mating for so many generations that members of the strain have become virtually homozygous for all histocompatibility genes apart from those represented in males but not in females evoke no allograft reaction when the donor is female or the recipient male, or when donor and recipient are of the same sex, and are termed *isogeneic;* a weak allograft reaction, due to so-called H-Y antigens, occurs, however, when either normal or neoplastic tissue is transplanted from a male donor to a female recipient.

Isogeneic transplants have proved of great value in studying the host reaction to tumors and the effect of different forms of treatment because a large number of similar transplants can be made at one time from one tumor, and further transplants of the same tumor can be made later if required. It is thus possible to compare the growth of the tumors in untreated isogeneic mice, in isogeneic mice treated in various ways designed to inhibit or potentiate homeostatic mechanisms, in F1 hybrids of the strain of origin and another inbred strain, and in congenitally athymic mice (5.523). Moreover, by locating the primary transplant on a limb it can be removed completely later, even when quite large, in order to study the effect of various procedures on the subsequent incidence of overt metastases (Schatten, 1958; Eccles and Alexander, 1975; Woodruff, 1975).

Tumors maintained *in vivo* by serial transplantation may change quite markedly, and this usually takes the form of an increase of the host range, i.e., an increased ability to grow in allogeneic animals (Barrett and Deringer, 1950, 1952; Barrett, Deringer, and Hansen, 1953). Sometimes the range is extended only to hosts of a particular genetic constitution, exemplified by tumors originating in F1 hybrids of two inbred strains becoming able to grow in one or both parent strains; sometimes, however, there is a general loss of strain specificity, so that the tumor will grow in virtually any animals of the species (E. Klein and Möller, 1963). This source of error can be virtually eliminated by storing frozen tumor cell suspensions in liquid nitrogen. If this is done it is usually wise to passage the tumor once more *in vivo* after thawing before using it in an experiment.

Tumor transplants may take the form of small pieces of tissue or cell suspensions. Cell suspensions have the advantage that the number of viable cells per unit volume of suspension can be determined with considerable accuracy and confidence limits can be calculated for this parameter; by making suitable dilutions any desired number of cells can therefore be inoculated subcutaneously, intramuscularly, intraperitoneally, intravenously, or by any other route in a standard volume of fluid. By using a range of doses the number of cells required to obtain tumors in 50 percent of animals inoculated, known as the TD50, can be determined. This varies widely with different tumors and also under different experimental conditions (Peters and Hewitt, 1974), and reported values range from 1 to 2 cells to more than 10,000 cells (Hewitt, Blake, and Walder, 1976). Experimental proof that a single cell may suffice to transmit one form of murine leukemia was reported many years ago (Furth and Kahn, 1937), and it is noteworthy that of the 27 murine tumors studied by Hewitt *et al.* (1976) the seven with the lowest TD50 values (1.2–9) were all of lymphoreticular origin.

When a tumor is growing in the so-called ascites form very little manipulation is required to prepare suitable suspensions; with solid tumors suspensions may be prepared by simple mechanical disruption of tumor tissue or with the help of proteolytic enzymes of various kinds including trypsin, pronase, and collagenase, together with a little deoxyribonuclease to break up DNA liberated from damaged cells. It is important in preparing suspensions to avoid applying shearing stress to cells, but even when great care is taken the proportion of non-viable cells in suspensions prepared without enzymes may be high and the total cell yield from tumors with a large amount of dense fibrous stroma may be small. This is common with many human tumors, for example, scirrhus carcinoma of the breast. When enzymes are used the proportion of non-viable cells may be less than 5 percent, but the procedure has the disadvantage that the surface of both neoplastic and normal host cells in the suspension may be modified in ways which affect the subsequent behavior of the tumor.

1.23 Choice of Animal Model

It is not surprising, in view of gross differences in size, life span, and other characteristics, that tumors in different species differ markedly in their anatomical distribution, rate of growth, and frequency of metastases. Because of these differences it is important to study a wide range of tumors in a variety of species, including spontaneous tumors as well as those which are induced experimentally, tumors which regularly metastasize as well as those which kill without metastasizing, and tumors which lack demonstrable tumor associated transplantation antigens as well as those which are manifestly highly "immunogenic" (G. Klein, 1959; Baldwin, 1976a; Martin, Stolfi, and Fugmann, 1977; Woodruff, 1977a).

It has been suggested (Hewitt, Blake, and Walder, 1976) that spontaneously arising tumors (and isogeneic transplants thereof) are the only appropriate models of human cancer, on the ground that human cancer is always spontaneous; this, however, ignores the fact mentioned previously (1.21) that the distinction between spontaneous and experimentally induced tumors is an operational one and does not necessarily reflect important biological differences. Indeed, the fact that tumor incidence in inbred strains can be manipulated by deliberate selection raises the converse possibility that tumors in some strains, including perhaps strains with a particularly low tumor incidence, may behave very differently from naturally occurring cancer (Woodruff, 1977b).

It would seem to be important to look for, or try to induce, animal tumors in particular tissues or organs in which human cancer is common, and, in view of the value of isogeneic transplantation, to do this in mice, rats, and other species of which inbred strains are available. Examples of such tumors which have not been very widely used and would seem to merit further study include chemically induced carcinoma of the intestine (M. S. Martin *et al.,* 1973) and radiation-induced osteogenic sarcoma in rats (Cobb, 1970), chemically induced carcinoma of the bladder in rats (Fingerhut and Veenema, 1975) and mice (Wahl *et al.,* 1974), and spontaneous astrocytoma which occurs in an inbred strain (VM) of mice (Fraser, 1971).

1.3 THE GROWTH OF HUMAN TUMORS IN ANIMALS

Many human tumors have now been successfully transplanted to animals by using immunologically privileged sites, or immunodeficient hosts, or both. Such transplants have been used mainly for assaying the effect of different chemotherapeutic agents, and it has been suggested (Berenbaum, Sheard *et al.,* 1974) that the best way to validate such assays is to set up animal transplants of human tumors whenever possible and observe in each case the response to whatever combination of drugs the clinician had decided to administer to the patient. Comparison of the effect of the same agents on the same tumor in patients and animals may also give some indication of the extent to which the reaction of the patient contributes to the therapeutic effect, but interpretation is difficult because the reaction of the animal host cannot be assumed to be negligible nor can its effect be accurately assessed. Further information about the reaction of the patient has been sought by transplanting cells obtained from macroscopically uninvolved regional lymph nodes with the tumor cells (Caldwell and Wright, 1966), but, once again, the results are difficult to interpret because the non-neoplastic cells may be selectively destroyed (G. Klein, Giovanella, Lindahl *et al.*, 1974).

Early successful attmepts to transplant human tumors to animals relied on (1) the use of special sites, notably the anterior chamber of the eye of guinea pigs, rats and rabbits (Smirnova, 1937; Greene, 1938, 1941, 1946, 1950, 1952; Greene and Lund, 1944; Masina, 1947; Schilling, Snell, and Favata, 1949; Snell, 1951) and the hamster cheek pouch (Chute, Sommers, and Warren, 1952; Handler, Davis, and Sommers, 1956; Toolan, 1953, 1954) and (2) x-irradiation or administration of cortisone, in association with transplantation to one of the special sites mentioned above or with subcutaneous transplants in weanling hosts (Toolan, 1951, 1953, 1954, 1958; Handler, Davis, and Sommers, 1956; Patterson, Patterson, and Chute, 1957; Buttle, Eperon, and Menzies, 1964; Williams, Evans, and Blamey, 1971). Another immunologically privileged site which has been used is the brain (Goldenberg, 1970), and as an alternative to administration of cortisone Richards and Klausner (1958) relied on the diminished immunological reactivity associated with pregnancy.

More recently human tumors have been transplanted subcutaneously, intramuscularly, intraperitoneally, and intravenously to animals immunosuppressed by thymectomy, usually combined with sublethal irradiation, lethal irradiation followed by isogeneic bone marrow transplantation, or administration of antilymphocyte globulin (Phillips and Gazet, 1970; Castro, 1972; Cobb, 1972, 1973; Detre and Gazet, 1973; Berenbaum, Sheard, Reittie, and Bundick, 1974; Mitchell, Rees, and Salsbury, 1974; Kelly, Snell, and Berenbaum, 1975; Double, 1975; Franks *et al.*, 1975), and to congenitally athymic mice (5.523) (Rygaard and Povlsen, 1969; Povlsen, Fialkow *et al.*, 1973; Giovanella, Stehlin, and Williams, 1974; Double, 1975). Mice congenitally devoid of both thymus and spleen have also been used as recipients of human leukemic cells (Lozzio *et al.*, 1976).

The proportion of animals in which the transplant takes, and the subsequent growth of the tumors, varies greatly with different tumors and different techniques. As a rule the transplanted tumors retain their general histological appearance even after repeated passage (Cobb 1972, 1973; Detre and Gazet, 1973; Berenbaum *et al.*, 1974) and a recognizably human karyotype (Visfeldt, Povlsen, and Rygaard, 1972; Cobb, 1973), but mitotic activity is sometimes markedly greater than in the original tumor (Cobb, 1973; Detre and Gazet, 1973). Some tumors continue to produce recognizable products such as hormones, melanin, and carcinoembryonic antigen (Visfeldt *et. al.*, 1972; Sordat *et al.*, 1974; Goldenberg, 1974). There is evidence that tumors in athymic mice may acquire C-type virus from the host (Achong, Trumper, and Giovanella, 1976).

Some transplants metastasize spontaneously in the new host (Cobb, 1972; Giovanella, Stehlin, and Williams, 1974), and the metastases may persist even though the primary transplant regresses. Metastasis has also been observed with a hamster tumor growing in athymic mice (Maguire *et al.*, 1976).

1.4 *IN VITRO* METHODS

The development of methods of tissue culture *in vitro*, pioneered by Harrison, Burrows, Carrell, Ebeling, W.H. and M.R. Lewis, and others (see Willmer, 1965), has proved a powerful tool in many areas of biomedical research. For many years interest centered on the cells which migrated from small pieces of tissue embedded in plasma clots, and the extension of this type of procedure to the study of small piéces of organized tissue, a technique which was named organ culture.

More recently techniques have been developed (see Willmer, 1965; Paul, 1975) for starting cultures with dispersed cells or even a single cell, and maintaining them either as a monolayer of cells on glass or plastic, or as a cell suspension. These techniques are currently widely used in cancer research, particularly in relation to the following topics which are discussed more fully in later chapters:

1. Comparison of normal and neoplastic cells with respect to their mobility and the extent to which they exhibit the phenomenon of density dependent inhibition of growth (3.1).
2. Study of tumor immunity, especially cell-mediated immunity (5.225, 5.226), and also cytotoxicity mediated by macrophages (5.43) and natural killer (NK) cells (5.44), using autochthonous tumor cells and established tumor cell lines as targets.
3. Studies of human tumor cell population kinetics (3.5).
4. Preparation of cell hybrids for use both *in vivo* and *in vitro* in the analysis of malignancy (3.113).
5. Screening of new chemotherapeutic agents (6.32).
6. Expansion of a tumor cell population for use in experimental active specific immunotherapy (8.252).
7. *In vitro* immunization of lymphoid cells for use in the study of adoptive immunization (7.413) and its therapeutic application (8.233).

It is difficult to make predictions which are valid *in vivo* from observations *in vitro* because of the absence *in vitro* of many factors which may stimulate or inhibit tumor growth in the living animal, and the consequent selection of clones of cells which are well adapted to grow in tissue culture but may be unrepresentative of the original tumor cell population (Sheard, Double, and Berenbaum, 1971; Lancet, 1972a; Berenbaum *et al.*, 1974). With animal tumors, however, behavior *in vitro* and *in vivo* can be compared experimentally, and some important correlations have been established, notably in respect of cytotoxicity mediated by T cells, macrophages, and NK cells. With human tumors *in vitro* studies are limited by ethical considerations, but when an animal tumor and a human tumor behave similarly *in vitro,* and there is good correlation between the behavior of the animal tumor *in vivo* and *in vitro,* it seems reasonable to postulate that this will hold good for the human tumor also, and to base further clinical investigations on this hypothesis.

2
Origin and Nature of the Cancer Cell

2.1 MECHANISMS OF CARCINOGENESIS

It is widely accepted that the primary event in the development of a tumor is a heritable change termed *transformation* in one or more cells, as a result of which the response of the cell, and the clone to which it gives rise, to factors which regulate the growth of normal cells is profoundly altered. Transformation may be triggered by chemical carcinogens, ultraviolet and ionizing radiation, contact with films of metal, plastic, or glass, and hormonal stimulation; it may also occur both *in vivo* and *in vitro* without demonstrable cause. Two general mechanisms have been proposed to account for the phenomenon: *mutation,* which implies a change in nucleotide sequence resulting from an alteration, deletion or rearrangement in the primary structure of cellular DNA, and *epigenetic change,* i.e., a heritable change in the expression of genetic information.

This view has been challenged by Smithers (1962a) on the ground that cancer is a disease of organization rather than of cells. In the light of this criticism, and the fact that one type of tissue may influence the growth of another not only during embryonic development but also during adult life (see Tarin, 1972), Burch (1970) has postulated that carcinogenesis begins with a mutation in one or more stem cells, the normal function of whose progeny is to control the growth of other cells by producing specific mitotic control proteins. As the result of such mutations a clone or clones of functionally defective growth control cells are produced, and the corresponding target cells, which are no longer restrained, proliferate and are eventually transformed to cancer cells. This hypothesis provides a plausible explanation of the bilateral or multifocal presentation of some human tumors (Smithers, 1960; Willis, 1960); it is, however, less easy to reconcile with the monoclonal nature of various animal and human tumors (3.114).

The suggestion that all or most cancer is initiated by somatic mutation appears to have been first put forward by Tyzzer (1916), and more recently has been strongly advocated by Burnet (1957) and others (Trosko and Chu, 1975).

In the most usual formulation of the hypothesis carcinogenesis is attributed to the direct action of some unidentified product of a mutant structural gene. An alternative

15

hypothesis proposed by Comings (1973) is that carcinogenesis is due to the action of a transforming gene which exists in normal cells but is suppressed by a diploid pair of regulatory genes. Carcinogens cause mutation of the regulatory genes and may thus lead to derepression of the transforming gene. As a rule mutation of both regulatory genes is required; in the case of autosomal dominant hereditary tumors such as retinoblastoma, however, one of the regulatory genes is hereditarily inactive and all that is required is a somatic mutation of the other.

Following the discovery that in eukaryotic organisms only a fraction of the total DNA can be accounted for as programming the synthesis of extranuclear protein, it has been suggested that some of the untranslated DNA may subserve a regulatory function of some kind. This line of argument has been developed by Burnet (1977), who has suggested that mutation in regulatory DNA, or to use his term *control DNA*, is the essential source of cancer and also of the morphological differences between closely related species.

Another hypothesis is that, under certain conditions, mitochondrial DNA (see Borst, 1972) gains entry to the nucleus and brings about neoplastic transformation. This derives from a suggestion of Handler, Daniel, and Platt (1971), and has been elaborated by H. Baum (1973), but must be regarded as highly speculative.

Except in the special case of the immune system, where the great diversity of antigen-sensitive cells can most easily be accounted for by mutation and selection (Burnet, 1959, 1970a), and perhaps also, as Burnet has suggested, in the development of receptors capable of responding to a great variety of olfactory stimuli, epigenetic change appears to play a major role in embryonic differentiation. This process would seem to require, in addition to mechanisms for activating and switching off structural genes, a system of feedbacks to signal the achievement of some phase of development (Burnet, 1977). In so far as carcinogenesis is epigenetic, it too requires some mechanism whereby an environmental change may bring about an alteration in gene expression (Horsfall, 1962; Gelboin, 1967; Dustin, 1972). The phenomenon of enzyme induction in bacteria provides an example of this process, and the underlying mechanisms have been analyzed in detail (see Goodwin, 1976) following the original description of the lac operon in *E. coli* by Jacob and Monod (1961). As yet, however, corresponding mechanisms have not been so clearly delineated in eukaryotic cells, and until this has been done the nature and role of epigenetic change in carcinogenesis seems likely to remain obscure.

Mutational theories derive considerable support from the fact that most carcinogens are also mutagens and *vice versa* (E. C. Miller and J. A. Miller, 1971; Ames *et al.*, 1973; Bartsch, 1976; Parke, 1977a), and that many tumors, both animal and human, show chromosomal abnormalities (Harnden, 1976), but this does not prove that tumors induced by exposure to such agents, or showing such abnormalities, have arisen as the result of mutation. There are, however, three sets of observations which, as Coggin and Anderson (1974), Ellison (1977), and Mintz and others (*vide infra*) have emphasized, are easier to account for on the basis of an epigenetic theory. Firstly, the cells of many tumors possess "phase-specific substances" (Manes, 1974) in the form of isoenzymes (Criss, 1971; Weinhouse, 1972), tumor-associated oncofetal antigens (5.23) and other proteins, and forms of transfer RNA (Yang, 1971) which are present in embryos at some stage of development, but not, or only in very small amount, in normal adult tissues. Tumors of viral origin do not constitute an exception, since, as will be discussed later (5.23), some virus-induced tumors have been shown to possess oncofetal antigens. Secondly, some human lung cancers and other tumors secrete "inappropriate" hormones (3.6). Thirdly, markers of mouse teratocarcinoma cells have been identified by Mintz and Illmensee (1975) and Papaioanno *et al.* (1975) in normal tissues of adult chimeric* mice which at the blastocyst stage had been injected with teratocarcinoma cells. These are powerful arguments, but mutation cannot be entirely ruled out. It is conceivable, for example, in respect of the mouse teratocarcinomas (Bouck and di Mayorca, 1976), that the phenotypic characteristics of malignancy were lost in the course of differentiation, or in consequence of fusion with a normal cell, while other characteristics used as markers persisted, and there is no obvious reason why, in a mutant lung cancer cell, the gene coding for a particular substance should be lost or incapable of being activated. Again, the absence of visible chromosomal damage does not exclude the presence of significant change in the DNA of the cell, whether as the result of direct damage, error of repair, or insertion of new material. The report that normal tadpoles may develop from eggs whose nuclei have been removed and replaced, not only by nuclei from normal cells of various kinds (see Gurdon, 1977) but also from cells of a renal carcinoma of the frog (King and DiBeradino, 1965), implies, if the donor cells were truly neoplastic and not stromal (3.1) cells, that no essential genetic information had been lost as the result of transformation, but it remains to be seen whether this is a special, or even a unique, case. The whole question may be resolved one day by nucleotide sequencing of tumor DNA; in the meantime available indirect evidence should be interpreted with caution.

Whatever the nature of the change from a normal cell to a cancer cell it seems almost certain that it is a multistage process, since it is difficult on the basis of a "one-hit" hypothesis to account for the steep dependence of human cancer incidence on age (J.C. Fisher and Holloman, 1951; Stocks, 1953; Armitage and Doll, 1954, 1957; Burch, 1965a, 1965b, 1965c; Ashley, 1969; Peto, Roe *et al.,* 1975). The various steps in the process may be brought about in different ways. Studies on chemical carcinogenesis, for example, to be considered in more detail later (2.11), have suggested that a distinction may be drawn between the *initiation* of a tumor and a later phase referred to as *promotion,* and Burch has postulated that initiation involves a series of mutations whereas promotion may be due to a change in gene expression. Another possibility is that promotors interfere with DNA repair mechanisms which might otherwise render the action of the initiating agent ineffective (Gaudin, Gregg, and Yielding, 1972).

Cairns (1975) has pointed out that the only mutations that accumulate during the life of an individual are those that arise in cells which themselves survive, or contribute descendants that survive, for the individual's lifetime, and he refers to such cells as "immortal" stem cells.[†] He has postulated that the class of mutation most likely to lead to cancer, which he terms a primer mutation, is a mutation in an immortal stem cell which increases the likelihood of further mutation and/or confers on the cell the ability to move out of its normal anatomical site. The histological diagnosis of carcinoma-in-situ in a biopsy specimen may be the first indication that a primer mutation has occurred. To account for the reported finding (2.15) that the lifetime risk of cancer of the breast developing in childbearing women is approximately linearly related to the

---

*Mintz and Illmensee refer to these mice as *mosaics,* but the terminology adopted by McLaren (1975), in which mosaic is used for a composite animal derived from a single fertilized egg and chimera for a composite animal in which there are different cell populations derived from more than one fertilized egg, seems preferable.

[†]The term stem cell commonly refers to a relatively undifferentiated cell which retains a wide range of developmental possibilities. This is not implied in Cairns' use of the term.

length of the interval between puberty and first pregnancy, Cairns has suggested that, whereas most epithelia probably establish their stem cells during intrauterine life, stem cells in mammary epithelium increase in number at puberty and then fluctuate in numbers with each ovarian cycle until the first pregnancy, whereupon the population stabilizes at a level that is no longer influenced either by the ovarian cycle or by further pregnancies.

How are the changes, genetic or epigenetic, that result in cancer brought about? If one looks at the whole spectrum of human cancer it seems clear that the genetic constitution of the host and environmental factors may both be concerned in its etiology. On the one hand, some individuals with specific chromosomal or Mendelian recessive genetic disorders show an increased susceptibility to certain kinds of cancer, while others have tumors associated with a single dominant gene (Knudson, 1973); in addition, with many cancers there is an increased family incidence which may be partly polygeneically determined. The incidence of some tumors, on the other hand, is associated with a history of exposure to agents which have been shown to be carcinogenic in experimental animals, or to cause transformation of animal or human cells *in vitro.*

Burnet (1974), taking as his starting point the importance of mutation in evolution, and also, as he has maintained, in the generation of diversity during development of the immune system, has argued that harmful mutations, including those concerned in carcinogenesis, are not due primarily to damage to DNA by an environmental agent but to errors produced in the course of DNA replication and repair. This hypothesis does not cast doubt on the importance of environmental factors, but it implies that by damaging DNA they increase the need for repair and so increase the probability of error.

As we have seen (1.211), it is common practice to label a tumor *spontaneous* when no external etiological agent has been identified, but this does not mean that no such agent exists or has contributed to the development of the tumor. Conversely, evidence of prior exposure to a known physical or chemical carcinogen does not suffice to establish its etiological role in any particular case, nor does association of a virus with a particular tumor, for, as Todaro (1972) has pointed out, viruses can multiply better, and proviruses become preferentially active, in cancer cells.

There is no obvious reason why only one factor should be involved in any given case. It may well happen, for example, as Burch (1965a) has suggested, that the first of a series of mutations culminating in the development of a tumor is inherited while later mutations are due to environmental causes.

During the period between the appearance of a malignant tumor in a patient and his death, the chance of another primary appearing seems to be greater than would be expected in the same period in another individual of the same age and sex who has not had a tumor. Thus of 37,850 patients with cancer studied at the Mayo Clinic, 1909 had two, 74 had three, 4 had four, and 1 had five consecutive apparently primary tumors (Moertel, 1966). Many other instances of multiple primary tumors were reported at an international congress held in 1973. Some of these data have been summarized by Ioachim (1976) as follows: (1) Among 158,000 cancer patients studied in Connecticut over a period of 30 years there were 5000 with multiple primary tumors (Schoenberg *et al.,* 1974). (2) At the Boston City Hospital, in 10,977 consecutive autopsies, 3008 malignant tumors were found in 2734 patients. Of the 249 patients with multiple tumors, 235 had two tumors and the others three or four tumors (Bauer and

Robbins, 1974). (3) In a study in Japan of 61,869 patients with cancer, 967 had multiple tumors (Miyaji, 1974).

Once again, however, the data are difficult to interpret. It is not always easy to exclude a metastasis, and, even when this can be done with confidence, the second or subsequent tumor, as Salaman (1976) has pointed out, could be (1) induced by the treatment given for the first tumor; (2) a manifestation of reduced resistance or increased susceptibility to cancer due to genetic or other causes; or (3) caused by the same environmental agent as the first tumor.

2.11 Carcinogenesis by Chemicals

Over 200 years ago Percival Pott (1775) suggested that the high incidence of carcinoma of the scrotum in chimney sweeps in England was due to prolonged contact with soot, but it was not until 140 years later that Yamagiwa and Ichikawa (1915, 1918) showed that skin cancer could be induced in experimental animals with coal tar. Some 15 years later Kennaway and Hieger (1930) succeeded in inducing cancer experimentally with a pure chemical substance, 1,2,5,6-dibenzanthracene, and shortly afterwards Cook, Hewett, and Hieger (1933) isolated 3,4-benzpyrene from coal tar and demonstrated its carcinogenicity. Since then many substances, both naturally occurring and synthetic, have been investigated, and in 1975 the International Agency for Research on Cancer (IARC) reported that 111 compounds were unquestionably carcinogenic in experimental animals, and that there was strong suspicion that 19 were carcinogenic in man.

In the earliest experiments epidermal carcinomas were induced by repeatedly painting an area of skin with the carcinogen, but it was soon found that some compounds induced local sarcomas when injected subcutaneously or intramuscularly, or carcinomas in the stomach or small intestine when given orally or by intragastric tube. It was also found that many locally acting carcinogens, including polycyclic aromatic hydrocarbons, when applied to the skin or injected subcutaneously, increased the incidence of tumors in remote organs and of leukemia, and that tumors in the liver and other organs could regularly be induced by oral administration of various azo and amino compounds.

The skin of newborn animals appears to be refractory to carcinogenesis by local application of methylcholanthrene, but this may be simply a matter of limitation of access of the carcinogen, due, for example, to the absence of hair, because when minced mouse embryo epidermis is mixed with an oily suspension of methylcholanthrene and injected into adult mice epidermoid cysts develop and rapidly become carcinomatous (Rous and Smith, 1945).

It is now known that many so-called chemical carcinogens are, strictly speaking, *procarcinogens;* i.e., they possess little or no carcinogenic activity themselves but become converted in the body by the action of microsomal enzymes to *proximal* and *ultimate carcinogens,* which bind covalently to cellular DNA, RNA, or protein, and, if the cell is not killed, as it may be (Tomatis, Mohr, and Davis, 1973), provide the stimulus for transformation (E.C. Miller and J.A. Miller, 1952, 1966; P.E. Hughes, 1965; Farber, 1968; van Duuren, 1969; J.A. Miller, 1970; Gelboin and Wiebel, 1971; Sims and Grover, 1974; Sarasin and Meunier-Rotival, 1976; Wood, Levin *et al.,* 1976; Parke, 1977a, 1977b, 1977c). Reaction of carcinogens with DNA may lead to single or double strand breaking, and mutations may result if these are inaccurately repaired (Sugimura, Otaki, and Matsushima, 1968; Sarma et al., 1973; Cox, Damjanov, and Irving, 1973; Stewart, Farber, and Mirvish, 1973; Sarasin and Meunier-Rotival, 1976) or not repaired at all. An important feature of the microsomal enzymes is that they may be induced by the substances on which they are acting and by other compounds (Sarasin and Meunier-Rotival, 1976). It is also important to note that enzymatic action may produce derivatives which are less reactive, as well as derivatives which are more reactive, than the original compounds. These chemical changes take place especially in the liver but can also occur in other sites including the lung, skin, intestine, and kidney.

The action of carcinogens has been studied *in vitro* as well as *in vivo*. It has been found that in fibroblast cultures over 50 percent of cells may be transformed (Heidelberger, 1973; Bevan and Trowbridge, 1976), so it seems clear that in this system carcinogens do not simply select pre-existing cells carrying a biochemical lesion of some kind, as suggested by Naha and Ashworth (1974), but actually transform normal cells.

It was observed by Rous and his colleagues that papillomas on rabbits' ears which regressed when painting with tar was discontinued reappeared when painting was resumed (Rous and Kidd, 1941), and also when non-carcinogenic chemicals were applied or holes were punched in the treated area (Friedewald and Rous, 1944). They concluded that carcinogenesis took place in two stages: an *initiating stage* during which normal cells were converted to "latent tumor cells," and a *promoting stage* during which the latent cells were stimulated to grow progressively. Confirmatory evidence was provided independently by Berenblum's studies of the co-carcinogenic action of croton oil with 3,4-benzpyrene on mouse skin, in which it was shown that when croton oil was applied after cessation of a brief course of applications of the carcinogen many more tumors developed than in mice treated with the carcinogen alone (Berenblum, 1941a, 1941b), whereas application of croton oil for several months before application of the carcinogen did not significantly alter the latent period or the tumor yield (Berenblum, 1941b). Further experiments (Berenblum and Shubik, 1947, 1949; Berenblum, 1954; Berenblum and Haran, 1955; Berenblum, 1969; Ryser, 1971) were consistent with the general hypothesis that there are two stages in carcinogenesis with different biological mechanisms, but interpretation was complicated by the fact that the agents used as initiators could act also to some extent as promotors and that croton oil alone is weakly carcinogenic. Attempts to find pure initiators and pure promotors have in the main been unsuccessful, though it has been reported (Salaman and Roe, 1953) that urethane, though capable of inducing lung tumors, and even skin tumors (Haran and Berenblum, 1956), when administered systemically, is completely non-carcinogenic when applied locally to the skin unless croton oil is applied subsequently; and in the case of methylcholanthrene, Burki and Bresnick (1975) have suggested that initiation of carcinogenesis is caused by alkylating epoxides produced from the original compound by the action of microsomal enzymes and promotion by methylcholanthrene itself. It would seem therefore that the distinction between initiator and promotor is not as clear cut as was originally thought.

This of course does not exclude the hypothesis of a multistage process requiring sequential somatic mutations, some or all of which may be chemically induced, or the involvement of a multiplicity of agents of various kinds in the process (Southam, 1963)—a phenomenon referred to as *cocarcinogenesis*. Green (1954, 1958) has suggested that the initiation stage may be the consequence of an immunological reaction to a chemical carcinogen and that promotion is due to a direct action of the carcinogen itself. This is in accord with the general concept of immunostimulation which will be discussed later (5.522), but there is insufficient evidence in support of Green's hypothesis for it to be regarded as more than an interesting speculation.

Opinions differ regarding the role of environmental chemicals in the etiology of human cancer, but there is growing support for the view that most human tumors are due to environmental causes, and in particular, to environmental chemicals (Kennaway and Lindsey, 1958; Magee and Barnes, 1967; Magee, 1974; Pelfrene, 1976; Preussmann, 1976; Doll, 1977). This hypothesis is based on the following considerations:

1. The high correlation between the incidence of particular tumors and the extent of exposure to known carcinogens—for example, the association between smoking and lung cancer (Doll and Hill, 1950, 1964a, 1964b; Doll, 1955, 1977; Doll and Peto, 1977; British Medical Journal, 1976c) and between various other tumors and carcinogens encountered at work or as the result of atmospheric pollution, diet (Hill, Crowther *et al.*, 1971) or medical prescriptions (Herbst, Ulfelder, and Poskanzer, 1971; Jick, 1974; Heinonen *et al.*, 1974; Armstrong, Stevens, and Doll, 1974; Sieber and Adamson, 1975; Armstrong, Skegg, White, and Doll, 1976; British Medical Journal, 1977b; Doll, 1977).

2. Differences in cancer incidence in different regions of the same country (Howe, 1971), and the fact that migrant populations tend to acquire the predominant cancer pattern of the host countries and lose that of their home country (Preussmann, 1976).

3. The fact that a large number of chemical substances known to be carcinogenic in animals exists in the human environment. Thus, according to the IARC (1975), human exposure to 106 of the 111 compounds reported as being unquestionably carcinogenic in experimental animals is known to have occurred, and, as already mentioned, there is strong suspicion that 19 of these compounds are carcinogenic in man.

2.12 Carcinogenesis by Radiation

Ionizing radiation is a powerful mutagen and can cause visible structural damage to chromosomes. It is also carcinogenic, as has been tragically demonstrated by the high incidence of various forms of cancer in many of the pioneers of radiology (Rowntree, 1922); in people employed in painting watch dials with luminous paint when this contained radium or mesothorium (Martland and Humphries, 1929); in patients given radium water as a tonic, or thorotrast for radiological visualization of the liver (see Southam, 1963), or x-ray therapy for ankylosing spondylitis (Court-Brown and Doll, 1957); in children irradiated *in utero* in the course of radiological investigations on their mothers, or subsequently for supposed pathological enlargement of the thymus, haemangiomas, or other conditions; and in people exposed to radiation as a result of the atomic bombs dropped on Hiroshima and Nagasaki (see Burch, 1965a).

The predominant type, and the overall incidence, of cancer depends *inter alia* on the age of the patient at the time of exposure, and on the dose and dose-rate of irradiation. Irradiation *in utero* appears to increase the incidence of all forms of childhood cancer, including leukemia, in approximately the same ratio; irradiation of the neck in children has resulted in cancer of the thyroid and also in leukemia; irradiation of adults has resulted mainly in various forms of acute leukemia and in chronic myeloid leukemia, but also in increased incidence of some solid tumors (see Duffy and Fitzgerald, 1950; Burch, 1965c; S. Graham *et al.,* 1966; A. Stewart, 1971; Kinlen, 1977).

As a tool for the study of carcinogenesis in animals, radiation has the advantage that its effect on cells is independent of permeability barriers, which may greatly influence the effect of chemical carcinogens and viruses.

The most striking results relate to the induction of leukemia with x-rays, and interest has centered on the possibility that irradiation may activate a latent virus (2.14), and on the dose–response curve which in mice flattens out at about 400 rad whole body irradiation, and above 600 rad falls so markedly that the incidence of leukemia may be considerably less in irradiated mice with a high natural incidence of leukemia than in unirradiated controls (Cole, Nowell, and Arnold, 1960; Upton *et al.,* 1960), probably because at higher doses more and more cells are killed. Irradiation may also cause an increased incidence of hepatomas and ovarian adenomas in mice (Upton *et al.,* 1960; Nowell and Cole, 1965), but although some of these tumors become very large Nowell and Cole (*op. cit.*) found no definite evidence of malignant transformation. The same authors have also reported that, for a given dose of irradiation, the incidence of tumors is greater at low dose rates of irradiation, whereas chromosomal damage was greater at high dose rates, and, while this might be explained entirely by high mortality among the cells with gross chromosomal damage, they have suggested that it may be due in part to indirect hormonal mechanisms.

Another type of experimental tumor, osteogenic sarcoma, has been induced in rats and other animals by feeding or injection of radioactive materials (see Finkel and Biskis, 1968) including bone-seeking isotopes like ^{90}Sr (Loutit and Carr, 1978), or by local implantation in the skeleton of radium (Ross, 1936) or polyvinylchloride discs impregnated with ^{32}P (Cobb, 1970).

Ultraviolet (UV) radiation, though non-ionizing, is also both mutagenic and carcinogenic. The carcinogenicity of this form of radiation is strongly suggested by epidemological studies which have shown that the incidence of basal cell and squamous cell carcinomas of the skin (Hueper, 1961; Segi, 1963; Keeler, 1963; Urbach, 1969), and probably also cutaneous melanoma (Lee and Merrill, 1970; Beardmore, 1972) is largely dependent on climatic and other factors which determine the amount of solar radiation which penetrates the skin, and it appears that radiation of a wavelength of 290–320 nm is likely to be responsible (see Gianelli, 1977). Studies of patients with the rare autosomal recessive hereditary disease xeroderma pigmentosum have clinched the matter and have thrown much light on the underlying mechanism. Patients suffering from this condition develop the same types of skin cancer as normal people, but much earlier and in much greater frequency (see Burnet, 1976); indeed, until the need for special protection from sunlight was realized, many such patients developed their first skin cancer before the age of 10 and died before the age of 20.

The explanation has emerged from study of the nature of the damage to DNA caused by UV irradiation and the extent to which this damage is repaired in normal people and in patients with the disease (see Burnet, 1976; Gianelli, 1977).

The main damaging effect of UV radiation on DNA is to cause the formation of dimers between adjacent pyrimidine bases (usually two thymines) on the same DNA strand and break the hydrogen bonds between the two DNA strands in the region of the dimer, and this interferes with the replication of DNA and translation to RNA. In normal cells the damaged DNA is efficiently repaired.* When only one strand is damaged the main process in mammals consists of excision of the dimer and a short piece of the affected DNA strand, resynthesis of a replacement for the piece excised using the other strand as template, and restoration of continuity, by the action of a series of enzymes (endonuclease, exonuclease, DNA polymerase, ligase); if dimers have formed in both strands the repair process, termed postreplication repair, is more complicated. In cells of patients with xeroderma pigmentosum, as was first shown by Cleaver (1968, 1969), the repair of DNA is defective. In the majority of patients the defect relates to the early stages of excision (Cleaver, 1968, 1969), but studies with hybrid cells formed by fusing fibroblasts from different patients have revealed a considerable degree of genetic heterogeneity, and such hybrids may, or may not, possess an effective repair mechanism. In a small proportion of patients excision occurs normally but postreplication repair is defective (Lehmann *et al.*, 1975). These findings, taken in conjunction with evidence that cells from patients with xeroderma pigmentosum are exceptionally prone to mutation following exposure to UV irradiation (Maher and McCormick, 1976), strongly support the hypothesis that the abnormal incidence of skin cancer in patients with this disease is the result of mutations caused by exposure to UV radiation, and that these mutations are caused by errors in the repair of DNA.

The relatively high incidence of skin cancer observed in Australia in kidney transplant recipients under treatment with immunosuppressive drugs (Marshall, 1974; Shiel, 1977; Kinlen *et al.*, 1979) raises the question of whether this may be due, at least in part, to a direct effect of the drugs used on DNA repair mechanisms, or perhaps even to the emergence of clones of cells which possess the same kind of defect as is inherited in patients with xeroderma pigmentosum, rather than to impaired surveillance (5.5) as is generally postulated. This suggestion would seem to merit consideration because there does not appear to be a comparable increase in the incidence of other types of cancer apart from the special case of tumors of the lymphoreticular tissues (5.523) in Australia, or of skin cancer in immunosuppressed patients in countries where exposure to solar UV radiation is on a much smaller scale than in Australia.

2.13 Effect of Trauma, and Contact With Films of Plastic, Metal, or Glass

The possible role of mechanical trauma in the etiology of human cancer has been hotly debated. So far as a single injury is concerned it seems likely that in most cases this has been coincidental and has done no more than draw the patient's attention to a previously existing but unnoticed lesion, though the possibility that it may sometimes play an etiological role cannot be definitely excluded (Auster, 1961; Pack, 1958; Stoll and Crissey, 1962). A possible special case is the reported predilection of breast cancer to recur in thoracotomy scars (Freund *et al.*, 1976). The role of recurrent trauma, particularly on epithelial surfaces, is more difficult to assess, and, despite current skepti-

---

*The fact that repair is occurring is easily demonstrated in cells from biopsy specimens by showing autoradiographically that non-scheduled (i.e., non-S phase) DNA synthesis is occurring (See Gianelli, 1977); to elucidate the mechanism is a much more difficult problem, and all that will be attempted here is to summarize briefly the results.

cism, the possibility that it may contribute to the development of cancer in sites such as the buccal cavity and the cervix uteri should probably not be dismissed, particularly in the light of Haddow's (1972, 1974) suggestion that carcinogenesis resembles wound healing in some ways and may perhaps be regarded as an aberration of this process. Experimental attempts to induce skin cancers by mechanical trauma have been unsuccessful, but when trauma is followed by regeneration associated with a marked increase in mitotic activity, as in the rat liver following partial hepatectomy, a situation is created in which the action of chemical carcinogens may be enhanced (Maini and Stich, 1961; Maini, Stich, and McCulloch, 1962).

The etiological role of injury appears more clear cut in the case of burns. Squamous cell carcinoma may develop in the burned area even before healing has occurred if this process is delayed, or years later in the scar. As Berenblum (1962) has pointed out, such tumors may occur in sites where tumors are extremely rare in the absence of injury; on the other hand, the overall incidence of cancer associated with burns is quite small despite the fact that burns are common.

Another method of carcinogenesis was discovered accidentally by Oppenheimer, Oppenheimer, and Stout (1948), who found that fibrosarcomas developed in rats whose kidneys had been wrapped in cellophane in the course of experiments on hypertension. Subsequently, the fact that inplantation of films of plastics of various kinds, and also of metals and glass, often leads to the development of tumors in the region of the foreign material has been confirmed by many observers in rats and other species (see Alexander and Horning, 1959). The effect does not seem to be due to the chemical nature of the material, since it occurs with films of very inert material such as polytetrafluoroethylene (Teflon), but not when plastics which in film form are carcinogeneic are implanted in powdered form (Oppenheimer et al., 1955). It seems possible, therefore, as Gelboin (1967) has suggested, that the effect is due to mechanical disturbance of cell-to-cell interactions which ordinarily maintain growth regulatory substances at normal concentration.

It is surprising, in view of the great variety of solid foreign material implanted in tissues for therapeutic reasons, that this form of carcinogenesis does not yet appear to have been described in man.

2.14 Viral Carcinogenesis

2.141 EXPERIMENTAL OBSERVATIONS

Before considering the possible etiological role of viruses in human cancer it will be helpful to review briefly the effects of oncogenic viruses in animals and some of their basic biological properties.

Members of a heterogeneous group of small DNA viruses, termed collectively *papova viruses,* are responsible for a variety of animal tumors. They include papilloma viruses, typified by the Shope papilloma virus, which are responsible for benign papillomas in rabbits and other species; polyoma virus (see Stewart, 1960), which causes a variety of tumors, including carcinomas of the parotid gland, mammary gland, and kidney, and subcutaneous fibrosarcomas, when injected into newborn mice, especially if these are thymectomized (J.F.A.P. Miller, Ting, and Law, 1964; Malmgren, Rabson, and Carney, 1964; Law, 1965) or treated with antilymphocyte serum (Allison and Law, 1968), but probably plays little if any etiological role outside the laboratory; and a monkey virus, SV40, similar in many respects to polyoma virus, which causes tumors when injected into newborn hamsters. Among larger DNA viruses, a herpes virus has been established as the cause of avian neurolymphomatosis (Marek's disease), which is a highly contagious neoplastic disease with some associated inflammatory features (Biggs and Payne, 1963; Purchase, Okazaki, and Burmester, 1971; Biggs et al., 1972; Biggs, 1973; Payne, 1977), and a similar virus has been shown experimentally to induce malignant lymphomas in monkeys (Ablashi et al., 1971; Ablashi, Easton, and Guegan, 1976).

In tissue culture, polyoma virus and SV40 multiply in some cells (termed permissive cells), and these are killed. Other cells (termed non-permissive cells), in which the virus does not multiply, may undergo a stable transformation (2.1), and in these cells viral DNA is integrated with the DNA of the cell; alternatively, they undergo an abortive transformation (Stoker, 1968) and after a few cell generations return to normal. It is noteworthy that SV40 can transform human cells in culture. Transformed cells are unaffected by crowding in culture and, unlike normal fibroblasts, do not enter the resting phase—commonly referred to as GO but termed by Dulbecco (1973) the holding (H-1) phase. In many non-permissive transformed cells the integrated viral DNA cannot replicate independently of the cell chromosome and generate infective virus, usually because it is incompletely transcribed, so the infection is latent. Integration may be reversible, and the detachment of viral from cellular DNA may be precise, yielding an infectious molecule, or imprecise (i.e., a segment of cell DNA may replace a segment of viral DNA), in which case the detached molecule is defective, and may be incapable of replicating, or may replicate only in cells co-infected with another virus which acts as a helper. Studies with temperature-sensitive mutants have shown that transformation by polyoma virus is controlled by two viral genes, a transforming gene which affects the growth regulation of the cell and another gene which probably affects integration, but the expression of the transforming gene is controlled by cellular genes. Herpes viruses also contain a transforming gene, but its expression may be masked because these viruses also possess genes which can block host macromolecular synthesis (see Dulbecco, 1973). It is of interest that fragments of viral DNA of less than (and sometimes much less than) genome size can transform cells in tissue culture and induce tumors in animals (Graham, 1977).

RNA viruses have been shown to cause leukemias in chickens, mice, cats, and cattle; sarcomas in chickens, mice and cats; and mammary carcinomas in mice. The sarcoma viruses (Levy and Leclerc, 1977) are, in the main, products of the laboratory, and may be of little or no significance in nature; this is not the case, however, with the leukemia viruses (Gross, 1961; J.F.A.P. Miller, 1961; Moloney, 1962), and it seems likely that most, if not all, leukemia in the species listed is of viral origin; moreover, an etiological role for RNA tumor viruses in other species is certainly not excluded (see Tooze, 1973).

The mouse mammary tumor viruses (MMTV) are morphologically of type B (Lyons and Moore, 1965; Hageman, Links, and Bentvelzen, 1968); all the other RNA tumor viruses are morphologically of type C, but differ in various ways (Aoki, 1974). The mouse sarcoma viruses (MuSV) readily cross species barriers and transform every cell they infect (Dulbecco, 1973). On the other hand, they do not possess RNA-dependent DNA polymerase (sometimes termed reverse transcriptase) and are present in infectious virions only after phenotypic mixing with infectious C-type virus (Hartley and Rowe, 1966; Temin, 1974). The mouse leukemia viruses (MuLV), which are morphologically indistinguishable from the MuSV, and the mouse mammary tumor virus (MMTV), can grow in many cells in an organism without appreciably altering their function, and transform only a very small proportion of the cells they infect (Dulbecco, 1973). They build at least one complete DNA replica of their genome in the cell by the action of RNA-dependent DNA polymerase (Baltimore, 1970), and these DNA replicas can integrate with cellular DNA as *provirus* (see Temin and Baltimore, 1972).

RNA oncogenic viruses may be transmitted in three ways:

1. Hereditarily, like ordinary cellular genes, through the ovum or sperm, in which case the virus is termed endogenous.
2. By infection of the embryo *in utero* from the mother or possibly from the father through the semen, or of the newborn via the milk.
3. By infection other than in the manner described under number 2.

The first two of these procedures are referred to as *vertical,* and the last as *horizontal,* transmission. The ability of the virus to infect new cells is limited by host specificities determined by cellular genes (Nandi, 1967; J. Klein, 1976), and the presence of endogenous virus may make a cell resistant to exogenous infection by a similar virus (Daams *et al.,* 1968; Gilden, 1975); it is, however, not uncommon for a virus to be able to transform cells from, and induce tumors in, more than one species (Rabotti *et al.,* 1966; Jarrett, Laird, and Hay, 1969; Theilen *et al.,* 1974).

The strain of MMTV originally discovered by Bittner (Bittner 1936, 1942, 1946; Dmochowski, 1953) is transmitted in the milk, but other strains of MMTV are transmitted hereditarily, or both hereditarily and via the milk (see Gross and Dreyfuss, 1967; Tooze, 1973), and perhaps also horizontally (Blair and Lane, 1974). In the cat, feline leukemic virus (FeLV), which is responsible for various forms of leukemia and other blood disorders, is transmitted horizontally (Jarrett *et al.,* 1973); cats also possess endogenous C-type RNA virus (Essex, 1975), but this is not known to be associated with any disease.

When mice of a strain with a low incidence of leukemia are exposed to sublethal irradiation (Krebs, Rask-Nielsen, and Wagner, 1930; Kaplan, 1947, 1950; Kaplan and Brown, 1952a, 1952b; Gross *et al.,* 1959), or lethal irradiation and rescue with bone marrow from mice with a high incidence of leukemia (Hays and White, 1964), or are injected with various chemical carcinogens (Irino *et al.,* 1963; Zilber and Postnikova, 1966; Ribacchi and Giraldo, 1966), the incidence of leukemia is increased. It has also been shown (Metcalf, 1964) that the incidence of leukemia and reticulum cell sarcoma in F1 hybrid mice is increased by transplantation of thymus from one of the parent lines (AKR) in which there is a high incidence of leukemia, and nearly all the neoplasms are of recipient origin.

The discovery (Leiberman and Kaplan, 1959) that filtrates from radiation-induced murine leukemia possess leukemic activity led Kaplan and his colleagues (Leiberman and Kaplan, 1959; Kaplan, 1967) to postulate that irradiation activates a latent virus, termed by Kaplan Rad LV, in the tissues of mice in which the incidence of leukemia is normally low. This hypothesis gains support from the discovery that the incidence of radiation-induced leukemia is reduced by prior thymectomy (Kaplan, 1950) and restored by a thymus graft as late as 8 days after the irradiation (Carnes *et al.,* 1956); and from the fact that C-type virus particles may be detected a few days after the irradiation, although the leukemia takes some months to develop.

The leukemias we have been considering appear to originate in the thymus, and spread later to other lymphoid tissues. The association of Rad LV with such neoplasms seems clear, but the question of causality is more difficult to resolve. Kaplan (1967) has argued on the following grounds that the virus plays a key etiological role: (1) when parental-strain thymus grafts are transplanted to thymectomized, irradiated F1 hybrid hosts, lymphomas of donor genotype develop (Kaplan and Brown, 1954; Kaplan, Carnes, Brown, and Hirsh, 1956; (2) a cell-borne antigen which develops in virtually all lymphomas induced by Rad LV in mice and W/Fu rats is also present in most radiation-induced lymphomas of C57 B1 and BALB/c mice; (3) by using the intrathymic route of injection for *in vivo* assay, leukemogenic activity can be consistently demonstrated; (4) infant W/Fu rats are highly susceptible to induction of lymphomas by Rad LV but not by radiation, suggesting that they lack the endogenous virus. This evidence is certainly persuasive, though it cannot be regarded as decisive.

Thymic lymphomas also develop in mice of susceptible strains (notably C57BL and Swiss) which are known to harbor a murine leukemia virus (Terracini and Stramignoni, 1967; Terracini and Testa, 1970; Joshi and Frei, 1970; Frei, 1970) after administration of methylnitrosourea (MNU)—a potent carcinogen which induces a variety of tumors in many species (see Denlinger *et al.,* 1973; Swenberg *et al.,* 1975; Terracini *et al.,* 1976). Although Frei, Iwasutiak, and Viragos (1973) observed no significant increase in C-type virus particles in the thymus and bone marrow of mice given a leukemogenic dose of MNU, this does not exclude the possibility that these lymphomas also result from virus activation.

Lymphomas of non-thymic type may also develop after irradiation; in particular, as a late event after whole body irradiation (Mole, 1958), and following injection of ^{90}Sr, ^{239}Pu, and ^{226}Ra to CBA/H and C3H/H mice and their F1 hybrids (Loutit and Carr, 1978). Intracellular virus particles, conforming to Dalton's (1972) Type A, are readily demonstrable in sections of lymphomas induced with these bone-seeking radionuclides, but Loutit and Ash (1978) have argued that the virus is a passenger and plays no etiological role on the ground that these tumors do not possess demonstrable tumor-associated transplantation antigens. This evidence loses some of its strength, however, from the fact that the tumors studied had been passaged many times.

Irradiation followed by administration of urethane can activate a latent provirus in some mouse strains like C57BL, which have a low incidence of mammary cancer, to produce a highly virulent MMTV (Timmermans *et al.,* 1969).

It has also been reported that chemically induced mammary carcinomas in the rat may be transmitted by cell-free preparations of tumor tissue (Scholler, Bergs, and Groupe, 1966), and this again points to activation of a latent virus by the chemcial carcinogen.

The discovery of endogenous RNA tumor virus led Huebner and Todaro (1969) to put forward their *oncogene hypothesis* (see also Todaro, 1972; Todaro and Gallo, 1973; Hill and Hillova, 1976), according to which the DNA of all somatic and germ cells of all animals contains the information necessary to specify the complete genome of an RNA tumor virus. The oncogenic information coded in this virus-specific DNA is normally repressed, but derepression can occur and is responsible for the development of many tumors. Various modifications of this hypothesis have subsequently been proposed (Temin, 1971a, 1971b; Bentvelzen, 1972). Todaro (1978) has suggested that the oncogenic information may play a role in embryological development, and also an evolutionary role as a conveyor of genetic information between species.

It was originally thought that endogenous virus would transform the cell in which it became activated, but transformation by this group of viruses is such a rare event that it seems more likely that, following activation in one cell, many other cells are infected exogenously and one or more of these undergoes transformation (see Dulbecco, 1973).

2.142   THE ROLE OF ONCOGENIC VIRUSES IN MAN

Direct evidence that a particular kind of human tumor is caused by a virus could only be obtained by totally unethical experimentation or as the result of an unfortunate accident in which an unexpectedly high incidence of tumors occurred in people who had been injected with a preparation which was later found to contain an active oncogenic virus. The case must rest therefore on circumstantial evidence, and the following criteria have been suggested (Tooze, 1973):

1. Infection with the virus precedes the development of cancer.
2. Products specified by the virus continue to be made in the tumor cells.
3. Viruses of the same group induce tumors in animals.
4. The virus can transform cells in tissue culture.
5. Vaccination against the virus reduces the incidence of the tumor.
6. The epidemiology of the tumor is similar to the epidemiology of infectious disease.

A papilloma virus very similar to the Shope virus is clearly associated with human warts and has been shown to transform human cells in culture, though with very low efficiency (Noyes, 1965). As these lesions are benign, however, they will not be considered further.

The criteria listed above are particularly difficult to establish in the case of herpes viruses (see Rapp, 1974), partly because these are so ubiquitous, and partly because they often persist throughout the life of an infected individual; it seems nevertheless that at present the strongest viral candidate for an oncogenic role in man is a member of the herpes group, namely, the Epstein-Barr virus, which is associated with Burkitt's lymphoma, and has also been proposed as the cause of nasopharyngeal carcinoma and carcinoma of the cervix uteri.

Burkitt's lymphoma is a rapidly growing tumor which is common in children in certain parts of Africa and typically involves the jaws; it is now known to be a B-cell lymphoma. It is common in areas where malaria is endemic, and this has prompted the suggestion that plasmodium, or some other parasite, plays an etiological role (O'Conor, 1961; Edington *et al.,* 1964). Burkitt (1962) suggested alternatively, on geographical and epidemiological grounds, that it was of viral origin and that the virus might be carried by an insect vector. The hypothesis of an insect vector has been discarded but the discovery by Epstein, Achong, and Barr (1964) of a herpes virus, now known as the EB (Epstein-Barr) virus, in a line of Burkitt's lymphoma cells in tissue culture, and the subsequent demonstration of EB virus in cultures of cells from many other Burkitt's lymphomas (Epstein, Achong, and Pope, 1967) lent support to the idea of viral etiology (see Epstein, 1970; Gunven *et al.,* 1970; Zur Hausen *et al.,* 1970). Further work has shown that even when EB virus cannot be recovered from Burkitt's lymphoma cells by cultivation or co-cultivation with susceptible cells, cells from virtually every biopsy of Burkitt's lymphoma, and all cell lines established from tumor tissues, that have been analyzed by DNA hybridization have been found to contain at least one copy, and often many copies, of EB virus DNA; moreover, antigens that are specific for EB virus can be demonstrated by immunofluorescence in or on the surface of Burkitt's lymphoma cells (G. Klein, Pearson, Nadkarni et al., 1968b), and T cells from a Burkitt lymphoma biopsy have been shown to kill not only cells of the autochthonous tumor but also cell lines carrying the EB virus (Jondal et al., 1975). Recent investigations of the state of the virus genome in the host cell have shown that non-integrated viral DNA is present in circular form and that, in addition, sequences of viral DNA are integrated with the cellular DNA (Kaschka-Dierich et al., 1976; Glaser et al., 1976).

EB virus is similarly associated with squamous cell carcinoma of the nasopharynx, which is common in Southern China and to a lesser extent in Malaysia, Indonesia, and parts of Africa (Clifford, 1970; Gunven et al., 1970; Nelson and Nelson, 1971; Kaschka-Dierich et al., 1976).

In parts of the world where Burkitt's tumor and carcinomas of the nasopharynx are rare, EB virus is associated with, and apparently causes, the common and benign disease known as infectious mononucleosis. If therefore, as seems likely, EB virus does play an essential role in the etiology of Burkitt's tumor and nasopharygeal carcinoma, some additional factor, genetic or environmental, must also be present for a tumor to develop. No such factor has as yet been clearly identified, but chronic malaria and malnutrition, which are both common in areas where Burkitt's lymphoma is common, may conceivably promote tumor development by weakening surveillance mechanisms (Burkitt, 1969). This suggestion gains support from the fact that infectious mononucleosis is a self-limited disease in which recovery is associated with a powerful humoral (Niederman et al., 1968) and T-cell-mediated (Steel and Ling, 1973; Nikoskelainen et al., 1978) immunological response to EB virus antigens or antigens which arise in EB virus-infected cells, and from the experimental observation that chronic malarial infection promotes the development of a viral-induced lymphoma in mice (Wedderburn, 1970). Moreover, there is evidence that, in patients with congenital immunodeficiency, infectious mononucleosis may progress to a malignant lymphoma (Bar et al., 1974; Purtilo et al., 1975).

It has been suggested that carcinoma of the cervix uteri is due to a venereally transmitted herpes virus (herpes simplex Type 2) on the grounds that women with carcinoma of the cervix have higher levels of antibody to this virus than matched controls (Naib et al., 1969; Rawls, Tomkins, and Melnick, 1969; Aurelian et al., 1970; Nahmias et al., 1970), and that the tumor occurs most commonly, though by no means exclusively, in women who are promiscuous or whose partners are promiscuous (Beilby et al., 1968). The serological evidence is, however, open to other interpretations; it is conceivable, for example, that the presence of carcinoma of the cervix increases the chance of infection by herpes simplex virus.

The possibility that an RNA virus might be concerned in human breast cancer (see Hollmann, 1973; MacMahon, Cole, and Brown, 1973) was suggested by the discovery in human milk of particles morphologically similar to the MMTV (Moore, Sarkar et al., 1969; Moore, Charney et al., 1971). The further discovery of reverse transcriptase in human milk containing virus particles (Schlom, Spiegelman, and Moore, 1971), and in human breast cancer (Axel, Gulati, and Spiegelman, 1972), appeared to reinforce this view, although the original report that B-type particles predominated, and were more frequent in milk from women with a family history of breast cancer, turned out on closer examination to be incorrect (Sarkar and Moore,

1972). It was also found that sera of women with breast cancer reduced the infectivity of MMTV in mice, though the effect was not very marked (Charney and Moore, 1971). Further evidence was provided by nucleic acid hybridization studies which showed that RNA from most mouse mammary tumors hybridized with DNA complementary to MMTV RNA synthesized *in vitro* by the action of reverse transcriptase, and that about two-thirds of human breast cancers examined also contained polysomal RNA that would hybridize with this complementary DNA (Spiegelman, Burney *et al.,* 1970; Axel, Schlom, and Spiegelman, 1972a, 1972b; Axel, Gulati, and Spiegelman, 1972), whereas RNA from normal human breast tissue and from tumors other than breast cancer did not hybridize with DNA complementary to RNA of the MMTV, nor did RNA from human breast tumors hybridize with DNA complementary to the RNA of oncogenic viruses other than MMTV. On the other hand, RNA from breast tissue affected by chronic fibroadenosis, which appears to be associated with a significantly increased risk of breast cancer (Warren, 1940; Foote and Stewart, 1945; Davis, Simons, and Davis, 1964; Black *et al.,* 1972; Wellings, Jensen, and Marcum, 1975; but see also E.R. Fisher *et al.,* 1975a), has not been found to hybridize with DNA complementary to the RNA of the MMTV, and there is no convincing evidence that women who were breast fed in infancy have an increased risk of breast cancer (Fraumeni and Miller, 1971).

Evidence of increased levels of specific antibody or increased cell-mediated immunity towards a particular tumor or type of tumor in household contacts of a patient with the tumor in question has been adduced as evidence that osteogenic sarcoma (Morton and Malmgren, 1968; Morton, Malmgren, Hall, and Schidlovsky, 1969; Priori, Wilbur, and Dmochowski, 1971; Byers *et al.,* 1975), soft tissue sarcomas (Eilber and Morton, 1970b), neuroblastoma (I. Hellstrom, K.E. Hellstrom, Bill *et al.,* 1970; Graham-Pole *et al.,* 1976), and carcinoma of the breast (Yonemoto, Fujisawa, and Waldman, 1976; Byers *et al.,* 1977) are horizontally transmitted and therefore of viral origin. This evidence is by no means conclusive, however, because normal people with no history of contact may possess antibodies or cells which react with various kinds of tumor tissue. It has also been reported that cell-free extracts of sarcoma tissue can induce sarcoma-specific antigen in normal human embryonic cells (Morton, Malmgren, Hall, and Schidlovsky, 1969), and that hamsters may develop sarcomas after inoculation of cell-free extracts of human osteogenic sarcoma (Finkel, Biskis, and Farrell, 1968; Pritchard, Reilly, and Finkel, 1971).

C-type virus particles have been demonstrated in various human sarcomas (Morton, Hall, and Malmgren, 1969), and also in Burkitt's lymphoma (Kufe *et al.,* 1973) and other tumors but may of course have been there as passengers.

The report by Fialkow *et al.* (1971b) of recurrence of leukemia in donor cells in a female patient with acute lymphatic leukemia who was treated by whole body irradiation and transplantation of bone marrow from her HL-A identical brother suggests either the activation of a virus in the donor cells or infection of the donor cells by a virus carried by the recipient. More direct evidence that C-type RNA virus is involved in human leukemia has come from three kinds of investigation. Firstly, baboon provirus sequences have been identified in the DNA of human leukemia cells (Wong-Staal, Gillespie, and Gallo, 1976). Secondly, antibodies which react with primate C-type virus proteins have been found in normal human sera (Prochnownik and Kirsten, 1976; Snyder, Pincus, and Fleissner, 1976; Kurth *et al.,* 1977). Thirdly, it has been reported by Metzgar, Mohanakumar, and Bolognesi (1976) that antisera prepared by immunizing rabbits and goats with purified glycoprotein of Friend mouse leukemia virus lysed leukemia cells from patients with some forms of leukemia but did not lyse leukocytes from normal donors, and also that sera from non-human primates immunized with human leukemia cells lost their toxicity for such cells when absorbed with Friend mouse leukemia virus antigens; the significance of these findings is difficult to assess, however, because absorption studies showed that the antigen on chronic granulocytic leukemia cells which reacts with antiserum to Friend virus is also present on normal human platelets and neutrophil polymorphonuclear leukocytes. Results generally similar to those of Metzgar *et al.* have been reported by Oliver and Pillai (1977), but, as these authors remark, "Critical absorption and biochemical studies are required to establish that the determinant on the leukemic cell is related to the oncorna virus protein," or, one might add, to refute this hypothesis.

2.15   The Effect of Hormonal Imbalance

In animals, endocrine deficiency may decrease or even abolish the incidence of tumors in response to chemical carcinogens. Examples include the inhibitory effect of hypophysectomy on the induction of fibrosarcomas in rats by methylcholanthrene (Moon, Simpson, and Evans, 1952) and on carcinoma of the liver in response to oral administration of an azo dye (Griffin, Rinfret, and Corsigilia, 1953); of thyroidectomy on the development of cancer of the liver in rats treated with 2-aminofluorine or its acetyl derivative (Bielschowsky and Hall, 1953); and of oophorectomy on the development of mammary cancer in rats treated with dimethylbenzanthracene (DMBA) (Huggins, Briziarelli, and Sutton, 1958; Dao and Sunderland, 1959). The effect of thymectomy in preventing the spontaneous development of leukemia in mice with a high incidence of leukemia (McEndy, Boon, and Furth, 1944; Law and Miller, 1950a), and of leukemia in response to irradiation (Kaplan, 1950), chemical carcinogens (Law and Miller, 1950b), and oncogenic viruses (Gross, 1959; Levinthal, Buffett, and Furth, 1959; J.F.A.P. Miller, 1959), may be similarly interpreted as reflecting the endocrine function of the thymus, though it seems more likely that it is due to the fact that these are, in the main, T cell lymphomas, and thymectomy acts by reducing the number of available target cells.

Carcinogenesis may also be inhibited by the presence of particular hormones. The incidence of mammary tumors in rats in response to oral administration of DMBA or methycholanthrene, for example, is inhibited by the administration of progesterone and estradiol, alone and in combination (Huggins, Grand, and Brillantes, 1961); and also by pregnancy starting before administration of the carcinogen, and by lactation (Dao and Sunderland, 1959).

Conversely, endocrine stimulation may lead to the development of a variety of animal tumors. It was shown, for example, many years ago that tumors develop in intrasplenic grafts of ovarian tissue in oophorectomized rats (Biskind and Biskind, 1944) because the estrogen secreted by the graft is destroyed in the liver and, as a result, the output of gonadotrophin from the pituitary is increased. Another example, among several discussed by Bielschowsky (1955), is the development of carcinoma of the thyroid in rats after administration of goitrogenic substances which stimulate the production of thyroid stimulating hormone (TSH) by the pituitary (Griesbach, Kennedy, and Purves, 1945; Purves and Griesbach, 1947; Sellers, Hill, and Lee, 1953). This effect can be potentiated by giving ^{131}I in a dosage which damages the thyroid but leaves enough viable thyroid tissue to respond to TSH (Doniach, 1953). As might be expected, ^{131}I hormonal imbalance affects the development of many other tumors of endocrine glands (see Meier, 1963). It has also been shown experimentally that a sustained high level of gonadotrophin increases, and injection of testosterone decreases, the incidence of various tumors including lymphosarcomas in response to 7,12-dimethyl-benzanthracene (DMBA) in female mice of some strains (Pierpaoli, Haran-Ghera, and Kopp, 1977).

Evidence of the etiological role of endogenous estrogens in human breast cancer is provided by the observation that the incidence of this tumor is decreased in women whose ovaries are removed prior to the natural menopause, and that the younger the patient at the time of operation the greater is this effect (Hirayama and Wynder, 1962; Feinleib, 1968). The inverse relationship between the incidence of breast cancer and the shortness of the interval between the menarche and the first pregnancy observed by MacMahon *et al.* (1970) and Henderson *et al.* (1974) also points to the operation of a hormonal factor and suggests that this operates early in life long before breast cancer normally develops. The mechanism responsible for the protective effect has not been established, but one suggestion is that it depends on the preponderance of estriol in relation to estrone and estradiol which is secreted during the latter half of pregnancy (see MacMahon, Cole, and Brown, 1973). A later study by Choi *et al.* (1978), in which great care was taken to ensure that the cancer patients and controls were matched in respect of socioeconomic status, has, however, not revealed any protective effect of early age at first pregnancy so that the question must be regarded as *sub judice,* and this applies also to the possible role of exogenously administered estrogen in human breast cancer.

It appears from the work of Metcalf (1973) that the development of granulocytes and monocytes is regulated by the interplay of a hormone-like humoral agent termed colony stimulating factor (CSF) and various CSF inhibitors; Metcalf's observations suggest further that a disturbance in the levels of these agents is concerned in the development and progression of acute and chronic myeloid leukemia, but do not of course exclude the possibility that C-type virus may be the initiating agent.

The question of hormone-dependence of established tumors will be discussed later (4.24).

2.16   Immunologically Induced Carcinogenesis

The hypothesis that immunological stimulation may play a role in the development of lymphomas and related tumors was suggested by three observations:

1. Injection of C57 B1/6 spleen cells to young (C57 B1/6 × DBA/2) F1 hybrids, which causes severe and often fatal graft-versus-host disease (GVH), results in the development of reticulum cell sarcomas in a high proportion of mice in which the severity of the GVH is mitigated by administration of amethopterin (Schwartz and Beldotti, 1965).
2. Injection of newborn mice of two congenic strains in which the incidence of leukemia is low, and which differ only at the weak H1 histocompatibility locus, with adult spleen cells of the opposite congenic strain, but not with cells of the same strain, results in a marked increase in the incidence of lymphomas (Walford, 1966).

3. There is a relatively high incidence of reticulum cell sarcoma and pleomorphic malignant lymphoma in an inbred strain of mice (NZB/B1) which spontaneously develop autoimmune hemolytic anemia and chronic glomerulonephritis (Mellors, 1966).

Subsequent investigations of the effect of the GVH reaction have shown that the development of tumors is preceded by activation of C-type RNA virus (Armstrong *et al.,* 1973) and progressive lymphoreticular hyperplasia (Gleichman, Gleichman, and Schwartz, 1972). In the early experiments most of the tumors appeared to have originated from host cells (Gleichman *et al.,* 1975a) and could not therefore be attributed directly to antigenic stimulation. More recently Gleichman *et al.* (1975b) have shown by using a variety of markers that the GVH reaction may lead also to the production of similar tumors which are clearly of donor origin; even in these experiments, however, about half of the tumors were of recipient origin. The precise mechanism remains *sub judice,* but it seems likely that the activation of latent oncogenic virus is involved, and Schwartz (1972) has suggested that this can occur not only as the result of a GVH reaction but, more generally, whenever normal feedback mechanisms regulating antibody production and T cell kinetics are disturbed in such a way as to promote excessive proliferation of B cells or T cells. This would account for the relatively high incidence of reticulum cell sarcomas in kidney graft recipients (5.523), and for the association of malaria with EB virus in Burkitt's lymphoma (2.142).

A somewhat similar hypothesis has been proposed by Salmon and Seligman (1974) in which they postulate that the first step in the emergence of B cell lymphomas of various kinds is triggered by specific antigen leading to expansion of a particular clone of cells, and that this is followed by a "second hit" of some kind which culminates in the development of a tumor.

The possibility that autoimmune disease in man may be associated with an increased incidence of cancer is illustrated by the high incidence of cancer of the stomach in patients with chronic atrophic gastritis, since this condition may be a manifestation of autoimmunity (Walker, Strickland *et al.,* 1971; Ungar, Strickland, and Francis, 1971; Strickland and Mackay, 1973).

2.17 Genetic Factors

Studies in inbred strains of mice and other laboratory animals, and in hybrids between such strains, in which precautions have been taken to exclude vertical or horizontal transmission of an exogenous virus, have established that the incidence of tumors of various kinds in animals may be greatly influenced by genetic factors. In mice, for example, it has been established that there are at least four non-linked loci which influence susceptibility to Friend mouse leukemia virus (Lilly and Pincus, 1974), and experiments with transplants of mammary tissue have shown that genetically determined factors in the gland itself influence susceptibility to mammary cancer both in the presence and in the absence of MMTV (Dux and Muhlbock, 1968).

In human populations it is more difficult to define the role of genetic factors unless the tumor happens to be associated with an abnormal karyotype or a known genetic marker.

The association of cancer with *specific* chromosomal disorders is exemplified by the presence of the Philadelphia (Ph[1]) chromosome in many patients with chronic myeloid leukemia (3.111), by the increased incidence of acute leukemia in children with trisomy 21 (Down's syndrome) (Heston, 1976; Kinlen, 1977), and by the increased incidence of breast cancer in XXY males (Kleinfelter's syndrome) (Harnden, MacLean, and Langlands, 1971).

Association with autosomal recessive disorders is exemplified by tumors in patients with xeroderma pigmentosum (2.12), with the syndromes of Fanconi and Bloom, and with congenital immune deficiency disease (5.523). It is noteworthy that in Fanconi's syndrome apparently random chromosome breaks are common, while in Bloom's syndrome there is a high incidence of chromatid exchanges between identical loci on homologous chromosomes and also a large increase in sister chromatid exchanges (see Harnden, 1976). Except in the case of immune deficiency disease, where impairment of surveillance mechanisms (5.5) may play a role, the increased incidence of cancer appears to be due to an increased risk of neoplastic transformation in response to environmental agents (Todaro and Martin, 1967; Knudson, Strong, and Anderson, 1973; Knudson, 1976).

A single dominant gene appears to be responsible for the occurrence of bilateral retinoblastoma, a highly malignant tumor of the eye which occurs in infants and young children, and in a small proportion of patients for unilateral tumors (see Heston, 1976). Congenital multiple polyposis of the colon, which carries such a high risk of colonic cancer that few if any untreated patients survive beyond the age of 50 (see Dukes, 1952; Burdette, 1970), is also associated with a single dominant gene.

Evidence from family and twin studies suggests that polygenic inherited predisposition is concerned in a significant proportion of patients with breast cancer (Macklin, 1959; Anderson, 1971; MacMahon et al., 1973; Lynch et al., 1976), especially when this develops before the menopause (Anderson, 1972), and perhaps also in patients with cancer of the stomach and lung (see Heston, 1976); other factors are also involved however, and the relative importance of genetic predisposition is uncertain (Knudson, 1976; Mulvihill, Miller, and Fraumeni, 1977).

2.2 EXPERIMENTAL INHIBITION OF CARCINOGENESIS

The following procedures have been shown to inhibit experimental chemical carcinogenesis, and in some cases other forms of carcinogenesis also:

1. *Administration of polycyclic hydrocarbons, phenothiazines, flavones, and other substances which are chemically similar to carcinogens but which are themselves noncarcinogenic or only weakly carcinogenic.* Some of these substances may compete with the carcinogen for cellular binding sites, but they appear to act mainly by inducing microsomal enzymes in the liver, gut, lungs, and other organs, which break down the carcinogen to products which are inocuous (see Gelboin, 1967; Wattenberg and Leong, 1965; Wattenberg, 1971). Chemically induced cancer of the liver and the mammary gland have been shown to be inhibited in this way.

2. *Administration of a variety of other substances,* including trace metals, vitamins A and E (Falk, 1971), and chlorpromazine (Levij and Polliack, 1970), whose mode of action has not been clearly defined, and substances which inhibit co-carcinogenesis. The antifungal agent griseofulvin is in the latter category; it interferes with the action of croton oil as a cocarcinogen on the skin (2.11), and appears to do so by arresting cell division (Vessilinovitch and Mihailovitch, 1968).

3. *Dietetic restriction* in the form of either a low calorie diet or a low protein diet (see Falk, 1971).

4. *Creation of endocrine deficiency or administration of hormones* (2.15).

5. *Administration of some immunosuppressive agents,* including methotrexate, actinomycin D, and 6-mercaptopurine, which have been shown to inhibit the development of leukemia in mice of strain DBA/2 treated by repeated painting of the skin with methylcholanthrene (Rubin and Ida, 1957; Rubin, 1962, 1971). This paradoxical effect has not been fully explained, but may be due partly to inhibition of a reaction which would otherwise destroy carcinogen–protein complexes, and partly to inhibition of the production of enhancing antibody (5.521) which would otherwise protect a developing tumor from cell-mediated immunological destruction.

6. *Repeated administration of specific antiviral serum* to mice or rats injected at birth with mouse sarcoma virus (Bubenik, Turano, and Fadda, 1969).

7. *Administration of non-specific immunopotentiating agents.* These will be discussed in detail in Chapter 7. Their effects may be highly complex, but their capacity to activate macrophages, and in some cases to stimulate T-cell-mediated immunity and to cause interferon induction, appear to be especially important. Another possible action is direct inhibition of neoplastic transformation. In the case of chemically induced transformation this has been demonstrated *in vitro* by Marquardt (1973) with a synthetic polynucleotide, polyriboinosinic-polyribocytidilic acid (Poly I:Poly C). Marquardt's suggestion that the effect might be due to inhibition of the action of reverse transcriptase would seem plausible if the transformation depended on chemically induced activation of a latent RNA oncogenic virus.

Treatment with BCG or BCG derivatives (7.51) has been reported to delay the appearance of tumors, or cause a modest reduction in the proportion of animals with demonstrable tumors at the termination of the experiment, in mice or rats given methylcholanthrene (Old *et al.,* 1961: Lavrin *et al.,* 1973), dibenzanthracene (Piessens *et al.,* 1970), urethane (Bekierkunst *et al.,* 1971) or ^{90}Sr (Nilsson, Revesz, and Stjernsward, 1965). Similar results have been obtained in mice treated with a killed vaccine of brucella (Le Garrec *et al.,* 1974) one week after injection of methylcholanthrene, or with Poly I:Poly C (Gelboin and Levy, 1970; Degre and Elgjo, 1971) when dibenzanthracene or methylcholanthrene was applied to the skin. On the other hand, prolonged treatment with Poly I:Poly C has been reported to increase the incidence of chemically induced thymic lymphomas in mice, though it reduced the incidence of radiation-induced lymphomas (Ball and McCarter, 1971).

Poly I:Poly C has also been shown to prevent the development of tumors in mice infected neonatally with mouse sarcoma virus, provided that the treatment was given 4–6 days after birth (Sarma, Shiu *et al.,* 1969; De Clercq and Merigan, 1971), and to retard the development of tumors in rats given polyoma virus (Vandeputte *et al.,* 1970). A naturally occurring ds (double stranded) RNA reduced the incidence of leukemia in mice infected with Friend virus when the treatment was given several days after the virus infection, whereas earlier treatment had the opposite effect (Pilch and Planterose, 1971).

The development of tumors in hamsters in response to benzpyrene was reported by Pinkerton (1972) to be inhibited by prior treatment of either pregnant or non-pregnant animals with *B. pertussis* vaccine or Freund's complete adjuvant, but in pregnant animals this treatment, or administration of live BCG, resulted in a greatly increased incidence of tumors in the progeny. It was suggested that this latter effect might be due to increased production of enhancing antibody (5.521) and passage of this antibody across the placental barrier.

Administration of a killed vaccine of *Propionibacterium acnes*, commonly referred to as *Corynebacterium parvum* or CP (7.52), which when injected intravenously or intraperitoneally causes widespread activation of macrophages (7.521) and inhibits the growth of various syngeneically transplanted tumors (7.522), has also been reported under certain conditions to delay or even prevent the development of tumors in response to both chemical carcinogens and oncogenic viruses.

Inhibition of methylcholanthrene-induced carcinogenesis, manifested by delayed development or reduced incidence of tumors, in mice which received subcutaneous injections of CP was reported by Baum and Baum (1974), who injected 0.7 mg CP 7 days before, and on the day of, injection of the carcinogen, and by Scott and Warner (1976), who gave 14 weekly injections of 0.035 mg CP, ending 8 days before injection of the carcinogen. The experiments of Baum and Baum were undertaken as part of a different study and are difficult to interpret in the present context because it is not clear whether the CP was injected at the same site as the carcinogen or subcutaneously at some other site. In the experiments of Scott and Warner the CP and carcinogen were injected at different sites. It seems surprising that subcutaneous injection had an inhibitory effect on the development of tumors in response to methylcholanthrene whereas intravenous injection did not, and it would be of interest to know whether this was due to the prolonged course of treatment which they adopted. It would also be interesting to know why subcutaneous injection of CP in a dosage which inhibited carcinogenesis by methylcholanthrene did not inhibit carcinogenesis by benzpyrene.

Treatment with CP has also been reported to protect mice against subsequent injection of Friend leukemia virus (Kouznetzova *et al.,* 1974), and to delay the development of tumors in newborn mice injected with Moloney sarcoma virus (Pazmino, Yuhas, and Milas, 1977).

The time of first administration of the protective agent may be highly critical. This was shown by Woodruff and Speedy (1978) in experiments with CP. A course of intravenous injections of this material starting 4 days before a single intramuscular injection of methylcholanthrene markedly delayed or prevented the development of fibrosarcomas in CBA mice, whereas similar treatment starting 4 weeks after injection of the carcinogen did not significantly alter the incidence of tumors. There seemed to be two possible explanations of these findings. Firstly, that treatment with CP might have inhibited activation or promoted degradation of the carcinogen by microphages. Secondly, that a transformational event occurs soon after injection of methylcholanthrene which results in the emergence of a clone of cells which are selectively liable to destruction by activated macrophages, but which, if not destroyed, multiply so rapidly that subsequent treatment fails to prevent, or even perceptibly delay, the appearance of a tumor. The second hypothesis gains support from the subsequent discovery that a single injection of CP 4 days before injection of the carcinogen has little protective effect, whereas repeated injection starting 42 days after injection of a smaller dose of the carcinogen has quite a marked effect, but the possibility that altered metabolism of the carcinogen also plays some part can not be ruled out.

8. *Injection of living or irradiated cells.* Some delay in the appearance of tumors has also been reported in mice given repeated injections of irradiated allogeneic cells (Oth and Liegey, 1975), or normal or irradiated syngeneic cells (Reiner, 1970), prior to injection of methylcholanthrene, due possibly in the case of the allogeneic cells to an overlap in the specificity of tumor-associated and H2 antigens (Invernizzi and Parmiani, 1975). More marked inhibition of carcinogenesis, attributed to the presence of common antigenic determinants on fetal and neoplastic cells, has been obtained by injecting irradiated syngeneic cells from 10–11 day mouse embryos 14 days prior to injection of methylcholanthrene (Castro *et al.,* 1974). Protection has also been achieved by injecting embryonal carcinoma cells (Sikora, Stern, and Lennox, 1977).

Later experiments have confirmed the earlier findings concerning the effect of injecting normal embryonic cells (Medawar and Hunt, 1978), and have shown further that, whereas injection of embryonic cells 7 to 14 days before administration of methylcholanthrene inhibits carcinogenesis, a similar injection at the same time as administration of the carcinogen, or 7 or 14 days thereafter, is much less effective. If the inhibition of carcinogenesis is indeed due to immunization by antigens common to embryonic cells and chemically induced fibrosarcomas, the findings suggest once again that a decisive transformational event occurs very soon after administration of the carcinogen. They also raise the possibility, as Medawar and Hunt suggest, that if, as has been claimed (2.15), the risk of breast cancer is reduced in women whose first pregnancy occurs soon after the menarche, this is an immunological rather than endocrinological phenomenon.

Inhibition of viral carcinogenesis by means of Freund's adjuvant or BCG has also been reported (Lemonde and Clode-Hyde, 1966; Berman, Allison, and Pereira, 1967; Sjögren and Ankerst, 1969). These results have been attributed to stimulation of cell-mediated immunity, but it seems possible that interferon induction may have contributed to the effect.

2.3 HOMEOSTATIC MECHANISMS TO PREVENT THE EMERGENCE OF CANCER CELLS

It would be surprising if the metazoa had not evolved homeostatic mechanisms to limit the emergence and multiplication of cancer cells, which constitute an important, though not unique, example of what Stoker (1972) has called *asocial cells,* i.e., cells which possess selective advantages in respect of their own survival but are disadvantageous as regards the survival of the organism of which they are a part.

This argument has often been challenged on the ground that many tumors develop after reproduction has ceased. But, although many species show a decline in reproductive function with age, there was until recently little evidence that a menopause occurs in species other than man. Cessation of menstruation in old females has now been observed in various nonhuman primates, although not convincingly in the chimpanzee (A.C. Hendrickx and R. Parker, personal communication). Therefore it would be rash to conclude that there has been no evolutionary drive to develop surveillance mechanisms. To develop the criticism it would be necessary to have data concerning the relationship between birth rate and parental age, at least for man and his more immediate ancestors. Moreover, even if it could be established that overt cancer has been largely confined to age groups which contribute a negligible fraction to the birth rate, this would still not exclude the possibility that many tumors are successfully aborted in early life.

The hypothesis that homeostatic mechanisms operate to limit the development of cancer in higher organisms including man is supported by the unexpectedly low incidence of spontaneous tumors in relation to the expected frequency of mutation, which has been estimated to lie between 10^{-5} and 10^{-6} per locus per cell generation both for germ cells *in vivo* in respect of mutations resulting in pathological traits, and for fibroblasts *in vitro* in respect of resistance to 8-azaguanine (Drake, 1970; Cavilli-Sforza and Bodmer, 1971; Albertini and De Mars, 1973). The average human adult has about 3×10^{13} cells, and allowing for the huge number of cells that are lost from the skin and intestinal epithelium, and in other ways, it has been calculated that between 10^{15} and 10^{16} cell divisions occur during the average human life span (Cairns, 1975); a plausible conservative estimate of the number of mutations which might be expected to occur throughout life is therefore in the region of 10^{10}. There is no obvious reason why a high proportion of these should be potentially carcinogenic, but unless this proportion is exceedingly small, or the process of carcinogenesis is somehow aborted, one would expect the incidence of cancer to be much greater than it is.

Some evidence concerning the ways in which the emergence of cancer cells may be prevented is provided by observations on the inhibition of experimental carcinogenesis discussed earlier (2.2), and by studies of DNA repair mechanisms. The following possibilities merit consideration:

1. An environmental chemical carcinogen is taken up by cells, possibly macrophages, which (1) lack the enzymes necessary to convert a procarcinogen into an ultimate carcinogen, or (2) possess or develop enzymes which render a carcinogen inocuous, or (3) do not divide and are eventually shed.

2. Either (1) viral carcinogenesis is prevented by an immunological reaction which prevents infection by an exogenous virus, or (2) the presence of latent non-transforming virus in a cell prevents infection and transformation by another virus (2.14). The first of these mechanisms might, however, be counteracted owing to the fact that many viruses which are known to be oncogenic in animals have immunosuppressive properties (Salaman and Wedderburn, 1966; Siegel and Morton, 1966; Ceglowski and Friedman, 1968; Salaman, 1970; Blair *et al.,* 1971).

3. Accurate DNA repair mechanisms prevent the occurrence of potentially dangerous mutations. The repair of DNA following damage by UV irradiation, and the high incidence of erroneous repair in patients with xeroderma pigmentosum, has been discussed earlier (2.12). Repair also occurs after damage by ionizing radiation (Elkind and Sutton, 1960) and chemical carcinogens (Liebermann and Forbes, 1973; Sarasin and Meunier-Rotival, 1976; Swann *et al.,* 1976), but the nature of the lesions and hence the repair mechanisms are different. The general biological significance of DNA repair has been discussed by Burnet (1976), who has pointed out that it became necessary at a very early stage in evolution to develop ways of protecting DNA from lethal damage by both ionizing and UV radiation, the environmental background levels of which were probably far higher than they are now. With the development of multicellular organisms the demands became

more exacting, since, as we have seen, inaccurate repair which is just sufficient to permit a somatic cell to survive and multiply, aptly referred to as "SOS repair," may give it a potentially dangerous survival advantage. It seems reasonable therefore to interpret those methods of DNA repair which are largely error-free as homeostatic mechanisms at the molecular level, evolved by the metazoa to prevent the emergence of asocial cells.

4. There is selective shedding of mutant cells. According to this hypothesis, which was put forward by Cairns (1975), when an "immortal" stem cell (2.1) divides to form another such cell and a "mortal" cell which is destined to be shed from the epithelium of the skin, bowel, or elsewhere, and a copying error has arisen during DNA replication in one strand, the abnormal strand goes selectively to the mortal cell.

5. Anatomical constraints limit the ability of stem cells, in Cairns' sense of the term (2.1), to escape into areas populated by other stem cells, so that competition between a potentially vigorous mutant and normal cells is limited.

Other evidence bearing on the questions of homeostatic mechanisms in relation to cancer, and in particular on mechanisms by which cancer cells may be recognized and destroyed, will be considered later (5.5).

3
Structure, Growth, and Functional Activity of Tumors

3.1 STRUCTURE OF TUMORS

Transformation, which we have postulated as the first decisive step in the development of a cancer cell from a normal cell (2.1), can occur *in vitro* as well as *in vivo,* and can be recognized as having occurred by changes in cellular morphology (Ambrose *et al.,* 1970), insensitivity to crowding manifested by loss of contact or density dependent inhibition of cell migration (Abercrombie *et al.,* 1957; Abercrombie and Ambrose, 1962) and replication (Stoker and Rubin, 1967; Dulbecco, 1970; Stoker, 1972), diminished serum requirement (Dulbecco, 1970), diminished surface charge (Abercrombie and Ambrose, 1962), diminished adhesiveness (Coman, 1944; Easty, Easty, and Ambrose, 1960), increased agglutinability by phytohemagglutinin and related lectins (Aub, Tieslau, and Lankester, 1963; Rapin and Burger, 1974), and changes in other cell surface properties (Borek, Grob, and Burger, 1973).

Contact inhibition of movement appears to be related to adhesiveness, and it has been suggested (Carter, 1965) that it occurs *in vitro* when cells are more adherent to glass than they are to each other. It is not exhibited by all transformed cells; indeed, as Macieira-Coelho (1967) has shown, transformed cells with an accelerated cell cycle may actually show evidence of decreased cell migration.

There appears to be a degree of specific recognition in contact inhibition of normal cells. It has been reported, for example (Eagle and Levine, 1967), that euploid human fibroblasts and animal cells both show contact inhibition of growth when cultured separately but do not inhibit each other in mixed cultures. Transformed cells in general show loss of contact inhibition by cells of the same kind. They may (Stoker, 1964; Borek and Sachs, 1966) or may not (Abercrombie *et al.,* 1957; Abercrombie and Ambrose, 1962) be inhibited by normal cells; they may also be inhibited by cells transformed by a different agent (Borek and Sachs, 1966), and may themselves inhibit normal cells (Borek and Sachs, 1966).

Normal cells treated with low concentrations of trypsin and other proteases may become as agglutinable by plant lectins as transformed cells and cease to be subject to contact inhibition (Burger, 1969, 1970); contact inhibition may also be lost as the re-

40

sult of treatment with neuraminidase (Vaheri, Ruoshlati, and Nordling, 1972). Conversely, contact inhibition is restored if transformed cells, which have been shown to have proteases on their surface (Borek, Grob, and Burger, 1973), are treated with protease inhibitors (Rapin and Burger, 1974), or if an artificial cover layer is provided by treating the cells with monovalent concanavalin A, which binds to the agglutinin receptor sites (Burger and Noonan, 1970). In the light of these findings it has been postulated (Burger, 1969; Burger and Noonan, 1970) that contact inhibition depends on the presence of a surface layer which is lost on transformation and can be removed by proteases, and that receptors for plant agglutinins happen to lie deep to this layer and become accessible only when it is lost. An alternative hypothesis (Singer and Nicolson, 1971), which gains support from observations of the surface distribution of ferritin-conjugated concanavalin A on normal and transformed cells (Nicolson, 1971), is that the agglutinin-binding sites are normally present in a distribution that does not favor agglutination (i.e., they are dispersed), but after exposure of the cell to proteases or transformation a redistribution (clustering) of the sites occurs which favors agglutination. The question of how a structural change on the cell surface causes a resting cell to resume DNA synthesis and cell division has been investigated by Mallucci (1972) by using metabolic inhibitors of various kinds. He has concluded that the cell surface change produced by exposure to proteases triggers protein synthesis dependent on pre-existing messengers, and swelling of the nucleus, and these changes in turn trigger DNA synthesis.

The fate of a transformed cell *in vivo* depends not only on the intrinsic properties of the cell but also on the reaction of the host. There are three possibilities, none of which can be excluded on the evidence available: (1) the cell is destroyed; (2) it is immobilized in the sense that it ceases, at least for a time, to divide; (3) it undergoes repeated division. Clearly if the number of newly formed cells exceeds the number lost the population will expand, and during this process further mutational and epigenetic change may occur with consequent selection of cells possessing a survival advantage. The members of this expanding population will be referred to as *cancer cells* or *tumor cells*. In the case of epithelial cells this population remains bounded for a time by the epithelial basement membrane, and while this is the case the lesion is termed *carcinoma-in-situ*.

The question of the extent to which homeostatic mechanisms operate at this stage, and later throughout the life history of a tumor, to destroy or immobilize tumor cells will be considered in the discussion of tumor cell population kinetics (3.5), and we shall return to it repeatedly in later chapters.

Without tumor cells there would of course be no tumor; a malignant tumor, however, except perhaps at a very early stage, is not just a collection of tumor cells. It is a highly complex ecosystem which contains, in addition to tumor cells, a supporting framework of vascular tissue, and a variety of other cells including lymphocytes and macrophages, the proportions of which differ in different tumors and at different times in the life history of the same tumor. These additional elements together constitute what is termed the stroma of the tumor.

Various markers have been used to identify the different kinds of cell and to trace their origin (3.11, 3.12); in addition, the kinetics of the populations which they represent have been investigated by methods described in a later section (3.5).

Different malignant tumors originating in the same kind of tissue may differ greatly in respect of the proportion of stromal tissues and the arrangement and cytological characteristics of the tumor cells. At one extreme a tumor may so closely resemble the normal tissue of origin that it may be difficult to decide on histological examination that the lesion is malignant. At the other extreme the appearance is so abnormal that it is not possible on morphological grounds to determine the tissue of origin, and such tumors are described as *anaplastic* or *undifferentiated.* Anaplastic tumors often show a high degree of *cellular pleomorphism;* i.e., the cells vary greatly in size and other characteristics. Tumors whose appearance lies somewhere between these extremes are described as well differentiated, moderately well differentiated, or poorly differentiated, according to their degree of morphological resemblance to normal tissue.

3.11 Tumor Cells

Cells obtained from tumors and then grown *in vitro* exhibit the same characteristics as cells transformed *in vitro. In vivo* they are relatively insensitive to the restraining effect of neighboring cells and of natural barriers such as the epithelial basement membrane and the walls of blood vessels. They do not, as a rule, cooperate normally with other cells to form organized functionally effective tissues, but sometimes quite considerable organization and functional activity is achieved (3.6).

3.111 CHROMOSOMAL ABNORMALITIES

Many cancer cells have an abnormal karyotype. The number of chromosomes may differ greatly from the normal diploid number; it is often close to, but seldom an exact integral multiple of, the normal haploid number. In addition, what are termed *marker chromosomes,* i.e., chromosomes which do not resemble any normal homologue, are often seen. Human marker chromosomes have been classified by Miles (1974) as (1) minute chromosomes; (2) fragments, i.e., paired chromatids about the size of minute chromosomes but without visible centromeres; (3) achrocentric chromosomes other than those which occur in the normal karyotype; (4) metacentric and submetracentric chromosomes larger than chromosome 1; (5) ring chromosomes; (6) dicentric chromosomes; and (7) multiradial chromosomes. The number of chromosomes in different cells from the same tumor is often fairly constant, but sometimes quite large differences are seen.

Studies of cells from a wide variety of human tumors have shown that the chromosomal abnormalities are by no means randomly distributed (see Miles, 1974). Deletions are most frequent in chromosomes of groups 4 and 5 and chromosome 1; gains in groups 6 to 12 and the X chromosome.

Some kinds of tumor show a remarkably consistent pattern of chromosomal abnormality. This is exemplified by the Philadelphia (Ph[1]) chromosome, which occurs in approximately 90 percent of patients with chronic myeloid leukemia (Whang-Peng *et al.,* 1968; Ezdinli *et al.,* 1970) and has been shown to be due to loss of most of the long arm of chromosome 22 (Caspersson *et al.,* 1970; O'Riordan *et al.,* 1971); by total or partial loss of the same chromosome in cells from many meningiomas (Zankl and Zang, 1971, 1972; Mark, Levan, and Mitelman, 1972); and by a structural abnormality of chromosome 14 in the cells of some patients with Burkitt's and other lymphomas (Fukuhara, Shirakawa, and Uchino, 1976). Many tumors, on the other hand, show no such uniformity. It has been postulated by Rowley (1974) that, when different individuals with the same type of tumor show the same chromosomal abnormality, a common etiological agent is involved, though the converse proposition, namely, that a particular agent always causes the same kind of abnormality, does not appear to be true.

3.112 CHANGES IN INTRACELLULAR AND SURFACE ANTIGENS

Cancer cells may show either a loss or an increase in the expression of normal cellular antigens.

Loss of tissue specific antigen has been demonstrated in various rat and mouse tumors, including chemically induced hepatomas (Weiler, 1959; Nairn et al., 1960; Baldwin and Barker, 1967a), skin carcinomas (Carruthers and Baumler, 1965) and muscle sarcomas (Fel and Taikarishvili, 1964) induced with methylcholanthrene, and kidney tumors induced with stilbestrol and x-irradiation (Nairn et al., 1960); and in a wide range of human neoplasms including carcinomas of the skin (Nairn et al., 1960), thyroid (Goudie and McCallum, 1963), and gastrointestinal tract (Nairn et al., 1962); myloid leukemia (Vulchanov, 1964); and astrocytomas (Vaheri et al., 1976). In general these tissue specific antigens are located within the cell and not on the surface. The antigen studied by Vaheri et al. occurs on the surface of normal fibroblasts and glial cells but is absent, or virtually absent, from the surface of transformed fibroblasts and cells derived from malignant astromytomas; it was shown, however, that the antigen, which has been termed fibroblast surface antigen (SFA) is produced in tissue culture by the tumor cells but rapidly lost from the surface.

Decreased expression of mouse H-2 histocompatibility antigens on the cell surface has been demonstrated in some forms of mouse leukemia (Boyse and Old, 1969), in sarcomas induced with methylcholanthrene (Haywood and McKhann, 1970, 1971), and in mouse cells transformed with polyoma virus (Ting and Herberman, 1971).

In contrast to these findings, the expression of Forssman antigens has been reported to be increased in chemically-induced guinea pig hepatomas (Crisler et al., 1966) and cells transformed with SV40 virus (Robertson and Black, 1969), and of HL-A histocompatibility antigens in some human leukemic cells (Peacocke, Amos, and Laszlo, 1966).

Tumor cells also often possess antigens, termed tumor-associated antigens (TAA), or tumor-specific antigens (TSA), which are not represented on normal cells (5.2).

Ting and Herberman (1971) have shown that there may be an inverse relationship between the extent to which the expression of normal cellular antigens is lost and new TAA are expressed, and they have suggested three possible reasons for this, namely, (1) that the two types of antigen share a limited topographical distribution of antigenic sites; (2) that steric interference limits access of antibody to the corresponding antigen; and (3) that with virus-induced tumors, or chemically induced tumors in which latent virus is activated, the integration of viral DNA into the cellular DNA stimulates the expression of new antigens but at the same time represses the synthesis of products of host genes including histocompatibility antigens.

3.113 CELL HYBRIDIZATION AND THE ANALYSIS OF MALIGNANCY

The development of methods of somatic cell hybridization in vitro by the use of inactivated Sendai virus, and more recently with polyethylene glycol, has provided a useful tool for analyzing some of the properties of tumor cells. Early reports that intraspecies hybrids of highly malignant and non-malignant or weakly malignant cells were tumorigenic in appropriate hosts (Barski and Cornefert, 1962; Scaletta and Eph-russi, 1965; Defendi *et al.,* 1967) suggested that malignancy behaves as a dominant character. Subsequently, however, Harris and his colleagues (Harris, Miller, Klein *et al.,* 1969; Harris, 1971; G. Klein, Friberg, Wiener, and Harris, 1973) showed that when a malignant mouse tumor cell was fused *in vitro* with a non-malignant mouse cell the resultant hybrid had little capacity to grow *in vivo* if, though only if, it retained something approaching the complete chromosome sets of both cells. Tumors which developed after the injection of hybrid cells showed a much lower number of chromosomes and were considered to have developed by selective overgrowth of cells from which some chromosomes had been eliminated. Since hybrid cells which had lost a similar number of chromosomes as the result of prolonged culture *in vitro* were not tumorigenic, it was concluded that the generation of malignant variants of hybrid cells requires not merely an overall reduction in chromosome number but the elimination of some particular chromosomes donated by the non-malignant parent cell. The expression of histocompatibility antigens can also be suppressed when a cell bearing particular antigens is fused with another cell that expresses them poorly, but the possibility that this might explain the apparent suppression of malignancy was excluded by the use of irradiated newborn mice, which are highly immunodeficient, as hosts in the tumor experiments.

The further observation that hybrids of cells from two different mouse tumors sometimes (Harris, 1971), though not always (Wiener, Klein, and Harris, 1973, 1974a, 1974b) grow less readily than cells from either one of the original tumors clearly mimics classical genetic complementation, and suggests that the fundamental lesion responsible for malignancy is associated with loss rather than gain of genetic (or stable epigenetic) information.

Studies of hybrids of two human tumor cell lines, and of a tumor cell line and either a senescent or a proliferating fibroblast line (Stanbridge, 1976), in (1) neonatally thymectomized mice treated with antilymphocyte serum, (2) thymectomized, irradiated, bone marrow reconstituted mice, and (3) congenitally athymic (nude) mice, have demonstrated virtually complete suppression of malignancy in tumor cell–fibroblast hybrids, though the hybrids with senescent fibroblasts, unlike the senescent fibroblasts themselves, had the capacity to proliferate indefinitely. In these experiments malignancy was not suppressed in the tumor–tumor hybrids, but this lack of evidence of complementation seems of little significance, since the tumor cell lines were both HeLa cell variants and therefore derived originally from the same tumor.

Hybrids of human epithelial cells which were derived from a HeLa cell line but showed contact inhibition, and Burkitt lymphoblastoid cells which expressed the EB viral genome and were not contact inhibited, were found by Glaser *et al.* (1977) to possess epithelial morphology but to be not subject to contact inhibition and to yield a higher proportion of tumors than the parent epithelial cell line when injected into athymic mice. It was concluded (Glaser *et al.,* 1977; Ablashi *et al.,* 1978) that if EB virus can enter a non-lymphoblastoid cell this cell may undergo malignant transformation.

The behavior of interspecific hybrids between human cells transformed with SV40 (2.141) and mouse macrophages is somewhat different in that these have been reported (Croce and Koprowski, 1974; Croce *et al.,* 1975) to be tumorigenic if, and only if, human chromosome 7 is retained in the hybrid, suggesting that the SV40 transformed phenotype is under some kind of positive control. Whatever the mechanism, it is clear from these and other experiments (see Ozer and Jha, 1977) that the expression of malignancy is suppressed when cells from a large variety of tumors, including chemically induced, RNA viral, and DNA viral tumors, are fused *in vitro* with a variety of normal cells, including fibroblasts, macrophages, lymphocytes, and cells passaged for a long time in tissue culture. There is now, in addition, convincing evidence, based on the identification of H-2 antigens and an easily recognisable marker chromosome (the T6 translocation), that mouse tumor cells injected into compatible hosts may fuse *in vivo* with host cells (Wiener, Femjo, Klein, and Harris, 1972), and further evidence which suggests that human tumor cells transplanted to the hamster cheek pouch may also fuse with cells of the heterologous host (Goldenberg, Bhan, and Pavia, 1971). These findings raise the question of whether hybridization with host cells is one form of homeostatic mechanism by which naturally occurring cancer cells are destroyed, or prevented from multiplying and disseminating.

3.114   EVIDENCE OF MONOCLONALITY

The question of whether a tumor has developed from one, or from more than one, cell has been investigated by looking for evidence of uniformity or heterogeneity in respect of (1) marker chromosomes; (2) production of specific immunoglobulin; (3) tumor-associated antigens (TAA); and (4) differences that occur in normal tissues in human females in consequence of random inactivation of one X chromosome.

The finding of the same chromosome abnormality in all the cells of a tumor is generally accepted as strong, though not conclusive, evidence that all these cells are the progeny of a single cell. The abnormality may conceivably arise at any stage in the development of the tumor, or may even antedate malignant transformation, as has been postulated in the case of the Ph[1] chromosome (Canellos and Whang-Peng, 1972), which is commonly found in patients with chronic myeloid leukemia (2.17) and has been interpreted as the marker of a clone of cells in which neoplasia is abnormally likely to arise. This implies that a considerable number of normal people have an occasional cell with the Ph[1] chromosome in their bone marrow (Harnden, 1976), but a large number of karyotypes would have to be examined to substantiate this hypothesis.

Immunoglobulin production is a characteristic of plasma cell tumors and B cell lymphomas, but these differ in that plasma cells, and the tumors arising from them, produce immunoglobulin in large quantity for export, whereas the small amount of immunoglobulin produced by B lymphocytes is retained as a cell surface marker.

It has now been established that plasma cell tumors, which can be readily induced in certain strains of mice with mineral oil, and occur spontaneously in various animals, and also in man in the form of multiple myeloma, produce a single immunoglobulin (Potter, 1972; Martensson, 1963; Abdou and Abdou, 1975), and this seems inconsistent with a multicellular origin. The study of cell-surface immunoglobulin points to a similar conclusion in respect of Burkitt's lymphoma (E. Klein, G. Klein, Nadkarni *et al.*, 1967; Fialkow, Klein, *et al.*, 1973) and chronic lymphocyte leukemia (E. Klein, Eskeland, Inoue *et al.*, 1970; Preud'Homme, Klein *et al.*, 1971; Aisenberg, Bloch, and Long, 1973).

The cells of many tumors, especially those caused by viruses and chemical carcinogens, possess surface antigens, known as tumor-associated antigens (TAA), which are not found on the surface of normal adult cells (5.2). Failure to identify populations of cells with distinct antigens is of no significance as evidence of monoclonality in the case of tumors of viral origin, since different tumors induced by the same virus typically have many antigens in common and unshared antigens may be difficult to demonstrate. The situation is different with chemically induced tumors, since different tumors, even if induced with the same carcinogen and in the same animal, are typically antigenically distinct and may indeed have no demonstrable TAA in common, but failure to demonstrate antigenically distinct populations does not prove conclusively that they do not exist, since particular antigens may be masked in the presence of specific antibody (5.521). On the other hand, if two or more antigenically distinct populations could be demonstrated, this would provide strong evidence of polyclonality. It is of interest therefore that, whereas Prehn (1970) had been unable to demonstrate any antigenic differences between cells obtained from different parts of the same chemically induced tumor, Pimm and Baldwin (1977a) found antigenic differences between primary methylcholanthrene-induced fibrosarcomas in rats and tumor recurrences at the site of surgical excision of the primary tumor. The explanation favored by Pimm and Baldwin is that the recurrent tumors developed from the proliferation of a previously dormant neoplastic cell, or a clone of dormant cells, of different provenance than the cells of the primary tumor; as a possible alternative they suggest that cells may have been transformed by residual carcinogen after the removal of the primary tumor.

The most generally applicable criterion of monoclonality is the last of the four listed above, which depends on the mosaicism in normal tissues in women caused by the random inactivation of one X chromosome in each somatic cell. Recognition of this mosaicism requires a marker of some kind which is the product of a gene carried on the X chromosome, and the enzyme glucose-6-phosphate dehydrogenase (G-6-PD), which exists in two forms, G-6-PD B and G-6-PD A, which can be easily distinguished by electrophoresis, has proved particularly useful for this purpose. Women who are heterozygous at the G-6-PD locus have two cell populations, one producing G-6-PD B and the other G-6-PD A, and both might be represented in polyclonal tumors, whereas only one of them should be represented in a monoclonal tumor.

According to this criterion (see Fialkow, 1972; 1974; Friedman and Fialkow, 1976), many human tumors, including uterine leiomyoma (Linder and Gartler, 1965), Burkitt's lymphoma (Fialkow, Klein et al., 1970; Fialkow, 1974), chronic myeloid leukemia (Barr and Fialkow, 1973; Fialkow, 1974) and carcinoma of the cervix (Park and Jones, 1968) have been found to be monoclonal, whereas neurofibromata in all specimens examined were polyclonal (Fialkow, Sagebiel et al., 1971).

The conclusion that a particular tumor is monoclonal on the ground of lack of evidence of mosaicism would be vitiated if there were any degree of clustering, i.e., if the two classes of cell which constitute the mosaicism of normal tissues were distributed in a non-random manner. This objection would fail if a larger number of tumors of a particular kind had been examined and none had been found to be mosaics. Except in the case of uterine leiomyoma, Burkitt's and other lymphomas, leukemias, carcinoma of the cervix, and neurofibroma, however, the number of specimens of each type of tumor examined has been small, ranging from one to six (see Friedman and Fialkow, 1976), so that generalizations must be viewed with caution. Conversely, evidence of mosaicism would not exclude the possibility that all the tumor cells arose from a single cell if the population studied included a significant proportion of stromal cells (3.1); indeed, failure to demonstrate mosaicism under these conditions would render the whole technique suspect.

Many pathologists with a wide knowledge of human cancer, and many clinicians, hold that tumors are often of multifocal origin (Cheatle and Cutler, 1931), or, as Willis (1960) has suggested, that they develop through a "field effect" which extends over an appreciable area of tissue. The demonstration by random biopsy in patients with breast cancer of multiple, apparently distinct areas of neoplastic tissue in addition to the palpable tumor (E. R. Fisher, Gregorio et al., 1975), supports the field hypothesis; it is, however, not entirely conclusive, because histological appearances may be deceptive, and malignant cells may migrate locally from their site of origin. Moreover, the rarity of overt separate tumors in the same breast, and of synchronous bilateral overt breast cancer, as compared with the incidence of a positive biopsy in the opposite breast to the one in which there is an overt tumor (Urban, 1967, 1969; Slack et al., 1973), suggests that small lesions diagnosable by biopsy do not necessarily progress to overt lesions and may actually regress (B. Fisher, Hanlon et al., 1978). A multifocal origin is not necessarily inconsistent with evidence of monoclonality, however, because a tumor which appears at a particular time in its life history to be monoclonal may have become so simply because one particular clone of cells outgrew all others. It is not surprising that some clones should be eliminated as the result of selection pressures of various kinds in the struggle for survival within a tumor cell population, but there is no obvious reason why one, and only one, clone should so regularly outgrow all others. This phenomenon would seem to merit more attention than it has received hitherto; one simple type of experiment which might throw some light on the matter would be to analyze tumors which develop when a suspension containing cells from two distinct tumors of the same kind is injected into an isogeneic animal, or, if the original tumors arose in the same animal, into another site in this animal.

Even when one clone clearly predominates, the presence of small minority populations, i.e., of cells not belonging to that clone, cannot easily be ruled out. Many tumors, both animal and human, as will be discussed later (3.34), contain dormant cells, and there is no obvious reason why these should all belong to the dominant clone; indeed, the observations of Pimm and Baldwin (1977a) cited earlier strongly suggest that cells which are both foreign and dormant can occur in *apparently* monoclonal experimental tumors, and may be responsible for local recurrence after treatment by surgical excision. The trauma of the surgical procedure, as these authors suggest, may have provided the stimulus which caused the dormant cells to proliferate; a further possibility to be considered, however, is the disturbance of an ecological balance resulting from removal of the bulk of the dominant clone. It seems reasonable to postulate that at least some of the dormant cells in human tumors are also foreign, and that they may be responsible in some patients for local recurrence, and also for the appearance of metastases, after surgical excision or radiotherapy. It should be possible to test this hypothesis by using appropriate cell markers.

3.12 Leukocytes and Macrophages

Infiltration of mononuclear cells has long been known to occur in malignant tumors of various kinds (Russell, 1908; Wade, 1908; Da Fano, 1912). These cells include lymphocytes, often in large numbers, plasma cells, monocytes, and mature macrophages. It is difficult to distinguish lymphocytes and monocytes on morphological grounds in conventional sections examined by light microscopy, so that an infiltrate described as lymphocytic may include an unspecified proportion of monocytes unless special methods of examination (*vide infra*) have been used. The degree of mononuclear infiltration is often relatively great in well-differentiated tumors; it is, for example, typically much greater in squamous cell cancer of the lung than in oat cell (small cell undifferentiated) tumors (Ioachim, 1976). Heavy infiltration is often seen in experimental tumors which are regressing, for example, tumors induced with murine sarcoma virus (Russell and Cochrane, 1974), and has also been described in the so-called halo nevus, a form of human melanoma which sometimes regresses spontaneously (Jacobs *et al.*, 1975).

J. B. Murphy (1926) held that lymphocytes play a key role in the resistance to tumors, and many subsequent investigators have claimed that there is a positive correlation between the degree of mononuclear cell infiltration and the prognosis in tumors of the same type (Black, Opler, and Speer, 1955; Berg, 1959; Takahashi, 1961; Keller *et al.*, 1968; Black and Leis, 1971; E. R. Fisher and B. Fisher, 1972; Lauder and Aherne, 1972; Barker *et al.*, 1975). This is by no means universally accepted (Willis, 1952; Tanaka, Cooper, and Anderson, 1970; Sarma, 1970; Champion *et al.*, 1972; Morrison *et al.*, 1973) even in the case of cancer of the breast where the evidence appears relatively strong, but recently the interpretation of lymphocytic infiltration as a manifestation of a defensive reaction evoked by tumor-associated antigens to a tumor has gained support from the observation of Ioachim (1976) that it occurs, independently of infection and necrosis, in close relation to carcinoma-in-situ (3.1) in various sites including the cervix uteri, the bronchial epithelium, the skin, and the breast.

It has been reported that some lymphocytes appear to have actually entered tumor cells. This phenomenon, which is termed emperipolesis (Humble, Jayne, and Pulvertaft, 1956), has been studied *in vitro* in organ cultures of tumor tissue (Richters and Sherwin, 1964), but its significance is not clear.

The lymphocyte population of mouse tumors has been shown to include T cells, B cells, and so-called null cells (Kerbel and Davies, 1974; Haskill, Yamamura, and Radov, 1975; Holden *et al.*, 1976); so far, however, little seems to have been done to characterize the lymphocytes which occur in human tumors other than those of lymphoreticular origin.

Plasma cells can be recognized fairly easily in sections stained with hematoxylin and methyl green pyronine (Unna-Pappenheim stain), and a positive correlation between the number of such cells and the amount of IgG in human mammary carcinomas has been reported (Roberts, Bass *el al.*, 1973).

It was reported by Evans (1972) that between 4 and 55 percent of the cells in chemically induced rat and mouse fibrosarcomas were macrophages, as judged by their morphological characteristics, capacity to adhere rapidly to glass and resist detachment by trypsin, and capacity to phagocytize carbon particles and tumor cells which had been pretreated with specific antiserum. Moreover, if a tumor cell suspension from which the macrophages had been removed was injected into a syngeneic animal, the resulting tumor quickly acquired the same proportion of macrophages as tumors which developed from inocula from which the macrophages had not been removed. Evans' work has been confirmed and extended, and it has been shown that the proportion of macrophages in a given fibrosarcoma remains fairly constant and is related directly to the immunogenicity of the tumor and inversely to its liability to metastasize spontaneously (Eccles and Alexander, 1974a). Kinetic studies using ^{3}H-thymidine suggest that macrophages within a tumor rarely divide (Alexander, 1974); it seems likely, therefore, that most of these cells enter the tumor from without, but the possibility that some arise by division of precursor cells, i.e., monocytes, within the tumor is not excluded.

Macrophages, monocytes, and lymphocytes of various kinds have on their surface receptors, termed Fc receptors, which bind antigen–antibody complexes and aggregated IgG. Cells bearing Fc receptors have also been demonstrated in both animal (Kerbel and Davies, 1974; Kerbel, Pross, and Elliott, 1975; Szymaniec and James, 1976) and human tumors (Tønder, Morse, and Humphrey, 1974). Some of these cells are also phagocytic, and it seems likely that most, if not all, of these are macrophages. The presence of macrophages in human tumors has also been demonstrated by enzyme histochemistry (Monis and Weinberg, 1961), and electron microscopy (Carr and Underwood, 1974; Carr, 1977), and by means of antimacrophage serum (Gauci and Alexander, 1975). Even when macrophages are present in quite large numbers, however, ultrastructural studies have failed to provide any evidence of cytotoxic interactions between macrophages and tumor cells (Carr, 1977), and their defensive role has not been established (Alexander, Eccles, and Gauci, 1976).

Neutrophil polymorphonuclear leukocytes may be present in large numbers in tumors in which secondary infection with pyogenic organisms has occurred as the result of ulceration or blood-borne infection, especially in association with areas of necrosis. Neutrophils are, however, sometimes quite conspicuous in both animal (Russell and Cochrane, 1974) and human tumors in which there is no evidence of infection, and in some tumors they may conceivably represent a component of the host reaction to the tumor. Eosinophils are found in some tumors (Marshall and Dayan, 1964), and these too may be a manifestation of the host reaction. Mast cells have also been identified in chemically induced fibrosarcomas in rats, but they disappeared when the tumors were transplanted syngeneically (Broom and Alexander, 1975).

3.13 Supporting Tissue. Angioneogenesis

Solid tumors all have a component of vascular connective tissue derived from the normal tissue of the host, but this varies greatly in quantity and vascularity in different tumors.

Studies of the vascular reaction to transplanted tumors in mice led Algire and Chalkley (1945) to conclude that tumor cells have the capacity to elicit the growth of new capillary endothelium, and subsequent studies of human tumors suggested that this is true also in man (Feigin et al., 1958). It was postulated by Chalkley (1948), and later by Warren and Shubik (1966), that the effect is due to a humoral substance produced by the tumor, and this was confirmed by experiments in which tumor transplants were isolated from host tissue by millipore membrane which allowed the free passage of fluid but not of cells. More recently Folkman and his colleagues (Folkman, Merler et al., 1971; Folkman, 1972, 1974) have isolated a diffusible factor which is mitogenic for capillary endothelium from animal and human tumor cells. They have termed this material tumor-angiogenesis factor (TAF), and have shown that it consists of RNA and protein and has a molecular weight of about 100,000 daltons. Several methods of bioassay have been developed to assess the potency of preparations of TAF, based on the study of angiogenesis in subcutaneous pouches prepared in rats, in the rabbit cornea, and in the chorioallantoic membrane of the chick embryo, and on the behavior of endothelial cells in culture (Folkman, 1974).

The capacity of tumor tissue to evoke angioneogenesis is abolished if the tumor cells are killed (Gimbrone et al., 1974; Folkman, 1974), but not if they are irradiated in a dosage (5000 R) which virtually abolished cell division (Auerbach et al., 1975).

A developing tumor must depend initially for its metabolic requirements on diffusion of nutrients and waste products. In the case of tumor cells growing in three-dimensional soft agar cultures *in vitro* a steady state is reached when the diameter of the colony is about 2 mm, and no further increase in diameter occurs however often fresh nutrient medium is added (Folkman and Hochberg, 1973); and it seems reasonable to postulate that the limiting size for a non-vascularized tumor *in vivo* is of the same order of magnitude. The development of a vascular stroma is therefore a critical step in the life history of a tumor. Moreover, subsequent growth is influenced by the extent to which the vascular supply is maintained, and it has been shown in kinetic studies that in a given tumor the probability of a cell entering mitosis varies inversely with its distance from the nearest capillary (Tannock, 1968, 1970).

It seems clear that a growing tumor stimulates the growth of host connective tissue (Vasiliev, 1958), as well as capillary endothelium. Sparck and Gross (1969) concluded from histological studies that host mesenchyme is not merely stimulated to grow but undergoes metaplasia and malignant transformation at the site of tumor transplants. They postulated that a similar phenomenon occurs during the development of autochthonous tumors, but there is no direct evidence of this, and in the case of predominantly monoclonal tumors it seems almost inconceivable.

3.2 PROGRESSION AND REGRESSION OF PRIMARY TUMORS

It is a familiar clinical observation in both human and veterinary medicine that the behavior of a tumor and its histological appearance may change throughout its life history, and similar changes occur also in experimental animal tumors. In patients the natural history of cancer is often profoundly modified by treatment, but information concerning the behavior of untreated tumors can sometimes be obtained by observations on patients who present late or refuse treatment, or in whom treatment is postponed for any reason (Bloom, Richardson, and Harries, 1962).

Most commonly a tumor exhibits what Foulds (1949, 1951, 1956a, 1956b, 1956c, 1956d, 1969) termed progression; i.e., it begins to grow more rapidly, becomes more invasive or less responsive to deprivation of hormonal stimulation, assumes a more anaplastic appearance in histological sections, or becomes more readily transplantable to a privileged site in a xenogeneic host or, in the case of animal tumors, to an allogeneic or isogeneic host (Greene, 1938, 1952; Browning, 1948; Kallman, Silini, and van Putten, 1967; Rees and Symes, 1971).

Foulds' studies of mammary tumors in mice, and more recently experiments in both mice and rats using the technique of transplantation of the mammary fat pad and fragments of the duct system (see Slemmer, 1974; Prehn, 1976a), have established that progression is associated with a fundamental change in the biological properties of tumor cells, and, in the case of predominantly monoclonal tumors (3.114), this implies the emergence of a new dominant clone of cells, either as the result of selection due to some change in the host environment favoring the growth of a particular clone of cells which was hitherto latent, or as the result of a new mutation or stable epigenetic change of some kind.

Progression may be halted at any stage, and sometimes there is a change in the opposite direction as shown by partial or even complete spontaneous regression of a tumor, i.e., regression either in the absence of any treatment or in the absence of treatment which, in the light of experience with similar tumors, might reasonably be expected to have any such effect.

Regression occurs not only with experimental animal tumors—for example, mammary carcinomas induced in rats with dimethylbenzanthracene (Young and Cowan, 1963) and sarcomas induced in mice with mouse sarcoma virus (Russell and Cochrane, 1974)—but also occasionally with human tumors, both primary and metastatic. The phenomenon has been discussed, and reported instances have been analyzed, by Handley (1909), Dunphy (1950), Boyd (1957, 1966), Gordon-Taylor (1959), Sumner and Foraker, 1960, Smithers (1962b), Fullerton and Hill (1963), Brunschwig (1963), and Everson and Cole (1956, 1966). In their later publication Everson and Cole listed 176 cases reported between 1900 and 1966 which they regarded as possible examples of partial or complete regression.

Regression of metastases will be discussed later (3.34); in this section we shall consider only regression of a primary tumor following biopsy or manifestly incomplete excision. There were 64 such cases in the series reported by Everson and Cole (1966). Some of these patients were alive and presented no clinical evidence of tumor; others had died and had been found at autopsy to be free of tumor. Others again showed only a small amount of recognizable tumor tissue at a subsequent operation. It is noteworthy that 19 of these patients were infants with neuroblastomas, 10 were patients with bladder cancer in whom a urinary diversion operation had been performed, 9 had soft tissue sarcomas, 5 had carcinomas of the colon or rectum, 4 had carcinomas of the stomach, and 2 had malignant hepatomas, while cancer of the larynx, lung, pancreas, and thyroid were each represented by a single patient. It is of interest that in 5 of the patients with neuroblastoma regression took the form of a change in histological appearance to that of benign ganglioneuroma—a phenomenon first reported by Cushing and Wolbach (1927). No cases of cancer of the prostate were included in this series, but it has been suggested (Franks, 1956a; Lancet, 1966) that this tumor often remains stationary for a long time, and probably sometimes regresses before it becomes clinically apparent, on the grounds that histological changes characteristic of cancer are often found at autopsy in the prostates of elderly men dying of other diseases—according to Franks (1956a) in almost 50 percent of men over the age of 80.

More recently Abbey Smith (1971) has reported complete regression with prolonged postoperative survival in three patients with lung cancer—two with squamous cell carcinomas and one with a tumor of mixed cell type—following resection which was noted to be incomplete at the time of the operation. Two of these patients died from other causes 7 and 15 years, respectively, after operation and no tumor tissue was found at autopsy; the remaining patient was alive and well 11 years after the operation. There have also been reports of regression of Burkitt's lymphoma (David and Burkitt, 1968), in one case in association with measles infection (Bluming and Ziegler, 1971), and further reports of regression of other primary tumors including melanomas (Cochran, Diehl, and Stjernsward, 1970; Stephenson, Delmez et al., 1971; Krebs et al., 1976).

It must be emphasized that even complete clinical regression does not necessarily imply that all tumor cells have been destroyed and that the tumor will not recur; moreover, the existence of disseminated malignant melanoma in the absence of a demonstrable primary tumor (Milton, 1969) suggests that regression of a primary tumor is not necessarily associated with a good prognosis (J. L. Smith and Stehlin, 1965).

The phenomenon is nevertheless of great biological interest and poses the question of the mechanism responsible, since, once again (cf. 1.211), the term *spontaneous* is used in an operational sense and implies only that the regression could not confidently be attributed to a defined cause. In some cases infection appears to play a role. This was first suggested by W. B. Coley, which led to the therapeutic use of bacterial toxins (see Nauts, Swift and Coley, 1946), and later to many other non-specific immunopotentiating agents (7.5, 8.24) in cancer patients. It has also been suggested that fever, irrespective of whether or not it is due to infection, may contribute to tumor regression (Bell, Jesseph, and Leighton, 1964). Finally, it seems likely that a change in hormonal balance is important in some cases, notably when regression occurs soon after parturition, as has been observed with malignant melanoma by Allen (1955) and others. In some cases, however, it is impossible from the data available to make even a plausible suggestion as to why regression occurred, and this highlights the need for detailed investigation *at the time* of all the factors which might conceivably have affected the patient's response to the tumor.

3.3 INVASION AND METASTASIS

Benign tumors displace but do not invade surrounding tissues. Malignant tumors may also displace neighboring structures, but they spread locally mainly by *invasion,* i.e., by a process of infiltration and destruction, of normal tissue. Malignant tumors may also give rise to secondary foci at a distance from the primary tumor. These secondary foci are termed *metastases,* and this form of spread is termed *metastasis.*

It is generally accepted that metastases are derived from viable cells which have come from either the primary tumor or from another metastasis (Roth *et al.,* 1976); it would seem wise, however, to keep an open mind concerning the possibility that some metastases are due to local transformation of cells by disseminated subcellular particles of some kind.

Metastasis is discussed in detail by Willis (1952, 1960) in a monograph which has become a classic. More recently Cole (1973) has discussed the routes and mechanisms involved, and the possibility of influencing the process, under three headings:

1. Metastasis via lymphatic vessels.
2. Metastasis via the bloodstream.
3. Metastasis by implantation of tumor cells on serous or epithelial surfaces, and in wounds.

3.31 Metastasis by Lymphatics

Tumor cells which gain entry to lymphatics may be carried as individual cells or small clumps to the regional lymph nodes. This is termed lymphatic embolism. Another process, termed lymphatic permeation, was described by Handley (1922), in which tumor tissue grows as a column within the lumen of lymphatic vessels, and continuity between the primary tumor and the growing tip of the column is subsequently broken as the result of an inflammatory reaction which destroys sections of the vessel and the tumor in its lumen. Lymphatic embolism is the more common mechanism, but permeation, though less important as a cause of metastasis than Handley supposed, does also occur.

Ever since Virchow (1863) postulated that lymph nodes filter out particulate matter of various kinds from lymph, it has been widely accepted that they constitute an effective, albeit often temporary, barrier to the passage of tumor cells. The first experimental evidence bearing on this question appears to be that by Zeidman and Buss (1952), who showed in rabbits that tumors regularly developed in the popliteal lymph nodes after injection of cells of the V2 carcinoma or the Brown-Pearce carcinoma to the afferent lymphatics, but rarely developed in more proximal nodes if the popliteal node was removed 1–42 days after the tumor cell injection. This, however, does not prove that the tumor cells were all arrested in the popliteal node, and subsequently B. Fisher and E. R. Fisher (1966a) found that when cell suspensions of the same tumors were perfused at low pressure into the afferent lymphatics of the rabbit popliteal node, or injected into the corresponding footpad, tumor cells could be demonstrated in the efferent lymphatic draining the node within an hour or two, and sometimes within 10 minutes. They showed also (B. Fisher and E. R. Fisher, 1966b) in rats that cell-bound label appeared in the lymph draining from a thoracic duct fistula 5–30 minutes after intravenous injection of living Walker carcinoma cells labeled with ^{51}Cr, whereas after injection of labeled dead cells only a small amount of label appeared in the course of the next 24 hours and this was cell-free. It seems clear therefore that, while tumor cells may be trapped in lymph nodes, they may also travel through nodes from the afferent to the efferent lymphatics, and thence via the thoracic duct to the blood stream.

More recently Hewitt and Blake (1975) have obtained evidence of a different kind which supports this conclusion. They found that when the axillary lymph nodes draining the site of a subcutaneous or intradermal transplant of an isogeneic mouse squamous cell carcinoma were transplanted subcutaneously to the same mouse or another mouse of the same strain, tumors developed in 40 percent of the recipients, whereas when the nodes were left *in situ* after radical excision of the primary tumor, tumors developed in only 4 percent of mice. They attributed the tumor-forming node transplants to tumor cells which, in small numbers, were in transit through the node and were destined to enter the blood stream.

When a node is invaded by tumor tissue, passage of lymph through the node may be prevented, but lymph and tumor cells may pass via connecting vessels to a more proximal node. Tumor cells may also invade veins, both small and large, in the vicinity of the affected node.

It is often stated that human carcinomas metastasize earlier and more frequently to lymph nodes than via the blood stream to other sites, whereas with sarcomas the reverse is the case. While there are many exceptions to this rule—some carcinomas, for example, metastasize early via the blood stream, and some sarcomas including osteogenic sarcoma, which commonly metastasize via the blood stream, may also metastasize to lymph nodes—there is no doubt that different tumors do differ in their pattern of metastasis, some showing a predilection for spread via the blood stream, others for spread to lymph nodes. Wallace and Hollenberg (1965) investigated possible reasons for this difference experimentally in rats by injecting cells of four different tumors either intravenously or into a testicular lymphatic vessel by the technique of Engeset (1959a, 1959b). They found that with two carcinomas, one of which was an isogeneic tumor, but not with a fibrosarcoma or a lymphoma, the number of animals which developed tumors (in lymph nodes) after intralymphatic injection was greater than the number which developed tumors (in the lung) after intravenous injection. They concluded that the nodes provided an environment which was particularly suitable for the carcinoma cells, but did not rule out the possibility that these cells enter the lymphatic system more readily than those of the other two tumors.

The bearing of these observations on the vexed question of whether or not the regional lymph nodes should be extirpated at the time of resection of a primary tumor will be discussed later (6.31).

3.32   Metastasis by the Bloodstream

Metastasis by the bloodstream is a complex process which involves invasion of the wall of a blood vessel or entry of tumor cells via the lymphatic system (3.31), the formation and arrest elsewhere of an embolus containing viable tumor cells, penetration of the vessel wall from within outwards, and the establishment and growth of a tumor with a stroma of vascular connective tissue at the new site. In the case of metastases in the liver the main vascular supply may be from the hepatic artery even when it seems clear *(vide infra)* that the route of metastasis was via the portal vein, but this is not always the case and the pattern of vascularization may change as the tumor grows (Bierman *et al.,* 1951; Healey, 1955; Ackerman, 1974). Similarly, metastases in the lung may derive their blood supply predominantly from the bronchial artery although the route of metastasis was almost certainly via the pulmonary artery (Noonan, Margulis and Wright, 1965); this is, however, possibly more the exception than the rule (B. J. Miller and Rosenbaum, 1967).

The venous channels within a tumor are more subject to invasion than the arteries. This is usually attributed to structural difference, and in particular to the thin walls of many of the venous channels, which in histological sections sometimes seem to be completely absent in places, but the difference in intraluminal pressure may also be important (Shivas and Finlayson, 1965). The susceptibility of the venous system to invasion is reflected in the fast that the common routes of blood-borne metastasis are (1) via the systemic venous system to the heart and thence to the pulmonary circulation, (2) to the liver from tumors whose venous drainage is to the portal system, and (3) to the spine and bones of the pelvis via the vertebral system of veins (Batson, 1940; Franks, 1953, 1956b) from tumors of the prostate gland. Tumor cells may be arrested in the capillary bed in the lungs or the liver, or elsewhere in the vascular system, and some of the cells so arrested may form metastases; it has, however, been shown that tumor cells can undergo sufficient deformation to pass through capillaries (Wood, 1958), and may also pass from the arterial to the venous side of the circulation via arteriovenous shunts in the liver, lungs, and elsewhere without having to pass through capillaries (Prinzmetal *et al.,* 1948).

Metastases develop occasionally in the placenta, and very occasionally in the fetus. It is of interest that in three of four reported cases of fetal metastasis the primary maternal tumor was a melanoma (Weber *et al.,* 1930; Holland, 1949; Dargeon *et al.,* 1950).

The presence of cancer cells in the bloodstream was reported by Ashworth in 1869. During the next 60–70 years further reports of this phenomenon were published, of which the most extensive is that of Pool and Dunlop (1934), who examined peripheral blood samples from 40 patients with advanced cancer and reported that 17 of them contained cancer cells. More recently, great interest was aroused by reports of cancer cells in the blood of patients with carcinoma of the colon or rectum by Engell (1955, 1959), and E. R. Fisher and Turnbull (1955), and these have been followed by many more reports of cancer cells in the blood of patients with colonic and other tumors (G. E. Moore *et al.*, 1957b; Roberts, Watne *et al.*, 1958; Roberts, Jonasson *et al.*, 1961; Pruitt, Hilberg, and Kaiser, 1958; Pruitt *et al.*, 1962; Sellwood *et al.*, 1964; Griffiths *et al.*, 1973).

Identification of cancer cells in blood samples requires care and experience if false positives are to be avoided, and there seems little doubt that in some cases megakaryoctes, monocytes, and other cells have been mistaken for cancer cells. Various techniques have been used to harvest as many tumor cells as possible and reduce the number of normal blood cells to a minimum. One of the simplest, described by Kuper *et al.*, (1961), involves removing the polymorphs with a magnet after adding carbonyl iron to the sample, lysing the erythrocytes with saponin, resuspending the remaining cells in saline, filtering the suspension through a millipore membrane, and staining the membrane either with Papanicolaou's stain or hematoxylin and eosin. This technique has been adapted to permit autoradiography of cells harvested from blood to which ^{3}H-thymidine has been added, and by this means Kuper and Bignall (1964) have demonstrated uptake of thymidine by cells in blood which morphologically appeared to be tumor cells.

Nuclear morphology is the main guide to the diagnosis of tumor cells (see Papanicolaou, 1954), but to avoid false positives it is wise to compare the appearance of cells harvested from the blood with those seen in imprints made with excised samples of the same tumor, and to base the diagnosis on the presence of small groups of atypical cells rather than on individual cells (see Sandberg and Moore, 1957; Alexander and Spriggs, 1960; Sellwood *et al.*, 1964; Griffiths and Salsbury, 1965; Griffiths *et al.*, 1973).

It might perhaps be expected that the demonstration of cancer cells in the blood would be associated with a poor prognosis and an increased probability of blood-borne metastases developing, but this is not necessarily the case. Engell (1959), in a series of patients followed for 5–9 years, found no difference in the survival of patients in whom cancer cells had been demonstrated in blood samples and those in whom they had not. Moreover, while Watne *et al.* (1960), in a study of patients followed for 18 months, observed a lower survival in patients in whom circulating cancer cells had been demonstrated, Roberts, Jonasson *et al.* (1961) observed a difference only in patients in whom showers of circulating cancer cells were demonstrated during the course of surgical removal of a tumor, and 10 of 22 patients with circulating cancer cells who did not show "showering," and in whom the resection was judged to be beyond the local limits of the tumor, were alive 2–4 years after operation. Even more remarkable is the finding by Griffiths and his colleagues of an inverse correlation between the demonstration of cancer cells in the bloodstream and the subsequent development of hepatic metastases in a study of over 200 patients with cancer of the colon or rectum with a 10 year follow-up period after operation (Griffiths *et al.*, 1973; White and Griffiths, 1976). It thus seems clear that many cancer cells which gain entry to the bloodstream spontaneously are destroyed; this is true also when tumor cells are injected intravenously in animals (Iwasaki, 1915; Warren and Gates, 1936; Zeidman *et al.*, 1950), and is reflected in the fact that the TD50 (1.22), i.e., the mean number of injected viable cells which causes tumors to develop in 50 percent of recipients, is much greater for intravenous than for subcutaneous injection. With an isogenic non-immunogenic mouse squamous cell carcinoma of spontaneous origin, for example, Hewitt and Blake (1975) found values of 7–25 cells (log mean 14 cells) and 2000 cells, respectively, for subcutaneous and intravenous inoculation.

What are the factors which determine whether tumor cells in the blood will give rise to metastases? Attempts have been made to answer this question by studying (1) the fate of tumor cells, in some cases carrying a radioactive label, injected to the systemic and portal venous systems, and also to arteries; and (2) spontaneous metastasis of both animal and human tumors. The main results, which are still far from providing a complete answer to the question, are as follows:

1. Many intravenously injected cells are trapped in the venous system and do not reach the lungs (van den Brenk et al., 1975). The proportion of trapped cells is increased by temporarily arresting the outflow from the vein, and decreased by administration of heparin (vide infra). Van den Brenk and his colleagues suggest that venous trapping plays a key role in the metastasis of human prostatic cancer via the vertebral system of veins (vide supra).

2. Most of the cells which reach the lungs are rapidly destroyed, and only a small proportion of them give rise to tumors. This is illustrated by the observation of Hewitt and Blake (1975) that minced lung tissue from mice killed within 90 minutes of intravenous injection of 200 viable cells of the isogeneic squamous cell carcinoma referred to above (i.e., about one-tenth of the TD50) usually gave rise to tumors when transplanted subcutaneously to mice of the same strain, whereas lung tissue from mice killed 20 hours or longer after injection of the same number of tumor cells never did. Clumps are more likely to give rise to tumors than single cells, but even with clumps the majority of cells are destroyed (Thompson, 1974).

3. Tumors commonly develop in sites in which spontaneous metastases are rarely seen if viable tumor cells are injected into an artery supplying the site in question (Coman, Eisenberg, and McCutcheon, 1949). This, together with the further observation that transplants of some tumors grow equally well in muscle, kidney, liver, and spleen (de Long and Coman, 1950), suggests that the distribution of metastases is not determined solely by differences in the capacity of different tissues to support tumor growth.

4. Surgical and other forms of trauma may encourage the development of tumors following intravenous injection of tumor cells, both at the site of the trauma (B. Fisher and E. R. Fisher, 1959a; Alexander and Altmeier, 1964; van den Brenk et al., 1974, 1976) and elsewhere (Robinson and Hoppe, 1962; van den Brenk et al., 1976), and rough handling or massaging of a tumor may increase the incidence of blood-borne metastases (Tyzzer, 1912; Romsdahl, 1964). It has also been reported that local trauma favours the survival of subcutaneous tumors (Vaitkevicius et al., 1965).

5. Various other experimental procedures may lead to an increase in the number of tumor nodules which develop in the liver after injection of tumor cells into the portal vein, including injection of homogenates of normal tissue (B. Fisher and E. R. Fisher, 1963), cirrhosis induced with carbon tetrachloride (E. R. Fisher and B. Fisher, 1960), increased liver blood flow (B. Fisher and E. R. Fisher, 1961a), and stimulation of reticuloendothelial function with Proferrin but not with BCG or endotoxin, possibly because Proferrin causes sinusoidal compression due to swelling of Kupffer cells (E. R. Fisher and B. Fisher, 1961, 1962).

6. The development of tumors after intravenous injection of tumor cells (Cliffton and Grossi, 1956; B. Fisher and E. R. Fisher, 1961b, 1967; Cliffton and Agostino, 1962, 1965; Rudenstam, 1968), and also of spontaneous metastases in animals (Wood, Holyoke, and Yardley, 1961; Ryan, Ketchman, and Wexler, 1968a) and man (Michaels, 1964), may be inhibited by administration of anticoagulants and

fibrinolytic agents. Moreover, clearance of intravenously injected cells from the bloodstream may be transiently delayed by administration of heparin (Stevenson and von Haam, 1966). Michaels' finding of an unexpectedly low incidence of metastases, but a normal incidence of primary tumors, in 540 patients receiving oral anticoagulants for thromboembolic disease seems particularly interesting, and small clinical trials of treatment with plasmin have been moderately encouraging (Larsen *et al.*, 1961; Hughes, 1964), but there is need for more extensive clinical studies of this kind. Another finding of interest in this connection is the discovery that episodes of increased fibrinolytic activity which may occur after operations on patients with cancer are associated with a high incidence of tumor cells in the blood stream (Salsbury *et al.*, 1973). This activity may be to some extent a general effect of trauma, but it may be due also in part to plasmin activator released by the tumor, since a high level of fibrinolytic activity has been demonstrated in tumors and in the venous blood draining from them (Newstead, Griffiths and Salsbury, 1976). The situation is complicated, however, because many tumors, like normal tissues, have also been shown to contain coagulant factors (O'Meara, 1958), and a clot-stabilizing factor allied to clotting factor XIII (Laki *et al.*, 1966).

7. With some tumors, after intravenous injection of viable cells, or, in the case of tumors which are known to metastasize, after subcutaneous transplantation, viable tumor cells can be demonstrated in only a restricted number of organs by transplanting fragments of the organs in question to other hosts, and tumors typically develop in these organs but not elsewhere. With other tumors, however, viable tumor cells can be demonstrated in many sites, though tumors commonly develop in only a few of these (Greene and Harvey, 1964).

8. In studies with variants of a mouse melanoma, Nicolson and Winkelhake (1975) observed a positive correlation between the number of spontaneous metastases which developed in the liver after subcutaneous tumor inoculation, the number of tumor nodules which developed in the liver after intravenous injection of cells of the same tumor, and the capacity of the tumor cells to form aggregates *in vitro* with cell suspensions prepared from normal lung tissue.

These findings suggest that the chance of metastases developing from circulating cells is small, and depends *inter alia* on (1) anatomical factors which influence the distribution of tumor emboli; (2) the properties of the sites at which such emboli are arrested and the extent to which they can satisfy the metabolic and other requirements of the particular tumor; (3) properties of the tumor including its capacity to produce plasmin-like enzymes; and (4) various factors which influence local and general resistance to the tumor and modify the complex process of metastasis in ways which, for the most part, remain to be elucidated. It seems likely that mechanisms which tend to prevent metastasis operate with particular efficiency in the lungs, as van den Brenk *et al.* (1975) have suggested, and also in the liver, since these organs trap a high proportion of circulating cells. The possibility is not excluded, however, that many cancer cells are killed in the bloodstream, though definite evidence of this is lacking.

3.33 Metastasis by Surface Implantation

Cancer cells implant readily on the endothelial surface of the pleura and peritoneum. When this occurs on an extensive scale it is almost invariably associated with an effusion of fluid containing tumor cells. Dissemination of cancer of the lung in the pleural cavity, and of cancer of the ovary, stomach, and colon in the peritoneal cavity, are familiar examples.

Cancer cells may also implant on epithelial surfaces; this occurs in the urinary tract from papillary carcinoma of the renal pelvis, and in the bladder from primary bladder tumors. It also occurs in the gastrointestinal tract, but appears to depend on a preexisting breach in the continuity of the epithelium.

Implantation of cancer in the subcutaneous tissue and in the wall of the colon may occur in the course of surgical operations (Cole, Roberts *et al.,* 1965; Cole, 1973) unless special precautions are taken to prevent this (Goligher, Dukes, and Bussey, 1958; Morgan and Lloyd-Davies, 1959; Southwick, Harridge, and Cole, 1962).

3.34 Dormancy and Regression of Metastases

Many years may elapse between apparently complete removal of a primary tumor and local recurrence or the development of metastases. This occurs particularly with carcinoma of the kidney, breast, and ovary, and malignant melanoma, and Everson and Cole (1966) collected almost 100 patients with such tumors in which local recurrence or metastasis was first recognized 10–50 years after removal of one of these tumors.

When metastases develop after a long, apparently disease-free, interval, they often grow rapidly. This change in behavior sometimes appears to be causally related to some definite event. This is illustrated by a patient (Woodruff, 1961) who developed a carcinoma of the breast 3 years after apparently complete excision of a melanoma on the foot, and was treated by radical mastectomy and postoperative radiotherapy. There had been no evidence of local recurrence or metastasis of the melanoma prior to treatment of the breast lesion, but 6 weeks after the mastectomy subcutaneous metastatic melanomatous nodules appeared, first in the field of irradiation and then elsewhere, and about 4 months later the patient was dead with melanomatous deposits in the lungs, liver, bone marrow, and brain. It seems clear that the change in behavior must have been due to some change in either the host environment or the dormant tumor cells, or both, caused by the radiotherapy or the trauma of the operation, and there is no knowing how long the residual melanoma cells might have continued to remain dormant had this not occurred.

Often, however, no cause for the sudden appearance of metastases can be discerned. This is illustrated by another patient (Woodruff *et al.,* 1976) who had a nephrectomy for a carcinoma of the left kidney and 4 years later was referred to the writer with a huge carcinoma in the right kidney. He was treated by right nephrectomy and transplantation of a cadaver kidney, and in the course of the nephrectomy it was observed that the tumor had invaded the renal vein. Despite this and the fact that the patient received routine immunosuppressive treatment with azathioprine and prednisone, he remained well without any evidence of local recurrence or metastasis for 7 years. He then began to lose weight, and a radiograph of the chest raised a suspicion of pulmonary metastases. Within a few months he was dead with numerous metastases in the lungs and liver. The sudden change in behavior of the tumor was not preceded by any change in routine treatment, or by any other event to which it could be attributed.

In many cases, even when there has been a delay in the appearance of metastases, it is possible with a little ingenuity to fit the data with a growth curve such as a Gompertz curve (3.4) for which the specific growth rate is a continuous function of time, but since there are no data in respect of the time before metastases became manifest, this appearance of continuity may be misleading. Indeed, in many cases the possibility is not excluded that the size of the tumor cell population remains constant for months or years, either because cell production is exactly balanced by cell loss, or because virtually all the tumor cells, while remaining potentially fertile, cease to divide. Cells which behave in this way may be described as *dormant* (Hadfield, 1954), *resting,* or *non-cycling* (GO) cells (3.4). These terms are also used in a less rigorous way to describe potentially fertile cells in which the cell cycle, though not completely arrested, is proceeding so slowly as to be imperceptible.

During the period between excision of a primary tumor and the development of local recurrence or metastases, a patient has *occult residual cancer* (Woodruff, 1972). This can, of course, only be diagnosed retrospectively, but the concept seems important because it is possible, from data concerning the incidence of metastatic disease following resection of tumors of various kinds, to assess the likelihood that a particular patient has occult residual disease which will eventually become manifest, and to take this into consideration when deciding whether or not to recommend further treatment.

Further evidence in support of the concept of disseminated but dormant tumor cells has been provided by animal experiments. B. Fisher and E. R. Fisher (1959b) found that when rats were given an injection of 50 Walker carcinoma cells into the portal vein they normally failed to develop tumors during the next 5 months. If, however, 3 months after the injection the rats were subjected to repeated laparotomy and examination of the liver at 7-day intervals, they all developed tumors within a few weeks. More recently Eccles and Alexander (1975) reported that only 10 percent of rats normally developed pulmonary tumors within 18 months of amputation of a limb bearing a subcutaneous transplant of a syngeneic fibrosarcoma. If, however, 1, 7, or 30 days post amputation the rats were exposed to 500 rad whole-body x-irradiation, or subjected to 7 days continuous drainage of thoracic duct lymph, there was a highly significant increase in the proportion which developed lung tumors during the 18 months period of observation. Eccles and Alexander described this finding as paradoxical because rats of the same strain were able to reject inocula of up to 10^7 cells of the same tumor when given intramuscularly.

An important question, which bears some relation to the question of dormancy, concerns the stage in the life history of a primary tumor when the cells which eventually give rise to overt metastases are disseminated. With some tumors, of which carcinoma of the breast and osteogenic sarcoma of the long bones in children are notable examples, postoperative metastases may develop even when the diagnosis has been made at the earliest possible time—i.e., within a week or two, or even a few days, of the patient first developing symptoms—and treatment has been undertaken without delay. In such cases dissemination leading to the development of metastases must have occurred either (1) prior to treatment, and probably prior to the onset of symptoms, or (2) at the time of operation or diagnostic biopsy.

It would be foolish to ignore the second of these possibilities and relax customary precautions to minimize the risk, but the demonstration of metastases in bone in a proportion of patients with untreated or apparently early breast cancer by sensitive scanning techniques using radioactive isotopes—initially ^{85}Sr, ^{87}Sr, and ^{18}F, and subsequently ^{90m}Tc—and a gamma camera (Gynning *et al.,* 1961; Galasko *et al.,* 1968;

Sklaroff and Charkes, 1968; Galasko, 1969, 1971, 1972, 1975; Galasko and Doyle, 1972; Citrin, Bessent *et al.,* 1974; Citrin, Furnival *et al.,* 1976; El-Domeiri and Shroff, 1976; C. J. Davies, *et al.,* 1977; see also British Medical Journal, 1977c), proves that metastasis, and *a fortiori* dissemination of viable tumor cells, may already have occurred when a patient is first seen, even when there has been no undue delay. Among 50 patients studied by Galasko (1975), 12 had positive scans and all developed overt metastases within 5 years, whereas only 8 of the 38 patients with negative scans developed metastases during this period. In a more recent study (Citrin *et al.,* 1976) of 75 patients with operable breast cancer, 49 of whom were classified as Stage I, (T_1NoMo or T_2NoMo) in the International Union Against Cancer Classification (UICC, 1960), and in whom repeated scans were performed, a routine x-ray survey of the skeleton when the patient was first seen revealed no evidence of metastasis, but the scan was positive in 11 patients, 6 of whom had been classified as having Stage I disease. Thirteen of the patients in whom the initial scan was negative, including 7 classified as Stage I, developed positive scans during the follow-up period, which ranged from 3 to 34 months. Nine of the 24 patients with positive scans died during the follow-up period, whereas all the patients whose scans remained negative were still alive when the report was published.

Another approach to the problem of when metastasis occurs is to plot the volume of pulmonary metastases, as estimated from radiographs, against time, fit some standard mathematical form of growth curve to the data, and extrapolate this curve back to the time when the estimated volume would have been approximately that of a single cell. This procedure, and the errors inherent in it, will be discussed later (3.4).

On several occasions the presence of unsuspected viable tumor cells in a healthy-looking kidney has been revealed when the organ was transplanted to another individual (see Penn, 1970). In most of these cases there were metastases in other organs in the donor and the risk of transmitting cancer was accepted because no other kidney was available and it was not possibly to treat the patient by dialysis. Today the presence of cancer, even without evidence of metastasis, except possibly in the special case of tumors of the central nervous system, is generally accepted as an absolute contraindication to using a deceased individual's organ as a transplant. If, however, dissemination of tumor cells can occur before a patient has any clinical evidence of cancer, the only way to exclude the risk of transmitting cancer with an organ transplant is to perform a full autopsy on the donor before transplantation is undertaken. This is impossible when organs are transplanted without a period of storage, and in other cases when permission for a full autopsy is refused.

It is of interest that one tumor transmitted with a kidney transplant, which only became apparent 3 years after the transplantation, metastasized in the recipient (Zukoski *et al.,* 1970). Immunosuppressive treatment was stopped and a month later the transplant was removed. The pulmonary metastases continued to enlarge for about 3 months but eventually regressed completely. This is of course a special case, since the tumor was an allograft, but regression of autochthonous metastases also occurs, usually, though not exclusively, after excision of the primary tumor, especially after nephrectomy for primary carcinoma of the kidney (Bumpus, 1928; Mann, 1948; Arcomano *et al.,* 1958; Hallahan, 1959; Jenkins, 1959; Kessel, 1959; Nicholls and Siddons, 1960; Buehler *et al.,* 1960; Samellas, 1961; H. C. Miller, Woodruff, and Gambacorta, 1962). Everson and Cole (1966) collected in all 106 examples, in which the primary tumors included carcinoma of the kidney (23 cases), neuroblastoma (19 cases), malignant melanoma (15 cases), chorion carcinoma (17 cases), malignant tumors of the testis (7 cases), carcinoma of the ovary (7 cases), and osteogenic sarcoma (3 cases), and further cases have been reported subsequently (Todd *et al.*, 1966; Stidolph, 1967). An interesting, and as yet unexplained, phenomenon, which occurs in patients with malignant melanoma who have multiple metastases in the subcutaneous tissue, and was demonstrated by Bodenham (1968) by the simple expedient of photographing his patients at intervals, is that some metastases regress completely while others are appearing, so that the observed rate of increase in the number of metastases represents the difference between the rates at which new ones appear and others disappear.

A question of considerable therapeutic importance is the extent, if any, to which metastases in lymph nodes regress. There is no doubt, from the cases cited by Everson and Cole (1966), and from the more recent reports of Edwards *et al.* (1972) and Murray *et al.* (1976) on the behavior of axillary lymph nodes in patients with breast cancer treated by simple mastectomy alone, that palpably enlarged nodes draining the region of a primary tumor may decrease in size and eventually cease to be palpable following removal of the primary tumor, but it is uncertain to what extent the nodes which disappeared were the site of metastatic tumor deposits, and to what extent their enlargement was simply a manifestation of the host reaction to the tumor. Edwards *et al.* (1972) took the view that they were enlarged because of a reaction to the tumor, and it seems likely that this is often the case; whether this is always so, however, is not known. Some indication should be obtainable by comparing the proportion of patients in whom palpable lymph nodes disappear after simple mastectomy with the proportion of patients with similar tumors who are treated by radical mastectomy and in whom no tumor deposits can be demonstrated in the axillary nodes. Unfortunately the reported incidence of node involvement in material obtained at operation depends very much on the assiduity of the pathologist who examines the specimen—the late H. S. N. Greene once told the writer, with perhaps a measure of hyperbole, that he could always find involved nodes if he tried hard enough—and before any firm conclusions could be drawn it would be necessary to obtain reliable figures based on a large number of specimens examined by a standardized procedure which included dissecting out and serially sectioning all identifiable lymph nodes. Such a task would be tedious and costly, but might be very instructive.

McWhirter (1955) criticized treatment of operable breast cancer by so-called radical mastectomy alone on the grounds that it leaves the internal mammary and supraclavicular nodes undisturbed, and advocated instead simple mastectomy combined with irradiation of an area which includes these nodes as well as those of the axilla. Subsequent trials have revealed little difference in the results of these two forms of treatment, however, and the proportion of patients whose death following radical mastectomy is attributable to involvement of the internal mammary nodes seems surprisingly small if, as Handley (1964) has reported, there are tumor deposits in the internal mammary lymph nodes in 40 percent of patients with deposits in the axillary nodes and in 10 percent of those in whom the axillary nodes are apparently not involved, unless regression occurs in an appreciable number of patients. Once again, it is doubtful whether enough reliable information is available to permit a firm conclusion to be drawn.

3.4 GROWTH CURVES

The volume of subcutaneous tumors in experimental animals is often estimated by measuring the linear dimensions of the tumor in three mutually perpendicular directions, two in a plane tangential to the skin surface and the third—sometimes referred to as the height measurement—in a direction perpendicular to this plane. The same procedure is applicable to some human tumors. The volume of tumors situated more deeply may also be estimated from three mutually perpendicular linear measurements if the tumor can be visualized radiographically. Alternatively, the mass of a tumor may be determined by excising it and weighing it, and from this the volume can be determined by density measurements based on the capacity of the tumor tissue to float or sink in solutions of known specific gravity.

The number of cells in a tumor may be estimated from its volume in the light of previous experience with similar tumors in which the mean number of cells per unit volume has been determined by counting cell suspensions made from a known amount of excised tumor tissue. For rat tumors Laird (1954) found that the mean number of cells per gram tissue was about 450×10^6, and this figure has sometimes been applied rather uncritically to other tumors. In the special case of ascites tumors (1.22) the number of cells constituting the tumor may be estimated from the number of cells per unit volume in samples of peritoneal fluid and the total amount of fluid which can be obtained by aspiration, on the assumption that all the tumor cells are growing in suspension.

These estimates are subject to many errors, to which it is often difficult to set plausible limits.

In the first place observer error may be considerable. With subcutaneous tumors the need to measure through a layer of skin affects all dimensions; in addition, the variable nature of the tissue underlying the tumor adds to the inaccuracy of height measurements, and it is sometimes better to assume that the height is proportional to the geometric mean of the other two measurements than to try to measure it directly. In measurements based on radiography a principal source of error is lack of sharpness of outline, as shown by the fact that different observers, or even the same observer on different occasions, may produce quite markedly different tracings of the same radiographic shadow (Gurland and Johnson, 1965).

Secondly, the calculated volume will depend on assumptions concerning the shape of the tumor. This is often assumed to be that of an ellipsoid, or alternatively a hemi-ellipsoid (Dethlefsen, Prewitt and Mendelsohn, 1968), but in practice may be decidedly irregular. Moreover, in the case of pulomary metastases, what appears to be a single tumor may in fact consist of multiple small closely packed, more or less spherical nodules (Breur, 1965).

Thirdly, the tumor may contain cysts and areas of hemorrhage which are virtually devoid of cells, areas in which there are large amounts of collagen but relatively few cells, and areas of necrosis in which many of the cells are dead.

Fourthly, tumors contain non-neoplastic cells (3.12), and the number of these may be considerable.

Nevertheless, in experimental animals and, in the case of pulmonary metastases, in man, the errors in serial estimation of volume, and even of cell number, in respect of the same tumor, may be reduced to a level which permits meaningful conclusions to be drawn, if all the observations are made by a single careful observer with previous experience of the type of tumor being studied; although with human tumors the period of observation before the tumor is removed, or growth is modified by treatment, may be too short to provide enough points to construct a growth curve.

Given reasonable serial estimates of the tumor volume or the total number of tumor cells, what form of growth curve may be expected to fit the data?

It has often been assumed in studies of human tumors (Collins, Loeffler, and Tivey, 1956; Garland et al., 1963; Welin el al., 1963; Spratt and Spratt, 1964; Spratt, 1965) that an exponential curve, expressed mathematically in the form

$$V = V_0 \exp{(-kt)} \tag{1}$$

will suffice, where V_0 is the volume at some chosen starting time, V is the volume at time t, and k is a constant. In theory this should hold good if the proportion of dividing cells and the generation time remain constant, and for those who prefer simplicity to accuracy the equation has the advantage that it yields a straight line when $\log V$ is plotted against time, or, what comes to the same thing, when V is plotted against time on semilogarithmic paper. In practice, however, except over short periods of time, it is likely to be highly erroneous (Brennan et al., 1962; Laird, 1964).

Mendelsohn and his colleagues (Mendelsohn, 1963; Dethlefsen et al., 1968) have proposed instead an equation of the form

$$\frac{dV}{dt} = kV^b \tag{2}$$

which leads on integration to

$$V^{1-b} = (1-b)(kt + c) \text{ when } b \neq 1 \tag{3}$$

and reduces to the exponential form when $b = 1$. In these equations V is the tumor volume at time t, k is a growth constant, c is proportional to the initial tumor volume, and b is a constant which varies from tumor to tumor and defines the mode of growth.

Dethlefsen et al. (1968) have shown that these empirical equations can be made to fit the observed growth curves of many experimental animal tumors, and have reported that the best value of b, based on a test of the linearity of regression and determined by an iterative procedure with the aid of a computer, is often in the region of 0.67. This corresponds to so-called cube-root growth, i.e., to the situation where the mean diameter of the tumor, or the cube root of the number of cells in the case of an ascites tumor, is a linear function of time. This conclusion is in conformity with much published work (Mayneord, 1932; Schrek, 1935, 1936a, 1936b; G. Klein and Revesz, 1953; Patt and Blackford, 1954). A possible reason for the relationship is suggested by the observation of Mayneord (1932) on transplants of the Jensen sarcoma in rats, in which he found that growth was confined to a rim of tissue on the periphery of the tumor, presumably on account of the ready availability of nutrient substances in this region.

Another type of growth curve, which has been found to fit many experimental tumors (Laird, 1964, 1965a; McCredie et al., 1965; Brenner et al., 1967) and some human tumors (Sullivan and Salmon, 1972), as well as human populations (Shyrock and

Siegel, 1973), embryos of various species including man (Laird, Tyler, and Barton, 1965; Laird, 1965b), and early postnatal growth in the rat (Laird, 1965b), is the S-shaped curve introduced for actuarial purposes by Gompertz (1825) over a century and a half ago. The essential property of this curve is that the specific growth rate

$$\frac{1}{V} \frac{dV}{dt}$$

decreases exponentially with time, presumably due to some form of feedback inhibition with increasing size, so that the final volume approaches a limit asymptotically. The equation of a Gompertz curve is thus given by the solution of two differential equations:

$$\frac{dV}{dt} = k_1 VG \tag{4}$$

$$\frac{dG}{dt} = -k_2 G \tag{5}$$

where, as before, V is the volume at time t, G is a function of t which indicates the growth rate at time t, and k_1 and k_2 are constants for a given tumor, though they vary from one tumor to another even when these are of the same type. The solution of these equations may be expressed in either of two forms:*

$$V = V_0 \exp \left(\frac{k_1}{k_2} G_0 [1 - \exp(-k_2 t)] \right) \tag{6}$$

$$\frac{dV}{dt} = AV - BV \ln V \tag{7}$$

where V_0 and G_0 are the initial values of V and G, respectively, $A = k_2 \ln Lt\ t \to \infty\ V$, $B = k_2$[†]

It has been shown that a Gompertz curve may be fitted satisfactorily to the observed growth curve of many experimental tumors, and that extrapolation of such curves backwards in time provides plausible estimates of the time when a tumor existed as a single cell (Laird, 1965a). For transplanted mouse tumors, Laird (1965a) found that, with one exception, this estimated time ranged from 1 to 6.4 days before transplan-

---

*An elementary knowledge of the exponential and logarithmic functions is all that is required to verify these relationships. A reader who lacks this must perforce take them on trust.

[†]The symbols used here for the various constants are those used by Norton et al. (1976), but we have used V (volume at time t) where he used $N(t)$ (number of cells at time t). Many authors, following Laird (1965a), write equation (6) in the form

$$V = V_0 \exp \left(\frac{A}{a} [1 - \exp(-at)] \right) \tag{8}$$

where a corresponds to k_2 of equation (6) and A to $k_1 G_0$. The letter A thus denotes different constants in equations (7) and (8).

tation, though it was considerably longer for transplanted rat tumors. With carcinogen-induced osteosarcomas (Finkel, Bergstrand, and Biskis, 1961) and hepatomas (Laird and Barton, 1961), the time was about 3 weeks before administration of the carcinogen.

If nothing is known *a priori* about the relationship between A and B in equation (7), observations over a long period of time are required to find the value of the constants for any given tumor, because the early growth pattern provides a good estimate of A but not of B, whereas the later pattern provides a good estimate of A/B but not of A alone. It was observed by Norton *et al.* (1976), however, that for two experimental tumors, the B-16 melanoma in BDF_1 mice and a rat mammary carcinoma, there was a linear relationship, with a very high degree of correlation, between the values of $\exp A$ and $\ln B$ obtained from observations of transplants of the same tumor in different hosts. If this relationship holds good not only for different transplants of the same tumor but also for different primary tumors of the same kind, equation (7), as Norton *et al.* (1976) point out, may then be rewritten in the form

$$\frac{dV}{dt} = AV - \exp \left(\frac{\exp A - n}{m} \right) V \ln V \qquad (9)$$

where n and m are constant for all tumors of the type in questions, and A, which is the only parameter which differs for different tumors of the same kind, can be estimated from a few measurements over quite a short period of time if m and n have already been determined by observations with other tumors of the kind in question.

For all these curves the specific growth rate, dV/dt, is a continuous function of time. There are no good reasons for assuming that this is always the case, and if there is a sudden change in specific growth rate it may be appropriate to fit two curves of the kind we have been considering, one describing the growth before the sudden change in growth rate and one after. A limiting case of theoretical importance arises if, initially, the tumor cell population is stationary, i.e., if all the cells are dormant (3.34).

When a Gompertz curve fits the observed growth of a human tumor, whether primary or metastatic, well over a fairly long time, it is plausible to extrapolate the curve to estimate the time of origin of the tumor and to predict its future course. Such estimates must be viewed critically, and are sometimes clearly inapplicable, for example, when there is a very long latent period followed by a phase of rapid growth. Generally speaking, however, they are much more reliable than estimates based on a simple exponential curve (McWhirter, 1966; White, 1966; Brenner *et al.*, 1967), which may seriously overestimate the time since the tumor originated.

Yet another form of growth curve has been proposed by Summers (1966), derived from the postulate that tumor growth is limited by the availability of nutrients supplied via the vascular bed, and from observed measurements of the volume of this bed in relation to the volume of the tumor. The equation of the growth curve thus derived takes the form

$$\ln V = t (k_1 - k_2 V) \qquad (10)$$

This curve has very similar properties to the Gompertz curve; in particular, it corresponds closely to an exponential growth curve when the tumor volume is small, and the final volume approaches a limit asymptotically. It is no easier to fit than a Gompertz curve, and its main interest is in relation to the extent to which the behavior of a tumor is determined by its blood supply.

3.5 CELL POPULATION KINETICS

Many cell populations, including the population of cells constituting a tumor, contain both proliferating and resting (dormant) cells. These subpopulations are not rigidly segregated, however, because cells which are proliferating may become dormant or be lost permanently, and dormant cells may resume proliferation.

It has been known for over 25 years that DNA is synthesized in proliferating cells during only a limited part of the interval between successive mitoses. The cycle of events (see Mitchison, 1971) therefore comprises a phase of mitosis (M), an interval or gap (G1), a phase of DNA synthesis (S), and a second interval or gap (G2). G1 + S + G2 constitute what is termed interphase. The terms interval and gap are perhaps ill-chosen; important events occur in the cell during these periods in preparation for the succeeding phases.

Measurement of the duration of these phases by methods which will be discussed briefly (*vide infra*) have shown that G2, M, and S are of relatively constant duration in many different cell populations; the duration of G1, and of the whole cycle, on the other hand, may vary widely even within a defined cell population, and the distribution curve for these times is not symmetrical but is skewed towards longer time intervals. To account for these findings J. L. Smith and Martin (1973) have proposed a new model in which the cell cycle is divided into two parts: the *A state,* which is entirely contained within G1, and the *B phase,* which consists of S, G2, M, and part of G1. Events in the B phase are highly coordinated and are interpreted on deterministic principles. In the A state, on the other hand, cells are not progressing towards mitosis, and transition from the A state to the B phase is interpreted stochastically; cells may remain in the A state indefinitely with the proviso that, under steady state conditions, the probability per unit time, termed the *transition probability,* of any cell leaving the A state and entering the B phase is constant for a given population under given conditions, but may be changed by altering the conditions, for example, by exposing the population to known mitogens (Brooks, 1976). This model seems to fit the observational data very well (Minor and Smith, 1974; Brooks, 1976), though the biochemical basis for the probability transition remains obscure (Shields, 1976). In the following discussion, however, we shall continue to refer to the older model, since this is used in the papers on tumor cell population kinetics which we shall be considering.

Among the various parameters used to characterize the behavior of tumor cell populations, the following are of particular import:

1. The duration of the cell cycle of proliferating cells, and its component phases.
2. The proportion of cells proliferating.
3. The extent of cell loss.

Methods for determining these both *in vitro* and *in vivo* have been developed (see Lamerton and Fry, 1963; Steel, Adams, and Barrett, 1966; Cleaver, 1967; Mendelsohn and Takahashi, 1971; Tubiana, 1971; Lamerton, 1973; Lala, 1971, 1977; Aherne *et al.,* 1977; Steel, 1977) and some of these have been used in the study of human tumors

(Clarkson *et al.,* 1965; Steel and Lamerton, 1966; Refsum and Berdal, 1967; Steel, 1967, 1977; Iversen, 1967; Frindel *et al.,* 1968; Shirakawa *et al.,* 1970; Iversen *et al.,* 1974; Britton *et al.,* 1975; British Medical Journal, 1976a; Tubiana and Malaise, 1976; Terz *et al.,* 1977; Straus and Moran, 1977).

The methods used are described in detail in the references cited. In brief, the duration of the cell cycle, and of the S phase, may be estimated from serial measurements of the frequency of labeled mitoses (FLM) on autoradiography after a single injection of ^{3}H-thymidine (see, e.g., Frindel *et al.,* 1968; Aherne *et al.,* 1977); or from measurements of the grain count per cell after repeated or continuous administration of the same material (Terz *et al.,* 1977). The duration of mitosis, and the rate of entry of cells into mitosis, can also be estimated by counting the proportion of cells in metaphase before, and on one or preferably several occasions after, administration of a stathmokinetic agent (i.e., an agent which arrests the cycle when a cell reaches metaphase) such as colchicine or vincristine (Iversen, 1967; Aherne *et al.,* 1977). The proportion of cells proliferating, commonly termed the *growth fraction,* may be estimated from the ratio of the proportion of labeled cells (termed the *labeling index* or *Is*) to the proportion of labeled mitoses 5 days after a single injection of ^{3}H-thymidine, as first shown by Mendelsohn (1962), or from repeated or continuous labeling as described by Steel, Adams, and Barrett (1966) and applied to human tumors by Shirakawa *et al.* (1970) and Terz *et al.* (1977). Attempts to measure cell loss directly by monitoring the disappearance of label from a cell population after administration of a single dose of ^{3}H-thymidine were frustrated by extensive reutilization of the labeled thymidine released by dead cells (Steel, 1967). More recently the possibility of using this type of procedure with iododeoxyuridine labeled with ^{131}I, ^{125}I, or ^{3}H, which behaves as a thymidine analogue but is much less readily reutilized, has been investigated (Hofer et al., 1969; Dethlefsen, 1971). This material is, however, more toxic than ^{3}H-thymidine, and a satisfactory technique has not yet been perfected. If the remaining problems can be solved the use of ^{131}I as a label would have the advantage that its rate of disappearance might be monitored by external scanning and so obviate the need for repeated biopsy. Alternatively, cell loss may be estimated indirectly by measuring the birth rate of cells within a tumor and comparing this with the rate of increase of the tumor cell population as estimated from the observed rate of increase in tumor volume. The cell birth rate may be estimated with a fair degree of accuracy by using stathmokinetic agents (*vide supra*) as described by Iversen (1967), Refsum and Berdal (1967), and Britton *et al.* (1975), or from the labeling index after administration of ^{3}H-thymidine, as described by Steel (1967); the error in the estimate of the rate of increase of the tumor cell population, and hence in the estimated cell loss, may, however, be quite large.

Systemic administration of stathmokinetic agents, and *a fortiori* of radioactively labeled thymidine or iododeoxyuridine, to human patients, raises difficult ethical questions. There is no doubt that such studies can provide information of great interest and potential practical importance, but what are the long-term risks? In the case of stathmokinetic agents, the risk, according to Iversen *et al.* (1974), is so small as to be acceptable in a patient over the age of 60 years with a malignant tumor. In the case of ^{3}H-thymidine it seems to be widely accepted that more stringent restrictions are needed, and that systemic injection, if used at all, should be confined to patients with advanced tumors and a short life expectancy. One possible alternative, discussed by Iversen (1967), which might be used with superficial tumors, is to inject ^{3}H-thymidine locally in the vicinity of the tumor. Another procedure, which eliminates the risk completely, is to label small fragments of excised tumor tissue with ³H-thymidine *in vitro*. This has been used by Cooper and his colleagues (Cooper, Frank, and Wright, 1966; Cooper, Peckham *et al.,* 1968; Levi, Cooper *et al.,* 1969) and by Iversen *et al.* (1974), and has been defended on the ground that with animal tumors labeling *in vivo* and *in vitro* have been reported to give very similar results (Helpap and Maurer, 1969). In recent years, however, *in vivo* labeling of human tumors has been used increasingly and seems to be generally accepted as more reliable.

Reported values of the cell cycle time for human tumors range from 1 to 7 days, and for rodent tumors from less than 1 day to nearly 3 days; the duration of the S phase has been within the range 6–21 hours for a wide variety of advanced solid human tumors, and 17–34 hours for malignant effusions. The duration of G1 was found to be virtually nil for the Ehrlich ascites tumor in mice (Lala, 1972), and about 16 hours for human Burkitt lymphomas (Iversen *et al.,* 1974). According to Lala (1977) the cycle time of experimental ascites tumors, and of some experimental solid tumors, increases with age, and this appears to be due mainly to prolongation of the S phase.

Reported values of the growth fraction range from 30 to 95 percent with experimental rodent tumors and from 10 to 90 percent with advanced human solid tumors. According to Lala (1977) the majority of noncycling cells in experimental ascites tumors appear to be arrested in G1. In a study of 6 patients with advanced tumors who received continuous infusions of ³H-thymidine for up to 21 days, Terz et al. (1977) distinguished four tumor cell compartments according to the rate of entry into the cycle, namely, (1) rapidly proliferating cells, comprising 10–40 percent of the tumor cell population, which synthesized DNA within 2 hours of starting the infusion; (2) slowly proliferating cells, comprising 55–85 percent of the cells which were not rapidly proliferating, which synthesized DNA within 21 days; (3) non-proliferating cells, comprising 5 percent of the tumor cell population, which failed to replicate within 21 days and were regarded as being in prolonged G1 or "real G0;" and (4) cells in mitosis which were unlabeled even after 21 days continuous exposure to ³H-thymidine, and were assumed to have been in G2 when the infusion was started and to have remained arrested in this phase. A small proportion of cells which remain unlabeled after prolonged continuous administration of ³H-thymidine has also been demonstrated in human leukemia (Maurer *et al.,* 1969) and in animal tumors (Post and Hoffman, 1969). Evidence of arrest in G2 has also been obtained by measuring the DNA content of the cells by cytophotometry (Bichel and Dombernowsky, 1973). It seems likely that some of these cells are sterile first-generation products of mitotic errors (Lala, 1977) and hence make no contribution to the G0 population, but evidence of resumption of cycling of animal tumor cells arrested in G2 has been observed following treatment with antilymphocyte serum or hydrocortisone (Decosse and Gelfant, 1967, 1968), partial excision of the tumor and transplantation (Bichel and Dombernowsky, 1973).

There is convincing evidence that non-proliferating cells may begin to cycle after incomplete excision of a tumor, or incomplete destruction by radiotherapy or chemotherapy. This has been shown with both experimental (Potmesil *et al.,* 1975; Simpson-Herren *et al.,* 1977) and human (Terz, Fu, and King, 1975) tumors. The experiments of Potmesil et al., which demonstrate transition in both directions, are particularly instructive. Working with a transplantable mouse mammary carcinoma in which proliferating and non-proliferating cells could be distinguished by nucleolar morphology (Busch and Smetana, 1970, 1974), they found that local irradiation (470–1880 rad) reduced the numbers of both types of cell, but especially of proliferating cells. The regenerative period started with a gradual increase in the number of proliferating cells but (in tumors treated with 940 or 1880 rad) a continued fall in the number of non-proliferating cells; later, however, the non-proliferating pool was replenished, apparently by transition from the proliferating pool.

The tumor cell birth rate, measured by using a stathmokinetic agent (vincristine sulfate), in 19 patients with rectal carcinoma and 10 patients with gastric carcinoma was found by Britton *et al.* (1975) to be lower in many (though not all) cases than the cell birth rate in the corresponding normal tissues. In this event, as the authors point out, a "tumoricidal" dose of chemotherapy or radiotherapy might well have at least as severe an effect on the cells of the normal gastrointestinal mucosa as on those of the tumor, and this may explain the poor response of many rectal and gastric carcinomas to these forms of treatment.

Cell loss, expressed as the ratio of the rate of cell loss to the rate of entry of cells into mitosis, has been reported to range from virtually nil to nearly 100 percent in experimental tumors. With human tumors it is said to be often more than 50 percent (Steel, 1967); the value in two patients with disseminated malignant melanoma was 70 percent (Shirakawa *et al.,* 1970), and in two patients with Burkitt's lymphoma, where the growth fraction was 90–100 percent, the value was 69 percent (Iversen *et al.,* 1974); as already mentioned, however, the errors in these estimates are likely to be considerable.

Cells may be lost by dissemination by any of the routes discussed earlier (3.3), or by cell death. Cell death may be preceded by a phase of reversible, followed by a phase of irreversible, damage, but it is difficult to study these processes except *in vitro*. It is often assumed that cell death is randomly distributed in respect of intrinsic factors such as the number of cell divisions which have occurred since transformation, the age of the cell (i.e., the time which has elapsed since mitosis), and the phase of the cycle in which it happens to be. It is difficult to determine to what extent this assumption is valid, but it does not seem to be universally true; with a mouse ascites tumor, for example, Lala (1972) observed an age-related elimination of non-cycling cells and a low death rate of cells in mitosis. Cell death may also be determined by extrinsic factors, notably by the extent to which the requirements of the cell in respect of oxygen and nutrient material are not fulfilled (Thomlinson and Gray, 1955; Tannock, 1968, 1970; see also Cooper, 1973) and by immunological and para-immunological homeostatic mechanisms (5.5).

It is important to remember that, as Cooper has emphasized (Cooper, 1973; Cooper, Bedford, and Kenny, 1975), while death of a multicellular organ or individual as a whole is a terminal event, programmed death and replacement of cells plays an important role in embryogenesis and also in adult organisms. It is clear from the preceding discussion that the death of even large numbers of tumor cells is not incompatible with progressive tumor growth, and may well be an important factor in promoting tumor survival in the face of host resistance or therapeutic attack by providing an opportunity for the emergence of a new clone or clones of cells of greater survival capacity.

The process by which cells are lost has aroused surprisingly little interest, but Kerr and his colleagues have described a two-stage mechanism of controlled cell deletion (Kerr and Searle, 1971), which has been termed *apoptosis* (Kerr, Wylie, and Currie, 1972). The first stage comprises nuclear and cytoplasmic condensation, and breaking up of the cell into a number of membrane-bound fragments termed apoptotic bodies. In the second stage these fragments are shed from epithelial-lined surfaces, or taken up by other cells, in which they are rapidly broken down. Kerr *et al.* (1972) have reported that apoptosis occurs spontaneously in untreated tumors and participates in at least some types of therapeutically induced tumor regression. It also appears to be involved in cell turnover in normal adult tissues and in the elimination of cells during embryonic development.

Dead tumor cells may also be engulfed by macrophages, or broken down by autolysis and absorbed.

In many papers dealing with tumor cell population kinetics there is no mention of the non-neoplastic component of the total population of cells which constitutes the tumor. In principle, it is possible to estimate the size of this component by counting neoplastic and non-neoplastic cell in histological sections of samples from different parts of the tumor, but in practice this is difficult and tedious. Unless this is done, however, and appropriate allowance made, the size of the growth fraction—which should relate specifically to the neoplastic cells population—is likely to be seriously overestimated, because most of the non-neoplastic cells do not proliferate in the tumor but are newly formed cells which have entered the tumor from the blood stream (Lala, 1974a, 1974c, 1976a, 1976b, 1977; Lala and Kaiser, 1976).

The question of whether immunological and paraimmunological mechanisms may influence cell proliferation in tumors as well as cell death will be discussed later (5.522).

3.6 FUNCTIONAL ACTIVITY OF TUMORS

Some tumors secrete or shed products which enter the blood stream in sufficient quantity to be detected by radioimmunoassay and other sensitive techniques. These include:

1. Immunoglobulins secreted by plasma cell tumors (3.114).
2. Tumor-associated antigens (5.2).
3. Hormones. These include hormones secreted by tumors arising from endocrine tissue which are characteristic of the tissue of origin, and so-called *ectopically produced* or *inappropriate* hormones (Liddle, Island, and Meador, 1962; Liddle *et al.,* 1969) which are produced by tumors of non-endocrine origin, or which, in the case of tumors of endocrine origin, are not characteristic of the tissue of origin.

In general, malignant tumors of endocrine origin seem to be less efficient hormone producers than benign tumors, but there are exceptions to this rule.

Ectopic hormone production appears to be restricted to the production of polypeptide hormones including adrenocorticotrophic hormone (ACTH), antidiuretic hormone, calcitonin, erythropoietin, gastrin, gonadotrophin, growth hormone, insulin, melanocyte-stimulating hormone, parathormone, serotonin, and thyroid-stimulating hormone (see L. H. Smith. 1975), but ectopically produced adrenocorticotrophic hormone (ACTH) or gonadotrophin may stimulate secretion of steroid hormones by the corresponding target organs. The following list shows some of the tumors in which ectopic hormone production has been demonstrated, and the hormones which have been identified:

1. Tumors of the lung producing ACTH (R.B. Cohen *et al.*, 1960; Strott *et al.*, 1968; Gabrilove *et al.*, 1969; J. E. Jones, Shane *et al.*, 1969; Sachs, Becker *et al.*, 1970; Upton and Amatruda, 1971; Corrin *et al.*, 1973; Olurin *et al.*, 1973; Gewirtz and Yalow, 1974; Rees, 1975), parathormone (Berson and Yalow, 1966; Sherwood *et al.*, 1967; Sealy, 1970), gonadotrophin (Fusco and Rosen, 1966; Faiman *et al.*, 1967; Dailey and Marcuse, 1969), antidiuretic hormone (Lipscomb *et al.*, 1968; W. B. Schwartz et al., 1975), growth hormone (Sparagana *et al.*, 1971), and calcitonin (Whitelaw and Cohen, 1973). It is noteworthy that secretion of gonadotrophin occurs mainly with large cell undifferentiated carcinomas, secretion of parathormone with squamous cell carcinomas, and secretion of ACTH with carcinoid tumors, adenocarcinomas, and small cell undifferentiated (oat cell) carcinomas.
2. Carcinomas of the kidney (Hodgkinson, 1964; Golde *et al.*, 1974b) secreting parathormone and gonadotrophin.
3. Hepatomas (Hung *et al.*, 1963; Knill-Jones *et al.*, 1970) secreting parathormone and gonadotrophin.
4. Tumors of the pancreas secreting ACTH (Corrin *et al.*, 1973), gastrin (Zollinger *et al.*, 1968; McGuigan and Trudeau, 1968), and vasopressin (Marks *et al.*, 1968).
5. Melanomas secreting ACTH (Carey *et al.*, 1973) and calcitonin (Milhaud *et al.*, 1974).
6. Thyroid carcinomas secreting ACTH (Anderson and Glenn, 1966; Donahower *et al.*, 1966; Williams, Morales, and Horn, 1968). Production of calcitonin by thyroid tumors is not classed as ectopic secretion because the normal thyroid gland contains cells which secrete calcitonin.
7. Parotid tumors secreting ACTH (Sherry *et al.*, 1963; Cox, Gourley, and Kitabchi, 1970).
8. Carcinomas of the stomach secreting growth hormone (Beck and Burger, 1972) and insulin (Miyabo *et al.*, 1968).
9. Carcinomas of the cervix secreting insulin (Kiang *et al.*, 1973).

The hormone secreted by a tumor may differ slightly from the normal hormone (Riggs *et al.*, 1971; Orth *et al.*, 1973). The ACTH secreted by tumors is often of greater molecular weight than normal ACTH and is probably a precursor; gonadotrophin secreted by tumors may lack the normal complement of carbohydrate. Secretion by the tumor may not be suppressed by procedures which suppress secretion by the normal gland (Linn *et al.*, 1967).

One hypothesis which has been put forward to account for ectopic hormone production is derepression of the genes coding for the hormones in question, and the association of particular hormones with particular types of tumors suggests that, if this hypothesis is correct, the gene derepression is non-random (E. D. Williams, 1969).

Many tumors which exhibit the phenomenon of ectopic hormone secretion arise from cells of the APUD (amine precursor uptake and decarboxylation) system, which are derived from the neural crest (Pearse, 1969; Pearse and Polak, 1971), and it has been suggested that the supposedly ectopic hormone secretion is due simply to the production in detectable amounts of substances which are synthesized in undetectable amounts by normal APUD cells (Shields, 1977). Other tumors which exhibit the phenomenon, including hepatomas, renal carcinomas, and tumors of connective tissue, do not appear to be derived from APUD cells (Levine and Metz, 1974) and it has been suggested (Warner, 1974) that the secretion is from hybrid cells formed by the fusion *in vivo* of malignant non-APUD cells with normal APUD cells. Many tumors of APUD-cell origin have been reported to secrete more than one hormone (Salama et al., 1971; Omenn, 1973). This is not necessarily inconsistent with a predominantly monoclonal composition (3.114) because, as Warner (1974) has pointed out, transcriptional control of multiple sets of genes by a common operator mechanism might result in simultaneous derepression of more than one structural gene.

Tumors may also secrete proteins such as mucin, which are neither hormones nor TAA and which may accumulate locally in considerable quantity.

The use of TAA, hormones, and other markers secreted by tumors in the diagnosis of primary residual cancer will be discussed later.

Another form of functional activity which some tumor cells have been reported to show is phagocytosis (Spivak, 1973), but it may be difficult to distinguish a phagocytic tumor cell from a macrophage.

4

The Relationship of Tumor and Host

4.1 THE CONCEPT OF ANTAGONISTIC SYMBIOSIS

Although tumors arise from host tissues it is customary to distinguish between the tumor and the host, and to describe the relationship between them as a form of parasitism or *antagonistic symbiosis.*[*]

This conceptual model is useful provided it does not obscure the fact that the asocial cells (2.3) which constitute the tumor cell population may be widely scattered in the host, and that the structure to which the term tumor is commonly applied is, as we have seen, a complex entity which contains both neoplastic and non-neoplastic elements (3.1).

The relationship may be further characterized as *obligate,* since a tumor has no independent existence apart from its host, although tumor cells may be maintained in tissue culture. Strictly speaking, therefore, it is absurd to describe a tumor as *autonomous,* but, as mentioned in the Preface, this qualification is often used in a more restricted sense which implies, firstly, that malignant tumors are unaffected by any of the factors which regulate the growth of normal tissues, and, secondly, that no homeostatic mechanisms, even of a rudimentary kind, have evolved to prevent the emergence of cancer cells or the subsequent development of a tumor. These dogmas merit critical appraisal.

4.2 RESPONSE OF TUMORS TO NORMAL CONTROLS

It seems clear that both local and systemic mechanisms are concerned in the maintenance of normal tissue equilibrium, which is manifested in such familiar phenomena as the orderly arrangement of cells within a tissue, the remarkably constant

---

[*]The use of the term symbiosis in a broad sense to include relationships which are antagonistic or neutral, as well as those which are mutually beneficial, has been adopted from a recent text on mycology (Cooke, 1977).

anatomical relationships between tissues of different kinds, and the process of controlled regeneration exemplified by regeneration of the liver after partial hepatectomy.

It is clear also that malignant tumors in general are, to say the least, relatively insensitive to these control mechanisms, and that tumor cells do not cooperate with other cells, in the way that normal cells do, to form tissues specialized for particular functions (Rapin and Burger, 1974). It should be noted, however, that cooperation between neoplastic and normal cells is essential for the development of a tumor (3.1), and while cooperation to produce a tissue having a specialized physiological function is the exception rather than the rule, some tumors, as mentioned previously (3.6), do exhibit functional activity in the form of hormone secretion.

Our understanding of the control mechanisms is so inadequate, however, that detailed comparison of the responses of tumors and normal tissues is not possible. The discussion will therefore be limited to some comments, mainly of a speculative kind, concerning local controls which depend on contact with neighboring structures and cells, chalones, and the possible significance of antigenic deletion exhibited by some tumors, and a more detailed examination of hormone-dependent tumors.

4.21   Contact With Neighboring Structures and Cells

Natural anatomical barriers, such as the epithelial basement membrane and the walls of blood vessels, are often breached by malignant tumors. The phenomenon of carcinoma-in-situ and the absence of vascular invasion in some tumors, particularly early in their development, suggest that these structures may exert a significant, but temporary, restraining influence.

Intercellular contact, as we have seen (3.1), profoundly influences the movement and replication of normal cells *in vitro;* transformed cells, on the other hand, are not subject to contact inhibition by cells of the same kind, though they may be inhibited by transformed cells of a different kind, and also by normal cells.

It is an open question whether contact inhibition plays a significant role in regulating the growth of normal tissues *in vivo* (Eagle and Levine, 1967). If it does not, then the behavior of tumor cells *in vivo* cannot be attributed to escape from contact inhibition. If, on the other hand, it does play such a role, two interesting questions arise. Firstly, is the movement and replication of tumor cells *in vivo* inhibited to some extent by contact with normal cells, as may happen *in vitro?* Secondly, is the predominantly monoclonal composition of some, perhaps indeed many, tumors (3.114) a manifestation of contact inhibition by the clone which is eventually dominant of cells belonging to different clones?

4.22   Chalones

It is claimed by Bullough and others that mitosis in normal tissues is controlled by negative feedback mediated chemically by mitotic inhibitors termed *chalones* which act specifically only on cells of the tissue in which they originate, and substances with these properties have been extracted from liver, kidney and epidermal cells, melanocytes, lymphocytes, and polymorphonuclear leukocytes (Bullough, 1965, 1975; Bullough and Rytömaa, 1965; Bullough and Laurence, 1968, 1970; Verly *et al.,* 1971; Paukowits, 1971; Mathé, 1972; Forscher and Houck, 1973; Houck *et al.,* 1973).

Whether or not chalones play an important role *in vivo,* however, must be regarded as still *sub judice.*

It has been postulated further that tumors escape from mitotic control either because they fail to respond to the chalone produced by the corresponding normal tissue or because the tumor cells do not synthesize chalone (Bullough and Rytömaa, 1965). In the former case control would be lost immediately; in the latter case control might be maintained by chalone produced by the surrounding normal tissue, either indefinitely or until such time as slow growth had resulted in a mass of tumor cells sufficiently large for the central region to be beyond the effective range of the inward-diffusing chalone. The second of these suggestions gains some support from experiments to be described later (6.4) in which the growth of various tumors in experimental animals was inhibited by intratumor injection of extracts prepared from the corresponding normal tissues but not by extracts from other tissues. These experiments raise interesting therapeutic possibilities but leave the question of whether chalones play an important physiological role still unresolved.

Another suggestion, due to Burch (1970), which has been mentioned earlier (2.1) is that tumors are permitted to develop as a result of the breakdown of local chemically mediated control mechanisms akin to those concerned in tissue induction—a process which occurs not only in embryos but also, under certain conditions, in adult organisms (see Woodruff, 1960; Tarin, 1972). At present, however, there does not appear to be any firm experimental evidence in support of this hypothesis.

4.23 Antigen Deletion

Tumor cells, as already mentioned (3.112), differ from normal cells in respect of cell surface structure, and, in particular, tumor cells often lack some of the antigenic determinants which are present on the corresponding normal cells. It has been suggested that tumors are insensitive to normal controls, at least partly as the result of this antigenic deletion (Burnet, 1957; Green, 1954, 1958; Nairn, Richmond *et al.,* 1960; Nairn, Fothergill *et al.,* 1962; Baldwin and Barker, 1967a). Until more is known about the role of surface antigenic determinants in the control of normal tissue equilibrium, however, this hypothesis must remain no more than a plausible speculation.

Tumor-associated antigens (TAA) may also be lost in the course of development of a tumor, but as these, by definition, are not represented on normal cells, this phenomenon will be considered later (5.521).

4.24 Hormone-dependent Tumors

Endocrine and secondary sexual organs whose functional activity is under hormonal control, including the pituitary, thyroid, adrenal, breast, ovary, uterus, testis, and prostate, may undergo hypertrophy or hyperplasia as a result of administration or increased endogenous production of the appropriate hormone, and atrophy as a result of hormone deprivation.

As we have already seen (2.15) the incidence of tumors in these organs and elsewhere may be decreased by endocrine deficiency or, alternatively, by administration of particular hormones. Conversely, endocrine stimulation may lead to the development of a variety of tumors in experimental animals and possibly also in man.

The question now to be considered is whether malignant tumors which have developed in organs which are normally subject to endocrine control may be influenced by hormones. It is important because an affirmative answer even for a restricted range of tumors—indeed, in strict logic, for a single tumor—would suffice to invalidate the dogma of autonomy.

In retrospect, the first evidence that a tumor may be hormone dependent was provided by Beatson's (1896) observation of the beneficial effect of oophorectomy in two women with cancer of the breast. Since this preceded the discovery of secretin and introduction of the concept of hormones by Bayliss and Starling (1902) by some six years and the isolation of estrogen from ovarian tissue (MacCorquodale *et al.*, 1936) by four decades, it is scarcely surprising that the significance of Beatson's observation was not appreciated at the time.

Convincing evidence that hormones may influence the growth of cancer was first obtained by Charles Huggins and his colleagues, who showed that orchidectomy or the administration of phenolic estrogens caused rapid shrinkage of prostatic cancer in dogs (Huggins and Clark, 1940) and regression of metastatic prostatic cancer in man as indicated by a fall in the levels of acid phosphatase and alkaline phosphatase in the patient's serum (Huggins and Hodges, 1941), whereas in untreated cases administration of testosterone resulted in more rapid growth of the tumors. Although some of Huggins' first 21 patients with prostatic cancer and advanced metastases treated by orchidectomy failed to respond, many showed marked regression with relief of pain and prolonged survival, and four patients survived for more than 12 years (Huggins, Stevens, and Hodges, 1941).

Huggins turned his attention next to mammary cancer. The beneficial effects of oophorectomy in some patients was confirmed, and it was found that when oophorectomy was ineffective, or was followed by relapse, remission might occur after adrenalectomy (Huggins and Bergenstal, 1952) or hypophysectomy (Luft, Olivecrona, and Sjögren, 1952). On the other hand, remissions also occurred in male patients after orchidectomy, as was first shown by Farrow and Adair (1942), and in some females after administration of stilbestrol (Haddow *et al.*, 1944).

Huggins set out to resolve experimentally what he called this "vexatious paradox." The mouse did not provide a satisfactory experimental model because in many strains mammary tumors which were large enough to be palpable were usually not hormone dependent. Mammary carcinomas induced in female rats by oral or intravenous administration of aromatic hydrocarbons (Huggins, Briziarelli, and Sutton, 1958), or by ionizing radiation (Huggins and Fukunishi, 1963), on the other hand, often disappeared permanently after oophorectomy or hypophysectomy. These tumors also often regressed following administration of large doses of estradiol and progesterone (Huggins, Moon, and Morii, 1962), and similar treatment induced remissions in some patients with disseminated mammary cancer. There was thus a high degree of concordance between the clinical and experimental findings, and taken together these clearly justify the conclusion which Huggins (1967) drew when reviewing this work in his Nobel lecture, that "cancer is not necessarily autonomous and intrinsically self-perpetuating. Its growth can be sustained and propagated by hormonal function in the host which is not unusual in kind or exaggerated in rate but which is operating at normal or even subnormal levels." Huggins asserted further that under conditions of hormone deprivation "cancer cells may die whereas their normal analogues in the same animal shrivel but survive," but this seems a much more controversial proposition.

Despite these great achievements, Huggins' vexatious paradox remained unresolved. The explanation has, however, begun to emerge following four important new discoveries which we shall now examine.

In the first place, there is evidence that breast cancer, not only in men but also in women, may be androgen dependent. Flax et al. (1973) demonstrated testosterone dependence in vitro in 14 of 130 women, of whom 13 were postmenopausal. The premenopausal patient had been treated with an androgen for several months before being tested, and 5 of the postmenopausal patients had also been treated with androgen or an anti-estrogen, and it was thought that this might have contributed to the subsequent androgen dependence, but the androgen dependence in the other postmenopausal patients could not be explained in this way. Four of the 14 patients responded well to estrogen administration and one to adrenalectomy. The tumor in one patient who failed to respond to estrogen administration appeared in vitro to be both androgen and estrogen dependent.

These findings, together with the fact that the capacity of the human adrenal to synthesize and secrete estrogen is extremely small (Baird et al., 1969; Cameron et al., 1969), suggest that the remissions which sometimes occur following adrenalectomy in postmenopausal patients with breast cancer are due not, as was once believed, to the elimination of adrenocortical estrogen production but to the elimination of adrenocortical androgen.

Secondly, it has been shown that the growth of mammary carcinomas may be promoted by prolactin (vide infra), growth hormone (De Souza et al., 1974), and placental lactogen (A. Barrett et al., 1975). Prolactin dependence has been demonstrated in rat tumors (O. H. Pearson et al., 1969; Nagasawa and Yanai, 1970; Lancet, 1972b; Turkington, 1974; P. A. Kelly et al., 1974), and also in human tumors by Salih et al. (1972), who found that 16 of 50 human mammary carcinomas tested were prolactin dependent in vitro. It seems likely, therefore, that some of the remissions after hypophysectomy are due, at least in part, to the elimination of prolactin secretion.

Thirdly, it has become apparent that normally the first step in the response of a hormone-sensitive cell is binding of the hormone to a receptor protein in, or on the surface of, the cell (Jensen et al., 1969). It was suggested by Jensen et al. (1967) that hormone receptors might be found on tumor cells in numbers corresponding to their degree of hormone dependence, and receptors for estrogen (Mobbs, 1966; Sander, 1968; Korenman and Dukes, 1970; Jensen et al., 1971; Olsnes and Pihl, 1974; McGuire, 1975; McGuire et al., 1975), androgen (Wagner et al., 1973; Engelsman et al., 1974; Bruchovsky et al., 1975), and prolactin (Turkington, 1974; Kelly et al., 1974) have been demonstrated in various animal and human mammary carcinomas. The presence of estrogen or other hormone receptors in or on a tumor cell does not necessarily imply that the whole hormone response mechanism is intact, but endocrine responsiveness would be established if a tumor was shown to produce a measurable product in response to hormonal stimulation (British Medical Journal, 1976b). The presence of progesterone receptors seems a possible marker for estrogen responsiveness because the synthesis of these receptors appears to depend on an intact response to estrogen (Horwitz and McGuire, 1975).

Fourthly, it has been shown that mammary carcinoma tissue may play a role in steroid biosynthesis, a property termed by Adams and Wong (1968) para-endocrine function. W. R. Miller and Forrest (1974, 1976) were unable to confirm the original report of Adams and Wong that microsomal preparations of breast carcinoma could convert testosterone to estriol, but they were able to show that tissue from all human breast cancers studied could convert testosterone into its active reduction products, and that some could synthesize estradiol-17β. In the light of these findings Miller and Forrest have suggested another explanation for the beneficial effects of adrenalectomy observed in some women, namely, reduction of circulating androgens of adrenal origin which, if available, can be used by the tumor as precursors for the synthesis of estradiol.

Hormone dependence is not confined to tumors of the breast and prostate. Carcinomas of the thyroid may be dependent on pituitary thyroid-stimulating hormone and may regress when production of this hormone is reduced as the result of administration of thyroxin (Balme, 1954; Crile, 1966a). In hamsters, carcinomas of the kidney may be induced with stilbestrol and caused to regress by administration of a progestational agent (Provera) and cortisone, and by orchidectomy or adrenalectomy (Bloom, Dukes and Mitchley, 1963; Bloom, Baker et al., 1963a). Regression of disseminated renal adenocarcinomas in patients has also been observed after treatment with Provera or testosterone (Bloom, Dukes, and Mitchley, 1963; Bloom and Wallace, 1964), but, as we have seen (3.34), these tumors do occasionally regress spontaneously. Various degrees of regression of human sarcomas of both soft tissues and bone has also been reported following administration of an agent (Melatonin) which inhibits secretion of growth hormone (Starr, 1969).

Tumors which are hormone dependent may lose this property on repeated transplantation (Bloom, Dukes, and Mitchley, 1963) and thus escape from hormonal control. It seems clear from experience of patients treated by endocrinological manipulations (6.33) that the property of hormone dependence may also be lost in the autochthonous host.

4.3 HOMEOSTATIC MECHANISMS

We have already discussed (2.3) mechanisms which may prevent the emergence of tumor cells. The question now to be considered is whether, when a tumor has developed, there are any homeostatic mechanisms which may help to prevent or limit its further growth and dissemination.

There are three lines of evidence which point strongly to an affirmative answer to this question, though it is clear that whatever mechanisms exist often fail to arrest the growth of the tumor or prevent it from killing the patient.

In the first place, the phenomena of progression, regression, and latency, which were discussed in Chapter 3, seem inexplicable except on the basis of homeostatic mechanisms of some kind which often break down but sometimes result in complete regression of a primary tumor (3.2) or its metastases (3.34), or in very prolonged periods of latency (3.34).

Secondly, kinetic studies (3.5) have shown that tumor cells are continually being lost, even from tumors which are increasing in size.

Thirdly, there is evidence that the behavior of tumors may be influenced by *immunological* reactions evoked by tumor antigens and dependent on recognition of these antigens on the surface of the tumor cell by specific antibody or by T lymphocytes bearing specific receptors coded for by V genes of the same kind as those which determine antibody specificity, and by other mechanisms, which we shall refer to as para-immunological. These para-immunological mechanisms are not necessarily triggered by specific antigens, and they are mediated by a variety of cells including macrophages, NK cells, and polymorphs, some of which also participate in reactions of a strictly immunological kind. This evidence will be discussed in Chapter 5.

4.4   THE DELETERIOUS EFFECT OF CANCER ON THE HOST

4.41   General Effects

As a general rule, malignant tumors which have developed sufficiently to be recognizable clinically grow progressively if they are not treated, and eventually kill the host unless death occurs at an earlier stage from some other cause. There are, as we have seen, (3.2, 3.34), exceptions to this rule, and the extent to which tumors are destroyed before they become recognizable is a matter of speculation.

Sometimes important damage to the host results from the local effects of the primary tumor or its metastases; familiar examples are obstructive jaundice and its attendant sequelae in patients with carcinoma of the ampulla of Vater or the head of the pancreas, raised intracranial pressure in patients with cerebral gliomas, secondary hemorrhage in patients with cancer of the tongue, and urinary tract infection in patients with cancer of the bladder. Often, however, tumors cause serious, and eventually fatal, systemic effects, manifested by such symptoms and signs as loss of weight, muscular weakness and wasting, anemia, and impairment of immunological and para-immunological responsiveness associated with increased susceptibility to infection and decreased resistance to the tumor. A curious observation which merits further investigation was reported by Azzarone et al. (1976), who found that fibroblasts from apparently normal skin of three patients with primary cancer of the lung and another patient with a plasmocytoma, unlike fibroblasts from normal people, underwent spontaneous transformation in tissue culture.

The mechanisms underlying these systemic effects have not been thoroughly elucidated, but they include competition between tumor and host in respect of their metabolic requirements (Mider, 1953; Begg, 1958); the production by tumors of hormones, enzymes, and other pharmacologically active substances which are deleterious to the host (Nakahara and Fukuoka, 1958), including substances with immunosuppressive properties (vide infra) which may weaken resistance to the tumor; secondary infection resulting from ulceration or impaired general resistance; and hemorrhage.

Another mechanism which has been postulated is the promotion of autoimmunity. It was pointed out many years ago by H. N. Green that the anemia associated with many types of cancer is hemolytic in character, and studies in patients and animals led him to conclude that it is due to the production of hemolytic antibody by the cells of the tumor in response to antigenic determinants on normal host cells which are not present on the tumor cells (Green, 1954, 1958; Green, Wakefield, and Littlewood, 1957). This hypothesis has been elaborated by Tyler (1962), who attributes both the high rate of proliferation of cancer cells and their deleterious effect on the host to loss of normal antigens from the cancer cells and, in consequence, the acquisition by these cells of the capacity to react against normal cells bearing these antigens. It seems unlikely that the behavior of tumors in general can be explained in this way, but it is conceivable that the proliferation of cancer cells is determined partly by antigenic deletion (4.22), and, in the special case of tumors of lymphoreticular origin, antibody production by the tumor may, as Kaplan and Smithers (1959) have claimed, contribute significantly to the deleterious effect on the host. With other tumors, however, it seems more likely that, when hemolytic anemia develops, it is due, as Friedell (1965) has suggested, to increased destruction of immature erythrocytes in the spleen as a result of hyperplasia of the reticuloendothelial system. Another systemic manifestation of cancer which has been attributed to autoimmunization is the severe neuromyopathy which sometimes develops, especially in patients with oat cell carcinoma of the lung. Burnet (1965), who put forward this suggestion, postulated that antigenic determinants on cells of the central nervous sytem, which are ordinarily "inaccessible" in the sense of not being capable of producing normal self-tolerance, become accessible by virtue of the fact that they are represented on the cells of the tumor.

There have been many reports of a high incidence of antibody to smooth muscle and antinuclear antibody in patients with a variety of lymphoid and non-lymphoid malignant tumors (Whitehouse and Holborow, 1971; Burnham, 1972; Whitehouse, 1973; Hodson and Turner-Warwick, 1975; Kumar and Taylor, 1975; Riesen *et al.*, 1975; Nelson, 1974, 1977); interpretation is difficult, however, because a high incidence of these particular antibodies has also been reported in patients with various non-malignant disorders of the skin, lungs, and cervix uteri. It is of interest in this connection that patients with one particular form of autoimmune disease, dermatomyositis, show an abnormally high incidence of tumors of various kinds, and removal of the tumor may be followed by improvement in the dermatomyositis (Williams, 1959). There is also a report of one case in which the clinical and immunological features of systemic lupus erythematosus disappeared after excision of a tumor and were still absent one year later (Kahn *et al.*, 1966).

4.42   Effect on Immunological and Para-Immunological Responsiveness

Impairment of immunological and para-immunological responsiveness has been observed in many patients with cancer, particularly in those with lymphoreticular neoplasms and advanced non-lymphoid tumors, but also in some patients with early carcinomas, and in tumor-bearing animals.

The main clinical findings are summarized below. Some of the methods used to assess immunological function in man have been reviewed by Forbes (1971) and Grob and Herold (1972), and the results obtained in patients with cancer by Burdick, Wells, and Herberman (1975). Since chemotherapy (Hersh *et al.*, 1971; Herberman, Rosenberg, and Halterman, 1972), and also radiotherapy even when only part of the body is irradiated (Stjernsward, Clifford, and Svedmyr, 1970), may be immunosuppressive, it is important to take into account the possible effects of treatment.

1.   Antibody formation.   Decreased primary or secondary antibody response to a variety of antigens has been observed in many patients with chronic lymphatic leukemia, lymphosarcoma, and multiple myeloma (Moreschi, 1914; Howell, 1920; Bernstein, 1934; Larson and Tomlinson, 1953; Shaw *et al.*, 1960; Barr and Fairley, 1961;

Cone and Uhr, 1964; Libansky, 1965), and in some patients with advanced carcinomas (Lee, Rowley, and Mackay, 1970); on the other hand, negative results have been reported in Hodgkin's disease (Aisenberg and Leskowitz, 1963), and in patients with a variety of other lymphomas and non-lymphoid tumors (Levin et al., 1970). It seems likely that some of the apparent discordance in the results is due to the use of different antigens by different investigators. Support for this suggestion is provided by the observation of Warr, Willmott, and James (1975), who found that the antibody response of mice bearing transplanted myelomas to alum-precipitated bovine serum albumin is consistently depressed, whereas the response to sheep erythrocytes in terms of splenic plaque-forming cells of IgM, IgGl, IgG2a, and IgG2b specificities is quite variable.

2. *Cutaneous hypersensitivity reactions.* More than half a century ago Rénaud (1926) reported that tuberculin sensitivity was lost in patients with cancer. Since then many studies of cutaneous hypersensitivity reactions have been undertaken using a variety of antigens. These may be subdivided broadly into two groups: *recall antigens,* i.e., antigens such as tuberculin, BCG, mumps vaccine, extracts of *Candida albicans* and *Trichophyton gypseum,* and Varidase (a mixture of the enzymes streptokinase and streptodornase), which many patients are likely to have been exposed to previously, and *newly encountered antigens* in the form of simple synthetic chemicals like 2-4-dinitrochlorobenzene (DNCB), which are unlikely to have been encountered previously. The recall antigens are injected intradermally; DNCB is applied to the skin.

Patients with Hodgkin's disease often show impaired responses to both types of antigen, and normal reactivity to newly encountered antigen is not restored by injection of lymphocytes or transfer factor from sensitized normal people (Kelly, Good, and Varco, 1958; Fairley and Matthias, 1960; Lamb et al., 1962; Aisenberg, 1965, 1966; Chase, 1966; Müftüoğlu and Balkur, 1967). Untreated patients with leukemia also often show moderately impaired reactions to recall antigens (Fairley and Matthias, 1960; Dupuy et al., 1971).

The reaction of patients with non-lymphoid solid tumors to DNCB is often impaired (Krant et al., 1968; Eilber and Morton, 1970a; Al-Sarraf et al., 1970; Pinsky et al., 1971; Wells et al., 1973a; Catalona and Chretien, 1973; Ketcham and Chretien, 1975; Duclos et al., 1977), including patients with primary intracranial tumors (Brooks et al., 1972). Their responses to recall antigens have been reported to be within normal limits by some authors (Logan, 1956; Lamb et al., 1962; Nelson, 1969; Wells et al., 1973b), whereas others have reported impaired responses to a variety of antigens (Solowey and Rapaport, 1965; Eilber and Morton, 1970a; Al-Sarraf et al., 1970; Roberts and Jones-Williams, 1974), especially to tuberculin (Hughes, 1965; Hughes and Mackay, 1965; Ashikawa et al., 1967; Israel, Mawas et al., 1967; Israel, Bouvrain et al., 1968). The results of Roberts and Jones-Williams are unusual in that they found an impaired response to Varidase in patients with breast cancer, including those in Stage I, whereas in other studies the reaction to this material in patients with tumors of various kinds has been normal (Lamb et al., 1962; Wells et al., 1973a).

Normal reactivity may be regained after successful excision of a tumor, but Twomey, Catalona, and Chretien (1974) reported that, as a rule, this did not happen in patients with squamous cell carcinomas.

3. *Number of circulating T lymphocytes.* Lymphocytopenia is common in patients with cancer (Zacharski and Linman, 1971) and has been reported to be asso-

ciated with a poor prognosis (Riesco, 1970; Papatestas and Kark, 1974). The discovery of markers for human T and B lymphocytes (see Papamichail, Holborow, Keith, and Currey, 1972; Brown and Greaves, 1974), in particular the capacity of human T cells to form non-immune rosettes (E rosettes) with sheep erythrocytes (Jondal, Holm, and Wigzell, 1972), and the presence on B cells of surface immunoglobulin and also of C3 receptors (demonstratable by the formation of EAC rosettes), has made it possible to determine the proportion and hence, from the total lymphocyte count, the absolute number of T and B cells in blood, and these techniques have been used in patients with cancer. Wybran and Fudenberg (1973) found that the proportion of T cells was reduced in many cancer patients to an extent which showed a good correlation with the clinical state of the patient. In patients with primary lung cancer, Anthony *et al.* (1975a) observed a reduction in the proportion of T cells in the majority of patients with oat cell tumors and also, though less frequently, in patients with squamous cell tumors; for some unexplained reason the reduction was of prognostic significance only in the patients with squamous cell tumors. The proportion of T cells increased significantly in some patients after pulmonary resection, palliative radiotherapy, or administration of BCG (Anthony *et al.*, 1975b). The proportion of T cells has also been reported to be below normal in patients with disseminated melanoma but not in those with melanoma apparently confined to the primary site (Silverman *et al.*, 1976), and in patients with *all* stages of breast cancer except locally advanced disease (Stage III) (Whitehead *et al.*, 1976), although in a previous investigation (Nemoto *et al.*, 1974) no change in T and B cell levels had been observed at any stage of the disease. These findings suggest that the population being estimated was a heterogeneous one and that the numbers of the various subclasses of T cell are reduced to a different extent at different stages in the progression of a tumor. An apparent reduction in the number of T cells might reflect decreased production or increased destruction; a third possibility, which Whitehead *et al.* (1976) favor on the ground that the proportion of E rosette forming cells in breast cancer patients increased after incubation of the cells *in vitro* with papain and fell again after reincubation in the patient's serum, is that there is a factor in the serum of cancer patients which can mask the E receptor site on the T cell.

The proportion of T cells in tumor-bearing mice, as indicated by the proportion of lymphocytes lysed by anti-Thy 1 (anti-θ) antibody plus complement, has also been found to be reduced (Takatsu *et al.*, 1972; R. T. Smith and Konda, 1973; Kilburn, Smith, and Gorezynski, 1974), though Smith and Konda found that the absolute number of T cells was increased.

4. *Functional activity of T cells.* The response of lymphocytes from patients with both tumors arising in lymphoreticular tissue (Bernard, Geraldes, and Boiron, 1964; Hershorn *et al.*, 1964; Quaglino and Cowling, 1964; Holm, Perlmann, and Johansson, 1966) and non-lymphoid tumors of various types (Israel, Bouvrain *et al.*, 1968; Gurrioch *et al.*, 1970; Stjernsward, Johansson *et al.*, 1970c; Whittaker, Rees, and Clark, 1971; Al-Sarraf *et al.*, 1972; Han and Takita, 1972; Catalona, Sample, and Chretien, 1973; Gillette and Boone, 1973; Guillou *et al.*, 1973; Twomey *et al.*, 1974; Golub *et al.*, 1974; De Gast *et al.*, 1975; Silverman *et al.*, 1976), and also from mice bearing chemically induced sarcomas (Adler *et al.*, 1971), to phytohemagglutinin (PHA) and other mitogens (see Elves, 1970; Mellstelt, 1975), has been reported to be diminished, but the results from different sources show a wide range of variation. Pos-

sible reasons for these differences, and ways of achieving greater uniformity, have been suggested by Teasdale *et al.* (1976).

It has been reported that lymphocytes from a patient with lung cancer were less stimulated by allogeneic lymphocytes in mixed lymphocyte culture than were lymphocytes from the patient's healthy identical twin (Stjernsward, Johansson *et al.*, 1970c).

The reaction produced *in vivo* by injection of lymphocytes from patients with lymphoreticular and non-lymphoid tumors to allogeneic (Aisenberg, 1965; Robinson and Hochman, 1966; Israel, Bouvrain *et al.*, 1968) and xenogeneic (Rees and Symes, 1973; J. J. Miller, Gaffney *et al.*, 1975; Salaman, Miller, and Brown, 1975) hosts has also been reported to be diminished as compared with that produced by lymphocytes from normal individuals.

5. Allograft rejection. Prolonged survival of allografts of skin, and also of tumor tissue, has been reported in patients with advanced cancer as compared with normal individuals (Grace and Kondo, 1958; Snyderman, Miller, and Lizardo, 1960; Gardner and Preston, 1962; Brunschwig *et al.*, 1965). Prolonged survival of skin allografts has also been observed in mice bearing autochthonous (Linder, 1962) and transplanted (McCarthy, 1964) tumors, and prolonged survival of second but not primary skin allografts in mice injected with cell-free peritoneal fluid from mice bearing an ascites tumor (McCarthy, Coffin and Gates, 1968).

It has also been reported that skin allografts from patients with cancer may survive considerably longer in other patients with cancer (E. Robinson *et al.*, 1965), and also in normal recipients (Amos, Hattler, and Shingleton, 1965), than grafts from normal donors. Similar findings have been obtained in mice (Marchant, 1966; Kaliss and Suter, 1968), but accelerated rejection of skin allografts from tumor-bearing animals has also been reported (Breyere and Williams, 1964; Svet-Moldavsky, Mkheidze, and Liozner, 1967; McCarthy and Russfield, 1968). Various explanations have been suggested in the papers cited to account for these phenomena, but none of them can be regarded as established.

6. Macrophage functions. Five criteria of macrophage function will be considered: (1) phagocytic activity *in vivo;* (2) response to chemotactic stimuli *in vitro;* (3) accumulation of macrophages at inflammatory sites *in vivo;* (4) resistance of animals to experimental infection; and (5) the level of serum lysozyme.

1. Phagocytic function in man has been assessed by measuring the rate of clearance from the bloodstream after intravenous injection of a variety of materials including lipid emulsions (Di Luzio and Riggi, 1964; Salky *et al.*, 1964, 1967), aggregated human albumin labeled with ^{125}I or ^{131}I (Iio *et al.*, 1963; Magarey and Baum, 1970), and ^{125}I-labeled polyvinyl pyrrolidone (Morgan and Soothill, 1975). Theoretical considerations and data from animal experiments relating to such assays are discussed by Cohen, Ingrand, and Caro (1968), and Di Luzio and Morrow (1971).

    Salky *et al.* (1967) found that the rate of clearance of lipid emulsion was increased in 48 of 53 patients with cancer as compared with normal controls, and decreased in only 2 patients. Magarey and Baum (1970), in a study of 160 cancer patients, found that reticuloendothelial activity, as judged by clearance from the bloodstream of intravenously injected aggregated human albumin, was greater than in patients with other chronic diseases, and the level of activity appeared to be directly related to the mass of the tumor. Accelerated clearance of colloidal carbon has also been observed in rats and mice bearing a variety of subcutaneous allogeneic tumor transplants (Biozzi et al., 1958; Kampschmidt and Clabaugh, 1964; El Hassan and Stuart, 1965). On the other hand, Stern et al. (1967) found that clearance of colloidal Cr ^{32}PO$_4$ was slower in mice with spontaneous mammary carcinomas and lymphomas than in tumor-free littermates; splenic, but not hepatic, uptake of ^{51}Cr-labeled sheep erythrocytes was also consistently less in the tumor-bearing mice. More recently Boak and his colleagues have reported that the uptake by the regional lymph nodes of technetium-labeled colloidal antimony sulfide injected in the vicinity of a tumor is diminished in patients with breast cancer (Boak and Agwunobi, 1977), and also in mice bearing isogeneic tumor transplants (Boak, Agwunobi, and Mosley, 1977), as compared with the uptake by the contralateral nodes following injection of the colloid at the corresponding site on the opposite side of the body.

2. Monocytes from the blood of patients with cancer may show diminished chemotactic responsiveness in vitro (Boetcher and Leonard, 1974; Snyderman, Dickson et al., 1974; Hausman et al., 1975), and this may improve after excision of the tumor (Snyderman, Pike, Meadows et al., 1975). Similar results have been obtained with peritoneal macrophages from tumor-bearing animals (Snyderman, Pike, Blaylock et al., 1976; Normann and Sorkin, 1976).

3. The accumulation of macrophages at a site of inflammation may be markedly reduced in tumor-bearing animals (Snyderman, Pike, Blaylock et al., 1976). This has been attributed in part to sequestration of macrophages within the tumor (Eccles and Alexander, 1974b). Since the blood monocyte count may be equal to or greater than normal (Eccles, 1977), however, other mechanisms may be involved, including suppression of responsiveness to chemotactic stimuli (Normann and Sorkin, 1977a, 1977b).

    A technique developed by Rebuck and Crowley (1955) which is applicable to man consists in abrading the surface of the skin, applying a coverslip to the raw area, and observing the accumulation of cells on the coverslip. It was reported by Dizon and Southam (1963) that accumulation of macrophages was deficient in patients with advanced cancer as compared with normal people and patients with conditions other than cancer, and further investigations have confirmed this observation (Goldsmith et al., 1965). A simple technique, recently developed in China (Chang, 1978, 1979), consists in raising a sterile blister by local application of cantharides to the skin and studying the cell content of fluid aspirated from the blister.

4. In mice, subcutaneous injection of viable tumor cells has been shown to cause marked, but short-lived, impairment of resistance to experimental infection with Listeria monocytogenes and Yersinia enterocolitica, followed by a prolonged period of enhanced resistance (North et al., 1976a, 1976b). These periods coincide with periods of decreased and increased resistance to fresh challenge with the tumor, and the conversion from decreased to increased resistance depends on the progressive growth of the primary tumor; the phase of increased resistance to tumor challenge is therefore characterized by so-called concomitant immunity (5.521). Since the only cells in the mouse that can destroy Listeria are macrophages, North et al. have argued that macrophages play a key role also in the resistance to tumors.

5. In the light of the observation (Currie and Eccles, 1976) that the level of serum lysozyme is increased in rats bearing syngeneic tumor transplants, due largely to lysozyme released from macrophages in the tumor and the draining lymph nodes, Currie (1976) studied serum lysozyme in patients with breast cancer. The level was increased in patients with localized, but not with disseminated, tumors, to an extent which corresponded with the degree of macrophage infiltration of the tumor, and *in vitro* studies showed that tumor macrophages could release large amounts of lysozyme.

7. Polymorph function. It has been reported (Henon *et al.,* 1977) that the phagocytic activity *in vitro* of neutrophil polymorphonuclear leukocytes from both normal people and patients with cancer is impaired when the cells are suspended in serum from patients with advanced cancer.

General comment. The mechanisms underlying these various manifestations of impaired immunological and para-immunological responsiveness in cancer patients are complex (Kerbel, 1974) and as yet far from fully elucidated.

The manifestations of impaired T-cell function have been attributed to substances released from tumors (Zoller *et al.,* 1976; Kamo and Friedman, 1977), including polypeptides (Glasgow *et al.,* 1974; Nimberg *et al.,* 1975), α_2 globulin (Ashikawa *et al.,* 1971), prostaglandins (Sykes and Maddox, 1972; Tashjian *et al.,* 1972; Plescia *et al.,* 1975), and steroid hormones (Amaral and Werthamer, 1976), and in mice to endogenous C-type virus, and to contaminants in the form of common viruses and mycoplasma (Bonnard *et al.,* 1976). Alternatively, it has been suggested that immunosuppressive polypeptides may be the products of fibrin degradation (Girmann *et al.,* 1976) or be released by macrophages (Kamo and Friedman, 1977), and that the production of excessive amounts of corticosteroids may be a manifestation of a stress reaction evoked by the tumor (Hilf *et al.,* 1960). Other possibilities are increased suppressor cell activity and increased lymphocyte trapping in lymph nodes (Kerbel, 1974).

There is evidence that the suppression of macrophage function in tumor-bearing animals may also be mediated by a humoral factor (Snyderman and Pike, 1976; Pike and Snyderman, 1976a; North *et al.,* 1976a, 1976b). North *et al.* showed that the serum of mice which had been injected with viable tumor cells contained a substance which caused impaired resistance to *Listeria monocytogenes* when injected to other mice. This substance was present in the serum even after the tumor-inoculated mouse had become resistant to Listeria and exhibited concomitant immunity with regard to the tumor. To account for this North *et al.* have suggested that the substance is produced by the tumor, and, while some enters the circulation, is present in sufficient concentration in the tumor to prevent its destruction by macrophages. Further evidence that tumors may produce substances damaging to macrophages is provided by the work of Nelson and Nelson (1978) on the inhibition of delayed-type hypersensitivity reactions by tumor extracts.

Non-specific immunosuppression and inhibition of macrophage function may help a tumor to escape destruction by homeostatic mechanisms of an immunological or para-immunological kind. There are, in addition, escape mechanisms which are immunologically specific, and these will be examined in the next chapter (5.521).

5
Immunological and Para-Immunological Mechanisms Affecting Tumor Growth

5.1 GENERAL CONSIDERATIONS

It was stated in the previous chapter that the behavior of tumors may be influenced by *immunological reactions* evoked by tumor antigens and by *para-immunological mechanisms* not necessarily triggered by antigen but mediated by macrophages and other cells, some of which may also play a role in mechanisms of a strictly immuno-logical kind. We shall now examine the evidence for this statement, and the possible role of such mechanisms in limiting the development and spread of tumors.

The evidence has come from animal experiments, studies in patients, and *in vitro* tests of many kinds. The situation *in vivo* is complex, and some of the variables on which the results depend may not be recognized. *In vitro* experiments are more easily controlled, but the results must be interpreted with caution because the demonstration that a particular effector mechanism can operate *in vitro* does not necessarily mean that it plays a significant role in the living animal or patient.

In the following discussion we shall make frequent use of the terms *cytotoxic* and *cytotoxicity,* especially in relation to *in vitro* tests. These will be used in a general sense to denote any process which results in reduced cell proliferation or cell death. The terms *cytostatic, cytocidal,* and *cytolytic* will be used to describe cytotoxic processes which are manifested by reduced proliferation without cell death, cell death, and cell death plus disintegration, respectively.

5.2 TUMOR-ASSOCIATED ANTIGENS

The history of tumor immunology, as Jacob Furth (1963) has pointed out, can be divided into three eras.

The first era began, as has already been mentioned (1.22), with the discovery by Hanau (1889) and Jensen (1903) that cancer could sometimes be transmitted from one animal to another by transplantation of tumor tissue. It was found subsequently that while some tumors—which characteristically acquired names like the Ehrlich mouse carcinoma and the Jensen rat sarcoma—regularly grew progressively and killed the host, many others appeared to grow for a time and then regressed completely.

A few years after Jensen's paper was published Paul Ehrlich (1906, 1907) reported that reinoculation of tumor cells to mice with an established tumor transplant often failed to produce a further tumor. This observation was confirmed and extended in many laboratories, but unfortunately, owing largely to the lack of genetically uniform strains of laboratory animals, and the failure to make, or take into consideration, comparable observations with transplants of normal tissues, many investigators thought that they were discovering something about tumors when they were in fact studying the laws of transplantation, and many erroneous conclusions were drawn. This period dragged on for years and has no precise end-point, but its death knell was sounded by Woglom in a pungently critical article published in 1929. In retrospect perhaps the most interesting observations during this period were those of J. B. Murphy of the Rockefeller Institute on the role of the lymphocyte in resistance to tumors, and his monograph on this and related subjects, published in 1926, is well worth studying.

The second era, which may be termed the era of immunogenetic analysis, was made possible by the development of inbred strains of animals, initiated by C.C. Little at Bar Harbor. In less than 20 years, as the result of the work of G.D. Snell, P. Gorer, P.B. Medawar, R.E. Billingham, L. Brent, N.A. Mitchison, and many other investigators (see Woodruff, 1960), the genetic basis of histocompatibility was firmly established, specific immunological tolerance and the graft-versus-host (GVH) reaction were discovered, and much was learned about the mechanisms of allograft rejection, methods of immunosuppression, and the chemical nature of transplantation antigens. This and subsequent work has had an enormous impact not only on tumor immunology, with which we are here concerned, but on immunology in general, genetics, and developmental biology.

During the third era, which overlaps with the second and was inaugurated by the publication in 1943 of a paper by Ludwig Gross, it has been established that tumors of various kinds possess cell surface *tumor-associated antigens* (TAA) which are not possessed, or are possessed to only a limited extent, by normal adult cells, and that the TAA of some tumors include a subset of cell-surface antigens termed *tumor-associated transplantation antigens* (TATA) which can evoke an immunological reaction in other animals isogeneic with the animal in which the tumor originated. It has also been shown that autotransplants of some tumors induce resistance in the animal in which the tumor originated. As G. Klein and Oettgen (1969) have pointed out, "this does not, in the strict sense, answer the question of whether, and to what extent, the primary host can mobilize a rejection response against its own tumor cells as they increase in number at their natural pace and at the site of origin." It has been shown further, however, that autotransplants of some tumors encounter stronger resistance than transplants in untreated isogeneic recipients, and this strongly suggests that such tumors possess what, for want of an appropriate short term, Klein and Oettgen (1969) have referred to as *tumor-specific antigens with a rejection-inducing potential in the autochthonous host* (TSARIPAH).

The rate of progress in this field during the last 20 years or so can be gauged from successive reviews which have been published (Zilber, 1958; Old *et al.,* 1961; Hirsch, 1962; Furth, 1963; Old and Boyse, 1964, 1966; Sjögren, 1965; Koldovsky, 1965; G. Klein, 1966a, 1968; Law, 1969; Sophocles and Nadler, 1971; Bagshawe, 1974; Old, 1977; Robins and Baldwin, 1977).

5.21 Tumor-associated Transplantation Antigens

It was reported by Gross (1943, 1945) that C3H mice which had been inoculated intradermally, in a dosage too small to produce lethal tumors, with cells of a sarcoma of recent origin induced with methylcholanthrene in a mouse of the same strain became resistant to subsequent challenge with the same tumor. These experiments, and others reported later by Foley (1953b) and Prehn and Main (1957) in which mice were shown to become resistant to rechallenge after a previous isogeneic transplant of a methylcholanthrene-induced sarcoma had been made to regress by ligating its blood vessels or had been removed surgically, strongly suggested that the tumors studied possessed TATA. The experiments of Gross and Foley were open to the alternative explanation that the resistance was due to antigens resulting from unsuspected genetic differences between the supposedly isogeneic donor and recipient, but this seemed very unlikely in the experiments of Prehn and Main because they showed that mice made resistant to the tumor would accept a skin graft from the tumor donor. The possibility of rejection due to unsuspected donor–host histoincompatibility was completely excluded by G. Klein et al. (1960), who showed that a mouse could be made resistant to its own methylcholanthrene-induced sarcoma by removing the tumor, injecting the original host on three occasions with irradiated tumor cells, and then challenging it with a small dose of viable cells. The feasibility of inducing resistance to isogeneic transplants of methylcholanthrene-induced sarcomas with cells exposed to ionizing radiation in a dose sufficient to prevent further division had been demonstrated previously by Revesz (1960).

There have been many subsequent studies of isogeneic tumor transplants in normal hosts of different ages (Forni and Comiglio, 1973), and in hosts previously injected with irradiated or mitomycin-treated (Wrathmell and Alexander, 1976) cells, or treated with non-specific immunopotentiating (7.5) or immunosuppressive agents, or placed in parabiosis with an isogeneic tumor-bearing partner (Feraci and Schour, 1974); and others, using what were originally called *neutralization tests* but are now commonly referred to as Winn assays, in which the tumor cell inoculum was mixed with serum (Winn, 1960a, 1960b, 1962) or lymphoid cells (Kidd and Toolan, 1950; E. Klein and Sjögren, 1960; Winn, 1961; Slettermark and Klein, 1962; Yoshida and Southam, 1963; Matsumoto, Otsu, and Komeda, 1966; Mikulska, Smith, and Alexander, 1966). Many criteria have been used to assess the host response. These include measurements of tumor growth; host survival; tumor cell population kinetics (Rajewsky and Gruneisen, 1972); the histological reaction in the tumor (3.12), the regional lymph nodes, and the spleen (Andreini, Drasher, and Mitchison, 1955; Woodruff and Symes, 1962a; Edwards, 1964; Mackay, 1965; Kruger, 1967; Blamey and Evans, 1971); adoptive transfer of increased resistance to an isogeneic animal with lymphoid cells (Mitchison, 1954, 1955; Koller and Doak, 1960; Old et al., 1962; Matsumoto, Otsu, and Komeda, 1966); *in vitro* evidence of a humoral (5.224) or cell-mediated (5.226) immune response; and the demonstration of skin hypersensitivity to tumor cells or derivatives (5.229). Since the *in vitro* and hypersensitivity tests are of particular interest in relation to the study of autochthonous tumors, the methods used will be discussed later, in the sections indicated.

In many transplantation experiments it has been found that a procedure which renders an animal resistant to subsequent challenge may have no apparent effect on an established tumor. This phenomenon, which is often referred to as *concomitant immunity,* will be discussed later (5.521).

The only way of making isogeneic tumor transplants in man is by using one of a pair of identical twins as donor and the other as host. This has been done occasionally, but it is not without risk and in the writer's opinion is ethically unjustifiable (1.12). Tests of cutaneous hypersensitivity (5.229), and for evidence of cytotoxic antibody (5.224), antibody-dependent cell-mediated immunity (5.225), and lymphocyte-mediated cytotoxicity (5.226) *in vitro,* have, however, been widely used in both patients and animals bearing autochthonous tumors.*

Another procedure applicable to both human and animal tumors, which derives largely from the work of Gorer and his colleagues (Gorer, 1956, 1961; Gorer, Tuffrey, and Batchelor, 1962), is to test the serum of allogeneic or xenogeneic tumor transplant recipients for antibody reactive against tumor tissue after absorbing the serum with normal donor tissue. The results on the whole have been disappointing. A modification of the procedure, which is theoretically attractive but difficult to achieve in practice with xenogeneic recipients (Levi, Schechtman *et al.,* 1959; Garb *et al.,* 1962; Sekla *et al.,* 1967; Billingham and Silvers, 1968), is to study serum from animals made immunologically tolerant of normal donor tissue before they received a tumor transplant.

In recent years there have also been many studies of the induction of tumor-specific immunity *in vitro,* with both murine (McKhann and Jagarlamoody, 1971a; Ilfield *et al.,* 1973; Lundak and Raidt, 1973; Wagner and Rollinghoff, 1973; Rollinghoff and Wagner, 1973a; Warnatz and Scheiffarth, 1974; Kuperman, Fortner, and Lucas, 1975; Kall and Hellström, 1975; Manson and Palmer, 1975; Burton, Thompson, and Warner, 1975; Chism, Burton, and Warner, 1975, 1976a; Glaser, Bonnard, and Herberman, 1976; Schechter, Treves, and Feldman, 1976; Treves *et al.,* 1976; Kedar, Unger, and Schwartzbach, 1976; Burton and Warner, 1977a, 1977b; Burton, Chism, and Warner, 1977; Kedar *et al.,* 1978b) and human (McKhann and Jagarlamoody, 1971b; Seigler *et al.,* 1972; Golub and Morton, 1974; Sharma and Terasaki, 1974) tumors. The procedure consists in incubating lymphoid cells with irradiated or mitomycin-treated syngeneic or autochthonous tumor cells for periods of up to 7 or 8 days, harvesting the lymphoid cells, and then determining their cytotoxicity for viable tumor cells by a chromium-release or other type of *in vitro* assay (5.226). The optimal conditions in respect of the number of tumor cells, the ratio of lymphoid to tumor cells, the requirement for 2-mercaptoethanol in the medium, and the time at which the cells are harvested are discussed by Burton, Thompson, and Warner (1975). The findings with particular types of tumor are discussed below. The use of lymphoid cells immunized *in vitro* in therapeutic experiments and trials are discussed in later chapters (7.413, 8.233); it is of interest in this connection that cell-mediated cytotoxicity of cells immunized *in vitro* may be greater than that of cells obtained by immunization *in vivo,* especially with only weakly immunogenic tumors (Schechter *et al.,* 1976).

Investigations of the kinds described have established that resistance may be induced not only to chemically induced tumors but also to tumors induced in other ways, and to some spontaneous tumors, and that this increased resistance is associated

---

*The term tumor-bearing will be used in a broad sense to describe not only hosts with manifest tumors but also those whose tumors have not yet become detectable, or have been partly, or even completely, destroyed.

with evidence of cellular or humoral immunity directed against tumor-associated antigens.

Some tumors appear to induce much greater resistance than others, and it is customary to describe these as strongly immunogenic; failure to demonstrate resistance, however, does not necessarily imply that a tumor is devoid of TATA, since it may evoke a reaction but be insensitive to rejection (Globerson and Feldman, 1964; Prehn, 1970; Oth, 1975), or be protected from attack by one of the escape mechanisms discussed later (5.521), or the host may lack the immune response (Ir) genes necessary for recognition of the antigens. This last mechanism may conceivably account for the failure of Moloney lymphomas to evoke a reaction in A-strain mice, since they do evoke a reaction in F1 hybrids of strain A and various other strains (Smith and Landy, 1976).

There are also important differences in the extent to which tumors induced by different types of carcinogen show cross-reactivity with other tumors induced by the same agent.

5.211   CHEMICALLY INDUCED TUMORS

Induction of resistance to syngeneic tumor transplants or other evidence of immunogenicity has been demonstrated in mice or rats with sarcomas (Prehn, 1960, 1962; Old et al., 1962; Pasternak, Horn, and Graffi, 1962; Boyse, 1963; Yoshida and Southam, 1963; Tuffrey and Batchelor, 1964; I. Hellström, K. E. Hellström, and Pierce, 1968; see also references cited in 5.21), mammary carcinomas (Prehn, 1962), and a cerebral glioma (Scheinberg et al., 1962, 1963) induced with various cyclic hydrocarbons including methylcholanthrene; hepatomas induced with azo dyes (Gordon, 1965; Baldwin and Barker, 1967b, 1967c, 1967d); Baldwin and Embleton, 1971); and other chemically induced tumors (Baldwin, 1973; Oth, 1975).

The degree of immunogenicity depends on various factors, including the carcinogen used, the latent period between the administration of the carcinogen and the appearance of a tumor, and the tissue or organ in which the tumor arises.

Tumors induced with urethane (Prehn, 1963b) and diethylnitrosamine (Pasternak, Hoffman, and Graffi, 1966) have been reported to be non-immunogenic or only occasionally immunogenic. These originated in the lungs, however, and lung tumors induced with methylcholanthrene have also been reported to be non-immunogenic (Prehn, 1963b), so that the target organ may be an important factor.

It was observed by Old et al. (1962) and Prehn (1963a, 1963b) that sarcomas which developed quickly in response to cyclic hydrocarbons were, as a rule, more immunogenic than those which developed slowly. Further investigation (Prehn, 1975) has shown that the dose of carcinogen is not important, except in so far as it affects the latent period, since tumors induced with high and low doses of methylcholanthrene, but selected because they had about the same latent period, differed little in respect of what Prehn termed the *antigenicity ratio*, i.e., the ratio of mean tumor size in control mice to mean tumor size in immunized mice, under defined experimental conditions.

A study of the behavior of isogeneic transplants of immunogenic tumors in hosts of different ages (Forni and Comiglio, 1973) showed good correlation between the number of viable cells needed to produce a tumor and the capacity of the host to mount a cell-mediated response to alloantigens.

It has been established that a tumor-bearing host (5.21) may become immunized by its autochthonous tumor *in situ,* as shown by the failure or slow growth of autotransplants despite rapid growth of transplants in untreated isogeneic hosts (Mikulska, Smith, and Alexander, 1966; Whitney, Levy, and Smith, 1974). Resistance has been reported to diminish when a tumor grows beyond a certain size but to increase again after complete surgical removal (Yoshida and Southam, 1963; I. Hellström, K.E. Hellström, and Pierce, 1968), and to a lesser extent after incomplete excision or destruction of the tumor *in situ* by irradiation (Vaage, 1971); increased susceptibility to rechallenge has, however, also been observed after excision of a primary transplant (Stjernsward, 1968).

Transplantation experiments have, for the most part, yielded no evidence of antigenic cross-reactivity between tumors induced with the same chemical carcinogen in different isogeneic animals (Prehn and Main, 1957; G. Klein *et al.,* 1960; Prehn, 1961, 1962; Old *et al.,* 1962; Pasternak, Horn, and Graffi, 1962; G. Klein and E. Klein, 1962; Basombrio, 1970), or even at different sites in the same animal (Globerson and Feldman, 1964; Rosenau and Morton, 1966), but exceptions to this rule have been reported (Prehn and Main, 1957; Stern, 1960; Pasternak, Horn, and Graffi, 1962; Globerson and Feldman, 1964; Takeda *et al.,* 1966; Reiner and Southam, 1967, 1969; Holmes *et al.,* 1971; Taranger *et al.,* 1972; Usubuchi *et al.,* 1972, 1973; Robert, Oth, and Dumont, 1973; Burton and Warner, 1978), including one instance of cross-reactivity between benzpyrene-induced tumors in rats and mice (Koldovsky and Svoboda, 1963). *In vitro* tests for humoral (McKhann and Harder, 1968; Harder and McKhann, 1968; I. Hellström, K.E. Hellström and Pierce, 1968; Tachibana and Klein, 1970; Burdick and Wells, 1973; Fritze *et al.,* 1976b) and cell-mediated (I. Hellström, K.E. Hellström, and Pierce, 1968; Forbes, Nakao, and Smith, 1975; Bataillon, Pross, and Klein, 1975; Kearney, Basten, and Nelson, 1975) immunity, including tests for cell-mediated immunity after immunization *in vitro* (Burton and Warner, 1978), on the other hand, have provided abundant evidence of cross-reacting antigens. Moreover, in the experiments of Burton and Warner (1978), in which there was evidence of cross-reactivity both *in vivo* and *in vitro,* the patterns of cross-reactivity suggested that the antigens detected *in vivo* were not identical with those detected *in vitro.*

It seems clear therefore that chemically induced tumors characteristically possess unique TATA, which are often strongly immunogenic, and common antigens which are only occasionally demonstrable by transplantation but are readily demonstrable by *in vitro* techniques. Some of these common antigens, termed oncofetal antigens (OFA), are found also in fetal tissues; these will be discussed in detail later (5.23). Others have been shown to be viral, or virus related (Hamburg, Loizner, and Svet-Moldavsky, 1966; Colnaghi and Della Porta, 1973; J.P. Grant *et al.,* 1974a), indicating either the activation of a latent oncogenic virus by the chemical carcinogen or the presence of passenger virus.

5.212 TUMORS OF VIRAL ORIGIN

It was found by Habel (1961), and Sjögren, Hellström, and Klein (1961a, 1961b) that polyoma virus-induced tumors contained a common group-specific TATA capable of inducing rejection responses in syngeneic hosts. This antigen was not present on the mature virion, and was present on polyoma-induced tumor cells whether they released virus or not (Sjögren, 1965). Cross-reactivity has been found to extend to polyoma-induced tumors of different histological type, and to occur also, as I. Hellström and Sjögren (1966) showed by colony-inhibition assay (5.226), between polyoma-induced tumors in mice and hamsters.

Analagous group-specific TATA have been demonstrated with many other tumors induced with DNA, and also with RNA, viruses; indeed in 1968 G. Klein stated that this was true of all the virus-induced tumor systems which had been investigated.

Examples of DNA virus-induced tumors include, in addition to polyoma tumors, SV40-induced hamster tumors (Defendi, 1963; Habel and Eddy, 1963; Koch and Sabin, 1963), tumors induced in mice and hamsters with human adenoviruses (Berman, 1967; I. Hellström and Sjögren, 1967) and variants of the Rous chicken sarcoma virus (Sjögren and Jonsson, 1963; Jonsson and Sjögren, 1965, 1966; Koldovsky and Bubenik, 1964, 1965; Koldovsky and Svoboda, 1965; Koldovsky, Svoboda, and Bubenik, 1966; Casey et al., 1966; Bellone and Pollard, 1970), and tumors induced in rabbits with Shope papilloma virus (C.A. Evans, Weiser, and Ito, 1962; Evans and Ito, 1966).

The RNA-virus tumors which have been most thoroughly studied are murine leukemias, sarcomas, and mammary carcinomas.

It has been shown that resistance to isogeneic transplantation or other manifestations of immunity in respect of Gross (G. Klein, Sjögren, and E. Klein, 1962; Slettermark and Klein, 1962; Alexrad, 1963), Moloney (E. Klein and G. Klein, 1964; Glynn, Bianco, and Goldin, 1964; Haughton, 1965; G. Klein, E. Klein, and Haughton, 1966), Graffi (Pasternak and Graffi, 1963; Pasternak, 1965), Friend (Old, Boyse, and Lilly, 1963; Wahren, 1963), Rauscher (Old, Boyse, and Stockert, 1964), and Rich (Rich, Geldner, and Myers, 1965) leukemias can be induced by immunization with the same or a closely related virus, allogeneic leukemic cells, viable isogeneic leukemic cells in low dosage, and irradiated isogeneic leukemic cells. More recent studies (see Sato et al., 1973; Bauer, 1974), using inter alia neutralization tests (Eckner and Stevens, 1972; Gomard, Le Clerc, and Levy, 1973), immuno-electron microscopy (Aoki, 1974; Aoki et al., 1974) and tests of cell-mediated immunity in vitro (Shellam et al., 1976) have demonstrated three kinds of TAA, namely, virus envelope antigens (VEA), which may be group, subgroup or type specific, virus structural antigens, which are present on the virion and in infected cells, and virus-induced surface antigens (VCSA). Among the VCSA there is a special group of antigens termed virus-induced cell surface differentiation antigens (VCSDA). The VCSDA are not truly tumor specific because, while they occur on cancer cells, they also occur on normal cells in some strains of mice; they include Gross cell surface antigen (GCSA), antigens of the TL system,* and another antigen specified by a murine leukemia virus termed GIX (MuLV), all of which occur on normal thymocytes of some mouse strains and on leukemic cells of mice of the same and other strains; and PCI, which occurs on some plasma cells and other normal cells. It is because tumors of viral origin may possess viral antigens and virus-specified antigens possessed by some normal cells, that the term tumor-associated antigen (TAA), which embraces these categories, has come to be used rather than the more restrictive term tumor-specific antigen (TSA). As we have seen, TATA constitute a subset of TAA, and virus-associated TAA, like other TAA, do not necessarily function as TATA (Chang, Law, and Appella, 1975).

Cells transformed by murine sarcoma viruses (MuSV) have also been reported to possess TAA demonstrable by isogeneic transplantation and a variety of in vitro tests (Fefer, McCoy, and Glynn, 1967; Law, Ting, and Stanton, 1968; Burstein, 1970). These antigens, however, cross-react completely with those of the corresponding MuLV (Chuat et al., 1969: LeClerc, Gomard, and Levy, 1972; Gomard, LeClerc, and

---

*There does not appear to be any direct evidence linking the TL antigen to a virus but an association is strongly suspected.

Levy, 1973; Kirschner *et al.,* 1976), and are demonstrable on MuSV-transformed cells only when the cells are producing infective virus as the result of phenotypic mixing with MuLV (McCoy *et al.,* 1972a, 1972b; Stephenson and Aaronson, 1972; Strouk *et al.,* 1972).

Early attempts to induce immunity to mouse mammary adenocarcinomas were inconclusive (Gross, 1947; Foley, 1953a), though it appeared from the work of Hirsch *et al.* (1958) and Weiss, Faulkin, and De Ome (1963, 1964) that they might be immunogenic even in the animal in which they arose. Reports then began to appear which suggested that isogeneic transplants of mammary carcinomas arising in mice bearing the mouse mammary tumor virus (MMTV) readily induced resistance in mice which did not bear the virus but failed to do so in those which did (Morton, 1962; Attia, De Ome, and Weiss, 1965; Lavrin, Blair, and Weiss, 1966; Suit and Silobrcic, 1967). It was concluded that these tumors share a common antigen (or antigens) possessed by, or induced by, the MMTV, but that animals which become infected with the virus during neonatal life become specifically tolerant of such antigens. Further investigations, using both transplantation and *in vitro* techniques, have confirmed this conclusion but have shown that some mouse mammary tumors possess in addition other tumor-specific antigens which are unrelated to the MMTV and make them immunogenic, though in general weakly immunogenic, in MMTV-infected mice (Vaage, 1968a, 1968b; Holmes and Morton, 1969; Morton, Miller, and Wood, 1969).

5.213 PLASMACYTOMAS

Plasma cell tumors can be induced readily in Balb/c, NZB, and (Balb/c × NZB) F1 mice, and less readily in some other strains, by injecting mineral oil; they also occasionally develop spontaneously (see Potter, 1972; also see 3.114). Their pathogenesis is not clear but it has been suggested that MuLV is involved.

The immunogenicity of mouse plasma cell tumors on syngeneic transplantation was reported by Lespinats (1969). Subsequent studies involving both *in vivo* (Williams and Krueger, 1972; Rollinghoff, Rouse, and Warner, 1973; McCoy *et al.,* 1974; Boyer and Fahey, 1976) and *in vitro* (Wagner and Rollinghoff, 1973; Burton and Warner, 1977a) immunization have shown that these tumors possess group-specific antigens which are common to tumors of the same (Williams and Krueger, 1972; Rollinghoff, Rouse, and Warner, 1973; McCoy *et al.,* 1974) or different (Burton and Warner, 1977a) mouse strains, and also unshared antigens (Wagner and Rollinghoff, 1973; Boyer and Fahey, 1976; Burton and Warner, 1977a). The shared antigens have been shown by serological tests and tests for cell-mediated immunity *in vitro* to include virion and virus-induced cell surface antigens (Hyman, Ralph, and Sarkar, 1972; Herberman and Aoki, 1972) and oncofetal antigens (5.23). The unshared antigens include, and may or may not be limited to, the idiotypic determinants of the immunoglobulins produced by different tumors (Eisen, Sakato, and Hall, 1975).

5.214 OTHER INDUCED TUMORS

It has been reported that Balb/c radiation-induced leukemic cells release C-type virus and possess leukemia-specific cell surface antigen (Sato *et al.,* 1973); these differ, however, from the cell-surface antigens on typical MuLV-induced Balb/c leukemic cells (Aoki, 1974).

With generalized lymphomas of non-thymic type induced in CBA and C3H mice with ^{90}Sr, ^{239}Pu, or ^{226}Ra, Loutit and Ash (1978) found no evidence of TATA in transplantation experiments in which attempts were made to immunize mice with sub-threshold doses of viable syngeneic tumor cells, large doses of viable allogeneic tumor cells, or large doses of killed syngeneic tumor cells, despite the fact that C-type and A-type viral particles were readily demonstrated in electron micrographs of the tumors. They suggested therefore that in these tumors the viruses were passengers and not causative.

Resistance to tumors induced by plastic films (2.13) has been demonstrated after previous isogeneic transplantation (Prehn, 1963a) or injection of irradiated syngeneic, but not autochthonous, tumor cells (G. Klein, Sjögren, and E. Klein, 1963); the antigenic properties of these tumors, however, have not been investigated in detail.

5.215   SPONTANEOUS TUMORS

The ambiguous nature of the term *spontaneous* in relation to tumors has been discussed earlier (1.211, 2.1). Here we shall consider tumors which have arisen, without any attempt having been made to induce them, in inbred strains of laboratory animals in which the incidence of tumors of the type in question is low.

Many tumors of this kind, including spontaneous mouse fibrosarcomas (Prehn and Main, 1957; Hewitt, Blake, and Walder, 1976), mammary carcinomas (Riggins and Pilch, 1964; Hewitt *et al.,* 1976), leukemias and other tumors (Hewitt *et al.,* 1976), and rat sarcomas, mammary carcinomas, and other tumors (Baldwin, 1966; Baldwin and Embleton, 1969b), have been reported to be non-immunogenic on syngeneic transplantation. This is not true of all spontaneous mouse and rat tumors, however, and some of the negative results can be attributed to using suboptimal techniques of immunization, or to challenging with pieces of tumor tissue or with too large a dose of cells in suspension. By using a variety of immunization procedures, among which administration of cells treated with mitomycin in low dosage appears to be particularly effective (Wrathmell and Alexander, 1976; Woodruff, Whitehead, and Speedy, 1978), and comparing the response of pretreated and non-treated hosts to challenge with viable cells at several dose levels, evidence of immunization may be obtained with tumors which under less stringent conditions appear to be non-immunogenic (Wrathmell and Alexander, 1976; Woodruff *et al.,* 1978). It is therefore an exaggeration to say that spontaneous tumors in inbred laboratory animals are always, or nearly always devoid of TATA. The proportion of such tumors shown to possess TATA is, however, decidedly smaller than is the case with chemically induced or virus-induced tumors. The extent to which this number will be increased by further changes in methods of immunization and assessment remains to be seen, but it seems clear that even when spontaneous tumors are immunogenic the response they evoke is often feeble. Indeed it has been suggested that when they do appear to be strongly immunogenic this may be due to viral contamination (Kieler *et al.,* 1972). Spontaneous tumors which are weakly immunogenic have been found not to cross-react with other tumors (Hammond, Fisher, and Rolley, 1967; Baldwin and Embleton, 1969b).

As mentioned earlier (2.11), it seems likely that some, and possibly many, tumors which are not deliberately induced are nevertheless due, or partly due, to accidental exposure to environmental carcinogens. This is not necessarily inconsistent with weak or even no demonstrable immunogenicity. Tumors induced chemically in laboratory animals are by no means always strongly immunogenic (Baldwin and Embleton, 1969a; Bartlett, 1972), especially if they develop slowly (Prehn, 1975), and chronic administration of small amounts of carcinogen, which seems the appropriate model for accidental exposure to environmental carcinogens, favors slow development, as compared with the common laboratory procedure of injecting a single large dose.

As we shall see later (5.4, 5.53), tumors which are non-immunogenic may nevertheless be influenced by para-immunological mechanisms.

5.22 Antigens of Primary Autochthonous Tumors

As we have seen (5.21), it has been established that many animal tumors possess TATA, and the discovery that transplants of some animal tumors may encounter stronger resistance in the autochthonous host than in syngeneic hosts (Mikulska, Smith, and Alexander, 1966; Whitney, Levy, and Smith, 1971) points strongly to the existence of antigens which, following Klein and Oettgen (1969), we have referred to as tumor-specific (or -associated) antigens with a rejection-inducing potential in the autochthonous host (TSARIPAH or TAARIPAH). While it is clear that TATA constitute a subclass, and possibly a small subclass, of TAA, it is an open question whether all, or only some, TATA are TAARIPAH.

With human tumors comparison of the behavior of autologous and isogeneic transplants is not possible except in the special case when the patient has an identical twin, and even when possible it is open to objection on ethical grounds. The existence of TAA in many human tumors is suggested, however, by accumulation of lymphocytes and plasma cells in the tumor stroma, the presence of immunoglobulin on tumor cells, and histological changes characteristic of an immunological reaction in the regional lymph nodes, and it has been established conclusively by the demonstration of antigenic differences between tumor cells and normal adult cells on xenogeneic immunization, and *in vitro* evidence of immunity to tumor cells or extracts mediated by the patient's serum or lymphocytes. It has been reported, moreover, that the results of some tests, in particular tests of lymphocyte-mediated cytotoxicity directed against tumor cells, show good correlation with the immunogenicity of animal tumors on isogeneic (I. Hellström *et al.,* 1969c; Forni and Comoglio, 1973) and autologous (Kikuchi *et al.,* 1972) transplantation, and with the growth characteristics of autochthonous human tumors (5.226), and this strongly suggests that these tests are detecting TATA and TAARIPAH.

5.221 HISTOLOGICAL EVIDENCE OF AN IMMUNOLOGICAL REACTION TO HUMAN TUMORS

Infiltration of lymphocytes and macrophages, and to a less extent plasma cells, occurs commonly in both animal and human tumors, including carcinoma-in-situ. As was mentioned in discussing this phenomenon (3.12), there have been many claims that heavy infiltration, particularly of lymphocytes, is associated with a high degree of differentiation, a tendency to spontaneous regression and a relatively good prognosis, though this is by no means universally accepted. In a study of lymphocyte and plasma cell infiltration in primary lung cancer of various histological types, Ioachim, Dorsett, and Paluch (1976) concluded that this represented a reaction to TAA, since it was associated with the presence in the tumor, and in pleural effusions, of immunoglobulin which reacted positively in indirect immunofluorescence tests with tissue cultures and also fresh suspensions of lung carcinoma cells, but not with cells of most non-pulmonary tumors in tissue culture, or with cell suspensions prepared from normal adult or fetal lung; it could not be interpreted as a reaction to necrotic or infected tissue, which evoked a polymorphonuclear, not a mononuclear, cell reaction. In breast cancer, however, Roberts (1974) found no correlation between the degree of lymphocytic infiltration and the capacity of an antigenic extract of the patient's tumor to evoke a delayed-type hypersensitivity reaction when injected intradermally.

It was claimed by Black and colleagues (Black, Kerpe, and Speer, 1953; Black and Speer, 1958) that the condition of *sinus histiocytosis,* characterized by distension of the sinusoids by large cells of the mononuclear phagocytic system, which is found quite often in the regional lymph nodes in relation to breast cancer, is associated with a relatively good prognosis. This claim has been the subject of much controversy, though the weight of evidence appears to be in Black's favor (for review see Anastassiades and Pryce, 1966; Berg *et al.,* 1973; Nathanson, 1977). Anastassiades and Pryce (1966) pointed out that different lymph nodes from the same patient often show different degrees of sinus histiocytosis but concluded from a study of 116 patients that marked sinus histiocytosis, especially when associated with mononuclear infiltration of the primary tumor, was associated with a reduced incidence of lymph node metastases. Hamlin (1968) devised an elaborate host defense factor (HDF) index based on the degree of mononuclear infiltration of the primary tumor, and of sinus histiocytosis and accumulation of pyroninophilic cells referred to as immunoblasts in the lymph nodes, and concluded from a study of 272 cases that a high value of the HDF was associated with a reduced incidence of nodal metastases. Tsakraklides *et al.* (1974, 1975) found that axillary lymph nodes with a high lymphocyte content and high ratio of T cells to B cells were associated with a relatively good prognosis, and lymphocyte-depleted nodes with a low ratio of T cells to B cells with a poor prognosis.

Sinus histiocytosis occurs also in nodes related to carcinomas of other organs (Black, Opler, and Speer, 1954, 1956) but has not been studied to the same extent.

In mice, increased trapping of intravenously injected ^{51}Cr-labeled normal isogeneic lymph node cells has been observed in the draining lymph nodes and the spleen following subcutaneous–intramuscular injection of MSV (Zatz, White, and Goldstein, 1973). It is of interest in relation to the observations of Tsakraklides *et al.* in patients that trapping was maximal at the time when the mouse sarcomas underwent spontaneous regression.

5.222 TUMOR-BOUND IMMUNOGLOBULIN

It has been shown by elution at low pH, binding of labeled anti-immunoglobulin, and detection of complement components that immunoglobulin (Ig) is present in many tumors, including Burkitt's lymphomas (E. Klein *et al.,* 1968; G. Klein, 1971; Nishioka *et al.,* 1968), sarcomas (Eilber and Morton, 1971), melanomas (Morton, Eilber, and Malmgren, 1971), carcinomas of the lung (Ioachim, Dorsett, and Paluch, 1976) and breast (Roberts *et al.,* 1973, 1975), and other human tumors (Anthony and Parsons, 1965) as well as autochthonous (Ran and Witz, 1970) and transplanted animal tumors. This may be bound in various ways to both neoplastic and non-neoplastic cells, but some at least is bound to antigenic determinants on tumor cells and eluted material has been shown to possess antibody activity in *in vitro* tests with cells of the same or similar tumors (see Witz, 1973, 1977 for review). With lymphomas, and possibly some other tumors, some Ig may persist on cells maintained in tissue culture, which would seem to indicate that it is produced by the tumor cells, but for the most part it disappears from cultured cells suggesting that *in vivo* it had been absorbed on the cell surface (E. Klein *et al.,* 1968; G. Klein, 1971; Witz, 1973, 1977). This adsorbed Ig may have been produced centrally, or at least in part, as Ioachim *et al.* (1976) and Roberts *et al.* (1973) have suggested, by plasma cells in the tumor stroma.

The possible effect of this Ig in protecting tumor cells from cell-mediated cytotoxicity will be discussed later (5.521); here the existence of Ig on tumor cells is presented simply as evidence of an immunological response to tumor antigens.

5.223 XENOGENEIC IMMUNIZATION

It was claimed by Björkland and his colleagues (Björkland and Björkland, 1957; Björkland, Graham, and Graham, 1957; Björkland, Lundblad, and Björkland, 1958; Björkland, 1961; Björkland, Björkland, and Hedlof, 1961), on the basis of studies of the cytotoxic effect of sera raised by immunizing horses with pooled human tumor tissue or cultured human tumor cells and cell lines that many human tumors share common TAA.

While there is no doubt that sera raised in these experiments were cytotoxic for a wide range of tumor cells, Björkland's work has been strongly criticized (see Grace and Lehoczky, 1959) on the ground that the evidence is not sufficient to establish the existence of antigens common to tumors but absent from normal adult cells. Zilber (Zilber, 1962; Zilber and Ludogovskaya, 1967), however, using adsorbed sera raised in rabbits, obtained evidence which pointed strongly to the existence of TAA in carcinomas of the stomach, and, as will be discussed in detail later (5.23), it has now been conclusively shown that there are a number of antigens, including α-fetoprotein (AFP) and *carcinoembryonic antigen* (CEA), which are present in some tumors, and in embryonic tissues, but not, or only in very small amounts, in normal adult tissues.

Xenogeneic sera have also provided evidence of TAA distinct from CEA in human acute leukemia (Mann *et al.,* 1971; Halterman, Leventhal, and Mann, 1972; Mann, Halterman, and Leventhal, 1973), Hodgkin's disease (Order, Chism, and Hellman, 1972; Order and Hellman, 1973), and squamous cell carcinoma of the lung (Veltri *et al.,* 1977). Mann *et al.* (1973) reported cross-reactivity between antigens in human cells injected with Rauscher leukemia virus and human acute leukemia cells, but it is difficult to assess the significance of this observation. Chechik (Chechik, 1968; Chechik and Gelfand, 1976), using Ig from the serum of rabbits immunized with human thymus and absorbed with immunoabsorbents prepared from human plasma and liver, claimed to have identified an antigen called H Thy-L which is common to leukemic cells and normal thymus.

Another approach has been based on the phenomenon of anaphylaxis *in vitro* known as the Schultz-Dale reaction. In the technique developed by Makari (1955, 1958, 1962) and Burrows (1962), which was intended as a diagnostic screening test for cancer, guinea pigs were sensitized to pooled antigenic human tumor extract. A strip of excised uterine smooth muscle was set up in a water bath, exposed to normal human plasma to desensitize it to normal antigenic plasma components, and then tested for sensitivity to plasma from patients with manifest or suspected tumors. It was claimed in the papers cited that the test was of diagnostic value, but this was denied by McEwen (1959).

A procedure which appears more promising so far as the demonstration of the existence of human TAA is concerned was used by Grace and Lehoczy (1959). They sensitized individual guinea pigs to extracts of one particular tumor, desensitized the excised uterine muscle *in vitro* with an extract of normal tissue from the patient from whom the tumor was obtained, and then tested the muscle for sensitivity to the original tumor extract. In a clear and admirably cautious paper they reported strongly positive results with 13 of 21 tumors tested, most of them being carcinomas of the gastrointestinal tract. It seems likely in retrospect that the test was detecting CEA.

5.224   *IN VITRO* TESTS FOR HUMORAL IMMUNITY

In vitro tests for humoral immunity in tumor-bearing animals or patients have included complement fixation, various tests based on the precipitin reaction, lysis of tumor cells in the presence of complement (Slettermark and Klein, 1962; Bubenik and Koldovsky, 1962; E. Klein and G. Klein, 1964; Old and Boyse, 1964), immunofluorescence on fixed cells (*vide infra*), membrane immunofluorescence (E. Klein and G. Klein, 1964; Pasternak, 1965; Aoki, Boyse, and Old, 1966), the indirect radioactively labeled antibody technique (Harder and McKhann, 1968; McKhann and Harder, 1968), immune adherence (Tachibana and Klein, 1970), the mixed antiglobulin reaction (Gillespie, 1968) and the related mixed hemadsorption test (Tachibana, Worst, and Klein, 1970) and inhibition of tumor cell mobility (Cochran *et al.,* 1972b). The standard complement (C) fixation test and immunofluorescence with fixed cells detect antigens within as well as on the surface of the cell; the modified C1a test (Borsos and Rapp, 1965; Borsos *et al.,* 1968) and membrane immunofluorescence, however, detect only cell surface antigens.

Reactivity of cancer patients' sera with intracellular antigen of their own or similar tumors, or cell lines derived therefrom, has been demonstrated by complement fixation (Graham and Graham, 1955; Armstrong, Henle, and Henle, 1966; Dore *et al.,* 1967; Gerber and Birch, 1967; Eilber and Morton, 1970b, 1970c), precipitin reaction with antigenic tumor extracts (Nairn *et al.,* 1963; Old *et al.,* 1966; Roberts, 1974), and immunofluorescence on fixed cells (Henle and Henle, 1966; Morton, Malmgren *et al.,* 1968; Morton and Malmgren, 1968; Morton, Malmgren *et al.,* 1969c; Muna *et al.,* 1969; E. Klein, 1970; Nairn *et al.,* 1971a, 1971b, 1972; Nelson, 1971, 1974) in respect of Burkitt's lymphoma, leukemias, sarcomas, melanoma, and carinomas of the kidney, colon, skin, nasopharynx, and cervix. There was, as a rule, evidence of widespread cross-reactivity between tumors of the same histological type, though there was also a suggestion of individual specific antigens in some carcinomas of the colon (Nairn *et al.,* 1971b).

Sera from many patients with Burkitt's lymphoma were found to react with Burkitt cell lines carrying detectable EB virus to an extent proportional to the number of virus-carrying cells, but not with lines free of detectable virus; moreover, immunofluorescence and virus particles have been demonstrated in the same cell (Zur Hausen *et al.,* 1967). It seems likely therefore, as E. Klein (1970) has argued, that the antigen detected on Burkitt lymphoma cells by this form of immunofluorescence is EB virus antigen.

Morton, Malmgren *et al.* (1968) reported that the sera of 20 percent of normal individuals gave positive immunofluorescence with melanoma cells; with osteosarcoma a positive reaction was obtained with 100 percent of sera from members of the patient's family, 85 percent of sera from associates of the patient outside his family, and 25 percent of sera from blood bank donors. They have claimed that this suggests a viral etiology for both these tumors.

Reactivity of patients' sera with tumor cell surface antigens has been demonstrated by membrane immunofluorescence of viable cells with Burkitt's lymphoma (G. Klein, Clifford *et al.,* 1966a, 1967; Osunkoya, 1967; Henle, Henle, and Diehl, 1968; G. Pearson *et al.,* 1969), leukemias (Dore *et al.,* 1967), melanoma (Morton, Malmgren *et al.,* 1968; Lewis *et al.,* 1969; Lewis and Phillips, 1972; Nairn *et al.,* 1972), and carcinomas of the colon (Nairn *et al.,* 1971b) and skin (Nairn *et al.,* 1971a), and by complement-dependent cytotoxicity with Burkitt's lymphoma (Herberman and Fahey, 1968), leukemias (Dore *et al.,* 1967), melanoma (Lewis *et al.,* 1969; Nairn *et al.,* 1972), sarcomas (Wood and Morton, 1970, 1971), and carcinomas of the colon (Nairn *et al.,* 1971b), skin (Nairn *et al.,* 1971a), and cervix (Byfield *et al.,* 1973). Two other tests have been used to demonstrate reactivity of patient's sera against cell surface antigens of leukemias and lymphomas, namely, immune adherence (Dore *et al.,* 1967; Nishioka *et al.,* 1968) and inhibition of tumor cell motility (Cochran *et al.,* 1972b, 1973a; Currie and Sime, 1973; Katz, Currie, and Oliver, 1977). Neutralization of MMTV (2.141, 5.212) by sera of women with breast cancer has been reported by Charney and Moore (1971).

In Burkitt's lymphoma cell surface antigens can be demonstrated by membrane immunofluorescence even on virus-negative cells (G. Klein *et al.,* 1968b; G. Pearson *et al.,* 1969); it appears therefore that membrane immunofluorescence is detecting antibody to cell surface antigens which are distinct from EB viral antigens, and this is confirmed by the observation that absorption with intact Burkitt lymphoma cells abolishes membrane immunofluorescence without significantly reducing the titer of antibody to EB virus. There is wide cross-reactivity of cell surface antigens from Burkitt lymphomas of different patients. It is of interest in relation to the role of EB virus in Burkitt's lymphoma and infectious mononucleosis that in the latter condition membrane-reactive antibody which reacts with Burkitt cell lines which are virus negative, and with cell lines from established cases of infectious mononucleosis, develops *pari passu* with antiviral activity of the patient's serum (Henle, Henle, and Diehl, 1968; G. Klein *et al.,* 1968a). In Burkitt's lymphoma correlation has been observed between the strength of the antibody which reacts with cell surface antigen and the durability of the response to chemotherapy (G. Klein, Clifford *et. al.,* 1966a).

There have been several reports of antibody cytotoxic for leukemic cells in the sera of relatives of the patient and unrelated normal people (Bias *et al.,* 1972; Santos *et al.,* 1973; Dore *et al.,* 1976), including in one case a multiparous pregnant woman (Cullen and Mason, 1974). This is clearly consistent with, though by no means proof of, the hypothesis that human leukemia is of viral origin and that some normal individuals become infected without developing leukemia.

In serial studies on patients with melanoma, Lewis, McCloy, and Blake (1973) found that the level of circulating antibody was not reduced by metastasis of the tumor to the regional lymph nodes but fell sharply when more distant metastasis occurred. They concluded therefore that circulating antibody in this disease "is important in protecting the bloodstream from blood-borne metastatic tumor."

5.225 *IN VITRO* TESTS FOR ANTIBODY-DEPENDENT CELL-MEDIATED CYTOTOXICITY

It has been shown that a variety of target cells may be lysed by cells from nonimmunized donors in the presence of specific antiserum or IgG antibody raised in xenogeneic and allogeneic animals, without the need for complement (Perlmann and Holm, 1969; Perlmann and Perlmann, 1970; MacLennan, Loewi, and Howard, 1969;

MacLennan, Loewi, and Harding, 1970; MacLennan and Harding, 1970; Fakhri and Hobbs, 1972). More recently, this phenomenon, which is termed *antibody-dependent cell-mediated cytotoxicity* (ADCC), has been demonstrated with antiserum from mice immunized with a syngeneic tumor and human effector cells (Gale and Zighelboim, 1975), and also with serum from mice bearing MSV-induced sarcomas and isogeneic effector cells (5.312), using the tumor cells as targets.

Various types of cell have been reported to function as effectors in ADCC, including lymphocytes lacking T-cell and B-cell markers, termed *null cells* or *K cells* (Harding *et al.*, 1971; Van Boxel *et al.*, 1973; Frøland and Natvig, 1973; Jondal, Wigzell, and Aiuti, 1973; De Bracco, Isturiz and Manni, 1976), monocytes (Greenberg *et al.*, 1973; Dennert and Lennox, 1973; Scornik and Cosenza, 1974; Cohen, Ehrke, and Mihich, 1975; Greenberg, Shen, and Medley, 1975), macrophages (Zighelboim, Bonavida, and Fahey, 1973; Evans, 1975, 1977; Haskill, Yamamura, and Radoff, 1975; Holden *et al.*, 1976; Russell and McIntosh, 1977), and polymorphonuclear leukocytes (Gale and Zighelboim, 1975), though in rats, according to Sanderson and Taylor (1976), macrophages do not participate in ADCC and may even play a protective role. These cells all possess Fc receptors (MacLennan, 1972; Gale and Zighelboim, 1975; Hersey, Edwards, and Edwards, 1976), and this appears to be an essential property. The early work on ADCC was concerned with IgG antibody, and this binds to receptors on null cells. More recently it has been shown (Lamon *et al.*, 1975) that IgM can participate in ADCC in association with B cells and also with T cells, and that subclasses of these two types of cell, but not null cells, possess receptors which can bind IgM–antigen complex (IgM Fc receptors). Still more recently Saal *et al.* (1977) have reported that lymphocytes with T-cell markers can cooperate with IgG antibodies in the lysis of human tumor cells *in vitro*.

5.226 *IN VITRO* TESTS FOR LYMPHOCYTE-MEDIATED CYTOTOXICITY

Three types of test have been used:

1. The *colony inhibition (CI) assay,* developed by Ingegerd Hellström (1967), in which the number of colonies which develop on tissue culture plates seeded with tumor cells as targets and lymphocytes as effector cells is compared with the number of colonies which develop on plates seeded with tumor cells only. A modification, termed the *cloning inhibition test,* in which the effector and target cells are incubated together in bulk before being seeded into microplates, has been developed by Amino and Degroot (1973) and Bataillon, Pross, and Klein (1975).
2. *Long-term (20–72 hour) cytotoxicity assays.* Several techniques have been developed, and these are discussed in detail by various contributors in a monograph edited by Herberman and Gaylord (1973). The microcytotoxicity assay of Takasugi and Klein (1970, 1971) is based on counting adherent target cells remaining in the wells of a microtest plate at the end of the period of incubation with effector lymphocytes; this is usually done visually under low magnification after staining the cells with Giemsa or some other stain, but Takasugi, Mickey, and Terasaki (1973a) have used an electronic method of counting the cells. Other techniques are based on labeling the target cells with ^{3}H-thymidine (Jagarlamoody *et al.*, 1971), ^{3}H-uridine (McKhann, Cleveland, and Burk, 1973), ^{125}I-iododeoxy-uridine

(^{125}IUDR) (Oldham *et al.,* 1973), or ^{3}H-proline (McBean *et al.,* 1973; Bataillon, Pross, and Klein, 1975). The assays are usually set up with several different effector to target cell ratios, ranging from 10 to over 1000, depending on the type of assay.

3. *Short-term (typically 4–8 hour) cytotoxicity assays* based on release of ^{51}Cr from labeled target cells. This method of labeling is unsatisfactory for long-term assays because of the relatively large amount of isotope lost from tumor cells incubated in the absence of effector cells.

Many patients with a wide range of tumors (I. Hellström and K.E. Hellström, 1971; I. Hellström *et al.,* 1971a), including neuroblastoma (I. Hellström *et al.,* 1968b, 1970), carcinomas of the ovary, thyroid, skin, and buccal cavity (I. Hellström *et al.,* 1971a; Nairn *et al.,* 1971a), colon (Nairn *et al.,* 1971b; Pihl *et al.,* 1975), breast (I. Hellström *et al.,* 1971a; Avis, Mosonov, and Haughton, 1974; Avis *et al.,* 1976), bladder (Bubenik *et al.,* 1970; O'Toole, 1973; Bean *et al.,* 1974; Bolhuis, 1977; Moore and Robinson, 1977), prostate (Avis *et al.,* 1975), and cervix (Vaseduvin, Balakrishnan, and Talwar, 1970; Disaia *et al.,* 1972), malignant tumors of the testis (I. Hellström *et al.,* 1971a), nephroblastoma (Diehl *et al.,* 1971), sarcomas (Cohen, Ketcham, and Morton, 1972, 1973), melanoma (Currie, Lejeune, and Fairlie, 1971; Nairn *et al.,* 1972), Burkitt's lymphoma (Chu *et al.,* 1967; Stjernsward *et al.,* 1968), acute leukemia (Leventhal *et al.,* 1972), and brain tumors including meningioma (Levy, Mahaley, and Day, 1972; Pees and Seidel, 1976) have been found to give positive reactions when their lymphocytes were tested in CI or long-term cytotoxicity assays with their own tumor, or with allogeneic tumors of the same type including established cell lines, and when both tests were used the results were similar.

Lymphocytes which are cytotoxic for autochthonous tumors have usually been found to be cytotoxic also for allogeneic tumors of the same type but not for tumors of a different type. While this clearly points to the existence of group-specific TAA, the existence of some antigens specific for individual tumors is not excluded, and there is evidence that these are possessed by some tumors. Some of the shared antigens may occur also in benign lesions; thus cross-reactivity has been reported between carcinoma of the breast and benign fibrocystic disease (Avis *et al.,* 1974, 1976) and between carcinoma and benign hypertrophy of the prostate (Avis *et al.,* 1975).

Lymphocytes from some close relatives of patients with acute leukemia have been reported to be cytotoxic for leukemic cells but not for normal cells (Rosenberg *et al.,* 1972; Levine, 1973; Santos *et al.,* 1973), again suggesting the possible involvement of an oncogenic virus in human leukemia. Cytotoxicity has also been observed with some tumor cell lines when the effector lymphocytes were obtained from normal donors (Takasugi, Mickey, and Terasaki, 1973b) or donors with tumors of a different kind; Skurzak *et al.* (1973), for example found that when lymphocytes from patients with gliomas were cytotoxic for allogeneic glioma cell lines they were also cytotoxic for an osteogenic sarcoma cell line. One possible explanation suggested by Skurzak *et al.* (1973) is sensitization of the lymphocytes *in vitro* during the course of the test.

In some cases a patient's lymphocytes cease to be cytotoxic when his tumor becomes widely disseminated (Byrne *et al.,* 1973); cytotoxicity may also be abolished in some cases by adding patient serum to the cultures. These effects will be discussed later (5.521). Lymphocytes from leukemic patients in remission do not easily become cytotoxic when cultured with irradiated autochthonous leukemic cells but may do so if a second target is provided in the form of irradiated allogeneic cells, apparently because the alloantigens stimulate proliferation of the responder cells whereas the TAA of the leukemic cells fail to do this (Zarling *et al.,* 1976).

Short-term cytotoxicity assays have given less consistent results, with more non-specific toxicity and often poor correlation with long-term assays (McCoy *et al.,* 1973; Peter *et al.,* 1975a, 1975b). Most of this work, however, has been done with allogeneic tumor cell lines, and such assays would seem to merit further study with autochthonous tumors.

5.227 MIGRATION AND LEUKOCYTE ADHERENCE INHIBITION ASSAYS

Migration inhibition assays are based on the discovery that sensitized T cells, on contact with the sensitizing antigen, liberate substances termed *lymphokines* which, *inter alia,* inhibit the migration of macrophages and leukocytes. Two types of assay have been developed: *direct assays* and *indirect assays.* In direct assays (Sorborg and Bendixen, 1967; Rosenberg and David, 1970) the migration of blood leukocytes is measured in the presence and absence of antigen; if sensitized T cells are present, the migration inhibition factor (MIF) they liberate inhibits the migration of other cells in the population which thus serve as indicators. In indirect assays (Thor *et al.,* 1968; Rocklin, Meyers, and David, 1970) lymphocytes are incubated with or without antigen, and the capacity of the culture supernatants to inhibit the migration of guinea pig peritoneal exudate cells is measured.

These tests, with various modifications, have been used to study cell-mediated immunity to tumor antigens in cancer patients.

Direct tests have been limited by the difficulty of achieving an effective concentration of tumor antigens while keeping the concentration of toxic substances in the tumor extracts to an acceptably low level (Rosenberg, 1973). The effect of non-specific toxicity is less apparent if neutrophils are removed from the leukocyte population (Bull *et al.,* 1973), and it should be possible to avoid it completely by using more highly purified antigens. Despite the technical difficulties, direct tests using antigenic extracts derived from autochthonous tumors and allogeneic tumors of the same type have yielded evidence of sensitization of lymphocytes to TAA in patients with carcinoma of the breast (Andersen, Bendixen, and Schrodt, 1969; Andersen *et al.,* 1970; Segall *et al.,* 1972; Cochran *et al.,* 1972c, 1973b; Black *et al.,* 1974, 1976; Jones and Turnbull, 1974) and colon (Bull *et al.,* 1973; Elias and Elias, 1975), malignant melanoma (Cochran, Jehn, and Gothoskar, 1972; Cochran *et al.,* 1973b), neuroblastoma (Graham-Pole *et al.,* 1976), and other tumors (Wolberg, 1971; Segall *et al.,* 1972).

Evidence of cross-reactivity with allogeneic tumors of the same type was found in 16 of 30 patients by Jones and Turnbull (1974). Black *et al.* (1974), however, using a modified technique in which the antigenic material took the form of a cryostat section of tumor tissue, found that leukocytes from patients with invasive breast cancer rarely showed cross-reactivity, whereas leukocytes from patients with carcinoma-in-situ often did. Segall *et al.* (1972) found cross-reactivity with five melanomas. In patients with carcinomas of the colon and rectum it was found by Bull *et al.* (1973) that the test often became negative after surgical "cure" of the tumor. Elias and Elias (1975) found no cross-reactivity with allogeneic tumors. In the case of neuroblastoma, Graham-Pole *et al.* (1976) found that leukocytes from 11 of 22 relatives, and 12 of

18 unrelated close contacts of patients, gave positive reactivity with preparations derived from one or more tumors.

Indirect assays would seem to be less liable to error and show good correlation with skin hypersensitivity tests with soluble protein antigens, but have been less widely used in studies of tumor immunity than direct tests.

Churchill and Rocklin (1973), in a small study, obtained positive results with autochthonous tumor antigens in four of seven patients but no definite evidence of sensitivity to carcinoembryonic antigen (5.232) in nine patients with carcinoma of the colon.

Field and his colleagues (Field and Caspari, 1970; Caspari and Field, 1971; Field, Caspari, and Smith, 1973) devised a modified test in which human blood lymphocytes are mixed with guinea pig macrophages, with or without the addition of antigenic material derived from human brain, sciatic nerve, or any of a variety of tumors, and the rate of migration of individual macrophages under the influence of an electric field is measured with a cytopherometer. After extensive investigation they came to the conclusion that lymphocytes from patients with a wide variety of tumors are sensitized to a basic histone-like protein which can be extracted from human brain and peripheral nervous tissue, and they suggested that this could provide a diagnostic test of malignancy. Although a considerable time has elapsed since this work was published, it does not appear to have been either independently confirmed or refuted.

Maluish and Halliday (1974) observed that blood leukocytes from patients with malignant melanoma, carcinoma of the breast, and carcinoma of the colon became less adherent to glass when incubated with extracts from a tumor of the same type, and they called this phenomenon *leukocyte adherence inhibition* (LAI). Serum from patients blocked the inhibitory effects of tumor extracts on the patient's leukocytes and on leukocytes from other patients with tumors of the same type. Grosser and Thomson (1975) reported that 40 of 47 patients with carcinoma of the breast, but only 2 of 32 patients with benign lesions of the breast, non-neoplastic disease, or malignant tumors of other kinds, showed significant LAI when incubated with antigenic extracts of breast carcinomas. LAI was less marked in patients with advanced disease and 2 weeks after treatment by surgery and/or radiotherapy. In contrast to Maluish and Halliday (1974), Grosser and Thomson (1975) were unable to demonstrate blocking of LAI by the patient's serum.

5.228 MIXED LYMPHOCYTE–TUMOR CELL CULTURES (MLTC)

Lymphocytes may be stimulated to increased DNA synthesis when mixed and cultured *in vitro* with isogeneic (Potter and Balfour, 1975) and autochthonous tumor cells. This has been shown with a wide variety of human autochthonous tumors including acute leukemias (Viza *et al.,* 1969; Fridman and Kourilsky, 1969; Bach, Bach, and Joo, 1969; Leventhal *et al.,* 1972; Gutterman *et al.,* 1973), Burkitt's lymphoma (Stjernsward *et al.,* 1968), carcinomas (Stjernsward *et al.,* 1970a; Deodhar, Crile, and Esselstyn, 1972; Mavligit *et al.,* 1973), sarcomas (Vanky, Stjernsward, and Nilsonne, 1971), and melanoma (Mavligit *et al.,* 1973) using lymphocytes from blood. In the case of solid tumors the tumor cells have been obtained from fresh biopsy specimens; with leukemias, blast cells have been obtained prior to the start of treatment or during a relapse and stored in liquid nitrogen until the patient was in remission and could provide non-neoplastic lymphocytes as the other component of the mixed culture. The tumor cells have often been treated with mitomycin C or irradiated to prevent further DNA synthesis; this does not seem to be necessary, however, since tumor cells are not as a rule stimulated by normal lymphocytes. Stimulation has also been demonstrated in lymphocyte cultures containing antigenic autochthonous tumor extracts instead of tumor cells (Savel, 1969; Jehn et al., 1970; Gutterman et al., 1973; Mavligit et al., 1973; Vanky et al., 1974).

Lymphocytes obtained from regional lymph nodes of patients with early breast cancer without evidence of lymph node metastasis were found by Deodhar, Crile, and Esselstyn (1972) to respond to a greater extent than blood lymphocytes in MLTC tests; regional lymph node cells from patients with extensive sarcomas, on the other hand, were found by Vanky, Stjernsward, and Nilsonne (1971) to be unresponsive. Lymphocytes from unrelated normal individuals have been shown to respond to tumor cells of various kinds but only rarely to antigenic extracts (Gutterman et al., 1973; Mavligit et al., 1973); lymphocytes from a healthy identical twin have also been shown to respond to lung cancer cells (Stjernsward et al., 1970c) and leukemic lymphoblasts (Han and Wang, 1972).

The addition of serum from the patient to MLT cultures may result in decreased stimulation (Vanky et al., 1973; Gutterman et al., 1973; Mavligit et al., 1973) as a consequence of non-specific or specific blocking activity (5.521). Increased stimulation may also occur (Gutterman et al., 1973; Mavligit et al., 1973); the reason for this finding is not known, but it has been reported to be associated with a good prognosis.

MLTC tests show good correlation with tests of hypersensitivity in vivo (5.229), and sometimes good inverse correlation with the extent of the tumor.

5.229   SKIN HYPERSENSITIVITY REACTIONS

Grace and Kondo (1958) tested five patients with breast cancer, one with Hodgkin's disease, and one with non-Hodgkin's lymphoma, selected because they showed evidence of an inflammatory reaction at the site of the tumor, with an intradermal injection of an extract of their own tumor. They reported that all showed positive immediate-type reactions and that sensitization could be transferred locally to other individuals by passive cutaneous anaphylaxis.

Delayed-type hypersensitivity reactions to crude cell-free autochthonous tumor extracts were demonstrated by Hughes and Lytton (1964), and similar findings were reported by Stewart (1969) and Stewart and Orizaga (1971) in about a quarter of the patients with cancer of the breast and other organs who were tested. There was no correlation with the degree of differentiation of the tumor (Hughes and Lytton, 1964) or with patient survival (Stewart and Orizaga, 1971). In discussing these reports Herberman et al. (1973a) have questioned the specificity of the response on the ground that extracts of normal tissue produced some positive reactions; the possibility of bacterial contamination of the extracts also has to be considered despite the fact that considerable care was taken to eliminate this.

Delayed-type hypersensitivity reactions have, however, been observed with autochthonous tumor extracts, in a dosage (expressed as protein content) which gave negative results with extracts of normal tissues, in patients with acute leukemia (Oren and Herberman, 1971; Char et al., 1973); Burkitt's lymphoma (Fass, Herberman, and Ziegler, 1970a; Bluming et al., 1971); carcinomas of the breast (Alford, Hollinshead, and Herberman, 1973; Roberts, 1974), colon (Hollinshead et al., 1970), lung (Wells *et al.,* 1973b), and cervix (Wells *et al.,* 1973b); melanoma (Fass *et al.,* 1970b); and sarcomas and other tumors (Vanky *et al.,* 1974). Reactions to extracts of allogeneic tumors of the same kind were also reported in some of the papers cited. In some series the extracts were sterilized by filtration; in others reliance was placed on negative bacterial cultures and negative tests for hepatitis-associated antigen. As a rule the tests showed good correlation with the clinical state of the patient; in acute leukemia, for example, hypersensitivity was usually demonstrable in patients in remission but not during relapse (Herberman *et al.,* 1973a), and in Burkitt's lymphoma 15 of 30 patients gave a positive test when in remission but only 1 of 16 when the disease was active (Bluming *et al.,* 1971); Roberts (1974), however, found no correlation in patients with breast cancer between skin hypersensitivity to tumor extracts and the degree of lymphocytic infiltration of the tumor. In patients with carcinoma of the colon Herberman *et al.* (1973a) obtained a fraction from tumor extracts which caused hypersensitivity reactions but was negative when tested by radioimmunoassay for the carcinoembryonic antigen (CEA) defined by Gold (5.232). They also obtained a fraction with similar properties from human fetal liver, and concluded that "the skin-reactive antigen in intestinal cancer appears to be a carcinoembryonic antigen different from the CEA of Gold." To reduce the risk of confusion we shall restrict the term *carcinoembryonic antigen (CEA)* to the antigen identified by Gold, and use *oncofetal antigen* in a general sense to include this and other antigens present in some tumors and embryonic tissue, but not, or only in very small amounts, in normal adult tissue.

Skin hypersensitivity tests are easy to perform but difficult to quantitate. The results depend on the antigenicity of the tumor and also the capacity of the patient to respond to tumor antigens; they are thus influenced by the general immunological responsiveness of the patient (4.42) and by specific abrogation of his response to tumor antigens (5.521).

What may be regarded as a modification of the skin sensitivity test was developed by Black and Leis (1971, 1973), who applied a cryostat section of autochthonous tumor tissue to an abraded area of skin ("skin window") in patients with breast cancer, and studied the cellular exudate which this evoked. They found that early tumors evoked a more marked response than advanced tumors.

5.23   Oncofetal Antigens (OFA)

It was reported by Schöne (1906) that mice which had been injected with fetal tissue subsequently rejected tumor transplants of a kind which were lethal in untreated mice or mice pretreated with normal adult tissue. The system was of course an allogeneic one, since inbred strains of mice did not then exist. Subsequently, many experiments have provided further evidence of the existence of what, following Alexander (1972), we shall refer to as *oncofetal antigens* (OFA),* i.e., antigens which occur in tumors and embryonic or fetal[†] tissue but not, or only in relatively small amounts, in normal adult tissues.

---

*Alexander (1972) says that "it seems necessary to coin this phrase because the more elegant description of carcinoembryonic antigen has been preempted to describe one class of these compounds."

[†]In gynecology the product of the human fertilized ovum is referred to up to a certain stage as an *embryo* and thereafter as a *fetus;* in dealing with a multiplicity of species, however, no common time can be assigned by which to separate these categories, and the terms embryo (or embryonic) and fetus (or fetal) are often used interchangeably. We shall follow this latter practice.

OFA may be subdivided operationally according to whether evidence of their existence has been obtained by immunizing xenogeneic, allogeneic, or isogeneic animals, or by demonstrating an immune response in the autochthonous host. There seems no reason why antigens demonstrated in isogeneic or autochthonous hosts should not be demonstrable in other categories of host, but the converse is not necessarily true.

OFA associated with tumors in mice and rats have been demonstrated by allogeneic immunization (see Coggin and Anderson, 1974). Various OFA associated with human tumors have been demonstrated by xenogeneic immunization, the best characterized being α-fetoprotein and carcinoembryonic antigen.

5.231 α-FETOPROTEIN (AFP)

It was shown by Abelev (Abelev, 1963; Abelev *et al.*, 1963), using immunodiffusion and immunoelectrophoresis against an antiserum raised in rabbits, that a chemically induced mouse hepatoma synthesized a protein which was antigenically indistinguishable from an α-globulin which was present in the serum of fetal and newborn mice but absent from the serum of adult mice. Soon afterwards Tatarinov (1964, 1966) found a similar protein in the sera of patients with primary hepatomas. This substance is termed α-fetoprotein (AFP), and sensitive methods have been developed for the quantitative estimation of AFP in serum by radioimmunoassay (Thomson *et al.*, 1969; Ruoslahti and Seppälä, 1971; Sell, 1973), and for its detection in tumor tissue by immunofluorescence (Nishioka *et al.*, 1972).

AFP levels ranging from less than $1\mu g/ml$ (i.e., below the limit detectable by gel diffusion, which is in the region of $1-3\mu g/ml$) to as much as 7 mg/ml have been reported in the serum of patients with primary malignant hepatoma (Purves, Bersohn, and Geddes, 1970; Abelev, 1971; Alpert *et al.*, 1971a). Levels tend to be higher in non-Caucasians, younger patients, and patients with advanced disease, but in individual patients seem to vary independently of other features of the disease and are of little prognostic significance. Raised AFP levels, sufficient to be detectable by gel diffusion, are also found in children, and to a lesser extent in adults, with testicular (Kohn *et al.*, 1976) and ovarian malignant teratomas, in patients with hepatic metastases from carcinoma of the stomach (Alpert, Pinn, and Isselbacher, 1971), and occasionally in patients with other tumors. Very low levels (2–16 ng/ml) have been detected by radioimmunoassay in the sera of normal individuals.

5.232 CARCINOEMBRYONIC ANTIGEN (CEA)

Gold and Freedman (1965) showed by immunodiffusion that rabbits immunized with human colonic cancer developed antibodies which reacted with extracts of fetal but not adult normal colonic mucosa, and concluded that there is an antigen, which they termed carcinoembryonic antigen (CEA), which is present in carcinomas of the colon and fetal colonic mucosa but not in normal adult tissue. By using an extraction procedure followed by radioimmunoassay, Thomson *et al.* (1969) detected low levels of CEA in normal human plasma, and elevated levels in 97 percent of patients with carcinomas of the colon and rectum and in some patients with carcinoma of the pancreas.

Subsequent investigations, using more sensitive assays which obviate the necessity for preliminary extraction procedures, have confirmed the presence of small amounts of CEA in normal serum (Kleenman and Turner, 1972; Chu, Reynoso, and Hansen, 1972) and have established that elevated serum levels of CEA may be found in patients with a variety of carcinomas, including not only carcinomas of the gastrointestinal tract but also carcinomas of the breast and, contrary to earlier reports, of the lung (T.L. Moore *et al.*, 1971; Lo Gerfo, Hansen, and Krupey, 1971; Lo Gerfo *et al.*, 1972; Reynoso *et al.*, 1972a, 1972b; Steward *et al.*, 1974; Tormey *et al.*, 1975). Levels may also be raised in patients with various non-neoplastic disorders such as cirrhosis of the liver, ulcerative colitis, pancreatitis, Crohn's disease, chronic lung disease, and myocardial infarction, and in heavy smokers (T.L. Moore *et al.*, 1971; Meriadec *et al.*, 1976; Williams *et al.*, 1977). On the other hand, in patients with small and non-disseminated tumors, levels of CEA may be within normal limits (Dhar *et al.*, 1972; Zamchek *et al.*, 1972).

CEA assays have not proved to be of much value for the diagnosis of primary cancer of the colon and rectum, but monitoring of CEA levels in serum may provide early evidence of recurrence after operation, and may also be a useful guide for controlling palliative treatment (Booth *et al.*, 1974; Herrera *et al.*, 1976, 1977).

5.233 OTHER HUMAN OFA DETECTED WITH XENOGENEIC OR ALLOGENEIC SERA

Various other OFA have been demonstrated in human tumors with xenogeneic or allogeneic immune sera. These include *fetosulfoglycoprotein,* found in the gastric juice of most patients with carcinoma of the stomach and in fetal gut, and occasionally in the gastric juice and gastric mucosa of adults in the absence of carcinoma (Hakkinen, 1966, 1972); γ-fetoprotein (γ-FP), which is found in a wide variety of benign and malignant tumors and various fetal tissues (Edynak *et al.*, 1972); unnamed antigens associated with leukemia (Viza, 1971), Hodgkin's disease (Katz *et al.*, 1973), malignant melanoma, Wilms' tumor, and nephroblastoma (Avis and Lewis, 1973); β-oncofetal antigen (BOFA), detected by rabbit antisera raised with human colon cancer extracts but present in carcinomas of various kinds (Fritsche and Mach, 1975); and colon-specific antigen protein (CSAp), which appears to be restricted to tumors of the gastrointestinal tract (Goldenberg *et al.*, 1976).

Antibody to γ-fetoprotein is found in some tumor-bearing patients; it was this property which led to its discovery, and human serum containing the antibody is used to assay γFP. The other antigens mentioned are assayed with immune rabbit sera.

5.234 OFA IMMUNOGENIC IN ISOGENEIC AND AUTOCHTHONOUS HOSTS

The evidence to be considered will be presented under the following headings:

1. Immunization with fetal tissue *in vivo.*
2. Immunization with tumor tissue *in vivo.*
3. Cytotoxicity of lymphoid cells from pregnant animals for tumor cells.
4. Immunization with fetal tissue *in vitro.*
5. Neutralization of isogeneic anti-embryo serum.
6. Skin hypersensitivity tests.

Immunization with fetal tissue in vivo. It was reported by Prehn (1967) that injection of fetal tissue protected mice to a slight or moderate extent against transplantation of an isogeneic methylcholanthrene-induced sarcoma. Coggin *et al.* (1971) found that the development of tumors in hamsters infected neonatally with SV40 or adenovirus was prevented in a proportion of animals injected intraperitoneally or subcutaneously at the age of 3–5 weeks with irradiated mid-gestational isogeneic fetal cells from primiparous females. Non-irradiated cells were ineffective when given intraperitoneally, though sometimes effective when given subcutaneously. Subsequent work (Herberman, Ting, and Lavrin, 1971; Hanna et al., 1972; Baldwin, Glaves, and Vose, 1972b, 1974; Baldwin and Vose, 1974; Bendich, Borenfreund, and Stonehill, 1973; Girardi et al., 1973; Grant, Lodisch, and Wells, 1974; Le Mevel and Wells, 1973; Menard, Colnaghi, and Della Porta, 1973, 1974; Menard and Colnaghi, 1975; Shah, Rees, and Baldwin, 1976), despite some negative reports (Ting, 1968; Baldwin, Glaves, and Pimm, 1971), has confirmed and extended these results and has shown that injection of isogeneic fetal tissue results in demonstrable immunity to a wide range of tumors of mice, rats, hamsters, and guinea pigs, including tumors induced by chemical carcinogens, and DNA and RNA oncogenic viruses, and tumors of spontaneous origin. In general, however, the strongest evidence of immunity has come from in vitro tests; protection against isogeneic tumor transplants has been feeble or not demonstrable at all (Ting, Rodrigues, and Herberman, 1973; Baldwin, Glaves, and Vose, 1974), and enhanced tumor growth may also occur (Castro et al., 1973; Chism et al., 1976).

It has been stressed by Coggin and Anderson (1974) that the fetal tissue should be obtained from primiparous animals and that the day of gestation may be critical; they and others (Herberman et al., 1971; Castro et al., 1974) have stated that it is essential to irradiate the fetal tissue, and have suggested that this is beneficial because it prevents further differentiation. It is of interest in this regard that it has subsequently been shown that immunization with the cells of an embryonal carcinoma cell line which do not differentiate in vivo or in vitro protects against challenge with a variety of methylcholanthrene-induced tumors of various degrees of immunogenicity (Sikora, Stern, and Lennox, 1977).

The OFA we have been discussing differ both from the individual-specific antigens which characterize chemically induced tumors (Baldwin, Glaves, and Vose, 1972b; Menard, Colnaghi, and Della Porta, 1973; Thomson and Alexander, 1973), and from the group-specific antigens of viral tumors (Ting et al., 1972; Kurth and Bauer, 1973). There may be cross-reactivity between OFA of different species (Ting et al., 1972; Salinas and Hanna, 1974).

Immunization with tumor tissue in vivo. Salinas and co-workers (Salinas, Smith, and Hanna, 1972; Salinas and Hanna, 1974) hyperimmunized mice with irradiated (5000 R) plasma cytoma cells and found that these mice developed fewer colonies in the spleen than controls when they were irradiated (750 R) and injected intravenously with isogeneic fetal cells. Confirmatory findings were reported by Chism et al. (1976b), but the effect was weak.

Cytotoxicity of lymphocytes from pregnant animals for tumor cells. Brawn (1970) reported that lymph node cells of inbred normal pregnant mice were cytotoxic for the cells of several distinct methylcholanthrene-induced sarcomas though not for normal fibroblasts. Subsequently, Girardi et al. (1973) showed that lymph node cells of pregnant mice were cytotoxic in vitro for tumors induced with SV40, polyoma virus, and adenovirus, and could also protect normal hamsters against transplants of SV40-induced syngeneic tumors. Cells from primiparous donors were much more effective than cells from multi parous donors. Serum from pregnant hamsters blocked the cytotoxic effect of lymph node cells from hamsters immunized with SV40-induced tumors on the cells of such tumors (Coggin and Anderson, 1972), and sera from multiparas had a greater blocking effect than sera from primiparas, suggesting that blocking antibody plays an important role in protecting the progeny of multiparous females from the consequences of maternal immunization resulting from previous pregnancies. Baldwin *et al.* (1972a), however, found that cell-mediated cytotoxicity to rat sarcomas was not blocked by pregnant rat serum.

Further evidence of the cytotoxicity of lymph node and spleen cells from pregnant mice on a variety of syngeneic tumor cells *in vitro* was reported by I. Hellström and K. F. Hellström (1975). The cytotoxic effect was decreased by treating the lymphoid cells with anti-Thy 1 serum and complement. Serum from pregnant mice reduced the cytotoxic effect of lymph node cells from pregnant mice but sometimes caused normal lymph node cells to show cytotoxic activity.

Immunization with fetal tissue in vitro. Evidence of the presence of OFA on a wide variety of murine tumor cells was obtained in a completely *in vitro* system by Chism, Burton, and Warner (1975, 1976). They cultured non-immune splenic lymphocytes with irradiated fetal liver cells and, at various times after setting up the cultures, tested for the presence of lymphocytes cytotoxic for tumor cells in a ^{51}Cr-release assay. Significant cytotoxic activity was regularly found, whereas only slight cytotoxic activity was generated in control cultures containing splenic lymphocytes and irradiated adult isogeneic spleen cells. Inhibition tests in which non-labeled cells of various kinds were added to the cultures showed that the reaction was inhibited by fetal and tumor cells, though not to the same extent by cells from different tumors; adult spleen cells, on the other hand, did not cause any inhibition. In the light of these findings Chism *et al.* suggested that the *in vitro* system permitted a more active response to OFA than that observed *in vivo*.

In further studies Chism *et al.* (1976b) compared the immunizing effect *in vitro* of irradiated and non-irradiated fetal liver cells. The irradiated cells were significantly more effective, and this was most clearly demonstrated at low effector to target cell ratios. On the other hand, Chism *et al.* found no consistent evidence that irradiated cells were more effective *in vivo*.

Neutralization of isogeneic anti-embryo serum. It was shown by Rees *et al.* (1975) that the serum of multiparous rats, which reacted with surface antigen on rat hepatoma cells as shown by indirect immunofluorescence, could be neutralized by the serum of hepatoma-bearing rats, due to the presence of the tumor-bearers' serum of hepatoma-associated OFA.

Skin hypersensitivity tests. As stated earlier (5.229), Herberman *et al.* (1973a) demonstrated skin hypersensitivity reactions in patients with colonic cancer following intradermal injection of extracts of fetal intestine and liver. Similar reactions were produced by intradermal injection of extracts of pooled allogeneic carcinoma tissue, and of a fraction of such extracts which was devoid of CEA, but not by injection of CEA. The reactions appear to be due therefore to OFA distinct from CEA.

General comment. The biological significance of OFA which are immunogenic in isogeneic and autochthonous hosts is not clear. The discovery by Menard and Colnaghi (1975) of a correlation between the growth capacity of tumors, assessed by the TD50 and the growth rate after inoculation of a standard dose of viable cells, and their level of expression of OFA, assayed by *in vitro* cell-mediated cytotoxicity tests and quantitative absorption of anti-embryo serum by the tumor cells, raises the question of whether immunostimulation (5.522) directed towards these antigens has a growth-promoting effect in fetal development (see also Hamilton, 1976) and in relation to tumors. The further discovery by these authors of the presence of cross-reacting antigens in adult testis has led them to postulate that OFA are related to a cell membrane function controlling mitosis rather than to a function specifically related to fetal or neoplastic status *per se.*

The reduced incidence of myeloblastic leukemia in women with three or more children, which Dausset *et al.* (1970) suggested might be due to immunization with HLA antigen, might alternatively be due to immunization against OFA, and this hypothesis would seem to merit further investigation.

Although OFA are relatively ineffective as TATA, and presumably therefore as TSARIPAH, they might nevertheless provide a point of attack for immunotherapy; this will be discussed in Chapters 7 and 8.

5.24   Antigens of Recurrent and Metastatic Tumors

It is sometimes assumed that locally recurrent and metastatic tumors will be antigenically identical with the original primary tumor, and those who hold this view are apt, when pressed, to defend it as a consequence of the proposition that tumors are monoclonal (3.114). As we have seen, however, the evidence underlying the conclusion that many tumors are monoclonal does no more than establish that they are *predominantly* monoclonal, i.e., it does not exclude the possible existence of small minority populations which under certain conditions might become predominant. Moreover, even if a particular tumor is strictly monoclonal, the possible emergence of mutant populations is clearly not excluded. Such minority populations may well be important sources of recurrent and metastatic tumors, since it seems likely that for a cell to survive and multiply as a local recurrence, or after being transported to a new site via the bloodstream or lymphatic channels, it will require special properties which are not necessarily of advantage to a cell growing as part of an established primary tumor. It would not be surprising if differences of this kind were sometimes accompanied by differences in cell surface antigens.

Evidence that this does occur has been reported by Pimm and Baldwin (1977a), who demonstrated by syngeneic transplantation that, with four methylcholanthrene-induced rat tumors, cell lines established from the primary tumor and from a local recurrence after incomplete surgical excision of the primary differed antigenically. Lines from two of the four primary sarcomas showed little or no immunogenicity, as assessed by rechallenge after injection of irradiated tumor cells or excision of a previous transplant, whereas cell lines from all four recurrent tumors were immunogenic. Moreover, immunization with the recurrent tumor line gave no protection against challenge with the primary tumor line, and *vice versa.*

It is clearly important to undertake similar investigations comparing recurrent, and also metastatic, tumors with primary tumors, not only by transplantation but also by *in vitro* tests which could be applied to human tumors.

5.25 Further Characterization of TAA

Many studies with both animal (Matsumoto, 1965; Oettgen *et al.,* 1968; McCollester, 1970; Baldwin and Moore, 1969; Baldwin and Embleton, 1970; Baldwin and Glaves, 1972; Baldwin, Harris, and Price, 1973; Davies *et al.,* 1974a; Pellis, Tom, and Kahan, 1974; Price and Baldwin, 1974, 1977; Laing et al., 1978) and human (Viza, Davies, and Harris, 1970; Viza *et al.,* 1970b; Gutterman *et al.,* 1972; Gentile and Flickinger, 1972; Hollinshead *et al.,* 1974; Watson, Smith, and Levy, 1974, 1975; Frost, Rogers, and Bagshawe, 1975) tumors have demonstrated TAA in membrane fractions of tumor cells, and in soluble form in preparations derived from whole cells or membrane fractions by extraction with hypertonic salt solutions or perchloric acid, pepsin hydrolysis, or sonication. Different antigenic components have been separated from such extracts by column chromatography and other procedures (Chang, Law, and Appella, 1975; Clemtson, Bertschmann, and Widner, 1976). TAA have also been isolated from the serum of tumor-bearing hosts by affinity chromatography with Sepharose-coupled antibody (Thomson *et al.,* 1973b) and by dissociation of antigen–antibody complexes at low pH (Bowen and Baldwin, 1976; Rao and Bonavida, 1977).

In general antigenic extracts have been found to be less active than intact tumor cells in protecting against subsequent tumor challenge, and more productive of humoral than of cell-mediated immune responses; as we shall see later, they have nevertheless been used in immunotherapeutic experiments (7.61) and also, on a small scale, in clinical trials (8.254).

Other methods of investigation which will not be reviewed in detail include the quantitative study of antibody binding to cell-surface TAA (Boone *et al.,* 1972) and the location of surface antigens in electron micrographs with hybrid antibody using ferritin or some other marker (Aoki *et al.,* 1970; Aoki and Takahashi, 1972). This last technique has been of particular importance in distinguishing the different categories of TAA possessed by viral tumors (5.212).

It has been suggested that some TAA, and in particular TAA of chemically induced tumors, are derepressed or mutationally modified histocompatibility antigens (Boyse, 1970; W.J. Martin *et al.,* 1973; R.T. Smith, 1975; Bowen and Baldwin, 1975) or determined by genes linked to those of the major histocompatibility system (Oth, Berebbi, and Meyer, 1975). This gains support from three sources—firstly, reports of an inverse relationship between the extent to which different methylcholanthrene-induced mouse sarcomas express TAA and H-2 antigens (Haywood and McKhann, 1971; E. Tsakraklides *et al.,* 1974); secondly, the discovery that H-2 isoantigenic loss variants obtained by passaging a sarcoma, induced in an F1 hybrid mouse with methylcholanthrene, in each of the parent strains possessed different antigenic specificities as shown by transplantation experiments (Oth and Barra, 1974); and thirdly, evidence of the existence on the cells of methylcholanthrene-induced sarcomas of H-2 specificities not represented on the normal cells of the strain of the tumor-bearing animal (Invernizzi and Parmiani, 1975; Parmiani and Invernizzi, 1975). On the other hand, as Davies (1975) has pointed out, TAA and histocompatibility antigens may be physically separable (Davies *et al.,* 1974a), and do not co-cap (Yefenof and Klein, 1974); moreover, studies with what G. Klein and E. Klein (1975) modestly refer to as a cytogenetically favorable somatic cell hybrid have established that the genetic determinants of the TATA of one particular methylcholanthrene-induced mouse sarcoma are not located on chromosome 17, which carries the mouse H-2 determinants.

The essential features of the system studied by Klein and Klein may be summarized as follows: The hybrid cells were derived from the fusion of an A strain (H-2a) ascites carcinoma (TA3Ha) and an A.SW strain (H-2s) methylcholanthrene-induced ascites sarcoma referred to as MSWBS. Tumor TA3Ha contributes two normal telocentric No. 17 chromosomes to the hybrid, whereas both No. 17 chromosomes of MSWBS are localized on readily identifiable translocations, and the No. 17 chromosomes of either parent strain, but not both, can be removed from the hybrid by selective passage in the opposite parental strain. It was found that unselected hybrids were as immunogenic in A.SW mice as MSWBS itself, as judged by their capacity to induce resistance to subsequent challenge with MSWBS. On the other hand, two strain A compatible, and two strain A.SW compatible, variants which had lost No. 17 chromosomes of the opposite strain showed a residual but weakened immunogenicity. Since there was no systematic difference between the reciprocal types, it was concluded that the genetic determinants of the TATA of tumor MSWBS are not located on chromosome 17, but that "a proper balance of this chromosome is required for the full expression of immunogenicity in the TATA system."

The expression of some TATA may be increased by treating the cells with neuraminidase. This phenomenon, and possible underlying mechanisms, will be discussed later in relation to immunotherapy (7.62).

5.26 Release of Antigen by Tumor Cells

Antigen may be released from cells when they are lysed. Surface antigen may also be released from viable cells, particularly in the presence of specific antibody, and it appears that this may occur either passively, when it is termed *shedding* or as the result of an active metabolic process involving protein synthesis, termed *antigenic modulation.*

In vitro antigen shedding is typically preceded by capping, i.e., a surface shift of antigen so that it accumulates in one particular region. Capping has been shown to occur also *in vivo* after intraperitoneal injection of specific antibody to mice bearing an ascites tumor (G. Klein, 1975a).

The term *antigenic modulation* was introduced by Boyse and his colleagues (Boyse, Old, and Stockert, 1965; Boyse, Stockert, and Old, 1967; Old, Stockert, Boyse, and Kimm, 1968) to describe a phenomenon which they discovered when mice were immunized against the TL antigen (5.22) and then challenged with a TL-positive leukemia. Contrary to expectation the leukemic cells were not rejected despite the presence of anti-TL antibody, and on investigation it was found that the leukemic cells had lost their TL antigenicity. It was shown that this change is not due to masking of antigen by blocking antibody or selection of TL negative cells but to loss of TL antigen from the cell surface. Since the phenomenon occurred *in vitro* at 37°C but not at 0°C, and was prevented by prior treatment of the cells with actinomycin D or iodoacetamide, it was concluded that an active metabolic process was involved. This is associated with synthesis of protein but not of RNA and DNA.

The demonstration of tumor antigens in various body fluids of tumor-bearing animals (Currie and Gage, 1973; Thomson *et al.,* 1973b; Baldwin, Bowen, and Price, 1973; Bystryn, 1976) and patients (Jehn *et al.,* 1970; Currie and Basham, 1972; Carrel and Theilkaes, 1973), and in the medium of tumor cells in culture (Bystryn *et al.,* 1974; Ben-Sasson, Weiss, and Doljanski, 1974), shows that TAA are commonly lost from tumor cells. It seems likely, as G. Klein (1975a) has postulated, that a state of equilibrium exists between antibody coating of tumor cells and loss of surface antigen, but the relative contribution of shedding and antigenic modulation in respect of a particular tumor is difficult to establish.

Evidence pointing to loss of TATA on repeated transplantation of a mouse tumor was reported many years ago by Woodruff and Symes (1962b). The possibility that the findings might be due to antigen masking was, however, not excluded.

The possible effect of antigen lost from tumor cells in protecting tumors from immunological destruction will be discussed later (5.521).

5.3 REGULATION OF THE IMMUNE RESPONSE TO CANCER

As we have seen, some tumors possess antigens which evoke reactions manifested by resistance of the host to autotransplants of the tumor (5.211), sensitivity of the host to intradermal injection of tumor extracts (5.229, 5.234), and manifestations of cytotoxicity when host sera or cells are used with tumor cell targets in Winn assays (5.21) or *in vitro* tests of various kinds. Moreover, as will be discussed later, the growth of tumors may sometimes be inhibited by passive immunization with serum (7.22, 8.211) or lymphoid cells (7.412, 8.233) from donors bearing tumors of the same kind, or which have been immunized with tumor tissue or antigenic extracts.

We must now consider the response to TAA of various kinds in the autochthonous host; the situation, however, is so complex that hypotheses must be based to a considerable extent on the analysis of simpler models provided by *in vitro* systems and transplantation. Clearly these will stand or fall on whether or not they are consistent with the observed behavior of autochthonous tumors *in vivo,* but critical assessment may be extremely difficult (see Levy and Leclerc, 1975).

Some of the reasons for the complexity are easy to discern.

Firstly, as with immunological responses to other antigens, cells of various kinds are involved which interact in a complex way (5.32), and regulation is further complicated by the fact that antibodies may themselves function as antigens. The antigenic determinants associated with the antigen binding sites of an antibody are termed *idiotypes,* and as Jerne (1972, 1974) first suggested, they provide the basis for a complex immunological network of antigen-binding sites that recognize sets of idiotypes and of idiotypes that are recognized by sets of antigen-binding sites (Richter, 1975; Hoffman, 1975; Raff, 1977). Moreover, if, as appears to be the case (see Eichman, 1978), T and B lymphocytes share at least some idiotypes, both these classes of cell will be involved in the network. Another lymphocyte network based on allotypes (i.e., antigenic determinants on Ig molecules which are unrelated to the antigen-binding site, and evoke a reaction in allogeneic recipients), and the possibility of others again based on Ig classes and determinants of the major histocompatibility complex (*vide infra*), are discussed by Raff (1977).

Secondly, cancer cells, except in the special case of chorioncarcinoma, are derived from normal host cells, and to be effective the immunological response they evoke must be damaging to the tumor but not cause serious damage to normal cells. The discovery of MHC restriction (5.333) has provided some clues as to how this may be achieved and suggests that, as the immune system has evolved, mechanisms for self-recognition have evolved which depend to a large extent on gene products of the so-called major histocompatibility complex* (Katz and Skidmore, 1977).

Thirdly, as will be discussed in detail later (5.521), the response of the host may be limited genetically by lack of the appropriate immune response (Ir) genes (see Benacerraf, 1973); impaired as part of a general reduction in immunological responsiveness caused by the tumor (4.42), associated disease, or senescence; or impaired specifically by a variety of suppressor mechanisms.

5.31 Cytotoxic Mechanisms

5.311   ROLE OF ANTIVIRAL AND CYTOTOXIC ANTIBODY

Passive administration of serum from tumor-bearing animals may have an inhibitory or, on the other hand, an enhancing effect on the growth of transplants of the tumor in isogeneic animals (7.22), and it seems likely that these effects can occur also with autochthonous tumors.

Inhibition has been observed mainly with tumors of viral origin, including mouse leukemias, MSV-induced sarcomas, and polyoma virus-induced tumors, but also with some chemically induced tumors; it has usually been found only with serum from animals with early tumors, but exceptions to this rule have been reported.

In the case of some viral tumors neutralization of the virus may contribute to the effect (Fefer, 1969; Pearson, Redmon, and Bass, 1973; Chesebro and Wehrly, 1976); other possible factors are complement-dependent cytotoxicity, antibody-dependent cell-mediated cytotoxicity (5.312), and unblocking effects which counteract the abrogation of cell-mediated immunity by blocking factors (5.521).

In the case of mouse leukemias and MSV-induced sarcomas, which are the models which have been most thoroughly studied, there has often been poor correlation between the levels of antiviral and cytotoxic antibody on the one hand and the behavior of the tumor (Fefer *et al.,* 1968; Lamon *et al.,* 1973a; Chesebro and Wehrly, 1976a). This suggests that neither antibody exerts a decisive influence, but Chesebro and Wehrly (1976a) have postulated that control of virus infections by antiviral antibody, though not sufficient, is a necessary step in the control of Friend virus leukemia.

Various reasons may be suggested to account for the ineffectiveness of cytotoxic antibody, including poor access and low cytotoxic efficiency of the antibody, low density of antibody receptor on the tumor cells, defects in the mechanisms for activating complement, and poor access of complement to parts of the tumor. Quantitative studies of cell lysis by antibody and complement have been concerned for the most part with lysis of sheep erythrocytes using anti-Forsmann antibody, and there is good evidence that in this system a single molecule of IgM may produce a lytic lesion, whereas in the case of IgG at least two molecules on adjacent sites are required. Studies of this kind with nucleated cells are difficult for a variety of reasons, but attempts have been made to measure the cytotoxic efficiency of radioactively labeled antitumor glob-

---

*In the writer's view the term major histocompatibility complex (MHC) should be changed because it fails to express the far-reaching biological importance of the system but tends to exaggerate its importance in relation to tissue and organ transplantation. The difficulty is to suggest a better name which would be applicable to the MHC of different species, for which, individually, the current labels HLA, H2, AGB, and so on are reasonably satisfactory. *Self-recognition system* would seem to merit serious consideration, although it fails to express the importance of the system in relation to the regulation of T-cell functions.

ulin and antilymphocyte globulin, this being defined as the reciprocal of the mean number of Ig molecules attached per cell under conditions in which 50 percent lysis occurs *in vitro* in the presence of optimal quantities of complement of an appropriate kind (Woodruff and Smith, 1970; Woodruff and Inchley, 1971a). These experiments were performed with IgG from sera raised in xenogeneic animals; the methods used, however, could be adapted to the study of antibody from a tumor-bearing host in conjunction with autochthonous tumor cells. The importance of the density of surface isoantigenic receptors was investigated in another way by E. Möller and G. Möller (1962), who compared the residual hemagglutinin titer of alloantiserum,* after absorption with known numbers of normal or neoplastic mouse cells, with the sensitivity of the cells to lysis by the serum in the presence of complement. It was found that different cell types differed with regard to their concentrations of antigenic surface receptors, and there was good correlation between cytotoxic sensitivity and the concentration of receptors. Confirmatory evidence of the importance of the density of reactive sites was provided by the discovery that tumor cells which were partly or completely resistant to a single antiserum might by lysed by a combination of sera directed against different sites.

It has been reported that cultured human lymphoid cells differ in their susceptibility to complement-dependent lysis by HLA antibodies, and heterologous antibodies directed to membrane antigens, at different stages of the mitotic cycle (Pellegrino *et al.,* 1974). These differences were not associated with differences in the capacity of the cell to interact with complement components or to activate the complement system through the classical or alternate pathways, and Pellegrino *et al.* have suggested that they are due to changes in the cell membrane, or in its ability to repair complement-induced damage, during the mitotic cycle. Further studies of this kind with host antibody and autochthonous tumor cells, with particular reference to the repair of lytic lesions, might be rewarding.

5.312   ANTIBODY-DEPENDENT CELL-MEDIATED
CYTOTOXICITY (ADCC)

In this section we shall consider three sets of observations which, taken together, suggest that ADCC may play a role in the resistance to some autochthonous tumors.

In the first place, it has been shown that spleen cells from tumor-bearing animals (Calder, Irvine, and Ghaffar, 1975; Ghaffar, Calder, and Irvine, 1976), and peripheral blood lymphocytes lacking a T-cell marker from patients with bladder cancer (O'Toole *et al.,* 1974) show K-cell activity in that they become cytotoxic for a variety of allogeneic and xenogeneic target cells in the presence of appropriate antibody.

Secondly, in studies with MSV-induced mouse sarcomas, many of which regress spontaneously, it has been shown that serum from animals with regressing tumors can render normal isogeneic lymphocytes cytotoxic *in vitro* for cells of the tumor (Pollack *et al.,* 1972; Skurzak *et al.,* 1972), and can also potentiate the cytotoxicity of immune lymph node cells (Skurzak *et al.,* 1972). Both IgG and IgM can cause these effects (Lamon *et al.,* 1975). The IgM appears to act in conjunction with both T and B cells, but not with macrophages or null cells. The question thus arises of whether IgM bound to T cells is concerned in cytotoxicity which appears to be due to T cells alone.

Thirdly, serum and immunoglobulin from patients with Burkitt's lymphoma (Jondal and Gunven, 1977) and melanoma (Saal *et al.,* 1977) have been shown to co-

---

*Referred to by Möller and Möller as isoantiserum, in accordance with the usual practice at the time.

operate with human blood lymphocytes in causing lysis of cell lines derived from the corresponding type of tumor. In the case of Burkitt's lymphoma, however, Jondal and Gunven found no correlation between ADCC and antimembrane activity or the behavior of the tumor, and suggested that the antibody concerned might be directed against EB virus-related antigens other than membrane antigens.

5.313   CELL-MEDIATED CYTOTOXICITY NOT DEPENDENT ON ANTIBODY

The effector limb of the cell-mediated response to TATA and other surface antigens may involve not only cytotoxic T cells (Tc) but other categories of T cells, non-T lymphocytes, and macrophages. Cytostasis and cytolysis may both occur, and the same effector cell may be involved in both processes; moreover, an early specific response may be followed by non-specific resistance (Currie and Gage, 1973; Owen and Seeger, 1973; Seeger and Owen, 1974; Kearney, Basten, and Nelson, 1975), and cells of the same type may be involved in both cases.

While cytotoxic T cells are generally considered to play a key (J.F.A.P. Miller and Osoba, 1967; J.F.A.P. Miller *et al.,* 1971; Cerottini, Nordin, and Brunner, 1970a, 1970b; Golstein *et al.,* 1972), though not exclusive (Lonai *et al.,* 1971; Scollard, 1975), role as mediators of target cell destruction in systems involving major histocompatibility differences, their role in the destruction of isogeneic and autochthonous tumor cells seems to be less paramount. Cells which are cytotoxic for syngeneic or autochthonous tumors *in vitro* have been demonstrated in suspensions prepared from lymph nodes or spleen, or in the thoracic duct lymph, from mice and rats with a variety of tumors, including chemically induced mouse sarcomas (Hellström, Hellström, and Pierce, 1968), MSV-induced sarcomas (Lamon *et al.,* 1972, 1973b, 1973c, 1974, 1975; LeClerc, Gomard, and Levy, 1972; LeClerc *et al.,* 1973; Plata *et al.,* 1974; Kiessling *et al.,* 1974), mouse mammary carcinomas (Roubinian *et al.,* 1976), Friend virus leukemia (Chesebro and Wehrly, 1976b), and a Gross virus-induced rat lymphoma (Tucker, Dennert, and Lennox, 1974). This activity may be reduced by treating the effector cells with anti-Thy 1 (anti-θ) serum and complement (Tucker *et al.,* 1974; Chesebro and Wehrly, 1976) and abrogated completely by neonatal thymectomy (Roubinian *et al.,* 1976), but while observations of this kind point to the involvement of T cells, they do not exclude participation by other kinds of cell. Moreover, in the case of MSV sarcomas, evidence of killing by non-T cells has been reported by various authors (Lamon *et al.,* 1973a, 1973b; Plata *et al.,* 1974), and in more recent studies (Lamon *et al.,* 1975) it has been shown that T-cell killer activity is a transient phenomenon which occurs only in animals with early regressing tumors, whereas B cell killer activity persists much longer.

Three stages have been distinguished in T-cell-mediated lysis *in vitro* (see Golstein and Smith, 1976), namely, (1) recognition of antigen on the surface of the target cell by receptors on T cells (Golstein, Svedmyr, and Wigzell, 1971; Berke and Levey, 1972), (2) a lethal hit of unknown nature resulting in irreversible target cell damage (Wagner and Rollinghoff, 1974; Martz, 1975), and (3) target cell disintegration. The last stage does not require the continued presence of viable effector cells at the target cell surface (Henney and Bubbers, 1973; Martz and Benacerraf, 1973; Miller and Dunkley, 1974; Wagner and Rollinghoff, 1974; Martz, 1975; MacDonald, 1975). There is evidence that an effector T cell can kill more than one target cell (Zagury *et al.,* 1975; Martz, 1976).

It has been reported that human lymphocytes may become non-specifically cytotoxic when cultured in the presence of PHA (Lundgren and Möller, 1969) and mouse lymphocytes when cultured in the presence of allogeneic fibroblasts (Shustik *et al.*, 1976). Shustik *et al.* suggested that the cells concerned were T cells because they were non-adherent to nylon wool and cytotoxicity was considerably reduced by treating the cell population with anti-Thy 1 serum plus complement, but it now seems likely that they were natural killer (NK) cells (5.44).

B lymphocytes and null cells may, as we have seen (5.312), kill antibody-coated cells. Lamon *et al.* (1972) have suggested further that membrane-bound Ig on B cells allows recognition of, and contact with, target cells, and that such contact may activate the B cell to lyse the target cell by some unknown mechanism. Denham *et al.* (1970) suggested that the killing of allogeneic tumor cells by large pyroninophilic radioresistant cells found in the efferent lymph from the draining lymph nodes 6–12 days after immunization with the tumor in question, which without obvious justification they refer to as lymphoblasts, might be due to the local production of specific antibody, but subsequent experiments (Denham, Wrathmell, and Alexander, 1975) failed to support this hypothesis in respect of allogeneic targets, though it did appear to apply to xenogeneic targets. It seems unlikely therefore that this mechanism would operate in an isogeneic system.

Macrophages may be armed by a factor secreted by sensitized T cells on contact with antigen, and such armed macrophages are activated and become cytotoxic when they encounter the same antigen on the surface of target cells (5.322). There is evidence that macrophages may also recognize, and exert a cytotoxic effect on, tumor cells by mechanisms which are not triggered by TAA and which fall in the category of what we have termed para-immunological mechanisms. This will be discussed later (5.43), and to avoid repetition we shall postpone further consideration of the mechanisms of macrophage-mediated cytotoxicity until then. We shall also postpone discussion of killing by NK cells, which may also be described as para-immunological, to a later section (5.44).

5.32 Helper Mechanisms

The type and intensity of the immune response to a variety of antigens are controlled by a complex series of interactions involving various subclasses of T cells,* B cells, and macrophages (see Cantor and Weissman, 1976; Cantor and Boyse, 1977). Regulatory substances secreted by T cells which influence the behavior of other subclasses of T cells, B cells, macrophages, and monocytes play an important part in these reactions (5.322; see also Tada, Taniguchi, and Takemori, 1976), which appear to be governed to a large extent by genes of the major histocompatibility complex (MHC) (see Miller and Vadas, 1977; David, 1979).

5.321   SUBCLASSES OF T CELLS

In the mouse three main subclasses of T cell can be distinguished on the basis of their cell surface antigens, in particular the Ly antigens discovered by Boyse and his colleagues (see Boyse and Old, 1978). These are T_H (Ly-1) or helper cells; $T_{C/S}$ (Ly-2,3) cells, which may be cytotoxic (T_C) or suppressive (T_S) of both humoral and cell-

---

*Here and elsewhere *T cell* and *B cell* denote *T lymphocyte* and *B lymphocyte*, respectively.

mediated immunity; and T_E (Ly-1,2,3) cells which, it is thought, may give rise to T_H and $T_{C/S}$ (Cantor and Boyse, 1977). There is evidence that Ly-1 cells may be further subdivided according to whether or not they possess Ia alloantigens (Vadas et al., 1976).

These properties were defined originally in studies of responses to alloantigens, and it was found that $T_{C/S}$ were activated in mixed cultures by H-2 differences in the K and D regions but not the I region, whereas T_H seemed to be stimulated by antigens (Ia) associated with I-region determinants. It has now been shown that T_C may also be generated after exposure to syngeneic cells expressing virus-specified (Zinkernagel and Doherty, 1975; Doherty, Blanden, and Zinkernagel, 1976) or chemically modified (Shearer, Rehn, and Garbarino, 1975) cell surface antigens, and to cells differing in respect of only minor histocompatibility antigens (Bevan, 1975), including HY (Gordon, Simpson, and Samelson, 1975); as will be discussed later (5.323), however, T_C generated in these ways manifest their cytotoxic potential only when the target cells express H-2K or H-2D phenotypes identical with those of the sensitizing cells. It appears, moreover, that T_H may be stimulated not only by allogeneic Ia but also by self-Ia that is associated with foreign determinants (Cantor and Boyse, 1977).

Reactions to isogeneic cells modified by viral infection or chemically seem likely to prove better models for immunological reactions to tumor cell surface antigens than reactions to strong alloantigens. It is of great interest therefore that recent studies (Glimcher and Cantor, 1978) have shown that T_E (Ly-1,2,3) cells play a central role in the generation of both cellular and humoral immunity to hapten-modified syngeneic or autologous spleen cells; in particular, they appear to be essential, probably as cytotoxic precursors, for the generation of Tc (Ly-2,3) cells cytotoxic for such targets, and can suppress the generation of specific antibody. This suggests that $T_E \rightarrow T_{C/S}$ is a maturation step which, with respect to reactivity to modified self-antigen, occurs only in the presence of the antigen, whereas $T_{C/S}$ operative against alloantigens may develop from T_E cells in the absence of the antigen. It thus seems reasonable to attribute the inability of spleen cells from aged mice to produce Tc after stimulation with hapten-modified syngeneic spleen cells to the fact that such mice possess fewer T_E cells and more T_H and $T_{C/S}$ cells than young mice (Cantor and Boyse, 1977), and to postulate further that a deficiency of analogous cells may develop with increasing age in man and other species, and contribute to the age-related incidence of cancer.

The study of subcategories of human T cells is at an early stage, but a start has been made and progress should be facilitated by the development of techniques for making monoclonal antibody (see Chess and Schlossman, 1977).

5.322   CELL COOPERATION

T cells regulate the multiplication of B cells and their differentiation to antibody-secreting plasma cells after antigenic stimulation. Evidence pointing to this conclusion accumulated over several years (see Playfair, 1971; Katz and Benacerraf, 1972), and it was definitely proved by Katz and Unanue (1973) in studies of the development of secondary antibody responses to hapten-protein conjugates in vitro. More recent studies (Cantor and Boyse, 1975a; Jandinsky et al., 1976) have shown that this helper function is mediated by Ly-1 cells. T_H Ly-1 cells can also amplify the generation of cytotoxic ("killer") T_C from prekiller cells in mixed cultures containing lymphocytes and allogeneic target cells, but they do not themselves contribute directly to the cytotoxic effect (Cantor and Boyse, 1975b; Cantor and Simpson, 1975). It has also been shown that the ability of thymectomized mice to mount a delayed-type hypersensitivity reaction to sheep erythrocytes can be restored by providing them with T_H Ly-1 cells but not with other subclasses of T cells (Huber *et al.,* 1976).

The generation of T_C in cultures of lymph node cells and allogeneic target cells has been reported to be greatly increased by the addition of spleen cells from congenitally athymic (nude) mice (Schilling, Phillips, and Miller, 1976). The T_C were shown to be derived from the lymph node cell population. The nature of the cooperating cells in the nude mouse spleen was not conclusively established, but the data were consistent with their being null cells.

Soluble products termed *lymphokines* (Dumonde *et al.,* 1969) are released by sensitized lymphocytes in the presence of antigen. Various names, including *macrophage migration inhibition factor* (MIF), *macrophage chemotactic factor* (MCF), *macrophage-activating factor* (MAF), and *specific macrophage-arming factor* (SMAF), have been given to lymphokines which affect macrophage function, but the degree of independence of the substances to which these labels are attached, and their roles *in vivo,* are uncertain. Moreover, confusion may result from the fact that some authors use MCF as an abbreviation for *macrophage cytotoxic factor,* which appears to be another name for macrophage-activating factor or specific macrophage-arming factor.

MIF, which has already been mentioned in connection with *in vitro* assays (5.227), appears to be a product of T_H cells, and is effective only if these cells and the macrophages are I compatible. MIF and MCF may play a role *in vivo* by promoting the local accumulation of macrophage at sites where T cells are in contact with antigen.

SMAF, it is generally agreed, confers a form of specificity on macrophages in that they subsequently become activated only on contact with the antigen to which the T cells which produced the SMAF had been sensitized (Evans and Alexander, 1972a, 1972b; Lohmann-Mathes and Fischer, 1973), but opinions differ as to whether, once activated, the macrophages are indiscriminately cytotoxic (Currie and Gage, 1973) or are cytotoxic only for the sensitizing cells (Lohmann-Mathes and Fischer, 1973). According to Meerpohl, Lohmann-Mathes, and Fischer (1976), not only mature macrophages, but also macrophage precursors in bone marrow, may be made cytotoxic by SMAF (termed by these authors *macrophage cytotoxicity factor*).

It has also been reported that B cells, with the help of T cells but not without such help, in the presence of soluble protein antigen produce a monocyte chemotactic factor (Wahl and Rosenstreich, 1976).

The macrophages of higher animals are the phylogenetic descendants of the phagocytic cells of invertebrate species which serve to eliminate foreign material. With the evolution of the immune system, macrophages have come to play a key role in a wide range of immunological reactions by destroying extracellular antigens which might otherwise inhibit the immune response, by processing antigen and presenting it to lymphocytes in an immunologically optimal form, and by secreting molecules that regulate lymphocyte differentiation and function (see Unanue, 1978). In addition they secrete a variety of other molecules including lysozomal enzymes and retain their capacity to phagocytose particulate material.

It has been postulated by Unanue (1978) that there are two pathways of antigen presentation to lymphocytes by macrophages. The first involves a molecule that is not extensively changed and is recognized by B cells. The second, which is concerned in the production of T_H cells (Erb and Feldmann, 1975), is subject to MHC restriction

(5.323), and appears to involve the release of a molecule containing antigen and an I-region gene product (see Benacerraf, 1978; Niederhuber, 1978). Since, in general, genetically determined failure to respond to a particular antigen is due to defective T-cell function rather than defective B-cell potential (Benacerraf, 1973), it has been suggested by Miller and Vadas (1977) that the I-region gene product concerned in T_H stimulation may be the product of the relevant immune response (Ir) gene. They have suggested further that antigen which is unable to associate effectively with the I-region gene product on the macrophage comes off and is available as soluble antigen to stimulate suppressor T cells (T_S).

Macrophages also play an important role in the non-specific stimulation of lymphocytes by mitogens, and appear to do this by binding the mitogen and presenting it in a stimulatory form (Rosenstreich, Farrar, and Dougherty, 1976; Rosenstreich and Mizel, 1978).

Regulatory molecules, both stimulatory and inhibitory, have been demonstrated in macrophage tissue culture supernatants (see Unanue, 1978), but their importance *in vivo* cannot as yet be assessed with confidence.

Stimulatory substances include mitogenic protein, which increases DNA synthesis in thymocytes and to a lesser extent in T and B cells; substances which promote the differentiation of immature thymocytes to mature T cells, and of primed B cells to plasma cells; and a substance which stimulates helper and suppressor T-cell activity, depending on the state of priming.

Substances secreted by activated macrophages which may inhibit lymphocyte responses include the nucleosides thymidine, adenosine, and guanosine; polyamine oxidase; complement components; prostaglandins; cyclic AMP; and interferons (see Nelson, 1976; Allison, 1978). The amount of thymidine may be sufficient to compete with radioactively labeled thymidine in cytotoxicity assays (5.226), and with some cells to result in a phenomenon termed *thymidine blockade,* in which the excess thymidine blocks the conversion of cytidilate to deoxycytidilate (Unanue, 1978). Unanue (1978) has postulated that the secretion of thymidine by macrophages is related to the fact that they lack the enzyme *thymidine kinase,* which, when present in a cell, phosphorylates thymidine and prevents it from escaping into the extracellular fluid. Whether or not the thymidine secreted by macrophages has any biological function is a matter of conjecture; it seems possible, however, that it may influence the behavior of tumors in which there is a large macrophage population.

Macrophages also secrete large amounts of the enzyme *lysozyme.* Since the secretion of lysozyme appears to be unaffected by the state of activation of the macrophages (Gordon, Todd, and Cohn, 1974), the amount produced may reflect the number of functioning macrophages, and, as Currie and Eccles (1976) have shown, serum levels of lysozyme can, under well defined conditions, be a useful marker of macrophage-mediated host responses to a tumor.

5.323   MHC RESTRICTION

As has been mentioned (5.321), mouse T_C derived by conventional immunization procedures and specific for virus-specified or chemically modified cell surface antigens and minor histocompatibility antigens are effectively cytotoxic only when the target cells, in addition to possessing the viral, haptenic, or minor histocompatibility antigens in question, express also the same H-2K or H-2D phenotypes as the sensitizing cells.

This limitation, which is termed *H-2 restriction* in mice and more generally *MHC restriction,* occurs also in relation to T-cell helper function, delayed-type hypersensitivity, and macrophage activation by T cells; but whereas the H-2 determinants restricting T_C activity are located in the K and D regions, those restricting other T cell functions are located in the I region (Katz and Benacerraf, 1975; Schwartz *et al.,* 1976; Miller and Vadas, 1977), except that K and D restriction may be involved in delayed-type hypersensitivity to contact chemicals such as dinitrofluorobenzene (see Miller and Vadas, 1977). There is, on the other hand, no evidence of H-2 restriction of B-cell functions or of their antibody products (Zinkernagel *et al.,* 1978a).

MHC restriction of T-cell functions is not confined to the mouse; it has been demonstrated in the guinea pig (Rosenthal, Lipsky, and Shevach, 1975) and rat (Zinkernagel, Althage, and Jensen, 1977), and also in man in relation to cytotoxicity of T cells for cells bearing the male (HY) antigen (Goulmy *et al.,* 1976) and proliferation of T cells in response to antigen presented by macrophages (Bergholtz and Thorsby, 1977).

Two hypotheses have been proposed to account for MHC restriction, namely the *dual recognition hypothesis,* according to which T cells recognize two distinct antigenic entities, self-MHC structures and foreign antigens (X), by means of separate receptors; and the *single receptor hypothesis,* which postulates that T cells possess one single receptor specificity that recognizes a neoantigenic determinant (NAD) formed either by a complex of self and X, by an antigen-specific modification of the self-MHC structure, or by host-specific modification of the foreign antigen (see Zinkernagel *et al.,* 1978a). Experiments in lethally irradiated mice reconstituted with bone marrow and irradiated thymus grafts (Zinkernagel *et al.,* 1978a, 1978b), have established that in the thymus precursor T cells develop recognition structures for self that are specific for the H-2, K, D, and I markers expressed by the thymic epithelium, since the restriction on virus-specific killing by T cells from chimeras was found to be determined by the H-2 antigens of the thymic graft irrespective of the H-2 antigens expressed by the T cells. Zinkernagel *et al.* have argued that this is readily compatible with dual recognition by T cells, though it does not formally exclude a single recognition model.

The possible significance of MHC restriction in relation to surveillance for neoplastic and other abnormal cells will be discussed later (5.53).

5.4 PARA-IMMUNOLOGICAL MECHANISMS

In this section we shall consider some tumor-inhibitory mechanisms involving lymphocytes and macrophages for which *immunological,* in the strict sense of the word (5.1), may be too narrow a label.

5.41 Allogeneic Inhibition

It was reported by Snell and Stevens (1961), and subsequently confirmed by K. E. Hellström (1963, 1964) and others, that tumors originating in an inbred (homozygous) strain of mice may grow better, as judged by the incidence of tumors and shortness of the latent interval, when transplanted to members of the strain than to F1 hybrids of the parent strain and another inbred strain. This phenomenon was termed the *hybrid effect* by Snell and Stevens but is now usually termed *allogeneic inhibition* (K. E. Hellström and I. Hellström, 1965) or *syngeneic preference.* It was reported initially that the effect was not increased by prior attempts to immunize the recipients against the tumor (Snell and Stevens, 1961), and was not abrogated (K. E. Hellström, 1963) by prior whole body irradiation (450 R). More recently, however, Oth and Burg (1970a) have reported that the effect is increased by prior immunization to an extent dependent on the strength of the TATA; they have suggested therefore that the phenomenon reflects a response to TATA, and occurs when, for genetic reasons, the hybrid is genetically able to respond more vigorously to these antigens than members of the parent line.

Further analysis has been based on Winn assays (5.21) and *in vitro* studies.

In Winn assays, Bergheden and Hellström (1966) found that lymphocytes from F1 animals in the presence of PHA were almost as effective as allogeneic lymphocytes in inhibiting tumor growth, and irradiation of the lymphocytes in a dose of 10,000 R did not abrogate the inhibitory effect. They reported that irradiated liver cells were also inhibitory. Inhibition by F1 lymphocytes did not occur, however, if their foreign H-2 antigens were covered by specific isoantibody (I. Hellström and K. E. Hellström, 1966). Subsequent investigations have shown that the effect, though relatively radioresistant, is less so than was originally thought, and may be weakened by exposing F1 lymphocytes to doses of 1000–5000 R (Oth and Burg, 1970b).

In vitro, it was shown by cytotoxicity and colony inhibition tests that tumor growth was inhibited by particulate antigenic extracts containing foreign H-2 antigens (K. E. Hellström, I. Hellström, and Haughton, 1964), and by F1 (or allogeneic) lymphocytes in the presence of PHA (E. Möller, 1965; K. E. Hellström, I. Hellström, and Bergheden, 1967). The killing was attributed to close contact with foreign H-2 antigens, and Möller (1965) suggested that it might be a manifestation of structural incompatibility. Support for this view was provided by the observation that lymphoid cells from A-strain mice which had been made neonatally tolerant of (A × CBA) F1 cells and were bearing a tolerated F1 skin graft killed both CBA and F1 embryo fibroblasts in culture (E. Möller, Lapp, and Lindholm, 1969). It was postulated that a similar mechanism might operate *in vivo.* As we shall see in the next section (5.42), however, other examples of radioresistant tumor inhibition have been described, and the hypotheses put forward to explain these, including cytotoxicity mediated by natural killer (NK) cells (5.44), may apply also to allogeneic inhibition.

5.42   Other Forms of Radioresistant Inhibition

It was reported by Boyse (1959), and confirmed by Cudkowicz and Stimpfling (1964a, 1964b), that transplanted normal hemopoietic cells from C57 mice grew less well in F1 mice than in the strain of origin, but that this was not the case with hemopoietic cells from A or C3H mice. Further investigations (Cudkowicz and Bennett, 1971a, 1971b; Lotzová and Cudkowicz, 1971, 1972, 1973, 1974; Rauchwerger *et al.,* 1973) have extended these findings and have shown that heavily irradiated F1 and homozygous mice of certain strains do not support the growth of isogeneic, allogeneic, and xenogeneic bone marrow, and that this is due to a host-antigraft mechanism mediated by cells which are destructive for stem cells, are highly radioresistant, can differentiate and mature even after neonatal thymectomy, and can destroy target cells *in vivo* within 1–4 days without prior sensitization. Radioresistant marrow rejection appears to depend on donor–host differences governed by multiple hemopoietic histocompatibility genes (Hh genes); these are distinguished from classical histocompatibility genes by non-codominant inheritance (Bennett, 1972), expression on bone marrow and lymphoid cells only, and in some cases lack of linkage with the MHC (Cudkowicz and Rossi, 1972).

The discovery by Lotzová and her colleagues (Lotsová and Cudkowicz, 1974; Lotzová, Gallagher, and Trentin, 1975) that the resistance of irradiated mice to hybrid, allogeneic, and xenogeneic bone marrow can be abrogated by treatment with silica or carageenan,* both of which are toxic for macrophages, led them to postulate that the resistance is due to a subpopulation of macrophages resident in the spleen and bone marrow. This is difficult to reconcile, however, with the fact that resistance is abrogated by intravenous injection of *Corynebacterium parvum* (Cudkowicz and Bennett, 1971a) but not by neonatal thymectomy (Lotzová *et al.,* 1975), and it was therefore suggested that an unidentified class of non-T lymphocyte might be involved. Recent work, which will be discussed later (5.44), supports this last suggestion and points to the natural killer (NK) cell as the lymphocyte in question.

The relevance of this phenomenon in relation to resistance to tumors is suggested by the observations that the growth of lymphomas, particularly in the spleen, is inhibited in both non-irradiated and irradiated congenitally athymic (nude) mice (Bonmassar *et al.,* 1975) and in irradiated conventional mice incompatible with the tumor for the D end of the H-2 complex (Bonmassar and Cudkowicz, 1976), and that in some strain combinations the inhibition of lymphoma growth in the spleen parallels the inhibition of bone marrow cells of the same genotype (Bonmassar and Cudkowicz, 1976).

5.43 Macrophage-mediated Cytotoxicity

The role of macrophages in ADCC (5.312) and their helper function in immune responses mediated by lymphocytes (5.322) have been discussed already. In this section we shall consider macrophage-mediated cytotoxicity which is not lymphocyte dependent. We shall begin by reviewing data provided by *in vitro* observations, and then discuss the extent to which this form of cytotoxicity may also limit the growth of tumors *in vivo.*

5.431 CYTOTOXIC EFFECT OF MACROPHAGES ON TUMOR
CELLS *IN VITRO*

Macrophages may or may not be cytotoxic for tumor cells *in vitro.* If they are cytotoxic this may be manifested as cytostasis or cytolysis. Cytotoxic macrophages typically cause cytostasis or cytolysis of tumor cells at effector–target cell ratios of about 1:1 or more (Tsoi and Weiser, 1968; Keller, 1973; Dullens and Den Otter, 1974; Gallily, 1975), but are not cytotoxic for normal cells (Hibbs *et al.,* 1972a, 1972c; Hibbs, 1974b; Cleveland *et al.,* 1974; Meltzer *et al.,* 1975b; Piessens *et al.,* 1975; Mansell and Di Luzio, 1976).

Macrophages from untreated mice are typically non-cytotoxic for syngeneic (Evans and Alexander, 1970) and allogeneic (Den Otter *et al.,* 1972) tumor cells *in vitro,* but sometimes show some degree of non-specific cytotoxicity (Evans and Alexander, 1972c; Keller, 1973; Hibbs, 1974a). A high background non-specific cytotoxicity seems to interfere with the production of immune macrophages and SMAF (*vide in-*

---

*Treatment with carageenan was tested with allogeneic and xenogeneic marrow only.

fra); in consequence, immune macrophages may appear to be non-specifically cyto-toxic (Boyle and Ormerod, 1976) and SMAF to be non-specific (Ziegler *et al.,* 1975; Kripke *et al.,* 1977).

Macrophages which show non-specific cytotoxicity for tumor cells *in vitro* are termed activated macrophages. As stated above, macrophages from untreated mice sometimes behave as activated macrophages. Activation may also be caused *in vivo* by infections of various kinds, including viral infection (Stott *et al.,* 1975; Rodda and White, 1976) and infection with intracellular parasites (Hibbs *et al.,* 1972a, 1972c; Krahenbuhl and Remington, 1974; Krahenbuhl and Lambert, 1975; Krahenbuhl *et al.,* 1976), and by administration of a variety of agents discussed in detail in relation to immunotherapy (7.5), including BCG (7.51), *Corynebacterium parvum* (7.52), bac-terial endotoxin (7.53), and double-stranded RNA (7.55). In mice, activated macro-phages which are cytotoxic for tumor cells may be generated not only in normal animals but also in congenitally athymic animals (Meltzer, 1976).

Activated macrophages may be cytostatic and also cytolytic.

As discussed earlier (5.322), macrophages may be armed by specific macrophage-arming factor (SMAF) released by immune T lymphocytes in the presence of antigen (Evans *et al.,* 1972). An important example of this phenomenon is arming by SMAF produced by immune T lymphocytes incubated with specific tumor target cells (Evans and Alexander, 1971, 1972a, 1972b; Pels and Den Otter, 1973, 1974). Macrophages armed with this material become activated on contact with cells of the tumor in ques-tion; *in vitro* this activation is manifested by a cytostatic effect on the tumor, or, if immune lymphocytes are also present, by cytolysis of the tumor cells (Zembala, Ptak, and Hanczakowska, 1973a, 1973b; Van Loveren and Den Otter, 1974). As we have seen (5.322), there appears to be a difference of opinion as to whether, once activated, the macrophages are indiscriminately cytotoxic or cytotoxic only for the specific tu-mor target cells. Despite this unresolved question, the term *immune macrophage* is sometimes used in an operational way to denote macrophages (usually from the peri-toneal cavity) from animals immunized with syngeneic (Evans and Alexander, 1970) or allogeneic (Granger and Weiser, 1964, 1966) tumors which are cytotoxic for tumor cells (see Den Otter *et al,* 1972; Lohmann-Matthes *et al.,* 1972; Temple *et al.,* 1973; Piper and McIvor, 1975; Gallily and Ben-Ishay, 1975; Den Otter *et al.,* 1977). It has been reported by Den Otter *et al.* (1974) that immunization with irradiated tumor cells results in cytostatic macrophages, whereas immunization with non-irradiated tu-mor cells results in cytolytic macrophages.

While the non-specific cytotoxicity of activated macrophages is readily demon-strable with a variety of tumor cell targets (Hibbs, Lambert, and Remington, 1972a, 1972b; Hibbs, 1973; Holtermann, Lisafield, and Klein, 1972; Holtermann, Klein, and Casale, 1973; Basic *et al.,* 1975; see also section 7.5), it may also occur, despite some reports to the contrary, with rapidly dividing embryonic (McLaughlin, Ruddle, and Waksman, 1972; Holtermann *et al.,* 1975) and non-transformed virus-infected (Gold-man and Hogg, 1977) cells. Close contact between the macrophages and target cells appears to be essential, and this may depend on particular surface properties of sus-ceptible cells (see Levy and Wheelock, 1974; Milas and Scott, 1977), which, according to Hibbs (1973), are not subject to contact inhibition of growth in tissue culture and are agglutinated by plant lectins. Cytotoxicity is blocked by inhibitors of protein syn-thesis and glycolysis (Keller, 1974).

Various mechanisms have been postulated to account for non-specific macrophage-mediated cytotoxicity; these fall under two main headings: phagocytosis, and release of a cytotoxic agent by the macrophage in the vicinity of the target cell. With "immune macrophages" (*vide supra*) cytophilic antibody may play an important role.

Phagocytosis does not necessarily imply complete engulfment of entire target cells; according to Chambers and Weiser (1969, 1972) the macrophage may pinch off bits of target cell membrane until repair ceases to be possible. Cytotoxic agents which it is thought may be concerned include lysozomal enzymes (Temple *et al.*, 1973), an unidentified "specific macrophage" cytotoxin (McIvor and Weiser, 1971), complement cleavage products (Schorlemmer *et al.*, 1977), and arginase (Kung *et al.*, 1977; Currie, 1978; Currie and Basham, 1978). The cytotoxic effect of arginase appears to be due to arginine deprivation and greater arginine dependence of susceptible cells, since it has been reported by Currie and Basham (1978) (1) that the cytotoxic effect of activated macrophages *in vitro* is abrogated by excess arginine, (2) that cells of human, rat, mouse, and hamster tumors require a higher concentration of L-arginine in the medium than corresponding normal cells with similar doubling times to maintain optimal proliferation, and (3) that addition of L-arginine after 24 hours deprivation allows normal cells to proliferate whereas the reproductive capacity of tumor cells is irreversibly impaired.

Macrophages often show little or no evidence of mitosis in tissue culture; they are able to divide under certain conditions, however, as has been shown with mouse peritoneal (More *et al.*, 1973) and alveolar (Soderland and Naum, 1973) macrophages and human alveolar macrophages (Golde, Byers, and Finley, 1974).

5.432 MACROPHAGE-MEDIATED CYTOTOXICITY *IN VIVO*

Macrophages, which were discovered and named by Eli Metchnikoff (see O. Metchnikoff, 1921), and which form an essential element of what Aschoff (1924) termed the reticuloendothelial system (RES), are widely distributed and occur in such sites as the spleen, lymph nodes, liver (Küppfer cells), pulmonary alveoli, serous cavities, and connective tissue, and also in inflammatory exudates. Connective tissue macrophages are sometimes termed histiocytes. As we have seen (3.12), macrophages occur also in tumors, including human (Carr, 1977) as well as animal tumors, sometimes in large numbers. While it is clear that macrophages subserve a wide range of functions, and that cells differing in respect of such properties as antigen-binding capacity, phagocytic activity, lysozomal enzyme content, density of membrane receptors for MIF, and radiosensitivity, can be separated or defined by density gradient and other experimental procedures, it is not known whether these differences reflect different stages of development or activation of a single type of cell or the existence of different cell populations arising from distinct precursor cells (see Walker, 1974; Stuart, 1977; Unanue, 1978).

Kinetic studies after labeling with ^{3}H-thymidine, and studies of chimeras, by Van Furth and his colleagues (Van Furth and Cohn, 1968; Van Furth and Diesselhoff-den-Dulk, 1970; Van Furth, 1970, 1977), following earlier work by Volkman (1966), point strongly to the conclusion that in normal tissues under physiological steady-state conditions, macrophages do not divide to a significant extent but are replenished by blood monocytes, which in turn are derived from premonocytes and monoblasts in the bone marrow. This conclusion has been challenged by Volkman (1976) and Shands and Axelrod (1977), but gains support from the demonstration that in human liver transplants in patients whose transplants had been obtained from a donor of the opposite sex and had survived for longer than three months, the Küppfer cells were of recipient karyotype (Porter, 1969; Portman *et al.,* 1976).

In inflammatory exudates monocytes accumulate from the blood and develop into macrophages, but within a day or two these cells then begin to divide (Spector and Mariano, 1975), and Spector (1977) has suggested that this proliferation *in situ* doubles or trebles the number of macrophages which would be present if migration alone were involved. Mitosis has also been demonstrated in peritoneal macrophages (Forbes, 1966) and Küppfer cells (More and Nelson, 1972) after rechallenging mice with an antigen with which they had previously been immunized.

There have been many studies of the macrophage content of tumors at various stages of their development (*vide infra*). The effect of a tumor on the production and distribution of monocytes has also been investigated. It has been shown that in animals with early syngeneic tumor transplants the capacity of the bone marrow to produce monocyte colonies *in vitro* (Baum and Fisher, 1972), and the blood monocyte count (Eccles, Bandlow, and Alexander, 1976), may be increased. It has also been shown (Gillette and Boone, 1974) that the distribution of intraperitoneally injected ^{51}Cr-labeled peritoneal cells is altered in tumor-bearing animals in a manner which depends on the stage of development of the tumor, though the significance of this observation is not entirely clear. The relative importance of monocyte infiltration and proliferation *in situ* in transplanted and autochthonous tumors has not been thoroughly investigated. It may well be, as Spector (1977) has postulated, that the steady-state physiological model is appropriate in the early stages of carcinogenesis, and the inflammatory exudate model in the later stages, but this clearly merits experimental study.

Analysis of the effect of activated macrophages on tumors *in vivo* is complicated by the fact that agents which cause macrophage activation may modify immunological responses in various ways. Experiments with a wide range of such agents which will be discussed in detail later (7.5), however, point strongly to the conclusion that activated macrophages can markedly inhibit tumor growth. Further evidence is provided by the observation of Bomford, Shand, and Christie (1975) that (CBA × C57B1)F1 hybrid mice in which a graft-versus-host (GVH) reaction had been induced by injection of parent line (CBA) spleen cells showed a transient resistance to intravenous injection of tumor cells at a time when there was macrophage activation associated with maximal immunosuppression.

Confirmation of the tumor-inhibitory effect of activated macrophages is provided by the demonstration that the growth of transplanted tumors may be inhibited by the injection of activated, but not inactivated, syngeneic or allogeneic viable macrophages (Alexander, Evans, and Mikulska, 1973; Fidler, 1974; Van Loveren and Den Otter, 1974; Dullens and Den Otter, 1973, 1974; Dullens, Kingma, and Den Otter, 1974; Dullens *et al.,* 1974b, 1975; Den Otter *et al.,* 1977; Keller, 1976, 1977). As a rule tumor inhibition occurred only when the macrophages were injected at the site of tumor inoculation, including under this heading intravenous injection of tumor cells and later of macrophages (Fidler, 1974); Keller (1976, 1977), however, has reported significant inhibition after injections at different sites.

The role of macrophages in the resistance to tumors in the absence of experimental procedures designed to cause activation is more difficult to assess. A critical experiment would be to compare the behavior of tumors in normal animals and in animals subject to chronic gross impairment of macrophage activity; normal animals, population, and so far it has not been found possible to induce such a state experimentally. Moreover, no strains of animals showing gross congenital macrophage deficiency have been discovered, and it seems possible that such a state would not be compatible with survival. Injection of materials such as silica and carageenan, which are selectively cytotoxic for macrophages, may cause enhancement of tumor growth especially when given on the day of tumor inoculation, and this effect is abrogated by administration of the lysozomal stabilizer polyvinyl-N-oxide (Keller, 1976d). Enhanced tumor growth has also been reported after injection of trypan blue, which inhibits macrophage-mediated cytotoxicity (Hibbs, 1975, 1976), and antimacrophage serum (Isa and Sanders, 1975). The macrophage-inhibitory effect of all these agents *in vivo* is short-lived, however, and they may evoke a complex compensatory host reaction (Levy and Wheelock, 1975; Keller, 1976), so that negative results are of little significance.

The macrophage content of different tumors varies greatly; it is often high in strongly immunogenic tumors and in tumors which rarely metastasize, and low in weakly immunogenic tumors and tumors which commonly metastasize (Birbeck and Carter, 1972; Eccles and Alexander, 1974a; Wood and Gillespie, 1975). With MSV-induced sarcomas, which regress spontaneously, the proportion of macrophages has been found to be higher in regressing than in progressing tumors (Russell, Doe, and Cochrane, 1976; Russell and McIntosh, 1977), but many other tumors grow progressively despite a high macrophage content. Macrophages or monocytes isolated from growing tumors may nevertheless show antibody-independent cytotoxicity for tumor cells *in vitro,* ranging from reversible cytostasis to irreversible lysis, usually but not invariably of a non-specific kind (Evans, 1973; 1977; Evans and Alexander, 1976; Van Loveren and Den Otter, 1974; Haskill, Yamamura, and Radov, 1975; Holden *et al.,* 1976; Russell and McIntosh, 1977), and may also participate in ADCC against the cells of the tumor (Evans, 1975; Haskill and Fett, 1976).

How do tumors grow progressively despite the presence of large numbers of macrophages which, at any rate *in vitro,* are cytotoxic? One suggested explanation (Evans, 1977), based on the fact that supernatants from cultures of both cytotoxic and non-cytotoxic macrophages may stimulate the growth of normal and neoplastic cells in culture, is that the cytotoxic effect is more than counterbalanced by direct stimulation of growth, and perhaps also by stimulation of vascularization of the tumor. Another possibility, suggested by the discovery that tumor cells *in vivo* secrete substances antagonistic to macrophages (Eccles and Alexander, 1974b; Nelson and Nelson, 1978; see also James, 1977), is that the expression of macrophage cytotoxicity is abrogated by substances of this kind produced locally in the tumor. A third hypothesis, which could be investigated experimentally by comparing the susceptibility of tumors with high and low contents of cytotoxic macrophages to macrophage-mediated cytotoxicity *in vitro,* is that cell populations which are relatively unsusceptible to macrophage attack emerge during the growth of a tumor. This question will be considered further in relation to the hypothesis of surveillance (5.52).

5.44 Cytotoxicity Mediated by NK Cells

It was discovered some years ago that lymphoid cells from normal untreated mice (Herberman *et al.,* 1973b, 1974; Herberman, Nunn, and Lavrin, 1975; Kiessling, Klein, and Wigzell, 1975b), rats (Holtermann, Klein, and Casale, 1973; Nunn *et al.,* 1976; Shellam and Hogg, 1977) and humans (Oldham *et al.,* 1973; Takasugi, Mickey, and Terasaki, 1973b; Rosenberg *et al.,* 1974) may be significantly cytotoxic *in vitro* for syngeneic and allogeneic tumor cells, and that the level of cytotoxicity in rodents depends on age, genetic background, and some not very clearly defined environmental factors (see Herberman and Holden, 1978). The cells which mediate this effect are generally referred to as *natural killer cells* or NK cells, and it has been shown that they may also be cytotoxic for cells infected with viruses and other agents, and some normal cells, notably thymocytes from young mice and bone marrow stem cells (see Cudkowicz and Hochman, 1979; Kiessling and Wigzell, 1979). In mice almost all studies of NK cell activity have been based on short-term ^{51}Cr-release assays, but in studies with rat and human cells both short-term and long-term assays (5.226) have been used, and recently Roder and Kiessling (1978) have developed a rosetting test, using mouse lymphoid cells and NK-susceptible target cells, which correlates well with the cytotoxic test.

The discussion which follows is based to a considerable extent on recent reviews by Herberman and Holder (1978) and Kiessling and Wigzell (1979).

5.441   NK-CELL ACTIVITY IN MICE

The mouse NK cell expresses H-2 K and D antigens, but has not been shown to possess surface Ig, Ia antigens, or complement (C3) receptors (see Kiessling and Wigzell, 1979), and is not lysed by antimacrophage serum plus complement (Ojo, Haller, and Witzell, 1978). It also lacks the Ly-1, Ly-2, and Ly-3 antigens which distinguish subclasses of T cells, but expresses one of two alleles coded for by another locus of the Ly system termed Ly-5 (Cantor *et al.,* 1979), and other antigens coded for by genes of a system termed Nk-1, the polymorphism of which, however, does not appear to be related to NK-cell function (Cantor *et al.,* 1979). It is generally held to lack the Thy 1 (θ) antigen characteristic of mature T cells, though Herberman, Nunn, and Holden (1978) have reported that a low density of this antigen can be demonstrated by repeated treatment with antiserum plus rabbit complement. The presence of Fc receptors is disputed, but the fact that NK cells can function as K cells in ADCC (5.225) would seem to indicate that these are present, although they appear to be of low avidity (Ojo and Wigzell, 1978).

Since lysis is the final step in a series of events which begins with recognition, Roder and Kiessling (1978) have developed a rosetting assay to assess the recognition phase. This has revealed two populations of cells which bind to NK-sensitive targets in the lymphoid tissues of non-immunized mice, but which differ in their capacity to adhere to nylon wool columns. The non-adherent cells, which have the appearance of small lymphocytes and do not show phosphatase or esterase activity, bind selectively to, and are able to kill a wide range of NK-susceptible tumor cell targets, but killing does not occur if binding is prevented by the addition of EDTA, and can also be prevented by sonicates of the target cells. The level of non-adherent cells correlates with NK activity, and is controlled by dominant genes linked to the H-2 region. The nylon adherent cells do not kill the target cells to which they are attached, and their level shows poor correlation with NK activity.

The level of NK activity has been found, both by lysis and by rosetting, to be highest in cells of the peripheral blood and the spleen, lower in lymph nodes, lower again in bone marrow, and absent in thymocytes (Kiessling *et al.,* 1975b), but, as Kiessling and Wigzell (1979) suggest, this may depend not only on the number of accessible NK cells but also on the presence or absence of other cells which suppress or augment NK activity. In the spleen, activity is maximal at the age of 6 to 8 weeks (Kiessling *et al.,* 1975a). The activity is typically greater in congenitally athymic (nude) mice than in the corresponding normal mice (Kiessling *et al.,* 1975b). It has been convincingly argued by Haller *et al.* (1977c) that mouse NK cells develop from a precursor cell in bone marrow, since lethally irradiated mice rescued with syngeneic marrow from mice of different ages, or allogeneic marrow from H-2 compatible mice, soon developed levels of NK activity characteristic of the marrow donor, although the marrow cells themselves showed little NK activity. B cells do not appear to be of any importance for the maturation of NK cells, since administration of IgM to mice from birth onwards, which markedly depresses B-cell numbers and function, has no effect on NK activity (Gidlund *et al.,* 1979).

In the light of the high level of NK activity in nude mice, and the discovery that such mice possess a plentiful supply of T-cell precursors (Pritchard and Micklem, 1973; Scheid *et al.,* 1973), it has been suggested by Herberman and Holden (1978) that the NK cell may be a precursor T cell which has not been processed in the thymus. This gains support from the fact that the Ly-5 gene product, which, as mentioned earlier, is expressed on NK cells, is also expressed on T cells (Komuro *et al.,* 1975) but not on mature B cells or macrophages. An alternative explanation of the high NK activity in nude mice considered by Herberman and Holden is that NK cells are non-T cells which are modulated by suppressor T cells, but they regard this as unlikely because they have shown that the NK activity of lymphoid cells from normal mice is not increased by specific depletion of T cells, nor is the high activity of nude mouse spleen cells decreased by adding normal spleen cells.

The recognition mechanism underlying NK cell-mediated cytotoxicity has not been elucidated, but, whatever its nature, it does not appear to be subject to H-2 restriction (5.323), since allogeneic and semisyngeneic target cells are lysed as readily as syngeneic targets (Herberman, Nunn, and Lavrin, 1975; Kiessling *et al.,* 1975c). NK cytotoxicity is blocked by anti-Ly-5 serum in the absence of complement, suggesting that the product of the Ly-5 gene is involved in the cytotoxic process (Cantor *et al.,* 1979). A further difference between killing by T cells and NK cells is that with T cells energy appears to be required for both binding and lysis, whereas with NK cells it is required for lysis only (see Kiessling and Wigzell, 1979). Herberman and Holden refer to the structures recognized by NK cells as antigens, but this seems unjustified at the present time. It was suggested by Herberman, Nunn, and Lavrin (1975) that NK cell activity is directed against C-type virus components expressed on the tumor cell surface because with various tumors they observed a correlation between NK sensitivity and release of endogenous C-type virus by the tumor cells. This hypothesis gained support from blocking experiments using cells of tumors associated with C-type virus (Herberman, Nunn, and Lavrin, 1975; Sendo *et al.,* 1975) or viral envelope glycoprotein (Lee and Ihle, 1977), but it now seems too restrictive in the light of reports that there appears to be no correlation between the expression of C-type cell surface virus proteins by various mouse lymphomas and their sensitivity to NK cell lysis (Becker, Fenyö, and Klein, 1976) and no consistent difference in the NK-cell sensitivity of human cell lines before and after infection with xenotropic mouse C-type virus (Kiessling *et al.,* 1978). Moreover, although tumors differ greatly in their susceptibility to lysis by NK cells, and in general tumors maintained *in vivo* are less susceptible than those maintained *in vitro* (Kiessling, Nunn, and Lavrin, 1975), it has recently been shown that some tumors which were thought to be completely insen-

sitive may be lysed by NK cells from animals treated with an interferon inducer, tilerone (Gidlund *et al.*, 1978), and it is conceivable that all tumors are susceptible to
some extent.

It has been claimed by Hcrbcrman, Nunn, and Lavrin (1975), as a result of inhibition assays, that NK cells are heterogeneous in the sense that particular clones recognize and lyse only a restricted range of NK-susceptible targets. Similar experiments
by Kiessling and Wigzell (1979), together with attempts to remove specific clones on
tumor cell monolayers, however, do not support this conclusion, and suggest that
mouse NK cells in general express one single specificity. These divergent views are
also reflected in the fact that work from Klein's laboratory (see Kiessling and Wigzell,
1979) points to the conclusion that the *relative* NK activity of different mouse strains
is independent of the target cells used, whereas work from Herberman's laboratory
(Herberman and Holden, 1978) points to the opposite conclusion.

Reference has already been made to the possible role of NK cells in allogeneic
inhibition (5.41) and rejection of parental bone marrow by F1 hybrids (5.42). This is
suggested (Kiessling *et al.*, 1977; Lotzová and Savary, 1977) by similarities between
these phenomena and non-T-cell rejection of tumors in respect of the distribution of
the effector cells in the various lymphoid tissues, the maturation of activity during the
fourth week of life, and the inhibition of activity by administration of rabbit anti-
mouse bone marrow serum or the bone-seeking radioactive isotope ^{89}Sr. One difference
has, however, been observed, namely, inhibition of NK activity, but not of hybrid resistance to parental marrow, by administration of cortisone (Hochman and
Cudkowicz, 1977).

NK activity in both normal and nude mice may be increased by prior inoculation
of tumor cells (Herberman *et al.*, 1977), allogeneic bone marrow (Herberman *et al.*,
1977), BCG (Wolfe, Tracey, and Henny, 1976; Herberman *et al.*, 1977), *C. parvum*
when given intraperitoneally (Herberman *et al.*, 1977; Ojo *et al.*, 1978a) but not intravenously (Savary and Lotzová, 1978; Ojo *et al.*, 1978a), Poly I:Poly C and Poly
A:Poly U (Gidlund *et al.*, 1978), and tilerone (Gidlund *et al.*, 1978). It has been suggested that all these agents stimulate NK activity by inducing interferon (Gidlund *et
al.*, 1978). Since tilerone greatly increases lysis but has no effect on the number of cells
which bind to NK-susceptible targets, it seems likely that interferon acts by increasing
the lytic potential of individual NK cells (Kiessling and Wigzell, 1979). It is noteworthy that the response of mice of different strains to interferon inducers varies considerably, but NK activity may be boosted by interferon even in a strain (AKR) which
does not respond to tilerone (Gidlund *et al.*, 1978).

NK-cell activity has been reported to be decreased temporarily in varying degree
by administration of silica (Lotzová, Gallagher, and Trentin, 1975), carageenan and
hydrocortisone (Cudkowicz and Hochman, 1979), *C. parvum* when given intravenously (Savary and Lotzová, 1978; Ojo *et al.*, 1978a), cyclophosphamide (Djeu, 1978), and,
in some strains, heterospecific anti-NK-cell serum (Glimcher, Shen, and Cantor,
1977). More prolonged inhibition follows irradiation of the bone marrow by ^{89}Sr. It
has been shown moreover (Cudkowicz and Hochman, 1979) that the spleens of infant
mice with low NK activity, and of mice treated with carageenan, hydrocortisone, or
^{89}Sr, contain suppressor cells which, when mixed with NK cells of high activity from
other mice, inhibit their cytotoxic effect. In these experiments two types of suppressor
cell were identified: a macrophage-like cell in mice treated with carageenan or hydrocortisone, and non-adherent cells in the spleens of infant and irradiated adult mice.

raises the question of whether NK cells are simply K cells which have been armed *in vitro* with natural antibodies. This hypothesis is considered unlikely by Kiessling and Wigzell (1979) because depletion of B cells has no apparent effect on NK activity, and suspensions of NK cells, freed as far as possible of T and B cells, which lose activity temporarily when treated with proteolytic enzymes recover when incubated at 37°C for 4 hours in the absence of such enzymes (Roder and Kiessling, 1978), but cannot be regarded as definitely excluded.

5.442   NK-CELL ACTIVITY IN OTHER SPECIES

Although NK-cell activity has been investigated most thoroughly in the mouse, there have been a number of studies in other species, notably in the rat and in man.

Rat NK cells, like those of the mouse, are non-adherent and non-phagocytic. They are the size of small lymphocytes, are moderately radiosensitive (Shellam, 1977), and lack the surface markers of mature T cells (Nunn *et al.,* 1976; Shellam, 1977; Oldham, Ortaldo, and Herberman, 1977) and surface Ig (Shellam, 1977). Absence of complement and Fc receptors has also been reported (Nunn *et al.,* 1976; Oldham *et al.,* 1977), but more recently Oehler *et al.* (1978a) have succeeded in demonstrating Fc receptors. Reactivity is abolished by treating the cells with papain but recovers on incubation at 37°C for 4–5 hours in the absence of enzyme (Shellam, 1977). NK-cell activity is greatest in the spleen and lymph nodes; peripheral blood lymphocytes and peritoneal exudate cells show some activity, and there are conflicting reports concerning the activity of thymocytes (see Herberman and Holden, 1978).

It was found by Shellam and Hogg (1977) that rat tumors induced by Gross or Moloney leukemia virus were susceptible to lysis by NK cells, whereas polyoma virus-induced tumors, non-viral tumors, and normal adult and fetal cells were not susceptible; it remains to be seen, however, whether apparently insensitive tumor cells can be lysed by NK cells from donors in which NK activity has been boosted experimentally. As with mouse tumors, cultured cells are in general more susceptible than cells from ascites tumors maintained *in vivo* (Shellam and Hogg, 1977).

Human studies have nearly all been concerned with peripheral blood lymphocytes; recently, however, Herberman and his colleagues have demonstrated activity in spleen cells, but little or no activity in cells from lymph nodes, tonsil, and thymus (see Herberman and Holden, 1978). As with other species, human NK cells are non-adherent and non-phagocytic (Hersey *et al.,* 1975; Peter *et al.,* 1975c; West *et al.,* 1977).

There are divergent views as to whether or not human NK cells possess T-cell markers (see Herberman and Holden, 1978). Although various authors claim that they do not, Saksela *et al.* (1979) concluded from cytotoxicity assays, and studies of cells eluted from Degalan beads coated with target cells and exposed to blood lymphocytes, that NK activity in human blood is mediated by large lymphocytes with cytoplasmic granules which form rosettes with sheep erythrocytes and possess esterases of a kind possessed by T cells; the possibility that a medium-sized lymphocyte might play a subsidiary role, however, was not excluded. In these experiments the targets were either human fetal fibroblasts or established human cell lines. The effector cells appeared to be of two kinds. One kind, which possessed high-avidity Fc receptors, killed both fetal fibroblasts and cell line targets; the other kind, which possessed fewer or less avid Fc receptors, did not kill fetal fibroblasts unless they had previously been exposed to cell line targets—a procedure which has been shown to result in the production of interferon—or interferon was added to the cultures.

The role of interferon has been studied in detail by Santoli and his colleagues

(Trinchieri and Santoli, 1979; Santoli and Koprowski, 1979). They have reported that, while viruses, virus-infected cells, and most tumor-derived cell lines stimulate lymphocytes to produce interferon, which *inter alia* enhances NK-cell activity, and NK cells can lyse not only neoplastic and virus-infected but also normal cells, interferon exerts a protective action on normal cells. This protection, they suggest, occurs not only *in vitro* but also *in vivo.*

There is also a divergence of views as to whether human NK cells all recognize the same targets or whether they are heterogeneous in this regard (see Herberman and Holden, 1978). Takasugi *et al.* (1977) have obtained evidence which suggests that the truth lies somewhere between complete non-selectivity and marked heterogeneity, and that most NK cells recognize one of two or possibly three targets, which they call TA1, TA2, and TA3, which are widely distributed on human tumor cells. There is also evidence that human NK cells may recognize and lyse some mouse tumor cells (Petranyi *et al.,* 1974; Pross and Jondal, 1975; Haller *et al.,* 1977b).

There is good correlation between the NK- and K-cell activity of human peripheral blood lymphocytes, but treatment with trypsin has been reported to inhibit NK activity only (see Herberman and Holden, 1978); the role of human NK cells in ADCC must therefore be regarded as *sub judice.*

5.443   ROLE OF NK CELLS IN RESISTANCE
TO TUMORS *IN VIVO*

There is a striking similarity in the genetic control of NK activity and resistance to a variety of syngeneically transplanted tumors (Kiessling and Wigzell, 1979). While this is not proof of a causal relationship, it suggests that NK cells may be concerned in the resistance to syngeneic tumors.

This hypothesis gains support from detailed studies with the A-strain lymphoma YAC which have established that lethally irradiated thymectomized F1 hybrids of strain A and various H-2-compatible strains showing either high or low NK activity, which were rescued with parental strain bone marrow, showed good correlation between NK cell activity *in vitro* and resistance to the YAC tumor *in vivo* (Haller *et al.,* 1977a). In other studies with the YAC tumor Cantor *et al.,* (1979) found that spleen cells depleted of Thy-1-positive cells and then subjected to a procedure which selected Ly5-positive, Ig-negative cells exerted a powerful antitumor effect in Winn-type assays.

Further support is provided by the observations of Warner, Woodruff, and Burton (1977), who found that Balb/c tumors which were lysed in short-term ^{51}Cr-release assays by spleen cells from nude Balb/c mice grew more slowly in nude mice than in heterozygous (Balb/c nu/+) littermates, whereas tumors which were not lysed *in vitro* by nude mouse spleen cells did not.

Attempts have been made to assess T-cell-independent resistance to the early survival and growth of tumor cells by measuring the uptake of ^{125}IUDR in various organs 3–5 days after intravenous injection of lymphoma cells to athymic or lethally irradiated mice (Campanile *et al.,* 1977; Riccardi *et al.,* 1978a; Iorio *et al.,* 1978), and more recently by measuring the amount of isotope in the spleen, liver, and lungs 4 hours after the intravenous injection of prelabeled lymphoma cells (Riccardi *et al.,* 1978b). These studies also showed considerable correlation between resistance to the tumor and NK-cell activity; most notably, there was markedly less radioactivity recovered at 4 hours in the spleen, liver, and lungs of young mice of strains with high NK activity than in older mice or mice of strains with low NK activity (Riccardi *et al.*, 1978b; Herberman *et al.*, 1979).

Stromal cells (3.1) from human tumors have been reported to show, as a rule, little cytotoxicity for tumor cell lines known to be sensitive to NK cells (Jondal *et al.*, 1975; Vose, Vanky, and Klein, 1977b, 1977c; Vose *et al*, 1977a; Saksela *et al.*, 1979), though they may be cytotoxic for fetal fibroblasts (Saksela *et al.*, 1979) and autochthonous tumor cells (Jondal *et al.*, 1975; Vose *et al.*, 1977a, 1977b, 1977c).

The possible role of NK cells in inhibiting experimental carcinogenesis and the development of spontaneous tumors will be discussed later (5.53).

5.5 SURVEILLANCE

The question now to be considered is whether, and if so to what extent, immunological and para-immunological reactions limit the incidence and development of primary tumors, local recurrence of tumors after treatment, and metastasis.

5.51   The Hypothesis of Thomas and Burnet

The notion that the incidence of cancer is limited by homeostatic mechanisms of an immunological kind seems to have originated with Paul Ehrlich (1909). Half a century later, Lewis Thomas (1959) suggested that the rejection of allografts, which by that time was widely accepted as immunological in nature but for which no convincing evolutionary explanation had been proposed, might be the consequence of a mechanism which had evolved to meet "the universal requirement of multicellular organisms to preserve uniformity of cell type and to prevent mutant cells from colonizing and flourishing," and he went on to say, "Perhaps, in short, the phenomena of homograft rejection will turn out to represent a primary mechanism for natural defense against neoplasia."

Thomas' suggestion was elaborated by MacFarlane Burnet into what he termed the concept of immunological surveillance (Burnet, 1964, 1967, 1970a, 1970b, 1971). This concept, according to Burnet (1970b), "is a broad one but it is part of the still broader concept of internal homeostasis within the mammalian body. It is not a specifically stated hypothesis susceptible to a precise experimental test, it is rather a tentative generalization which would give some logical unity to a wide range of observable phenomena."

Despite this disclaimer, we shall refer to Burnet's "concept" as a hypothesis. This seems justifiable, firstly, because, even in its general form, as Burnet himself shows, it is not inaccessible to experimental investigation, and, secondly, because, as was perhaps inevitable at the time, Burnet committed himself explicitly to the readily testable proposition that surveillance is mediated almost solely by the thymus-dependent system of immunocytes, with antibody-producing cells, and, by implication, other categories of cell which he does not mention, playing an almost negligible role.

Burnet's hypothesis quickly became widely accepted (see Smith and Landy, 1970) because it appeared to provide a satisfactory explanation of many otherwise puzzling phenomena, including the evolution and persistence in higher animals of the capacity to reject allografts and to react immunologically to various kinds of autochthonous tumor (5.22); the age incidence of cancer (2.1) in relation to immunological status;

the occasional spontaneous regression of tumors (3.2) and the high frequency of histological features of malignancy found at autopsy in some organs, particularly the prostate, in relation to the incidence of clinical cancer; the increased incidence of some forms of cancer in congenitally immunodeficient and immunosuppressed patients; and the increased susceptibility of neonatally thymectomized mice to tumor induction by polyoma virus. The hypothesis is, moreover, consistent with the fact that many carcinogens, including cigarette smoke (see Thomas *et al.*, 1974), are immunosuppressive (see Stjernsward, 1969); and offers an explanation (Steel and Ling, 1973), though as we shall see later (5.53) not the only one, of the association of EB virus with Burkitt's lymphoma in some patients, and with a benign condition, infectious mononucleosis, in others.

What is more important than its wide acceptance, however, is that the hypothesis has generated much critical discussion, based partly on old data and partly on data which have become available since Burnet's (1970b) book was published.

5.52   Criticism and Countercriticism

Criticism of Burnet's hypothesis has been based on five main grounds (see G. Möller and E. Möller, 1976; Woodruff, 1977a):

1. Many tumors grow progressively and kill their hosts, so that either there is no such thing as effective surveillance, or the tumors that behave in this way constitute a special class of tumors which somehow manage to escape.
2. An immunological reaction against a tumor may stimulate mitosis of tumor cells.
3. The predicted higher incidence of tumors in immunodeficient animals and patients has been only very partially confirmed.
4. Many spontaneous tumors are non-immunogenic or very weakly immunogenic, including, in particular, tumors arising in cells in tissue culture or in diffusion chambers where selection against immunogenicity cannot operate.
5. The reported monoclonality of many tumors.

5.521   ESCAPE FROM SURVEILLANCE

The fact that many people and animals die of cancer does not necessarily invalidate Burnet's hypothesis.

In the first place, there may be tumors, possibly many tumors, which are destroyed before their presence is detected. The fact that active growth may be preceded by a long period in which the condition appears to merit the label *premalignant,* or takes the form of carcinoma-in-situ (3.1), is sometimes cited as evidence to the contrary, but proves only that lesions of this kind *may* develop into aggressive tumors and not that they always do.

Secondly, some tumors which grow progressively may be completely, or almost completely, devoid of antigens of the kind we have referred to as TAARIPAH (5.22); and for the rest, as the writer pointed out many years ago (Woodruff, 1964), one can postulate, and indeed demonstrate, a variety of mechanisms by which they may escape from surveillance.

The following classification of escape mechanisms, which does not claim to be either exhaustive or free of overlapping categories, includes some which have been demonstrated with animal or human tumors, and others which are postulated on theoretical grounds:

1. *The TAARIPAH behave as weak antigens,* i.e., they evoke only a weak rejection reaction.

2. *The tumor cells cease to be antigenic due to shedding of antigen or antigenic modulation (5.26).* This refers primarily to TAARIPAH, but the phenomenon of MHC restriction (5.323) raises the possibility that loss of MHC antigens (H-2 in the mouse, HLA in man, and corresponding antigens in other species) may also constitute an escape mechanism.

3. *The immunological responsiveness of the host is generally impaired* owing to the presence of the tumor (4.42) or by an oncogenic virus with immunosuppressive properties (2.3).

4. *There is specific abrogation or impairment of the immunological response to the tumor.* This may be the result of blocking by antigen, antibody, antigen-antibody complexes, or suppressor cells; sequestration of effector cells in lymph nodes while the primary tumor is *in situ* (Alexander and Hall, 1970) or in the tumor itself (Field and Caspari, 1972); failure of cytotoxic antibody, complement, and cells mediating the effector side of the immune response to gain access to the tumor owing to poor vascularization or other causes; intrinsic properties of the tumor; and a process termed *sneaking through* (*vide infra*). It may also be congenital, due to specific immunological tolerance of a vertically transmitted oncogenic virus (2.141), such as the MMTV (Morton, Goldman, and Wood, 1969), or possibly, as Laroye (1974) has suggested, to an inherited selective defect of the immune response associated with the absence of particular Ir genes.

The role of various categories of blocking factor, intrinsic properties of the tumor, and sneaking through will be considered in detail.

Blocking by antigen. Antigen released from either dead or living tumor cells competes as a target with antigen on tumor cells (Currie and Basham, 1972; Currie and Alexander, 1974; Thomson *et al.,* 1973a, 1973b, 1973c; Thomson, 1975). Evidence suggesting that this mechanism may be important has been obtained in both clinical and animal studies. The *in vitro* cytotoxicity of lymphocytes from patients with cancer for autologous tumor cells or allogeneic tumor cells of similar histological types was found by Currie and Basham (1972) to be markedly increased by washing the lymphocytes and decreased by subsequently adding serum from the patient, but not serum from normal individuals or patients with other types of tumor, to the system. The factor in the serum responsible for this effect appeared to have affinity for the effector cells but not for the target cells, suggesting that it was tumor antigen. In animals bearing isogeneic transplants of chemically induced fibrosarcomas, loss of resistance to further challenge with the same tumor was found to coincide with rising levels of circulating tumor antigen determined by radioimmunoassay (Thomson *et al.,* 1973b; Thomson, 1975).

Blocking of CMI by antibody and complexes. Blocking of CMI *in vitro* by antibody and antigen–antibody complexes has been repeatedly demonstrated with both animal (I. Hellström and K. Hellström, 1969; I. Hellström *et al.,* 1969b; K. Hellström and I. Hellström, 1971, 1974; Pearson, Redmon, and Bass, 1973; Bowen and Baldwin, 1976; Rao and Bonavida, 1977; Jennette and Feldman, 1977; Höffken *et al,* 1978) and human (I. Hellström and K. Hellström, 1971; I. Hellström *et al.,* 1971b; Cohen, Ketcham, and Morton, 1972; Höffken *et al.,* 1977) tumors, and there is evidence that the level of circulating immune complexes demonstrable by *in vitro* tests increases during the early stages of tumor growth (Bansal and Sjögren, 1973; Jennette and Feldman, 1977; Höffken *et al.,* 1978). It has also been shown in rats that the growth of isogeneic transplants of a polyoma virus-induced tumor may be enhanced by the injection of specific antiserum or tumor eluates (Bansal, Hargreaves, and Sjögren, 1972). In these last experiments the enhancement seems to have been due to either a central or an efferent type of block* because the cytotoxicity of lymphocytes from the treated animals for the tumor cells *in vitro* was unimpaired.

While these findings do not provide direct evidence that specific antibody and immune complexes inhibit cell-mediated resistance to autochthonous tumors, they do at least suggest this possibility. This suggestion gains some support from the observation of Höffken *et al.* (1977) that patients with breast cancer showed raised levels of circulating immune complexes prior to mastectomy, and that subsequent levels showed good correlation with prognosis, being high in patients with detectable residual disease and almost normal in other patients without detectable residual disease and whose prognosis was thought to be good. Since the tumor-specific nature of the complexes was not established in this investigation, however, the findings must be interpreted with caution.

We have been discussing so far blocking by antibody which reacts with tumor antigens. There is now evidence (Moroni and Schumann, 1977) that antibody directed against endogenous C-type virus may also block antitumor CMI.

Blocking of humoral immunity by antiideotype antibody. Some years ago Lewis *et al.* (1971) postulated that the disappearance of demonstrable antitumor antibody from the serum of patients with melanoma when dissemination of the tumor became apparent might be due to "a specific antibody against the tumour specific antibody," and they obtained some evidence in support of this hypothesis. This work attracted little attention at the time, but in the light of further evidence (Hartmann *et al.,* 1974; Lewis, Hartman, and Jerry, 1976), and the development of network theories of the regulation of the immune response (5.3), the possibility that antiideotype antibody plays a role in permitting tumors which are susceptible to inhibition by humoral mechanisms to escape from surveillance seems highly plausible.

Blocking by suppressor cells. It was observed many years ago by Mitchison and Dube (1955) that the growth of subcutaneous transplants of an allogeneic tumor was enhanced in C57Bl mice which received at the time of tumor transplantation an intraperitoneal injection of a large number of lymph node cells from isogeneic (C57Bl)

---

*The concept that an immunological reaction may be blocked at afferent, central, and efferent levels was introduced by Billingham, Brent, and Medawar (1956). According to their definition, afferent inhibition results from direct inactivation of antigen or some process which prevents release of antigen or its access to a seat of response; central inhibition affects the machinery of antibody formation or some equivalent immunological process; and efferent inhibition prevents the effectors of the immune reaction from exercising their function.

donors which had previously been treated by repeated injections of a cell-free tumor supernatant followed by a transplant of viable tumor tissue. Further evidence of enhancement when lymphoid cells from "immunized" donors and allogeneic tumor cells were injected at different sites or mixed together was reported from other laboratories (E. Klein and Sjögren, 1960; Batchelor and Silverman, 1962; Hutchin, Amos, and Prioleau, 1967; Irvin and Eustace, 1970, 1971; Prehn, 1972).

In retrospect these findings point to the existence of lymphocytes able to suppress the activity of other lymphocytes, but the claim that T cells can function in this way was first advanced by Gershon and Kondo (1970, 1971). Since then the capacity of suppressor T cells (T_S) to inhibit both humoral and cell-mediated immune responses has been demonstrated in many different experimental systems (see Gershon, 1975; Dutton, 1975); and the role of T_S in homeostatic regulation of the immune response (Baker, 1975), in the immunosuppression generated by the graft-versus-host reaction (Shand, 1975), and in some forms of immunological tolerance (Kölsh, Stumpf, and Weber, 1975; Nachtigal, Zan-Bar, and Feldman, 1975; Weigle et al., 1975) has been more clearly delineated.

Evidence from various sources points to the ability of T_S to enhance the growth of isogeneic tumors in vitro and in vivo.

It was reported by I. Hellström et al. (1976) that lymphocytes from tumor-bearing mice did not kill cells of the tumor in question if they had previously been cultured with tumor cells for 6 days, whereas they did if tested without being cultured with tumor cells, or if they had been cultured together for only 3 days. Mixtures of lymphocytes from tumor-bearing mice which had been cultured with tumor cells for 6 days, and lymphocytes from tumor-bearing mice which had not been cultured in this way, were not cytotoxic, suggesting that some suppressor cell function was involved.

Treves et al. (1974) showed that T cells from mice bearing a syngeneic tumor could suppress the resistance of other syngeneic mice to the same tumor.

Umiel and Trainin (1974) showed local growth of the Lewis lung carcinoma after subcutaneous inoculation was more rapid, and metastases were more numerous, if the spleen cells from mice which had been inoculated with the same tumor 2 weeks previously were mixed with the tumor cell inoculum, whereas spleen cells from untreated donor mice had no such effect. Further experiments using spleen cells from thymectomized, irradiated mice repopulated with either syngeneic thymocytes or syngeneic bone marrow strongly suggested that the cells responsible for the enhancement were thymus derived. More recently, Small and Trainin (1976) have succeeded in separating lymphoid cells from mice immunized with a syngeneic tumor into two fractions, one of which enhanced, and the other inhibited, the growth of transplants of this tumor in other mice.

Intrinsic properties of the tumor.   The tumor cells may be resistant *ab initio* to destruction by humoral or cell-mediated mechanisms, or cells which are susceptible to immunological destruction may be replaced by a clone of resistant cells.

It seems likely that the emergence of clones which are resistant to natural or therapeutic attack constitutes a major escape mechanism. The progress which has occurred in recent years in elucidating and preventing the development of antibiotic resistance in bacteria suggests that more intensive study of the development of resistant tumor cells might prove rewarding and might lead to the development of methods of preventing this from happening.

Sneaking through. The term *sneaking through* was coined to describe a phenomenon first observed by Old *et al.* (1962), namely, the growth of an isogeneic tumor transplant from a small cell inoculum when a larger inoculum of the same tumor was destroyed. When applied to an autochthonous tumor it implies that this has survived for essentially the same reason—whatever that may be. Old *et al.* suggested that a small inoculum succeeds because the immune response develops slowly and the tumor becomes established, and relatively invulnerable, before the host defences are effectively mobilized. There is thus, as G. Klein (1966b) put it, a discrepancy in timing which happens to favor the tumor rather than the host. Sneaking through thus seems akin to the persistence of an allograft despite the rejection of a subsequent allograft of the same kind, a phenomenon first reported by Ehrlich (1906) in relation to tumor allografts and named by Bashford *et al.* (1908a, 1908b) *concomitant immunization.* This, however, may not be the whole story because, as Prehn and Lappé (1971) have pointed out, a small inoculum may sometimes favor tumor survival even in preimmunized recipients.

Some years ago the writer (Woodruff, 1959), in discussing concomitant immunity and related phenomena, introduced the term *graft adaptation.* This was used in a purely operational sense; in particular, it did not imply, though it did not necessarily exclude, a stable, heritable change in the antigenic constitution of the cells of the graft. While such changes were considered unlikely in allografts of normal tissues, they may well occur in rapidly expanding tumor cell populations, and may be one way, perhaps indeed the main way, in which sneaking through occurs.

Whatever the explanation, it may be, as G. Klein (1966b) has suggested, that sneaking through, though the least spectacular, is the most important escape mechanism.

5.522 IMMUNOSTIMULATION

In 1971 Prehn put forward what he termed an immunostimulation theory of tumor development, according to which "although specific immune reactivity may sometimes be adequate to control a neoplasm, lesser degrees of immune reactivity may promote the growth of nascent tumors" (Prehn, 1971; Prehn and Lappé, 1971). This was proposed as "complementary rather than antithetical" to the hypothesis of immunological surveillance, but as it has developed (Prehn, 1972, 1976b, 1977) it has led Prehn to ask whether tumors, and in particular tumors of low immunogenicity, grow *because* of the immune response of the host, and to call into question "the more widely held assumption concerning the efficacy of immunological surveillance."

Prehn cites many observations of his own and of others which support his claim that, under certain conditions, specific antibody (Shearer, 1973; Biddle, 1976) and sensitized lymphocytes (Fidler, 1973) can stimulate tumor target cells, and that immunostimulation may be followed by progressive growth of a tumor and death of the host (Jeejeebhoy, 1974). But is this outcome inevitable? This question is not discussed by Prehn, but it merits serious consideration. The writer does not know of any decisive evidence to justify a negative answer, but it would seem unwise to ignore this possibility in the light of the discovery by Heslop and Little (1976) that rat skin grafts transplanted across an H-Y barrier, i.e., from male donors to female recipients of the same inbred strain, which evoke a weak immunological reaction show early evidence of immunostimulation manifested by much greater proliferation of epidermal cells and dermal fibroblasts than occurs in strictly isogeneic (female to female) grafts, but are always eventually rejected (median survival 50 days, range 27 to 130 days), whereas the isogeneic grafts survive indefinitely.

Insofar as immunostimulation enhances tumor growth it might be expected that under certain conditions growth would be retarded in immunodeficient hosts. As will be seen in the next section (5.523), this prediction has been confirmed, but the findings can also be explained, and in some cases more readily explained, in other ways.

5.523　TUMORS ARISING IN IMMUNODEFICIENT HOSTS

In this section we shall examine the effect of oncogenic viruses and chemicals, and the incidence of spontaneous tumors, in thymectomized, ALS-treated, and congenitally athymic animals, and the incidence of tumors in patients suffering from congenital immunodeficiency or subjected to prolonged treatment with immuno-suppressive drugs.

The use of athymic mice in this and other fields of immunology stems from the discovery by Pantelouris (1968) that a hairless mutant mouse, which had been de-scribed a year or two previously by Flanagan (1966) and shown to be dependent on an autosomal recessive gene (nu), lacked a thymus, and the subsequent development by backcrossing of inbred mice bearing the nu gene on a variety of genetic back-grounds.*

An essential property of these so-called nude mice is that they show virtually no evidence of any functional activity attributable to T cells, although they possess T-cell precursors and also cells bearing the Thy 1 (θ) antigen, albeit in low density (Raff and Wortis, 1970; Raff, 1973; Loor and Roelants, 1974; Loor et al., 1975); observa-tions on the incidence of tumors might therefore be expected to provide important, and perhaps decisive, evidence for or against the hypothesis of T-cell mediated sur-veillance. In the event, however, the nude mouse, though an important witness, has not entirely resolved the controversy.

Viral oncogenesis.　Neonatal thymectomy increases the susceptibility of both rats (Vandeputte et al., 1963; Vandeputte and De Somer, 1965) and mice (J.F.A.P. Miller, Ting, and Law, 1964; Mori, Nomoto, and Takeya, 1964) to oncogenesis by polyoma virus. Moreover, C57B1 mice, which are normally highly resistant to oncogenesis even when inoculated with polyoma virus at birth but become susceptible as a result of neo-natal thymectomy, become resistant again if, after thymectomy, they are given an in-jection of syngeneic adult spleen cells (Law, 1965). Repeated administration of ALS† beginning at or just before the time of inoculation of polyoma virus has a similar effect to neonatal thymectomy in mice (Allison and Law, 1968) and an even greater effect in rats (Vandeputte, 1968). More recently it has been reported that congenitally athy-mic nude mice *(cide infra)* are highly susceptible to polyoma virus oncogenesis

---

　　*An authoritative account of the discovery, physiology, and husbandry of these mice, and of their use in various fields of research, will be found in Fogh and Giovanella (1978). Nude mice are sometimes derived from (nu/+)×(nu/+) matings. As Stutman (1978) has pointed out, the non-nude progeny then include both heterozygous nu/+ mice, and are phenotypically similar +/+ mice which lack the nude gene, and the term heterozygous littermates is sometimes loosely applied to both nu/+ and +/+ raised in this way. It is preferable to obtain litters consisting solely of nu/nu and nu/+ by mating male nu/nu and female nu/+.

　　†ALS is used to include heterologous antisera raised with thymocytes (referred to by some authors as ATS) as well as those raised with lymphocytes from blood, thoracic duct lymph, spleen, or lymph nodes.

Allison, Monga, and Hammond, 1974; Stutman, 1975a). Neonatal thymectomy and treatment with ALS have also been reported to increase the incidence of tumors in mice inoculated with adenovirus type 12 (Allison, Berman, and Levy, 1967).

The incidence of lymphomas* in response to Moloney leukemia virus (MLV) is also increased by injection of ALS starting before inoculation of the virus (Allison and Law, 1968; Law and Chang, 1971). Similar results have been reported with Gross leukemia virus (Vredevoe and Hays, 1970). In their early experiments, Allison and Law (1968) found that the majority of tumors in the ALS-treated mice were reticulum cell sarcomas which developed at the site of ALS injection; later, however, Law and Chang (1971) reported an increased incidence of leukemia. The incidence of lymphomas in response to Moloney leukemia virus is not increased by thymectomy (Moloney, 1962), nor are nude mice susceptible to Gross and Moloney virus-induced leukemia; this, however, is not surprising in view of the fact that T lymphocytes are the main target for transformation by these viruses (Allison, 1977a).

Normal adult mice inoculated with Moloney sarcoma virus (MSV), as we have seen (5.312), develop sarcomas which frequently undergo spontaneous regression. The proportion of progressively growing tumors is greater in young mice (Fefer, McCoy, and Glynn, 1967; Law, Ting, and Stanton, 1968) and in mice immunosuppressed by irradiation (Fefer et al., 1967) cortisol (Schachat, Fefer, and Moloney, 1968), cyclophosphamide (Fefer, 1969), ALS (Law, Ting, and Allison, 1968) or thymectomy (Law, Ting, and Stanton, 1968; East and Harvey, 1968). The effect of thymectomy can be reversed by grafting isogeneic thymus to a site beneath the kidney capsule, but not by a thymus graft enclosed in a diffusion chamber which prevents the escape of cells (Collavo et al., 1974); it seems clear therefore that T lymphocytes are necessary for regression to occur. Confirmatory evidence is provided by the discovery that tumors develop earlier in nude mice inoculated with MSV and never regress (Stutman, 1975b).

While, as we have seen (vide supra), the non-susceptibility of athymic mice to viral leukemogenesis can be attributed to the dearth of target cells, this cannot explain the reduced incidence of mammary carcinomas in neonatally thymectomized mice bearing the MMTV, first reported by Martinez (1964). Subsequent experiments (Yunis et al., 1969) have shown that the effect of thymectomy is reversed by transplantation of thymus from compatible MMTV-positive or -negative donors, and of spleen cells from MMTV-negative, but not from MMTV-positive donors. In the light of these findings, Yunis et al. have postulated that the development of mammary carcinomas in MMTV-positive mice is due not to tolerance of the virus, as has sometimes been suggested, but to breakdown of tolerance permitting the development of an immunological situation which somehow favors tumor development. This suggestion, which antedates Prehn's theory of immunostimulation (5.522), would seem to merit further investigation.

Chemical oncogenesis. Studies of the effect of neonatal thymectomy and administration of ALS on chemical carcinogenesis have yielded conflicting results. According to some reports neonatal thymectomy hastens the appearance of skin tumors in response to topical application of benzpyrene (J.F.A.P. Miller, Grant, and Roe, 1963;

---

*As stated in the Preface, the term lymphoma is used throughout the book to include lymphatic leukemia as well as solid lymphomas.

Grant, Roe, and Pike, 1966) and dibenzanthracene (S. Johnson, 1968b), of sarcomas in response to intramuscular injection of methylcholanthrene (Grant and Miller, 1965; S. Johnson, 1968a), and of mammary tumors in response to dimethylbenzanthracene (S. Johnson, 1968b), but Balner and Dersjant (1966) and Allison and Taylor (1967) found on the other hand that this procedure had little effect on methylcholanthrene oncogenesis. It was reported by Woods (1969) that administration of ALS hastened the development of tumors in the hamster cheek pouch following topical application of dimethylbenzanthracene and also increased the number of tumors. Moreover, Balner and Dersjant (1969), Cerilli and Treat (1969), and Rabbat and Jeejeebhoy (1970) all reported that the susceptibility of mice to methylcholanthrene oncogenesis was increased by administration of ALS, but this was not confirmed by J.C. Fisher, Davis, and Mannick (1970) or Wagner and Haughton (1971). The incidence and latent period for the development of tumors in response to subcutaneous injection of weight-adjusted doses of methylcholanthrene at birth or 30 days of age has been reported to be the same in athymic nude mice, whether derived from heterozygous [(nu/nu)×(nu/+)] or homozygous [(nu/nu)×(nu/nu)] matings, as in immunologically normal controls (Stutman, 1974, 1979). This has also been found to be the case with germ-free nude mice which, at the age of 4 to 8 weeks, received subcutaneous implants of millipore membrane impregnated with methylcholanthrene dissolved in molten paraffin wax (Outzen *et al.*, 1975). When methylcholanthrene was administered in low dosage to older "conventional" nude mice, the incidence of tumors was lower than in normal mice of the same age (210 or 360 days).

Spontaneous animal tumors.   Sanford *et al.* (1973) found that neonatal thymectomy did not alter the overall incidence of tumors in Balb/c mice, though there appeared to be a wider variety of tumors in the thymectomized animals with a lower incidence of mammary and pulmonary tumors.

Simpson and Nehlsen (1971) studied the incidence of tumors in mice which received a subcutaneous injection of rabbit anti-mouse ALS or normal rabbit serum (NRS) and in untreated control mice. Tumors developed in 54 of 130 mice which received ALS but in neither of the other groups. Two of the tumors were lymphomas, but the other 52, comprising mammary and renal carcinomas, osteosarcomas, and mixed salivary tumors, were attributed to the accidental presence of polyoma virus in the ALS. Hattan and Cerilli (1971), however, observed four reticulum cell sarcomas, of which three were at the site of ALS injection, in 28 mice which received injections of ALS and rat antigenic tissue extract over a period of more than 100 days and which carried surviving rat skin grafts.

Studies of the incidence of spontaneous tumors in athymic nude mice have been complicated by the fact that, unless special precautions are taken to avoid infection, the life span of these mice is much shorter than that of normal mice, averaging in different colonies from a week or two to between 3 and 6 months. It may therefore be of little significance that only one spontaneously developing tumor—a lymphoma detected in a 156-day-old host—has been reported in nude mice reared under conventional conditions (Custer *et al.*, 1973). Under specific pathogen-free (SPF) conditions the life span is commonly 8–10 months and may be considerably longer. Rygaard and Povlsen (1974a, 1974b, 1976), in a large study of 15,700 nude mice observed for an average period of 4.3 months, did not find any spontaneously occurring tumors and argued that this provided strong grounds for rejecting Burnet's hypothesis. Under germ-free conditions, however, where the survival of nudes approached that of normal mice, Outzen *et al.* (1975) recorded 22 lymphoreticular tumors, which appeared after a mean latent period of 57 weeks, but no other tumors in a population of 261 germ-free nudes (Balb/c background) as against a total of 2 lymphomas among 308 germ-free heterozygous littermates. At first sight this strongly suggests that the incidence of lymphomas is higher in nude mice than in non-nude mice provided that they live long enough. Stutman (1978) has pointed out, however, that the reported incidence of lymphomas in normal Balb/c mice ranges from 1 to over 20 percent, and that in the absence of more information concerning the degree of inbreeding of the mice used by Outzen *et al.* it would be unwise to conclude that a real difference in incidence exists. His own very carefully controlled studies suggest that "the incidence and type of spontaneous tumor development in nude mice is basically comparable to that of the immunologically normal controls, and that it follows rather strictly the tumor incidence and type which is observed in the inbred strain into which the nude gene has been inserted."

Tumors in children with primary immunodeficiency disease. The incidence of malignant neoplasms in children and young adults with primary immune deficiency disease is 100 or more times greater than the incidence in children of the general population, and all the main forms of primary immune deficiency disease, namely, sex-linked (Bruton's) agammaglobulinemia, isolated deficiencies, severe combined immunodeficiency, Wiskott-Aldrich syndrome, ataxia telangiectasia, and common variable late-onset immunodeficiency, contribute to this increase (see Kersey, Spector, and Good, 1973a, 1973b; Good, 1975, 1977; World Health Organization, 1978). The distribution of tumor types in children with primary immunodeficiency, however, differs markedly from that seen in the general population. Thus among patients recorded in the immunodeficiency registry, 67 percent had lymphoreticular tumors and 25 percent had leukemia, whereas the corresponding figures derived from death certificates of over 29,000 children in the United States were 8 percent lymphoreticular tumors, 48 percent leukemia, and 44 percent other tumors. The distribution of subgroups of lymphoreticular tumors is also abnormal, 78 percent in the immunodeficient patients being B-cell tumors as compared with about 18 percent in the general population (see Good, 1975, 1977).

Tumors in immunosuppressed organ transplant recipients. Tumors in organ transplant recipients may have been present, though as a rule unrecognized, as primary tumors or metastases, or be transmitted in the transplant, or arise *de novo* after the transplant operation.

No firm conclusion concerning the effect of organ transplantation and immunosuppression on residual cancer can be drawn from the data available. Patients with carcinoma of a solitary kidney treated by nephrectomy and renal transplantation may die of metastatic disease within a few weeks or months, or after many years in which there is no clinical evidence of residual disease; they may also die as the result of graft failure or other cause and show no evidence of residual tumor at autopsy. Prolonged survival with eventual death from metastases is illustrated by a patient of the writer's (Woodruff *et al.,* 1976), referred to previously (3.2), who remained well and clinically free of residual tumor for 7 years after nephrectomy and renal transplantation for a huge hypernephroma in his only kidney, and then developed obvious metastases and died within a few months. It seems therefore that renal transplantation and immunosuppression does not necessarily cause rapid growth of residual tumor, but the number of cases is too small to permit a comparison to be made of the incidence and behavior of metastases after nephrectomy for hypernephroma in transplant recipients and patients with a remaining functioning kidney. Moreover, even if such a comparison could be made, it would be necessary to determine whether or not the immunosuppressive drugs had any direct effect on the tumor before valid conclusions could be drawn. No such comparison is possible in the case of patients with primary malignant hepatoma, since if total hepatectomy is performed the patient will necessarily be given a transplant. In Starzl's series, 25 of 40 patients followed postoperatively for 2 to 90 months developed locally recurrent or metastatic disease, and this sometimes progressed very rapidly (Starzl, 1969; Penn, 1978); one of Calne's patients, on the other hand, who survived for 5 years died of cholangitis, and no residual tumor was found at autopsy (Calne, 1978).

Tumors transmitted in a transplant are of interest in relation to the time at which cancer cells become disseminated (3.34), but because they are allografts their behavior in the recipient has no direct bearing on the question of immunological surveillance.

Reports of lymphomas of a particular kind developing in kidney transplant recipients began to appear in 1968 and 1969 (Doak *et al.,* 1968; Penn *et al.,* 1969; Woodruff *et al.,* 1969). Since then there have been numerous reports of tumors arising *de novo* in immunosuppressed recipients of kidney, liver, and heart transplants, notably by Penn and by Hoover and Fraumeni, who have collected cases from many countries (Penn, 1970, 1974, 1978; Penn, Halgrimson, and Starzl, 1971; Penn and Starzl, 1972; Hoover and Fraumeni, 1973), by surgeons in Australia (Marshall, 1973, 1974; Sheil, 1977), and most recently by Kinlen *et al.* (1979), representing a large group of collaborators in the United Kingdom and Australia.

These studies have established that immunosuppressed organ allograft recipients have a 6 percent risk of developing tumors *de novo* at some time after transplantation, corresponding to a frequency 100 times that in the general population in the same age group (Penn, 1978). The relative frequency of tumors of different types is, however, strikingly different in the transplant patients, who show (1) a much higher incidence of non-Hodgkin's lymphomas, in particular of reticulum cell sarcoma, the incidence of which is 350 times that of the general population; (2) a high incidence of premalignant and malignant lesions of the skin, with a preponderance of squamous cell carcinomas as compared with basal cell carcinomas; (3) a high incidence of *in situ* carconoma of the cervix; and (4) a decreased incidence of carcinomas of the lung, prostate, colon, rectum, and female breast. The increase in lymphomas is remarkable not only for its magnitude but also because of the high proportion of patients showing involvement of the central nervous system, and for the short induction period, indicated by the fact that increased risk of developing a lymphoma is demonstrable within 6 months of transplantation.

Immunosuppressed non-transplant patients.   It would clearly be of interest to compare critically the incidence of tumors in immunosuppressed transplant recipients and non-transplant recipients who received immunosuppressive treatment for autoimmune and other disorders. The data available are insufficient for this purpose, but, in addition to reports of small numbers of cases, there are a few reports of larger series of personal (Symington, Mackay, and Lambert, 1977) or collected (Penn, 1978; Kinlen *et al.,* 1979) cases which, taken together, suggest that there may be some increase in the incidence of non-Hodgkin's lymphomas and skin cancers in non-transplant patients receiving immunosuppressive treatment for 3 months or longer, but that this is much less marked than in the transplant recipients. Symington *et al.,* in 133 patients treated in Australia with azathioprine (mean duration of treatment 1.9 years, mean duration of observation 3.8 years) or cyclophosphamide (mean duration of treatment 0.7 years, mean duration of observation 4.6 years), combined with steroids, observed only two skin cancers (both squamous cell carcinomas), though two more skin cancers developed after the study was closed. Kinlen *et al.* (1979), in a study of 1151 patients treated in the United Kingdom, reported four non-Hodgkin's lymphomas as against an expectation of 0.28 (corresponding to a probability $p=0.0002$), and four skin cancers as against 1.80 expected ($p=0.082$). Clearly many more cases are needed, but even if these were available comparison would still be difficult because, firstly, in non-transplant patients, the level of immunosuppression is likely to have been less in consequence of a different therapeutic regime and the absence of pre-treatment uremia which may cause significant immunosuppression in patients who subsequently receive renal transplants, and secondly, in non-transplant recipients, the development of a tumor may be a consequence of the condition for which the patient was treated.

General Comment.   Various explanations of the high incidence of lymphoma in various categories of immunodepressed host have been proposed. Burnet (1976) has suggested that cells of the immune system are exceptionally prone to malignant transformation but are normally protected by a highly efficient surveillance mechanism, but this *ad hoc* addition to his hypothesis does not explain why there is no increase in the incidence of many other kinds of tumor. This objection is met by the plausible suggestion that the lymphomas concerned are of viral origin (Hirsch *et al.,* 1973), and that viral tumors are especially, or perhaps uniquely, subject to T-cell surveillance (G. Klein and E. Klein, 1977). Schwartz (1972), in a hypothesis which he said was not intended to compete with the theory of immunological surveillance but to extend it, postulated that these lymphomas were due to activation of a latent oncogenic virus, and that this was prevented in normal, but not in immunosuppressed, individuals by a mechanism dependent on feedback loops controlling the immune system. Others have suggested that the development of these tumors has nothing to do with breakdown of surveillance and attribute it to an oncogenic effect of the immunosuppressive drugs themselves, or of partial immunosuppression, combined, in the case of transplant recipients, with antigenic stimulation (see Penn, 1970).

Only a small proportion of the transplant patients who developed lymphomas had received ALS. The fact that one of these patients developed a reticulum cell sarcoma at the site of ALS injection (Deodhar *et al.,* 1969) is noteworthy in relation to the occurrence of similar tumors at the site of ALS injection in mice which also received MLV (Allison and Law, 1968) and in rats which received ALS and allogeneic tissue extract (Hattan and Cerilli, 1971), but the mechanism underlying this phenomenon has not been elucidated.

5.524 NON-IMMUNOGENIC TUMORS

It has been argued by Hewitt, Blake, and Walder (1976) that many tumors which arise spontaneously, i.e., without the deliberate administration of known oncogenic agents, in inbred laboratory animals lack demonstrable TATA (5.21) and hence that human tumors, which are also spontaneous, will be equally lacking in TATA (and *a fortiori* what we have termed TAARIPAH), and therefore will be beyond the reach of T-cell-mediated surveillance. As we have seen (5.215), however, even if the premise were completely true the conclusion would not necessarily be valid, because the antigenic structure of a tumor does not depend on whether or not it was deliberately induced but on the nature of the agents which contributed to its induction, and there is strong evidence that physical, chemical, and probably also viral oncogens, all of which may induce strongly immunogenic tumors in animals, play a considerable role in the etiology of human cancer (2.11, 2.12, 2.142).

A more plausible argument applicable to chemically induced tumors is that in animals those which develop slowly tend to be less immunogenic, as revealed by excision and rechallenge assays, than those which develop quickly (Prehn, 1975), and that human tumors such as lung cancer, which appear to be chemically induced, may not appear until many years, or even decades, after the first exposure to the carcinogen. Since there is no possibility of assessing the immunogenicity of human tumors by excision and rechallenge, the only evidence by which to judge the validity of this criticism will be that provided by the behavior of tumors in immunosuppressed patients, discussed in the previous section (5.523), and by their response to specific immunotherapy, which will be discussed in Chapter 8.

5.525 MONOCLONALITY AND IMMUNOSELECTION

While the dogma that nearly all tumors are monoclonal goes further than the evidence warrants, there are, as we have seen (3.114), good grounds for concluding that some, and possibly many, types of tumor are predominantly monoclonal. It has been claimed by G. Möller and E. Möller (1976) that this tells strongly against the immunological surveillance hypothesis.

Möller and Möller consider three possible explanations of monoclonality.

The first, namely, that carcinogens affect only rare susceptible variants, is, they argue, highly unlikely in the case of tumors induced by chemical and physical carcinogens and RNA viruses because the frequency with which transformation occurs *in vitro* is too high to be compatible with this explanation; it might, however, apply in the case of a cytopathic DNA virus like SV40.

The second possibility, that of immunoselection, they reject on the ground that it is inapplicable to any tumor whose cells all possess the same TATA, which they say is true not only of viral tumors but probably also of chemically induced tumors. In the case of non-viral tumors this generalization rests on very limited experimental evidence, but, even supposing that it is correct, the Möllers' argument is unconvincing because it fails to consider the possibility of selection of cells for properties other than the array of antigens they possess, for example, their capacity to resist destruction by immunological effector mechanisms.

Möller and Möller make the further point that if monoclonality depends on immunoselection it should not occur in tumors which develop *in vitro* or in diffusion chambers, where they are not exposed to cell-mediated immunoselection, or in immunodeficient hosts, and such tumors might be expected to be more immunogenic than those which develop in normal hosts. There is no direct evidence as to whether tumors arising in immunodeficient hosts are monoclonal or not, but this criticism gains support from reports that tumors induced *in vitro* (Heidelberger, 1973), or which develop "spontaneously" *in vitro* or in diffusion chambers (Parmiani, Carbone and

Prehn, 1971), either show the same range of immunogenicity as unprotected tumors induced *in vivo* or possess little or no immunogenicity; and it may well be, as Kieler *et al.* (1972) have suggested, that occasional reports of high immunogenicity in such tumors are due to contamination with passenger virus. It has, however, been reported that tumors induced with methylcholanthrene in thymectomized mice grow more slowly, and evoke a more intense cellular reaction, than tumors induced in normal mice, when transplanted to normal syngeneic hosts (Nomoto and Takeya, 1969), and immunoselection is the only plausible explanation proposed for Prehn's (1975) finding of an inverse relationship between the time taken for chemically induced sarcomas to appear and their immunogenicity. It would seem desirable to investigate the matter further by comparing the immunogenicity of tumors induced with a variety of agents in homozygous athymic (nu/nu) mice and their heterozygous (nu/+), T-cell-competent, littermates.

The third possible explanation of monoclonality, namely, that carcinogens only accelerate the appearance of rare genetic changes leading to neoplasia, is the one favored by Möller and Möller. There seems no reason, however, why this should be regarded as incompatible with any form of surveillance hypothesis.

5.53 A More General Hypothesis

It seems to the writer that two general conclusions may be drawn from the criticisms and countercriticisms of the immunosurveillance hypothesis which we have discussed in the preceding section (5.52).

Firstly, there are no compelling reasons for rejecting the general hypothesis that surveillance mechanisms have evolved for the elimination of cancer cells, and that these are to some extent effective.

Secondly, while T-cell-dependent mechanisms may play some part, their role is decidely more limited than was envisaged by Burnet.

We shall therefore now consider the hypothesis that surveillance involves both strictly immunological and para-immunological mechanisms, and make some suggestions concerning their respective contributions.

As G. Klein and E. Klein (1977) have argued, the data concerning the development of tumors in normal and immunosuppressed hosts (5.523) is consistent with the proposition (G. Klein, 1975b) that T-cell-mediated surveillance plays an important role in promoting the rejection of cells transformed by ubiquitous oncogenic viruses such as polyoma virus in rodents, herpes virus saumiri in monkeys, feline leukemia virus in cats, the virus of Marek's disease in chickens, and Epstein-Barr virus (2.142) in man, though non-T-cell mechanisms may also be concerned, especially perhaps in relation to feline leukemia (Essex *et al.,* 1975).

It seems reasonable to postulate also that T-cell-mediated surveillance eliminates some immunogenic tumors induced by environmental carcinogens. It seems likely that many human tumors induced by such agents escape because of the emergence of nonimmunogenic clones, but it is an open question whether many, or a few, or no tumors are successfully aborted before this happens.

It has been suggested by Rapaport (1974, 1975) that T cells which are cytotoxic for tumors may result from immunization by cross-reactive bacterial and other antigens.

A possible surveillance role for naturally occurring antibody is suggested by the discovery (Martin and Martin, 1974, 1975) that mouse sera, including sera from a-thymic nude mice, contain antibody, predominantly IgM, which, in the presence of rabbit complement, is cytotoxic for a variety of mouse lymphoid and non-lymphoid tumor cell lines.

The hypothesis that K cells (5.312), macrophages (5.43), and NK cells (5.44) are concerned in surveillance against human cancer is plausible in the light of the evidence discussed in the sections indicated that these can all promote the destruction of human tumor cells *in vitro,* and a variety of animal tumors *in vivo,* but at present one can only speculate about their relative importance. Until recently the macrophage was considered to be the strongest candidate, because the cytotoxicity of NK cells appeared to be confined to targets bearing C-type virus, but this restriction seems no longer valid (Kiessling and Wigzell, 1979). The data concerning the incidence of tumors in athymic nude mice (5.523), often cited as evidence that surveillance by T cells is a figment of the imagination, may also be interpreted as showing that, in these mice, effective surveillance may be provided by NK cells.

Insofar as para-immunological mechanisms are concerned in surveillance they seem likely to be limited by the emergence, through selection, of clones of cells resistant to the mechanism in question, and this might well be a fruitful field for investigation.

We have been considering so far surveillance in relation to the development of primary tumors. It may, however, also be postulated that surveillance operates to limit metastasis and the recurrence of tumors after partial ablation by therapy of one kind or another. This gains support, so far as metastasis is concerned, from the experimental observation of Eccles and Alexander (1975) that immunosuppressive treatment in the form of sublethal whole body x-irradiation or chronic thoracic duct drainage, initiated 1, 7, or 30 days after excision of a syngeneic sarcoma transplant and the related lymph nodes, resulted in a highly significant increase in the number of metastases which developed in the lungs; and by the fact that metastases in patients may remain dormant for years and then suddenly begin to grow rapidly (3.34). While the experiments of Eccles and Alexander suggest a T-cell-mediated mechanism, an earlier experiment (Proctor, Rudenstam, and Alexander, 1973b), in which metastasis of relatively non-immunogenic tumors was facilitated by thoracic duct drainage followed by replacement of the cells but not of the lymph, suggests that other mechanisms are also concerned. The factor in lymph which was responsible was not definitely identified, but Proctor *et al.* suggested that it might be SMAF (5.322, 5.431).

It was suggested by Prehn and Lappé (1971), and the suggestion was described by Möller and Möller (1976) as important, that immunological surveillance is a theory in which we all passionately wish to believe. If this means that many people have been attracted by the elegance and economy of the hypothesis, then it is undoubtedly true. If, however, it means, as some have taken it to mean, that our fear of cancer makes us want to believe in the theory, then it is not true. For surely no one with sufficient knowledge and understanding to grasp what the surveillance hypothesis is about can believe that, if it were proved today to be false, the statistics concerning the incidence and curability of cancer would be any different tomorrow. Polemical arguments of this kind, however, are no substitute for rigorous testing and for the generation of new hypotheses to replace those which can be shown to be false, without which there can be no scientific progress.

6
Therapeutic Implications of the Host Reaction

6.1 INTRODUCTION

The data we have been discussing concerning the host reaction to cancer have important therapeutic implications. Firstly, they suggest that the general physical and psychological state of an individual may affect his liability to develop cancer, and the course of the disease if it does appear. Secondly, they raise the question of whether conventional methods of treatment, designed primarily to attack the tumor directly, may modify the host reaction either favorably or unfavorably. Thirdly, they point to the possibility of augmenting or supplementing host resistance by immunological and para-immunological manipulations, and of using such procedures therapeutically, either alone or in conjunction with other methods of treatment which act more directly on the tumor, and possibly also prophylactically.

These considerations have prompted a reappraisal—to some clinicians an agonizing reappraisal—of current methods of treatment, and extensive study of immunotherapy in animals and also in man.

6.2 THERAPEUTIC OBJECTIVES

The ideal is to destroy a tumor completely without causing significant harm to the patient. If this is not possible, the aim should be to prolong useful and enjoyable life, and to alleviate pain and mental anguish during the terminal stage of the disease. As Rodney Smith (1970) has put it, "All of us are going to die and, travelling in the same direction through life, each one of us does indeed 'nightly pitch his moving tent a day's march nearer home.' When a patient has a serious ailment and seeks our help what we are trying to do, surely, is to see that he does not, on this journey, take some short cut he would rather avoid, and also that the terrain over which he travels shall be as smooth and as agreeable as possible." The fact that a patient dies therefore does not necessarily imply that treatment has failed; it has failed if he died prematurely or alternatively if, during its terminal stages, the patient's life became a painful and intolerable burden.

There is no valid criterion of absolute cure in any given case. It would, however, be unduly restrictive to abandon the term cure, and we shall use it in an operational way if any of the following criteria are fulfilled:

1.   The patient is alive with no clinical or laboratory evidence of recurrence n years after treatment was stopped, where n exceeds a value N such that the likelihood of future recurrence is considered to be small in the light of available data concerning recurrence (the term recurrence here includes both local recurrence and the development of recognizable metastases) in other patients with tumors of the same type.

2.   The patient died n years after treatment was stopped, where n exceeds N. During his life there was no clinical or laboratory evidence of recurrence. No autopsy was performed, but death could reasonably be attributed on clinical grounds to some cause other than recurrence of the tumor.

3.   The patient died n years after treatment was stopped, where n exceeds N. There was no evidence of recurrence while the patient was alive or at autopsy.

Opinions will differ regarding the value which should be assigned to N when applying one of these criteria to a given kind of tumor. In the writer's view it should rarely be less than 5 years and never less than 3 years. With some tumors, such as chorioncarcinoma and malignant hepatoma, sensitive biochemical or immunological markers are available for detecting recurrence (Bagshawe and Harland, 1976; Robins and Baldwin, 1977), and if these are used the value assigned to N may be reduced. The value may also be reduced with tumors such as basal cell carcinoma of the skin, which rarely recur after a long latent interval, and should be increased with tumors such as hypernephroma and carcinoma of the breast, which quite often recur late.

In assessing the cure rate of a population of patients treated in a given way the most valid procedure is that of Haybrittle (1964), namely, to determine the proportion of patients surviving when the survival curve for the patients first becomes parallel to that of an age-matched control population, since at that time the risk of death in the patient and control populations is the same.

It is important to recognize that treatment may be unsuccessful either because of failure to make proper use of available knowledge and resources, or because currently accepted methods of diagnosis and treatment are inadequate. Here, however, we need consider only failure due to inadequacy of current methods of treatment.

6.3   LIMITATIONS OF CURRENT METHODS OF TREATMENT

In this section we shall discuss the achievements and limitations of surgery, radiotherapy, chemotherapy, and endocrine manipulations in the treatment of cancer, the extent to which the host reaction contributes to the success of these procedures, and their possible deleterious effect on this reaction.

6.31   Surgical Treatment and Radiotherapy

By surgical treatment we mean excision of a primary tumor, with or without its lymphatic extensions, and of metastases, and ablation of tumors by such procedures as electrocoagulation (Crile and Turnbull, 1972), cauterization, laser beam surgery (Goldman, Siler, and Blaney, 1967), and cryosurgery (Fraser and Gill, 1967). Under the heading of radiotherapy we shall consider external ionizing irradiation and the surgical insertion of radioactive material in, or in the vicinity of, a tumor. The administration of radioactive isotopes orally or by injection will be included under the heading of chemotherapy (6.32).

The surgical approach to the treatment of cancer, insofar as it aims at cure as distinct from palliation, is, or until quite recently used to be, based on two premises: firstly, that cancer begins as a localized disease, and usually remains localized for a considerable time after the appearance of the primary tumor; and secondly, that recurrence will occur, provided the patient lives long enough, unless every cancer cell has been removed or destroyed. It follows that the possibility of increasing the proportion of patients cured depends on the development of improved methods of diagnosis that will allow for both treatment and more radical operations to be undertaken earlier.

It is a tautology to say that, if a tumor is localized and is removed completely, the patient will be cured in an absolute sense of that particular tumor. It is also an empirical fact that surgical operations are successful in many patients with cancer, and may also result in cure, in the sense in which we have defined these terms, and that delay in treatment may be disastrous. Basal cell and squamous cell carcinomas of the skin provide striking illustrations of the possibility of cure by early treatment. With cutaneous malignant melanoma it is difficult to compare survival rates reported from different centers because the prognosis varies greatly according to the type and location of the tumor and the age and sex of the patient, but the danger of delay is again apparent. The best evidence of this comes from Brisbane (Australia) where, according to Davis (personal communication), the overall age-adjusted 5 year survival in over 1100 cases reviewed in 1975 was 81.6 percent. This is much higher than figures published from other centers, or from Brisbane 4 years previously, where the corresponding figure was 69 percent (McLeod et al., 1971), and it seems likely that, as Davis has suggested, the difference is due to the fact that, in the state of Queensland, both the public and the doctors have been made aware of the danger of neglecting pigmented spots.

Timely surgical intervention also offers the best prospect for long survival or relief of symptoms to many patients with cancer in other sites including the breast, gastrointestinal tract, esophagus, lung (with the possible exception of undifferentiated tumors), kidney, and bladder. The value of surgical treatment has sometimes been questioned, particularly in respect of cancer of the breast, because, it is claimed, the outcome in any given case depends solely on the biological properties of the tumor. This nihilistic proposition, which carries the implication that delay in seeking treatment will have no effect on the outcome, appears to gain support from reports that patients may survive for many years without any treatment (Bloom, Richardson, and Harries, 1962; MacKay and Sellars, 1965), and that the prognosis is much the same in women who present within 3 months of noticing a lump in the breast or other relevant symptoms as in those who delay for a year (Bloom, 1965). The evidence concerning patients who refuse treatment is, however, of doubtful value because of the lack of histological confirmation of the diagnosis of cancer, and uncertainty concerning the extent to which tumors in this self-selected group can be regarded as representative of those in the population as a whole, and in Bloom's series the proportion of tumors regarded on histological grading as being of relatively low malignancy was significantly greater in the patients who presented late than in those who presented early. While there is no doubt of the importance of the biological properties of the tumor, the suggestion that treatment makes no difference to survival is therefore unconvincing. Formal proof that the suggestion is false could be obtained only by a prospective randomized clinical trial; in practice, as Baum (1976) has stated, no control group of untreated women with early breast cancer could possibly be included in such a trial.

Radiotherapy offers an alternative to surgical excision which is sometimes less mutilating and easier to apply. Its scope has been increased by the development of supervoltage x-ray therapy, and may perhaps be further increased by the use of radiosensitizing agents (Adams et al., 1976) and by fast neutron therapy (Caterall, Bewley, and Sutherland, 1977; Parker et al., 1977). Radiotherapy is, for example, widely used in the United Kingdom as an alternative to surgery for the treatment of squamous cell carcinoma of the lip, tongue, buccal cavity, and cervix, and in combination with simple mastectomy as an alternative to more radical surgery for carcinoma of the breast. Moreover, radical radiotherapy has improved the prognosis in Hodgkin's disease (Fairley and Freeman, 1974), even when lymph nodes in more than one region are involved, to the point where 90 percent of patients in Stages I and IIA (i.e., with disease confined to nodes on one side of the diaphragm, and not associated with general symptoms such as fever, night sweats, and weight loss) may be cured if an adequate dose of irradiation is given within a few weeks to all existing tumors (Wintrobe et al., 1974).

Despite the great achievements we have been considering, it is nevertheless becoming increasingly clear that there are limits to what can be expected from earlier diagnosis, or at any rate from earlier use of currently available diagnostic methods, and radical surgery or radiotherapy.

One reason for this limitation is that tumors may originate in, or spread locally at an early stage to, vital structures that cannot be removed without destroying not only the tumor but the patient. Improvements in technique, and developments in the surgery of replacement, have advanced the frontier a little further, but this is still often a major limiting factor with, for example, carcinomas of the pancreas, gall bladder, lung, and cerebral gliomas.

There is, however, another limitation of an even more intractable kind. This arises from the fact that, as we have seen (3.32), many tumors metastasize early, and, if widespread dissemination has occurred by the time the patient presents for treatment, part of the tumor cell population will be beyond the reach of surgery and radiotherapy. As already mentioned, the prognosis in cutaneous malignant melanoma can be improved considerably by prompt treatment of early tumors. Some patients, however, die as the result of metastases which first appear months or even years after excision of the primary tumor. It seems clear that during the interval, though apparently tumor-free, they were in fact harboring occult residual metastatic disease. The same phenomenon occurs with many other tumors. For example, about one-quarter of all patients with early (Stage I) cancer of the breast who are treated by so-called radical mastectomy, or by simple mastectomy and radiotherapy, die within 5 years of operation, and about one-quarter of the remainder within the next 5 years, and most of these deaths are due to distant metastases. With osteogenic sarcoma the situation is even worse, and the majority of patients with this tumor die from metastases irrespective of whether, or when, or where an amputation is performed, unless they are salvaged by some form of adjuvant therapy (6.322).

Radiotherapy is subject to the further limitation that the tumor must be sufficiently radiosensitive to respond to doses which the patient can tolerate. Even when confined to part of the body, irradiation may cause recognizable chromosomal damage (Kingston *et al.,* 1971) and impaired responsiveness to PHA and other mitogens (Stjernsward *et al.,* 1972; Braeman and Deeley, 1973; Campbell *et al.,* 1973) in peripheral blood lymphocytes, and also, as discussed earlier (2.11), leukemia and, in children who receive irradiation to the neck, carcinoma of the thyroid.

While there is clearly a risk of overt recurrence in patients with occult residual cancer after surgical treatment or radiotherapy, this should not be regarded as inevitable. Conversely, when treatment by surgery or radiotherapy is successful, it does not necessarily mean that every single cancer cell has been removed or destroyed in the course of the procedure. As we have seen, regression of macroscopic residual tumor after incomplete excision (3.2), and regression of metastases after apparently complete excision of the primary tumor (3.34), both occur very occasionally, and it seems reasonable to postulate that regression of occult residual tumor occurs no less, and probably more, frequently. Moreover, even if the residual cells are not all destroyed they may remain dormant throughout the rest of the patient's life. This, in the writer's view, is the justification for surgically removing overt metastases in the lung, liver, bones, brain, and other sites in selected patients when only one, or a small number, can be demonstrated, and the explanation of the success of this procedure in some patients with primary melanoma, hypernephroma, carcinoma of the colon and rectum, and other tumors (Creech, 1951; Gliedman, Horowitz, and Lewis, 1957; Brown, 1973; Leditsche, 1964; Thomford, Woolner, and Clagett, 1965; Edlich *et al.,* 1966; Johnson and Lindskog, 1967; Borrie, 1969; Gottlieb, Frei, and Luce, 1972; Cahan, 1973; Morton *et al.,* 1073; Schulten, Heiskell, and Shields, 1976).

An important and controversial question which we must now consider is whether, when a primary tumor is treated surgically or by radiotherapy, the regional lymph nodes should also be excised or irradiated, since there is evidence that lymphadenectomy may weaken immunity to syngeneic transplants of some animal tumors (B. Fisher and R. Fisher, 1972).

In theory we can distinguish four mutually exclusive possibilities:

1. The tumor is completely localized, i.e., there is no spread to lymph nodes or distant sites. All that is then required to achieve a complete cure is to excise the primary tumor completely without spilling viable cancer cells. It will make no difference so far as eliminating the tumor is concerned whether lymphadenectomy* is performed or not, though this procedure may add to the morbidity of the operation.
2. The regional lymph nodes contain viable tumor cells but are fulfilling the function ascribed to them by Virchow (3.31) of providing an effective temporary barrier to further dissemination of the tumor. The tumor may have extended locally to in-

---

*Lymphadenectomy means, literally, excision of lymph nodes. In the present discussion it will be used to denote excision of lymph nodes in relation to a tumor. The qualification *en bloc* or *block dissection* implies that an attempt is made to remove the primary tumor and its lymphatic extensions in continuity.

volve neighboring tissues, but there are no disseminated tumor cells apart from those in the regional nodes. This is the model which prompted the development around the end of the nineteenth century of "radical mastectomy" for carcinoma of the breast by Halsted (1891), block dissection of the cervical lymph nodes in patients with carcinomas of the head and neck by George Crile (Senior) (1906), block dissection of lymph nodes in patients with cutaneous malignant melanoma, based on the work of W. S. Handley (1907), and radical operations for cancer of the stomach, colon, and rectum by Robson and Moynihan (1904), Miles (1908), and other surgeons, and the subsequent development of even more extensive operations, such as the supraradical mastectomy of Urban and Baker (1952), radical esophagectomy involving block dissection of mediastinal lymph nodes, and extensive operations for cancer of the pelvic viscera.

Insofar as the primary tumor, the draining nodes, and the lymphatic connections between them are removed in continuity, the operation should completely eradicate the tumor if the model correctly represents the clinical situation. If, on the other hand, viable cells are left behind, the mechanical effect of lymphatic obstruction, resulting from removal of lymph nodes, may facilitate further dissemination (Pack, Scharnagel, and Morfit, 1945; Burn, 1973).

The following comment by Harold Ellis (1973) sets the work of Halsted and others concerned in the development of lymphadenectomy in perspective: "There is no doubt that these great pioneers made immense contributions to our understanding and management of the major killing cancers, but their teachings became enshrined like religious beliefs rather than accepted as scientific hypotheses which might be modified by further research and thought." The next model to be examined provides the basis on which these long-accepted beliefs have been challenged.

3. Spread of the tumor has extended beyond the regional lymph nodes as the result of metastasis by the bloodstream or other routes (3.3), but homeostatic mechanisms have not completely broken down. In this case the host reaction may well be increased if the tumor burden is greatly reduced by excising the primary tumor. On the other hand, insofar as the regional lymph nodes are contributing to the host reaction, their removal may well be harmful rather than beneficial, and the harmful effect may be increased if viable cells escape into the surrounding tissue in the course of the operation.

4. Spread of the tumor is as described for the previous model but homeostatic mechanisms, insofar as they exist at all, have broken down irrevocably. Under these circumstances no surgical treatment can be regarded as other than palliative.

In practice, while the situation may be only too clear in patients with locally inoperable tumors, gross involvement of lymph nodes, or manifest blood-borne metastases, it may be impossible in less advanced cases, where the choice of treatment can be crucial, to determine which model corresponds to the condition of the patient. Histological examination of lymph nodes removed in a preliminary biopsy or in the course of an operation (Cant, Shivas, and Forrest, 1975; Forrest et al., 1976) and lymphangiography (1.112) may provide evidence of lymph node metastases, and bone scans (1.112) may reveal skeletal metastases which are not evident on ordinary radiological examination, but when these and other diagnostic procedures are negative or equivocal the uncertainty remains.

Since any reasonable form of treatment will be effective if the first model represents the clinical situation, and no surgical treatment will be more than palliative if the fourth model applies, the critical question is whether to plan treatment on the basis of model two or model three.

For many years, as we have seen, surgical thinking was dominated by model two. Today we have moved from an era of dogma to an era of lively, though not always enlightened, controversy. This is perhaps most clearly illustrated by the controversy concerning the management of breast cancer.

Halsted's operation, as he himself realized, is open to the criticism that it does nothing about the supraclavicular and internal mammary nodes, which may also contain metastatic tumor. In 1898 he reported that his house surgeon, H. W. Cushing, later to become famous for his pioneering work in neurosurgery, had in three cases cleared out the anterior mediastinum (where the internal mammary nodes are located) on one side to deal with recurrent tumor, and he envisaged the possibility of undertaking this as part of the primary procedure. Many years later the concept of an extended Halsted operation was developed further by Urban (Urban and Baker, 1952; Urban, 1956; Urban and Castro, 1971), but these extensive procedures have not found favor with many surgeons.

A more serious challenge to the Halsted operation came from a radiotherapist, Robert McWhirter (1955, 1957), who persuaded, at first a few and later many, surgeons that operable breast cancer should be treated by simple mastectomy (i.e., removal of the whole breast but not the axillary or other lymph nodes), followed by radiotherapy directed to the axillary, supraclavicular, and internal mammary nodes. McWhirter based his proposal on the grounds that, in patients with operable breast cancer and involvement of the axillary lymph nodes, it appears, from the work of Andreassen and Dahl Iversen (1949), that the probability of supraclavicular node involvement also is about 33 percent, and, from the work of R. S. Handley (1952), that the probability of involvement of the internal mammary nodes is about 48 percent. This is an overall figure. As Handley (1964) reported later, the probability is greater with tumors in the inner half (51 percent) or central region (59 percent) of the breast, and less with tumors in the outer half (28 percent).

In practice, while the Halsted operation, and the pectoral-muscle-conserving modification (Patey and Dyson, 1948; Madden, Kandaloft, and Bourque, 1972), on the one hand, and McWhirter's procedure, on the other, both have their enthusiastic supporters and opponents (see, e.g., Haagensen, 1974), data from many centers, including the results of a number of clinical trials (Brinkley and Haybrittle, 1971; Wise, Mason, and Ackerman, 1971; Burn, 1974; Forrest et al., 1974; Hamilton, Langlands, and Prescott, 1974; Hayward, 1974; Crile, 1975; V. Peters, 1975), suggest that it makes little or no difference, so far as survival is concerned, which type of procedure is adopted.* Moreover, in a well-controlled double-blind trial, Paterson and Russell (1959) found that radiotherapy after radical mastectomy had no effect on survival or local recurrence rates in patients with axillary lymph node involvement, and appeared to shorten the survival of those whose nodes were not involved. It would seem therefore that minimal metastatic deposits in the supraclavicular and internal mammary nodes may remain quiescent, or even regress, after the Halsted type of procedure; or,

---

*These trials differ considerably in the extent to which they conform to the requirements laid down in section 1.113, and therefore in respect of the weight to be attached to the findings, but they all point to the same conclusion.

alternatively, that the beneficial effect of destroying metastases in the supraclavicular and internal mammary nodes in some patients by irradiation is counterbalanced by the harmful effect of destroying reactive but tumor-free nodes in other patients, or by some harmful systemic effect of the irradiation.

Clearly neither the Halsted nor the McWhirter procedure conforms to the theoretical requirements of patients for whom our third model is appropriate. This has led Crile (1961b, 1964, 1965, 1966b, 1968, 1972) to treat patients with clinical Stage I breast cancer (i.e., with a primary tumor of limited extent and without palpable axillary lymph nodes or evidence of spread elsewhere) by simple mastectomy alone. Both the 5 year survival and the 5 year disease-free survival were reported (Crile, 1968) to be slightly longer than for patients treated by either radical mastectomy (with or without irradiation) or by simple mastectomy plus irradiation, but the trial was not a randomized one and the difference cannot be regarded as significant.

Another approach, which has been studied in a randomized multicenter trial organized in the United Kingdom (Baum, Edwards, and Magarey, 1972; Murray, 1974; Murray *et al.,* 1976), is to perform simple mastectomy only in the first instance, but to keep the patient under close observation and undertake lymphadenectomy or radiotherapy if lymph nodes become palpable in the axilla, or lymph nodes which were palpable prior to operation fail to disappear, or at least to become significantly smaller, in the course of a few weeks. In the trial referred to this regimen was compared with simple mastectomy and radiotherapy. Caution is required in interpreting the reported results because of the authors' unwillingness to distinguish between local recurrence properly so termed, i.e., the appearance in the axilla of palpable and presumably tumor-involved nodes which were not present before the operation, and the failure of nodes which were palpable to disappear—a finding for which the appropriate term would seem to be *persistence,* though it is included under the general heading of recurrence. Although at an early stage it began to look as if routine radiotherapy might be disadvantageous, it appears from the 5 year follow-up that it is neither harmful nor beneficial as regards survival or prevention of distant metastases, though it does significantly reduce the incidence of "local recurrences" when this term is used in the idiosyncratic way referred to above. In other words, a palpable axillary node is more likely to disappear if it is irradiated than if one merely watches it. This is scarcely surprising, and gives no indication of the underlying pathology. Doubtless many of the disappearing nodes in non-irradiated patients were enlarged as the result of sinus histiocytosis (5.221), but did some of them contain tumor metastases? The trial under discussion provides no answer to this important question. The answer might be sought by comparing the proportion of patients with Stage II breast cancer (i.e., operable tumors with palpably enlarged axillary nodes but no evidence of metastasis elsewhere) in whom the axillary nodes disappear clinically after simple mastectomy, with the proportion of similar patients treated by radical mastectomy in whom tumor metastases can be demonstrated histologically in the excised axillary nodes, and in particular in those axillary nodes which are sufficiently enlarged to have been clinically palpable; so far as the writer is aware, however, no study of this kind has ever been undertaken. It was reported by Huvos, Hutter, and Berg (1971) that among 227 patients treated in the Memorial Sloan-Kettering Cancer Center (New York) by radical mastectomy, 62 had no demonstrable lymph node metastases, and 40 of the remaining 125 patients had only "micrometastases," i.e., metastases less than 2 mm diameter. It is also of interest that the survival of patients with micrometastases only confined to the lower axillary nodes was not significantly different from that of patients without demonstrable metastases. These data, however, do not provide an answer to our question because it is not recorded which patients had clinically palpable axillary nodes prior to operation.

The question of whether, and if so in what circumstances, lymphadenectomy (or node irradiation) should be undertaken in patients with cutaneous malignant melanoma (see Bodenham, 1968; Hiles, 1973; Westbury, 1977; Milton *et al.*, 1977), head and neck cancer, and other tumors has also been hotly debated. The principles we have been discussing in relation to carcinoma of the breast apply *mutatis mutandis* to malignant tumors of all kinds, but the problem of determining which theoretical model corresponds to the situation in a particular patient may be even more intractable when the tumor and the regional lymph nodes are located in sites such as the abdomen, the thorax, or the retroperitoneal area.

6.32   Chemotherapy

6.321   CHEMOTHERAPY AS THE PRIMARY OR SOLE PROCEDURE

It is conceivable that chemotherapy will one day provide a complete solution to the cancer problem. This goal still seems remote, but important advances have been made. Not many years ago chemotherapy provided at best a modest degree of palliation and at worst merely added to the patient's misery; today it is claimed to be curative, when appropriate combinations of drugs are used, in a proportion of patients with trophoblastic chorioncarcinoma (Hammond *et al.* 1967; Bagshawe, 1969; Elston and Bagshawe, 1973; De Vita, Young, and Canellos, 1975), Burkitt's lymphoma (Ziegler, 1972; Nkrumah and Perkins, 1973), and acute lymphoblastic leukemia (ALL) and Hodgkin's disease (De Vita *et al.*, 1975), and of substantial benefit in patients with a variety of other tumors.

If the term *cure* is used as suggested earlier (6.2) these claims seem reasonable. In chorioncarcinoma, according to De Vita *et al.*, the expected cure rate is over 70 percent, even if the tumor is widely disseminated; in Burkitt's lymphoma, on the other hand, cures seem to be largely restricted to patients with localized tumors (Nkrumah *et al.*, 1977). In children with ALL, for whom the median survival in 1957 was about 4 months, it is now nearly always possible to induce a complete remission, and in a recent trial (Hardisty, Kay *et al.*, 1977) 50 percent of those who subsequently received irradiation to the central nervous system and intrathecal injection of methotrexate, followed by courses of maintenance therapy over a period of 3 years, were still in first remission 6 years after the start of treatment. In adults with ALL Clarkson *et al.* (1975) obtained complete remission in 78 percent of cases, but the median duration of remission was only 2 years. In acute myeloid leukemia (AML) and related non-lymphoblastic acute leukemias, remission can be induced in over 50 percent of patients but relapse usually occurs within 1 or 2 years; a few patients, however, have remained in remission for over 4 years, and Clarkson *et al.* suggest that some of these may have been cured. In advanced Hodgkin's disease chemotherapy is the treatment of choice, and with the most effective drug combinations complete remissions have been reported in 80 percent of cases, with a median survival of 8 years (De Vita *et al.*, 1975; Peckham *et al.*, 1975).

As with surgery and radiotherapy, however, success is limited by the difficulty of achieving an adequate antitumor effect without causing undue damage to normal tissue.

Many of the agents used act by impairing the reproductive function of cells. The tissues mainly at risk are therefore those with a high rate of mitosis, notably the bone marrow, the lymphoid tissues, and the epithelium of the gastrointestinal tract. The possible consequences of damage include the induction of tumors and, in the case of the lymphoid tissues and bone marrow, of immunosuppression with consequent impairment of cancer homeostasis. The risk of inducing another tumor appears to be much greater with alkylating agents than with antimetabolites.

Attempts have been made to increase the damage to the tumor and protect the host by administering the drug into a main artery supplying the tumor. One procedure is to infuse an antimetabolite, methotrexate, through an intraarterial canula, and later treat the patient with citrovorum factor to counteract drug not fixed in the tumor (Djerassi, Kim, and Suvansri, 1974; Djerassi and Kim, 1976; Tattersall and Tobias, 1976). Another procedure, applicable to metastatic cancer of the liver, is to inject the drug into the hepatic artery (Murray-Lyon *et al.*, 1970). This procedure has been used as an alternative to, or in conjunction with, hepatic artery ligation. The rationale is that much of the blood supply of metastatic tumors in the liver is derived from the hepatic artery. A third procedure, which is most readily applicable to tumors of the limbs and has been used mainly for the treatment of malignant melanoma (Krementz and Ryan, 1972; Stehlin *et al.*, 1975), is to connect the main artery and vein to a pump–oxygenator, isolate the circulation to the part with a pneumatic tourniquet or in some other way, and introduce the drug into the system at a controlled rate.

Attempts have also been made to counteract damage to bone marrow by removing and storing autologous marrow before starting treatment and replacing it later (Woodruff, 1961; Kurnick, 1964), or by infusing syngeneic (Klemperer *et al.*, 1976) or allogeneic marrow. Reinfusion of autologous marrow has the disadvantage that, if the tumor has already become disseminated to bone marrow, viable tumor cells may be reintroduced into the circulation when the marrow is replaced. Infusion of syngeneic and allogeneic marrow avoids this complication but raises other important questions and will be discussed later (8.231).

A more general approach to the problem is to try to find drugs and combinations of drugs, and schedules of administration, which are therapeutically efficient, i.e., which have a powerful antitumor effect but cause only minimal complications. The agents studied include not only cytotoxic drugs but also substances which cause asynchronously proliferating cells to accumulate in the phases of the cell cycle in which the cytotoxic drugs chosen are likely to be most effective (H. O. Klein, 1972). Dose–response curves showing the effect of different types of cytotoxic drugs, and of individual drugs of each type, on both tumor and normal cell populations provide a useful basis for designing new protocols (Berenbaum, 1969b), though the final assessments must of course be based on clinical trials. The tumor dose–response curve also has an important bearing on the theoretical probability of killing all the tumor cells (Berenbaum, 1968). Dose–response curves based on killing *in vitro* may be misleading because they do not take into account the possible effect of the host reaction; an approximate value for the fractional kill *in vivo* in response to a given dose of a drug can, however, be calculated from the observed growth rates before, during, and after treatment (Berenbaum, 1972).

The dose–response curves for alkylating agents, as for ionizing radiation, are often exponential or nearly so (Levis, 1963; Berry, 1964; Skipper, Schabel, and Wilcox, 1964, 1965; Madoc-Jones and Bruce, 1967), i.e., the logarithm of the fraction of cells surviving after administration of a single dose of the drug is proportional to the dose (the constant in this relationship is of course negative); whereas with antimetabolites, as Berenbaum (1969a) has pointed out, the dose–response curve is approximately hyperbolic, i.e., the proportion of cells surviving is proportional to a power of the dose.

6.322   ADJUVANT CHEMOTHERAPY

With both exponential and hyperbolic dose–response curves the expected proportion of cells killed is related to the dose but independent of the absolute number of tumor cells. This relationship, which is commonly referred to as first-order kinetics, appears to hold good in practice for most chemotherapeutic agents (Shapiro and Fugmann, 1957; Skipper, Schabel, and Wilcox, 1964; Schabel, 1968, 1969); it seems reasonable to postulate therefore that chemotherapy would be more effective if the bulk of the tumor to be treated was first reduced by surgery or radiotherapy. This has prompted the study of what has come to be called *adjuvant chemotherapy* in association with surgical treatment for a variety of solid tumors (Schabel, 1975; Burchenal, 1976).

Carcinoma of the breast.   A large-scale trial of adjuvant chemotherapy in breast cancer was begun in 1957 and, according to Burchenal (1976), was based on the belief which then prevailed that postoperative recurrence was due largely to cancer cells which entered the circulation during the operation as a result of manipulation of the tumor. Patients with operable breast cancer were therefore allocated by randomization into two groups: a "chemotherapy group" who were treated by radical mastectomy and administration of thiotepa during the operation and on each of the first two postoperative days, and a "control group" who were treated by radical mastectomy with or without administration of a placebo (B. Fisher *et al.,* 1968; B. Fisher, 1971). Data from 826 patients who were followed for at least 5 years showed no significant difference between the two groups in respect of either the incidence of recurrence or survival. Detailed analysis showed that premenopausal patients with four or more positive axillary lymph nodes (i.e., axillary nodes in which tumor metastases were demonstrated histologically) who received chemotherapy had a lower incidence of recurrence 18 to 36 months after operation than those who did not, but by 48 months there was no longer a significant difference. In a second trial designed to compare the value of thiotepa and 5-fluorouracil (5-FU) for short-term adjuvant chemotherapy, the effect of thiotepa was even less than in the first trial, while 5-FU had no apparent antitumor effect and caused unacceptable local and systemic complications (B. Fisher, 1971). Various other trials of this kind have been undertaken (see Hines and Williams, 1975) but, despite some early optimistic reports, do not provide any convincing evidence of the value of short-term adjuvant chemotherapy.

More recently, prospective randomized trials of prolonged adjuvant chemotherapy after radical mastectomy in patients with operable breast cancer and at least one positive axillary lymph node have been set up in the United States by B. Fisher (B. Fisher *et al.,* 1975a, 1977) and in Italy by Bonadonna (Bonadonna *et al.,* 1976, 1977). The results merit careful study. They draw attention to the fact that patients with breast cancer are a heterogenous population, and that treatment which is advantageous for some may be of no value for others; they show also that in premenopausal patients postoperative recurrence may be delayed by adjuvant chemotherapy. As yet, however, there is no evidence that survival is increased by the chemotherapy, and the view expressed by Carter (1977) and others that these trials have been "dramatically successful" seems unjustified.

In Fisher's initial trials a single drug, phenylalanine mustard (L-PAM), was used. One year after mastectomy there was an overall fall of 50 percent in the incidence of treatment failure* in the patients who received chemotherapy, but by 2 years this was only 5 percent and the overall difference between these patients and those who received a placebo was not significant; there was, however, a marked significant difference in treatment failure at 2 years in the case of premenopausal patients with one to three positive axillary nodes, and a smaller difference in those with four or more positive axillary nodes. At 2 years the proportion of surviving patients in the chemotherapy group was greater than in those who received a placebo, but it remains to be seen whether there will eventually be a significant difference in the median survival times. About two-thirds of the patients experienced some degree of nausea and vomiting, and in half of these it was classified as moderate or severe. Alopecia occurred in 5 percent of patients and stomatitis in 4 percent. In later trials the chemotherapy patients received either L-PAM, L-PAM plus 5-FU, or L-PAM plus 5-FU plus methotrexate. The combination of L-PAM and 5-FU has resulted in a reduction of treatment failures at 12 months which is reported to be "as good or better than that observed with L-PAM," but the incidence of cytotoxic symptoms has been somewhat greater.

Bonadonna *et al.* used a combination of cyclophosphamide, methotrexate, and 5-FU. At 12 months after operation treatment failure was significantly reduced in all categories of patient who received chemotherapy, but thereafter the difference was significant only in premenopausal patients. At 3 years there was no significant difference in the survival of all patients who received chemotherapy as compared with all those who did not. At this time there was also no statistical difference in the mortality rates for premenopausal and postmenopausal patients. Toxic effects were greater than in Fisher's trial of L-PAM; they included prolonged nausea and loss of appetite, and loss of hair of varying degrees in more than two-thirds of the patients.

Carcinoma of the lung. Short-term adjuvant chemotherapy with nitrogen mustard, cyclophosphamide, or a combination of these drugs, in association with pulmonary resection for operable tumors, has been reported to be of no benefit (Dolton, 1970; Higgins, 1972; Shields *et al.,* 1974), except possibly in patients with undifferentiated tumors who received cyclophosphamide (Higgins, 1972). Long-term adjuvant chemotherapy with a variety of drugs and drug combinations has been variously reported to prolong survival, especially in patients with undifferentiated tumors (Katsuki *et al.,* 1975), to be of no benefit (Shields, Robinette, and Keehn, 1974; Stott *et al.,* 1976), or to hasten recurrence and shorten survival (Brunner, Marthaler, and Müller, 1973).

The trials conducted by Shields *et al.* were randomized and included in all 2348 patients. Every patient had what was regarded as a potentially "curative" resection, and 1176 received in addition adjuvant chemotherapy. The accumulated 5 year and 10

---

*Defined by Fisher as "the presence of tumor in local, regional, or distant sites, confirmed by biopsy when possible or by acceptable clinical, pathological, or radioisotopic evidence."

year survivals were 24.8 percent and 13.5 percent for those who received chemotherapy and 26.2 percent and 16.3 percent for those who did not; the differences were
not statistically significant.

Colorectal cancer. In colorectal cancer administration of thiotepa (Dixon,
Longmire, and Holden, 1971) or 5-FU and related drugs (Higgins *et al.*, 1971, 1976;
Rousselot *et al.*, 1972; Dwight *et al.*, 1973; Lawrence *et al.*, 1975; Grage *et al.*, 1975;
A. J. Hill *et al.*, 1976), in association with supposedly curative resection, has on the
whole been of little benefit, though in some series recurrence has been delayed. Rousselot *et al.* (1972) and Hill *et al.* (1976) reported prolonged survival in some categories
of patients; Lawrence *et al.* (1975), however, in a well-controlled study reported no
benefit from the adjuvant therapy. It is of interest, in the light of these results, that the
chemotherapeutic regimens used by Rousselot *et al.* and Lawrence *et al.* both included
intraluminal administration of 5-FU during the operation and intravenous administration postoperatively, but that Lawrence *et al.* followed this treatment with five courses
of oral administration of the drug.

Other tumors in adults. Trials of surgery plus chemotherapy for the treatment
of various other solid tumors in adults have been set up (Kenis, 1971; Hill *et al.*, 1976;
Salmon and Jones, 1977), but so far, with two exceptions, they have proved disappointing. The first exception is osteogenic sarcoma. This occurs occasionally in older
patients, but since the main incidence is in children and adolescents, it will be considered below. The other exception is Burkitt's lymphoma with involvement of lymphoid
tissue in the abdomen. Chemotherapy alone is decidedly less effective in patients with
this pattern of disease than in those whose tumor is entirely extraabdominal, but the
chances of long-term remission are markedly improved if the abdominal tumor is excised nearly completely (Magrath *et al.*, 1974). Here, however, as Magrath *et al.*
points out, "there has been a reversal of roles, with surgery in effect being used as a
relatively minor adjunct to chemotherapy."

Tumors which occur mainly in children and adolescents. In contrast to the rather unimpressive results we have been considering, adjuvant chemotherapy has dramatically improved the results in children with Wilms' tumor and Ewing's tumor.
Thus in Wilms' tumor, where the cure rate with surgery and radiotherapy is about 20
percent, a cure rate of 80 percent was reported by Farber (1966) in patients treated by
surgery, radiotherapy, and repeated courses of actinomycin D. In Ewing's tumor,
where treatment by radiotherapy alone suffices to destroy the primary tumor but is
followed in 80–90 percent of patients by death from metastases, prolonged disease-free
survival has been reported in 55–70 percent of patients who also received adjuvant
chemotherapy (Hustu, Pinkel, and Pratt, 1972; Rosen *et al.*, 1974).

Considerable, though less dramatic, benefit has been observed in children with
rhabdomyosarcoma (Malpas *et al.*, 1976), and in children and young adults with osteogenic sarcoma, treated with cytotoxic drugs in addition to amputation (Cortes *et
al.*, 1974; Jaffe *et al.*, 1974; Sutow *et al.*, 1974; Douglas *et al.*, 1975; Burchenal, 1976;
Ivins and Pritchard, 1976; Gehan *et al.*, 1978; Miké and Marcove, 1978), in the form
of delayed recurrence and prolonged survival. Similar improvement has also been reported in patients who received long-term anticoagulant therapy after amputation
(Hoover *et al.*, 1978).

General comment. The dominant concept in the development of adjuvant chemotherapy has been to reduce the tumor cell population sufficiently to render it susceptible to total destruction by cytotoxic drugs. The possible contribution of the host reaction seems to have been underestimated and at times ignored. It is conceivable—indeed, in the writer's view, likely—that better results would be obtained if chemotherapy were planned with this factor in mind, and if additional procedures (6.4) were used to counteract the inhibitory effect of the chemotherapy on the reactivity of the host.

6.33 Endocrinological Procedures

The discovery that some tumors are hormone dependent (4.24) opened the way to the use of endocrinological manipulations for the treatment of cancer. Subsequent developments in endocrinology, including the discovery of cell hormone receptors (see Jensen *et al.,* 1971; Humphrey, 1976; British Medical Journal, 1976b), have made it possible to use these procedures in a more discriminating way.

The methods used are administration of hormones or hormone antagonists, and endocrine ablation. The main applications at present are as follows:

1. Administration of estrogens, and bilateral orchidectomy, as the primary treatment for cancer of the prostate. Administration of stilbestrol or related substances, sometimes combined with orchidectomy, has been the usual practice in the United Kingdom, but this policy is being challenged on the grounds of the cardiovascular complications of prolonged estrogen administration, the extent to which the results may depend on the natural history of the disease, and the response to radical prostatectomy which has been widely used in the United States, interstitial radiation, and combined hormonal therapy and chemotherapy (British Medical Journal, 1977d).
2. Various procedures for the palliative treatment of advanced breast cancer. These include oophorectomy, oophorectomy and adrenalectomy, various forms of pituitary ablation, and administration of estrogen antagonists such as nafoxidine or tamoxifen which compete for estrogen receptors in younger patients; and administration of stilbestrol in older patients.
3. Administration of estrogen, and orchidectomy, for the treatment of disseminated cancer of the prostate when these procedures have not been used as the primary treatment.
4. Administration of progestogens for the treatment of disseminated endometrial and ovarian cancer.
5. Bilateral orchidectomy for the treatment of disseminated cancer of the male breast.
6. Administration of thyroxin in high dosage to prevent or control recurrence after radical surgery for cancer of the thyroid. This is given not only as necessary replacement therapy but in higher dosage to suppress production of thyroid stimulating hormone by the pituitary.

Oophorectomy has been tried as an addition to mastectomy in younger patients with operable cancer of the breast, but was found in a randomized trial to be of no benefit (Ravdin *et al.,* 1971; B. Fisher, 1971). A trial of an estrogen antagonist, tamoxifen, is in progress (Baum, 1977).

Endocrinological manipulations may cause unpleasant, and sometimes dangerous, complications. Prolonged administration of stilbestrol in patients with prostatic
cancer, for example, was found to be associated with a significant increase in cardiovascular deaths, and this led to a general reduction in the dose employed. These manipulations may also modify immunological and para-immunological responses; in
particular it has been shown in various experimental models that T-cell activity is reduced not only by administration of cortisone but also, to a lesser extent, by administration of estrogens (Graff, Lappé, and Snell, 1969) and androgens (Kappas, Jones,
and Roitt, 1963), and according to Prentice et al. (1976) by hypophysectomy, but may
be increased by orchidectomy (Castro, 1974c) and adrenalectomy (Castro and Hamilton, 1972), whereas macrophage activity is stimulated by estrogens (Magarey and
Baum, 1971). As Castro (1978) has pointed out, these effects may weaken, augment,
or possibly in some cases be wholly responsible for the therapeutic response of cancer
patients to endocrinological procedures.

6.4 NEW APPROACHES TO PROPHYLAXIS AND
TREATMENT

Increased understanding of the role of genetic and environmental factors in carcinogenesis increases the possibility of more effective prophylaxis by genetic counsel-
ing, and by reducing exposure to environmental carcinogens. The search for more
sensitive markers of malignancy and premalignancy, if successful, should lead to the
development of better, and more generally applicable, non-invasive procedures for
screening large populations, and hence to earlier treatment. The discovery of homeostatic mechanisms points to the need for continuous monitoring of the effect of treatment on the host reaction and for devising treatment schedules which are
therapeutically efficient (6.321), and provides a basis for research into new methods of
prophylaxis and treatment.

It seems likely that for many solid tumors surgical excision of the primary tumor,
and in some cases also of macrometastases, will continue for a long time to play a major role, but that it will often be combined with adjuvant chemotherapy, based on efficient drug combinations and regimens of administration, and with measures to
promote a favorable host reaction and counteract the inhibitory effect of other forms
of treatment on this reaction.

Possible new therapeutic, and in some cases also prophylactic, procedures include
administration of antiangiogenesis factor (Folkman, 1972; see also 3.13) and chalones
(4.22), and a variety of immunologicol and para-immunological manipulations.

As we have seen (4.22), it has been postulated that the proliferation of normal
cells is regulated by inhibitory factors termed *chalones* which are specific for the type
of cell in question, and, secondly, that a chalone may also inhibit proliferation of neoplastic cells of corresponding type. If these hypotheses are true—and at present there
is some evidence in their favor and none which tells decisively against them—administration of the appropriate chalone might be useful ancillary treatment for cancer. The
chalone would, *ex hypothesi,* inhibit the proliferation of normal as well as neoplastic
cells, but, as Rytömaa (1976) has pointed out, the effect on the tumor would be additional to any inhibition caused by other forms of treatment or by homeostatic mechanisms. Experimental evidence is scanty, but it has been reported that extracts

containing granulocyte chalone may be effective in treating chloroleukemia in rats (Rytömaa and Kiviniemi, 1969, 1970), and also active against human myleoid leukemia (Rytömaa *et al.,* 1976), and extracts containing melanocyte chalone in treating melanomas in mice and hamsters; as will be seen later (7.53), however, it has been suggested that contamination of the extracts with Clostridium spores may have been responsible for some of the therapeutic effects.

It is tempting to dismiss chalones as a figment of the imagination because of the lack of definite evidence of specificity, and the fact that they have not been isolated in chemically pure forms. In the writer's view this would be a mistake, though it remains to be seen whether or not the chalone hypothesis will turn out to be important in relation to biology in general and the biology of cancer in particular.

The search for immunological and para-immunological methods of treatment and prophylaxis, which has intensified greatly in recent years, will be discussed in detail in the next two chapters.

7
The Experimental Basis of Immunotherapy

7.1 INTRODUCTION

In this chapter we shall consider possible forms of immunotherapy, using this term in a broad sense to include all immunological and para-immunological manipulations used to control tumor growth, and the experimental study of immunotherapy in animals bearing autochthonous tumors or syngeneic tumor transplants. Observations in patients will be mentioned only insofar as they help to elucidate the mode of action of the procedures used, since clinical trials will be discussed in the next chapter.

The procedures used may be classified as shown below, with the proviso that the distinction between passive and active immunotherapy is not entirely clear cut. Passive immunotherapy implies only that antibody, cells, or cell products able to participate in a reaction directed against the tumor are provided from an extraneous source; it does not exclude participation of the host in this reaction, or modification of the host reaction as a result of the treatment.

1. Passive immunotherapy.
    (1) Passive immunization with serum, plasma, or immunoglobulin.
    (2) Immunochemotherapy (i.e., the use of antibodies as carriers for chemotherapeutic agents).
    (3) Passive immunization, with cells and cell products (sometimes termed adoptive immunization).
    (4) Passive immunization with both antibody and cells.
2. Active immunotherapy.
    (1) Non-specific immunopotentiation.
    (2) Specific immunization.
    (3) Combined non-specific and specific procedures.
3. Combined passive and active immunotherapy.
4. Procedures to eliminate blocking factors and suppressor cells, or promote access of cells, antibody, and complement to the tumor.

When immunotherapy is used in combination with surgical excision, radiotherapy, or chemotherapy, it will be referred to as *adjuvant immunotherapy*. In this context, as in the analogous term adjuvant chemotherapy (6.322), adjuvant means something added and has no technical immunological connotation. An alternative usage adopted by some authors is to refer to courses of treatment in which chemotherapy and immunotherapy are both used as *chemoimmunotherapy* or *immunochemotherapy*. A term is needed, however, to denote the use of chemotherapeutic agents coupled chemically to tumor-specific antibody, and we shall use *immunochemotherapy* in this restricted sense. We shall use the term *combined immunotherapeutic procedures* to denote courses of treatment in which two or more different forms of immunotherapy are used, irrespective of whether or not other methods of treatment are used as well.

Immunotherapy involves the risk that under certain conditions tumor growth may be enhanced rather than suppressed; it has been suggested, however, that specific immunotherapy should be relatively free of other complications. It has also been suggested (Fefer, 1973) that the effect of immunotherapeutic procedures on a cell should be the same at all stages in the cell cycle, and should not be limited by the so-called first-order kinetics rule; i.e., a given procedure should destroy a certain number, not a certain proportion, of tumor cells.

In the discussion which follows we shall consider the extent to which these predictions have been verified.

7.2 PASSIVE IMMUNIZATION WITH SERUM, PLASMA, OR IMMUNOGLOBULIN

7.21 Mechanisms of Tumor Inhibition and Stimulation

There have been many studies of the effect of serum or Ig from isogeneic, allogeneic, and xenogeneic donors immunized with tumor cells or extracts on the growth of tumors in experimental animals. Useful reviews have been published by Wright *et al.* (1976) and Rosenberg and Terry (1977). The effects of sera which react with plasma cells, B cells, and suppressor T cells have also been studied, but this work will be considered later (7.82).

Knowledge of how antitumor serum or Ig might inhibit or stimulate tumor growth *in vivo* has increased greatly since many of these experiments were planned, and the following possibilities have now to be considered:

7.211 INHIBITION OF TUMOR GROWTH

1. Complement-dependent cytotoxicity (5.311) mediated by antibody in the serum directed against tumor antigens, and complement provided by the tumor-bearing host, or present in inactivated serum or injected as an additional procedure.
2. Antibody-dependent cell-mediated cytotoxicity mediated by antibody in the serum and host cells (5.312).
3. Unblocking effect (5.521) of antibody in the serum.
4. Arming or activation of host macrophages or uncommitted lymphocytes by soluble factors other than immunoglobulin in serum from isogeneic donors (5.4).

5. Antiviral activity of naturally occurring antibody in serum from isogeneic or allogeneic donors.
6. Increased immunogenicity of the tumor cells caused by bound antibody from xenogeneic donors ("xenogenization") (7.63).
7. Non-specific immunopotentiation by serum protein from xenogeneic donors (7.5).
8. Non-immunological mechanisms due to agents such as hormones (4.24, 6.33) and chalones (4.22, 6.4).

If the antitumor antibody in the serum is non-cytotoxic or only weakly cytotoxic, it may nevertheless be possible to obtain an antitumor effect by administering first the specific serum or immunoglobulin and then a heterologous antiglobulin antibody (7.24), or by coupling the specific antibody to a chemical cytotoxin or radioactive substance (7.3).

Antibody directed against cell surface antigens may also potentiate the cytotoxic effect of chlorambucil and some other chemotherapeutic agents with which they are not coupled, and of x-irradiation, both *in vitro* (Rubens and Dulbecco, 1974; Rubens, Vaughan-Smith, and Dulbecco, 1975) and *in vivo* (7.23). The mechanism has not been elucidated, but on the basis of their *in vitro* studies Dulbecco *et al.* excluded (1) increased uptake of the drug in the presence of antibody; (2) increase in the rate of mitosis due to the antibody which, if it had occurred, might have made the cells more sensitive to the drug; and (3) lysis of the cells by the drug at concentrations which do not cause lysis in the absence of antibody. It does not of course necessarily follow that these exclusions are universally valid. It has been shown, for example, that non-cycling Ehrlich ascites carcinoma cells may be stimulated to divide by exposure to heterologous antilymphocyte serum (Decosse and Gelfant, 1968) under conditions in which lysis does not occur, and the same may well be true of other tumor cells on exposure to specific antibody. Such stimulation might well bring resting cells resistant to radiotherapy and chemotherapy (Sarna, 1974) into cycle, and thus increase their susceptibility.

7.212 STIMULATION OF TUMOR GROWTH

1. Specific enhancement due to blocking antibody.
2. Immunostimulation by small amounts of antibody which in larger amounts would be cytotoxic (5.522).
3. General immunosuppression due to the presence of antilymphocytic antibody.
4. Non-immunological mechanisms due to agents such as hormones (4.24, 6.33) and angiogenesis factor (3.13, 6.4).

7.22 Isogeneic and Allogeneic Donors

It was reported by Gorer and Amos (1956) that C57B1 mice were protected against inoculation of the EL4 lymphoma by prior injection of serum from allogeneic mice immunized with this tumor, and that injection of immune serum 2 days after inoculation of the tumor had a slight protective effect. It has been shown subsequently that mice may be protected in varying degree against other tumors, including lymphomas (Amos and Day, 1957; Alexander, Connell, and Mikulska, 1966; Alexander, 1967; Wahren, 1968; G. Pearson, Redmon, and Bass, 1973; G. Pearson, Redmon, and Pearson, 1973), chemically induced fibrosarcomas (Möller, 1964), and Moloney sarcoma virus (MSV)-induced tumors (Bubenik and Turano, 1968; Bubenik, Turano, and Fadda, 1969; Pearson, Redmon, and Bass, 1973) by immune serum raised in isogeneic or allogeneic animals and administered at the time of tumor inoculation or up to a few days after virus inoculation of newborn animals. On the other hand, administration of serum from tumor-bearing or immunized animals starting before tumor inoculation has been found in some experiments to have no effect (Forni and Comoglio, 1974), and in others to enhance tumor growth (Möller, 1964; Bubenik and Koldovsky, 1965; Bubenik, Ivanyi, and Koldovsky, 1965; Attia and Weiss, 1966).

An appreciable therapeutic effect has also been observed in animals with minimal residual disease following surgery or chemotherapy. Koldovsky (1962) reported that administration of immune serum of isogeneic origin after not quite complete surgical excision of a transplanted isogeneic tumor reduced the incidence of recurrence. Pearson, Redmon, and Pearson (1973) reported that the proportion of long-term surviving Balb/c mice with Moloney lymphomas treated by chemotherapy only was 34 percent. Additional treatment in the form of repeated injection of normal (Balb/c × DBA)F1 serum increased this figure to 54 percent; a single injection of immune serum raised by immunizing (Balb/c × DBA)F1 mice with C57B1 Moloney lymphomas raised it to 79 percent, and repeated injection of immune serum raised it to 95 percent.

With established tumors treatment with immune serum alone has usually been ineffective, but two exceptions to this rule have been reported.

It was found by Fefer (1969) that small but palpable primary MSV-induced tumors in Balb/c mice regressed completely in 30 to 40 percent of animals treated with serum from Balb/c or (Balb/c × DBA)F1 mice which had been inoculated with virus when they were more than 30 days old and whose tumors had regressed spontaneously. *In vitro* studies (I. Hellström and K. Hellström, 1969; Fefer, 1969; G. Pearson, Redmon, and Bass, 1973) have shown that serum from regressor mice contains complement-dependent cytotoxic antibody, unblocking antibody, and lymphocyte-dependent antibody, but their relative importance *in vivo* is undetermined. Inactivation of virus by the serum may also contribute to the therapeutic effect in this system since MSV-induced tumors release infective virus, and this, if not inactivated, may transform previously unaffected cells.

Bansal and Sjögren (1972, 1973) showed that polyoma virus-induced kidney tumors in W/Fu rats underwent complete or partial regression after splenectomy and repeated injection of isogeneic immune serum, whereas regression did not occur in tumor-bearing rats treated with normal serum. It was shown in previous experiments (Bansal and Sjögren, 1971) that the immune serum eliminated blocking activity from the serum of tumor-bearing rats *in vitro,* and caused tumor regression after temporary growth when injected intraperitoneally 1 hour after subcutaneous inoculation of polyoma-induced tumor cells; there was moreover good correlation between the unblocking effect and the antitumor effect *in vivo.*

7.23 Xenogeneic Donors

There have been many reports of increased survival of mice bearing transplanted leukemias and lymphomas treated with serum from rabbits immunized with the leukemia in question, or with pooled cells from a variety of murine leukemias, or with normal mouse lymphocytes, either alone or combined with chemotherapy (Mohos and Kidd, 1957; Schabel *et al.,* 1966; Bremberg, Klein, and Stjernsward, 1967; D.G. Miller *et al.,* 1968; Reif and Kim, 1969; Mempel and Thierfelder, 1970; Siegel and Morton, 1970; Hill and Littlejohn, 1970; Hill, 1971; Shirato *et al.,* 1972; Hersey, 1973; Drake, Ungaro, and Mardiney, 1973; Drake and Mardiney, 1974; Drake *et al.,* 1975; Davies and O'Neill, 1973; Davies *et al.,* 1974b, 1974c).

Such sera may be highly toxic but become much less so after absorption with mouse erythrocytes (Reif and Kim, 1969); they may also be immunosuppressive even when raised with leukemic cells (Witz, Yagi, and Pressman, 1968b), but this is not always the case (Sloboda and Landes, 1969).

It was found by Miller *et al.* (1968) that, when injection of antiserum was begun 2–4 hours after leukemia inoculation, the length of survival was inversely proportional to the logarithm of the number of tumor cells inoculated; in this system, therefore, contrary to the suggestion of Fefer (1973) mentioned earlier (7.1), the first-order kinetics rule did apply.

The therapeutic effect has usually been slight when injection of serum was started even 1 day after tumor inoculation, though somewhat greater when serum was given before this, but Reif and Kim (1969) obtained a few permanent survivors among C3H mice injected intraperitoneally with 10^5 Gardner lymphosarcoma cells and treated on days 1, 2, and 3 after tumor inoculation with Ig from a potent antiserum.

Davies and his colleagues (Davies and O'Neill, 1973; Davies, 1974; Davies *et al.,* 1974b, 1974c) found that chemotherapy followed by administration of immune globulin gave much better protection than either treatment alone and were able to protect all mice completely when treatment was begun up to 48 hours after tumor inoculation. Chemotherapy followed by injection of normal rabbit serum gave slightly better protection than chemotherapy alone, and this was attributed to the toxicity of rabbit sera for mouse cells in general. It has been shown however (Witz, Yagi, and Pressman, 1968a) that there is a component of normal rabbit IgG which has a special affinity for the cells of the L1210 mouse leukemia, and it is conceivable that it may also have an affinity for the EL4 leukemia used by Davies *et al.*

Reference has been made to the immunosuppressive property of some of the sera used. This may be particularly marked with sera raised with normal lymphocytes, and it is not surprising that such sera may either inhibit or promote the growth of transplanted leukemias (Bremberg *et al.,* 1967). This ambivalent effect may also occur with sera raised with tumor cells. Thus Yutoku, Grossberg, and Pressman (1974) found that administration of antisera raised in rabbits to Balb/c myelomas, starting the day after tumor inoculation, inhibited the growth of some myelomas but stimulated the growth of others.

In some of the experiments referred to, complement was administered as well as antiserum; this will be discussed in the next section (7.24).

Old *et al.* (1967) raised serum by immunizing (W/Fu $\times$ BN)F1 hybrid rats with a W/Fu leukemia originally induced by wild-type Gross virus from C58 mice and showed that this protected C57Bl/6 mice completely from a C57Bl/6 leukemia bearing the G (Gross) antigen when given up to 3 days after inoculation of the leukemia; the same serum, however, did not protect C57Bl/6 mice against inoculation of a radiation-induced isogeneic leukemia which did not bear the G antigen.

A modest, and often rather variable, therapeutic effect of early treatment with immune xenogeneic serum (or Ig) has also been observed with non-lymphoid tumors including mammary carcinoma (Woodruff and Smith, 1970), melanoma (Hill and Littlejohn, 1971), and ovarian carcinoma (Order *et al.,* 1973, 1974). In some experiments a slight therapeutic effect also occurred when normal rabbit serum was given (Order *et al.,* 1973, 1974; Mizejewski and Allen, 1974). With chemically induced fibrosarcomas, however, stimulation has been observed with antitumor serum or globulin, and it was considered that this was due to the immunosuppressive effect of the material used (Woodruff and Smith, and Smith, 1970).

7.24 Reasons for Failure. Attempts to Overcome Them

We shall now consider possible reasons why passive immunotherapy has had such a limited success, and various attempts which have been made to make it more effective.

1. The amount of immunoglobulin which reaches the tumor is insufficient in relation to the tumor mass.

This may occur because the dose administered was too small, or because the immunoglobulin did not localize in the tumor (Witz, Klein, and Pressman, 1969), owing to poor blood supply to parts of the tumor or other causes (*vide infra*).

It was shown in quantitative studies with a C3H strain murine lymphoma and antibody in the form of ascitic fluid from isogeneic mice immunized with cultured tumor cells in complete Freund's adjuvant that the antibody was equally effective in suppressing freshly injected tumor cells and the same number of established tumor cells (Shin *et al.,* 1976a, 1976b). When the tumor burden ranged from 10^5 to 10^6 cells the amount of antibody required to suppress 50 percent of the tumor cells was directly proportional to the number of cells present; above this level the effectiveness of passive immunization diminished markedly. In this particular model the antibody was reported to be mainly in the IgG1 fraction, and it is to be hoped that similar studies with other tumors and other types of antibody will be undertaken.

2. The antibody is of low titer or affinity, insufficiently specific, or of a kind which does not contribute to cytolysis.

Various immunization schedules have been used with the object of obtaining potent antisera, including injection of tumor cells to the footpads of mice in complete Freund's adjuvant and intraperitoneally without adjuvant on one occasion followed 4 weeks later by subcutaneous and intraperitoneal injection without adjuvant (Woodruff and Smith, 1970, 1971); repeated intravenous injection of viable tumor cells (Kim and Reif, 1971); and initial intravenous injection of cells (preceded by intraperitoneal injection of cyclophosphamide 4 hours earlier), followed by subcutaneous and intraperitoneal injection of cells 7 and 14 days later (Baker and Taub, 1973b). The subject has been approached in a rather empirical way, and more systematic study might prove rewarding.

Antibody which is insufficiently specific may fail to localize in the tumor (Witz, Klein, and Pressman, 1969) and may damage normal cells. The problem of activity against normal tissues does not arise with sera from isogeneic donors, and is greatest with xenogeneic sera. Various methods have been used to obtain more specific material.

Firstly, the serum or Ig may be absorbed with normal cells after being inactivated by heating to 56° C. Absorption with erythrocytes is necessary if much hemolytic or hemagglutinating antibody is present, and this does not, as a rule, result in significant loss of antitumor activity. If immunoglobulin fractions are first prepared it may obviate the need for this absorption, or greatly reduce the number of erythrocytes required, because the bulk of the antitumor and antierythrocyte antibodies may be found in different Ig classes or subclasses. The serum or Ig may also be absorbed with whole tissue or nucleated cells *in vitro,* or *in vivo* by injecting the material, after inactivation, into an animal isogeneic with the ones to be treated and harvesting its serum some hours later (Shigeno *et al.,* 1968). These procedures may result in considerable improvement in specificity, but some loss of antitumor activity is almost inevitable, and the loss may be large. It may thus be difficult or impossible to end up with a product which retains significant antitumor activity but is not immunosuppressive or harmful in other ways.

Secondly, a more defined antigen may be used to raise the serum. This may take the form of cell plasma membranes (Wolf, Barfoot, and Johnson, 1972), partly purified antigen (Order *et al.,* 1974), or products of tumor cells which are not secreted by normal adult cells, or are secreted in small quantity. Sedallian and Triau (1968) suggested using normal embryo cells, and tested serum raised in this way in mice inoculated with an allogeneic tumor. More recently Mizejewski and Allen (1974) immunized rabbits with α-fetoprotein (AFP) prepared from the amniotic fluid of C57B1 mice in Freund's complete adjuvant, and showed that treatment with serum raised in this way slowed the growth of an AFP-secreting C57B1 hepatoma *in vivo.* Stevenson, Elliott, and Stevenson (1976) suggested that, in the special case of B cell lymphomas and lymphocytic leukemias, antibody reacting with the ideotypic determinants (Id) of the immunoglobulin on the surface of the tumor cells might be of therapeutic value. They investigated this by raising a serum in sheep against the Id of the guinea pig L2C leukemia. These leukemic cells exhibit cell surface IgM, and two different antigenic materials were used in raising sera. One was prepared by detaching Fab fragments containing Id by treating the tumor cells with papain and recovering these Fab on immunoabsorbent particles; the other consisted of α chains recovered from the urine of tumor-bearing guinea pigs. Both gave rise to antibody which reacted specifically with IgM on the surface of the leukemic cells. Both could promote complement-dependent and lymphocyte-dependent cytotoxicity *in vitro,* and a single dose given to animals inoculated with the leukemia increased survival to an extent which suggested that 90 percent of the cells in the inoculum had been killed.

Thirdly, an attempt may be made to make the prospective serum donor specifically tolerant of normal tissues of the animals to be treated prior to immunization with tumor cells or antigen. The first step towards this goal was taken by Zilber *et al.* (1958), who made rats tolerant of normal fowl tissue and then immunized them with the Rous sarcoma. The serum gave a positive complement fixation test with Rous sarcoma extract but not with normal tissue extract. It was reported subsequently by Levi *et al.* (1959) and Levi and Schechtman (1963) that the serum of rabbits made tolerant by neonatal injection of normal mouse tissue homogenate (which contained, however, many intact cells) and later immunized with cells of the Ehrlich mouse ascites carcinoma was much less toxic, and therapeutically more effective, in mice inoculated with the Ehrlich tumor than serum raised in non-tolerant rabbits. Although two inbred strains of mice were used as recipients in these experiments the Ehrlich tumor was certainly not isogeneic with either of them, and doubts have also been raised about the efficacy of the procedure used to induce tolerance. It has been shown, however, by Koldovsky and Svobody (1962) that antiserum from rats made tolerant by neonatal injection of tissue from 18-day-old A-strain mouse embryos and later immunized with a chemically induced A-strain sarcoma markedly inhibited tumor growth when administered to A-strain mice 1, 3, and 5 days after inoculation of this tumor, whereas serum from non-tolerant rats immunized with the tumor had little effect. It is not clear why embryo cells were used to induce tolerance in these experiments. In view of the possible existence of antigens common to the tumor and normal embryo tissue this might well have been disadvantageous.

Fourthly, sera have been raised by immunization with tumor cells or antigen mixed with antibody to normal cells (Motta, 1970; Ungaro et al., 1972; Weiner, Hubbard, and Mardiney, 1972; P. J. Smith, Robinson, and Reif, 1974). It has been reported that such sera may possess various degrees of antitumor activity but are relatively non-toxic, and any antibody reacting with normal cells can be easily absorbed.

Antibody, however specific, may be ineffective because it is of a kind which does not contribute to cytolysis.

Although IgM is much more efficient than IgG in promoting lysis of erythrocytes by complement, it does not necessarily follow that it is more efficient in promoting lysis of nucleated cells in vitro (5.311). In vivo, while IgM is perhaps more likely to promote cytolysis and IgG to cause enhancement, it is clear that IgM may enhance, and IgG inhibit, tumor growth (Chard, 1968; Fuller and Winn, 1973). Were this not the case passive immunotherapy with serum might well have been even less effective because it has been found that most of the activity of antilymphocyte serum raised by repeated immunization resides in the IgG, and it seems likely that the same is true of much of the antitumor serum which has been used. Clearly if antibody does not bind complement it will not promote complement-dependent cytolysis, but IgG subclasses which do bind complement may nevertheless under certain conditions cause enhancement of tumor growth (Irvin, Eustace, and Fahey, 1967; Takasugi and Hildemann, 1969).

The cytotoxic efficiency of antilymphocytic and antitumor IgG in vitro may be augmented, though not to the same extent as antierythrocyte IgG, by exposing the target cells first to the specific antibody raised in rabbits and then to antiglobulin in the form of IgG2 from guinea pigs immunized with rabbit IgG (Woodruff and Inchley, 1971a). The possibility of using this type of procedure in vivo does not seem to have been explored.

3.   *Complement components are not available in sufficient quantity or fail to gain access to the tumor.*

Host complement components may be depleted when the tumor burden is large (Hartveit, 1964; Yoshikawa, Yamada, and Yoshida, 1969; Drake, Le Gendre, and Mardiney, 1973), or following administration of heterologous serum (Turk and Willoughby, 1969). Host complement may also be ineffective in association with the antibody used for treatment. Thus some strains of mice (Nilsson and Muller-Eberhard, 1967) and other laboratory animals have an inherited deficiency of C5, and even when, as is usually the case, mouse complement contains all the recognized factors of the complement system, it exhibits little overall hemolytic activity, probably mainly due to a low level of activity of C2 and C3 (Borsos and Cooper, 1961), and is much less effective than rabbit or guinea pig complement in lysing nucleated cells in the presence of cytotoxic antibody in vitro (Drake, Ungaro, and Mardiney, 1973). There is also evidence that with immune sera of allogeneic origin, guinea pig complement may be less effective than rabbit complement in lysing tumor cells *in vitro* (Young-Rodenchuk and Gyenes, 1975), though it does not necessarily follow that the same is true *in vivo*.

It would seem desirable therefore, when passive immunotherapy with serum is undertaken, to monitor complement activity throughout the course of treatment, and to attempt to compensate for the lack or ineffectiveness of host complement by administering exogenous complement. There is evidence that this may be of value (Motta, 1971; Negroni and Hunter, 1973; Drake and Mardiney, 1974). It has been suggested (Drake and Mardiney, 1974; Drake *et al.*, 1975) that to avoid increasing the avidity of antitumor serum for normal tissue antigens, and to obtain the maximum antitumor effect, the antibody should be injected first to allow for preferential binding to tumor cells, and the complement should be injected later.

4. *Host lymphocytes are unable to participate effectively in antibody-dependent lymphocyte cytotoxicity.*

In theory this situation might be met by providing exogenous K cells as well as antibody.

5. *The tumor cells are resistant to complement-dependent cytotoxicity or antibody-dependent lymphocyte cytotoxicity.*

As mentioned above, complement-fixing IgG may cause either inhibition or enhancement of tumor growth. There is evidence that an important factor in determining the outcome is the density of antigens on the surface of the target cells, which affects both the extent to which complement-fixing sites are generated and the efficiency with which such sites are converted to actual lesions in the cell membrane (Linscott, 1970a, 1970b).

7.3 IMMUNOCHEMOTHERAPY

The use of antibodies as carriers for cytotoxic drugs appears to have been initiated by Mathé, Loc, and Bernard (1958), who conjugated methotrexate with antibody raised in guinea pigs to the mouse L1210 leukemia by diazotization. Treatment of mice inoculated with the leukemia with this material resulted in longer survival than treatment with either methotrexate or antibody alone, or both together but unlinked, but the effect was not very great.

Encouraged by the report of Israels and Linford (1963) that chlorambucil could be bound to plasma proteins without losing its alkylating activity, Ghose and Nigam (1972) conjugated chlorambucil with heterologous antitumor globulin active against the Ehrlich mouse ascites tumor by non-covalent linkage, and showed that this material concentrated selectivity in the tumor and inhibited its growth *in vivo*. Ghose *et al.* (1972) showed further that treatment of C57B1/6 mice, 2, 24, 72, or 120 hours after inoculation of the EL4 lymphoma, with chlorambucil-bound antibody directed against this tumor was much more effective than treatment with either chlorambucil or antibody alone. In these experiments Ghose *et al.* did not include a group of mice treated with unconjugated chlorambucil and antibody together. Davies and O'Neill (1973) conjugated chlorambucil with Ig from allogeneic mice or xenogeneic animals (rabbits) immunized with either the EL4 C57B1/6 lymphoma or the SB1 Balb/c lymphoma, either at pH 3.5 by a slight modification of the procedure of Ghose *et al.* (1972) or at pH 8, which yielded a compound less prone to dissociate *in vivo*. They confirmed that repeated injection of chlorambucil conjugated antibody starting 6–24 hours after tumor inoculation was more effective in inhibiting development of the tumor than either chlorambucil or antibody alone, but found that it was not more effective than the same amounts of drug and antibody unconjugated provided that the drug was given an hour before the antibody. It was concluded that the drug and antibody acted in a synergistic way, and it was suggested that exposure to the drug made the cells more susceptible to the action of antibody.

Despite this synergistic effect it was decided to continue to try to develop stable covalently linked drug-antibody compounds, on the ground that such compounds would not damage cells which did not bind the antibody, and side effects of the drug would therefore be eliminated. Davies and O'Neill (1974) produced a compound of this kind by conjugating phenylenediamine mustard (PDM) to antibody by the carbodiimide method. PDM conjugated to Ig from rabbits immunized with the EL4 mouse lymphoma proved more effective than either drug or antibody alone in protecting mice inoculated with the lymphoma 24 hours previously. Treatment with the compound was also compared with treatment with both the drug and antibody unconjugated, but the results of this comparison are not given in the paper cited. Large amounts of conjugated material were required because the degree of drug substitution was limited by the fact that conjugation caused physicochemical changes resulting in diminished antibody activity and reduced water solubility of the compound. To overcome this problem Rowland, O'Neill, and Davies (1975) first conjugated PDM with polyglutamic acid (PGA), and then coupled the PDM-PGA to the antibody. PDM coupled in this way to Ig from rabbits immunized with the EL4 lymphoma proved highly effective when given on four successive days to mice inoculated with 5×10^4 viable EL4 cells 24 hours before the first dose. Five of five mice treated in this way were alive 60 days later and the median survival time was more than 100 days, whereas the median survival time of mice given four daily injections of Ig and of PDM-PGA unconjugated was 38 days, and that of untreated controls 13 days.

Before studying conjugates of chlorambucil, Ghose et al. (1967) coupled ^{131}I to immunoglobulin (Ig) from rabbits immunized with the Ehrlich mouse ascites carcinoma and showed that mice inoculated with tumor cells which had been incubated with this material did not develop the tumor. The development of highly radioactive ^{125}I-labeled antilymphocyte globulin by Dresser (1971) and Basten et al. (1971), whose preparations had activities of 3.2 μCi/μg and 150–170 μCi/μg, respectively, and of ^{32}P-conjugated antibody by Spence et al. (1968), seemed to point the way to the use of heavily labeled antitumor Ig in therapeutic experiments, but interest in this approach has waned as methods of making drug–antibody conjugates have improved.

7.4 PASSIVE IMMUNIZATION WITH CELLS AND CELL PRODUCTS

The possibility that tumor growth might be inhibited by the transfer of immunoreactive cells is suggested by the following considerations:

1. Some tumors possess tumor associated transplantation antigens (TATA) (5.21).
2. Lymphocytes play a crucial role in the rejection of grafts of normal allogeneic tissues (see, e.g., Woodruff, 1960) and immunogenic tumors (5.313).

3. Resistance to transplants of immunogenic tumors may be transferred to other animals of the same inbred strain with cells from lymphoid tissues (Potter, Taylor, and MacDowell, 1938; MacDowell et al., 1938; Brncic, Hoecker, and Gasic, 1952), including the lymph nodes draining the site of the tumor transplant (Mitchison, 1954, 1955), and bone marrow (Koller and Doak, 1960).
4. Lymphocytes and macrophages under certain conditions inhibit the growth of tumor cells in vitro (5.226, 5.431).
5. Antibody-dependent cytotoxicity (5.312) may be mediated by lymphocytes.
6. Natural killer (NK) cells inhibit the growth of some tumors in vitro and probably also in vivo (5.44).

It has long been known that the development of radiation leukemia (2.12) in C57B1 mice may be prevented by shielding either one femur or the exteriorized spleen during radiation (Kaplan and Brown, 1951, 1952a, 1952b), or by the injection of non-irradiated isogeneic bone marrow after irradiation (Kaplan, Brown, and Paull, 1953); and more recently Cole (1964) has reported that the incidence of spontaneous leukemia in susceptible mice is markedly reduced if the mice are lethally irradiated and rescued with syngeneic bone marrow or spleen cells. It has been suggested that the protective effect is due to the replacement of susceptible thymic cells by less susceptible bone marrow or spleen cells. It seems likely, however, that restoration of immunological competence is an important factor, and this suggestion is consistent with Cole's further observation that the incidence of spontaneous leukemia is lower in mice subjected to high sublethal irradiation (690 R) followed by infusion of spleen cells from young isogeneic donors than in mice subjected to irradiation alone in the same dosage.

The first attempts to treat transplanted tumors by transfer of cells involved the infusion of bone marrow, and were undertaken primarily to see whether experimental leukemia which could not be eradicated by sublethal whole body irradiation could be successfully treated by giving a dose of irradiation which would ordinarily cause lethal damage to bone marrow and then rescuing the animal by transplantation of marrow from an isogeneic or allogeneic donor (Lorenz and Congdon, 1955; Barnes et al., 1956; Barnes and Loutit, 1957; Trentin, 1957). It was, however, envisaged by Barnes et al. that if allogeneic marrow was used "the colonizing cells might retain the capacity of the donor to destroy by the reaction of immunity . . . residual leukemic cells—and perhaps also the host." Since then, not only bone marrow but also spleen cells, lymph node cells, peripheral blood lymphocytes, thoracic duct lymphocytes, peritoneal exudate cells, and materials derived from them, from isogeneic, allogeneic, and xenogeneic donors, and also autochthonous cells, have been used in therapeutic experiments. The cells used have been of four types: non-immune unstimulated cells, cells from immunized donors, cells specifically immunized or armed in vitro, and cells non-specifically stimulated in vitro.

It is useful to have a generic term to include lymphocytes other than those present in cell suspensions prepared from bone marrow and thymus. The term lymphoid cells, which otherwise seems redundant, will be used for this purpose. Peritoneal exudate (PE) cells, which include both macrophages and lymphocytes, are sometimes referred to as peritoneal macrophages, but we shall restrict this label to purified cell suspensions from which most of the lymphocytes have been removed.

A general problem which arises when viable lymphocytes are transferred is that, as in the case of treatment with antibody, tumor growth may be stimulated instead of being inhibited. This phenomenon, which was referred to earlier (5.521) as cell-mediated enhancement, is due to the action of suppressor T cells. It has been observed particularly after transfer of isogeneic cells (Treves *et al.,* 1974; Small and Trainin, 1976), but may also follow transfer of allogeneic cells (Prehn, 1972; Shand, 1975). Another problem, which occurs only when allogeneic or xenogeneic lymphocytes are transferred and which will be discussed later (7.42), is the development of graft-versus-host disease (GVH).

Injection of macrophages has been ineffective except, as we shall see, when the macrophages were cytotoxic for the tumor *in vitro* and were injected with, or at the site of, the tumor—including the case where tumor cells and macrophages were both injected intravenously (Fidler, 1974; Kaplan and Morahan, 1975; Den Otter *et al.,* 1977).

Two types of material derived from tumor-immune cells have been used in tumor-bearing recipients, namely, extracts containing RNA (referred to as immune RNA or I-RNA) and transfer factor (TF or, because it is dialyzable, TF_D). In this chapter, however, we shall consider only I-RNA. Discussion of transfer factor will be postponed to the following chapter (8.234) because it has been used only in clinical trials and not for the treatment of tumors in experimental animals. The reason for this apparent anomaly is that while, as Lawrence (1955) showed long ago, delayed-type hypersensitivity can readily be transferred from one person to another with leukocyte extracts, it has proved difficult to do this in experimental animals. This has, however, now been achieved in a variety of experimental models (Lawrence, 1974), so that interest in the use of transfer factor in experimental tumor immunotherapy may be expected to increase.

7.41 Isogeneic and Autochthonous Cells

7.411 NON-IMMUNE UNSTIMULATED CELLS

The results of treatment with non-immune unstimulated isogeneic cells have been surprisingly variable.

Barnes *et al.* (1956) reported prolonged survival in 20 out of 25 mice with transplanted leukemia treated by 1500 R whole body irradiation and bone marrow from isogeneic non-immunized donors. With a smaller dose of irradiation (800–850 R) combined with bone marrow infusion, DeVries and Vos (1958), Mathé and Bernard (1959a, 1959b), and Fefer (1973) observed little or no benefit; when spleen cells were given as well as bone marrow, DeVries and Vos (1958) reported significant benefit and some cures.

Floersheim (1969) obtained a 50 percent cure rate in CBA mice bearing a transplanted CBA Moloney virus-induced leukemia treated by chemotherapy and infusion of normal isogeneic bone marrow and spleen cells, but Fass and Fefer (1972) observed only slightly increased survival in experiments of the same kind but with a different chemotherapeutic agent.

Blamey (1966) observed inhibition of growth of primary sarcomas in mice given infusions of non-immune spleen and lymph node cells without either irradiation or chemotherapy, but others have reported no benefit from this treatment in animals with established tumors (Delorme and Alexander, 1964; Borberg et al., 1972).

7.412 CELLS FROM IMMUNIZED OR TUMOR-BEARING DONORS

Various degrees of tumor inhibition have been observed when lymphoid cells from immunized or tumor-bearing isogeneic donors were mixed with a tumor inoculum (Bubenik, 1965; Rosenau and Morton, 1966; B. Fisher, Saffer, and Fisher, 1974a), but tumor growth may also be enhanced by this procedure (Bubenik, 1965; Umiel and Trainin, 1974). When lymph node cells from the nodes draining the site of a tumor were used they were found by Fisher et al. to be effective even when they were harvested as long as 2 months after removal of the tumor.

Treatment with immune isogeneic lymphoid cells has also been shown to prevent the development of autochthonous leukemia in mice made susceptible by the induction at birth of tolerance to Gross virus (Sparck and Volkert, 1965).

In animals treated after tumor inoculation, including some with manifest tumors, administration of immune isogeneic lymphoid cells in the absence of other treatment may result in prolonged survival and even complete regression (Borberg et al., 1972; H.G. Smith et al., 1977), but often has little or no effect (Fefer, 1969, 1974). Treatment with isogeneic immune lymphoid cells after radiotherapy (Koldovsky and Lengerova, 1960), or partial excision of solid tumors (Delorme and Alexander, 1964), or reduction of the tumor burden by chemotherapy in the case of both lymphomas (Mihich, 1969; Vadlamudi et al., 1971; Fefer, 1971; Fass and Fefer, 1972; Fefer et al., 1976) and other tumors (Fefer, 1969, 1973; Gotohda et al., 1974) has proved more effective and many instances of complete regression have been reported.

A technique described as specific activation of T cells rather than immunization was used by J.F.A.P. Miller (1973), based on previous work with allogeneic skin grafts (Sprent and Miller, 1972). Thymus cells from CBA mice were injected intravenously to lethally irradiated Balb/c mice, and 3 days later lymphocytes, which were shown to be of CBA origin and were referred to as CBA T.TDL, were collected by thoracic duct drainage. These, when mixed with mastocytoma cells and injected into neonatally thymectomized CBA mice, completely suppressed growth of the tumor.*

Alexander, Evans, and Mikulska (1973) collected adherent peritoneal exudate cells from DBA/2 mice which had been immunized with a syngeneic lymphoma on a film of collagen and then separated them with collagenase. Intraperitoneal injection of 5×10^5 of these "immune macrophages" (5.431) to DBA/2 mice 2 days after intraperitoneal injection of viable lymphoma cells resulted in significantly increased survival.

7.413 CELLS IMMUNIZED OR ARMED IN VITRO

As stated previously (5.21), T cells specifically cytotoxic in vitro for a variety of tumor cells can be induced by incubating normal animal or human lymphoid cells in vitro with cells or extracts of the tumor in question. Cells sensitized in this way have also been used in in vivo experiments and clinical trials (8.233).

---

*The mastocytoma used in these experiments originated in strain DBA/2, not Balb/c, but these strains are of the same H2 type ($H2_d$).

In what appear to have been the first experiments of this kind, Koldovsky (1966a) showed that lymph node or spleen cells which had been incubated with a cell-free supernatant of homogenized tumor tissue prevented, or markedly inhibited, growth of the tumor in isogeneic mice when injected prior to, or mixed with, the tumor inoculum.

Rollinghoff and Wagner (1973b), in a somewhat complicated model, showed that *in vitro* sensitized isogeneic lymphocytes protected lethally irradiated bone-marrow-reconstituted mice against an allogeneic plasmacytoma. Subsequently Burton and Warner (1977b), in an entirely syngeneic system, showed that spleen cells which had been incubated *in vitro* with a Balb/c murine plasmacytoma inhibited tumor development in isogeneic mice when mixed with the tumor cells inoculum, even in a ratio of two lymphocytes to one tumor cell, though they were only marginally effective when the tumor cells were injected subcutaneously and the sensitized lymphocytes intravenously on the same day in ratios of up to 100 lymphocytes per tumor cell. Treves, Cohen, and Feldman (1975), however, obtained a modest degree of protection against lethal pulmonary metastasis following resection of a primary murine tumor by intravenous injection of lymphocytes immunized *in vitro*.

Trainin and his colleagues (Ilfeld *et al.,* 1973; Small and Trainin, 1975) found that syngeneic lymphocytes which had been cultured on monolayers of murine sarcomas were cytotoxic *in vitro* for the corresponding tumor; *in vivo,* however, they caused enhancement of growth when mixed with a tumor cell inoculum, slight inhibition of growth when injected intravenously, and neither inhibition nor enhancement when injected subcutaneously separately from the tumor. Allogeneic lymphocytes sensitized *in vitro* in the same way also caused enhancement *in vivo* when mixed with tumor cells. Addition of a partly purified extract of calf thymus to the cultures during sensitization resulted in increased cytotoxicity of the lymphocytes *in vitro* (Carnaud *et al.,* 1973), reduced enhancing activity when mixed with the tumor cell inoculum, and increased tumor inhibition when injected intravenously.

Kedar *et al.* (1978b) found that syngeneic lymphocytes mixed with murine leukemic cells (the EL4 leukemia of C57Bl/6 mice and YAC leukemia of A strain mice) to which they had been sensitized *in vitro,* inhibited tumor growth strongly when the mixture was injected subcutaneously (sc), and to a slight extent when the mixture was injected intraperitoneally (ip) or intravenously (iv), and there was good correlation between the cytotoxicity of different cell preparations *in vitro* and their effectiveness *in vivo.* Intravenous, and to a less extent ip, injection of *in vitro*-sensitized lymphocytes 24–48 hours after sc, ip, or iv injection of a lethal dose of viable leukemia cells resulted in significant prolongation of survival but only a few complete cures. When mice which had been inoculated with a lethal dose of leukemia cells were treated 1 or 3 days later with a partially curative dose of cyclophosphamide (80–140 mg/kg) followed by ip or iv injection of *in vitro*-sensitized syngeneic lymphocytes 16–24 hours later, however, 80–100 percent of the mice survived over 100 days and were regarded as cured, whereas with cyclophosphamide alone the cure rate ranged from 20 to 60 percent (Kedar *et al.* 1978a).

Mokyr *et al.* (1978) compared the capacity of spleen cells from normal and tumor-bearing mice which had been incubated *in vitro* with isogeneic plasmacytomas to inhibit tumor growth *in vivo* when mixed with a tumor cell inoculum, and found that the spleen cells from tumor-bearing animals were at least as effective, and usually more effective, than cells from normal animals, whereas the latter showed the greater cytotoxicity *in vitro.* These authors suggested that autochthonous *in vitro*-activated cells from tumor-bearing animals might prove effective in therapeutic experiments and possibly clinically.

Cohen and his colleagues (Treves and Cohen, 1973; Livnat and Cohen, 1975a, 1975b) concluded that T cells sensitized *in vitro* by isogeneic or allogeneic embryo fibroblasts and injected into the mouse footpad did not themselves differentiate into effector cells but recruited effector T cells within the draining lymph nodes, because adoptive immunization in this system was prevented by irradiation of the recipient animal but not by irradiation (200 rad) of the transferred cells. Recruiting ability appeared to depend on the intrinsic metabolic function of the initiator lymphocytes and not merely on the presence of passively absorbed antigen carried over into the recipient mouse, because, although it was lost when the cells were treated with trypsin, it returned after a further 4 hours incubation in trypsin-free medium in the absence of contact with the sensitizing cells, and this recovery could be blocked with cyclohexidine. It was suggested that the specific information transferred in recruitment might involve RNA, transfer factor, or a specific immunoglobulin produced by T cells.

Van Loveren and Den Otter (1974) prepared activated armed macrophages (5.431) by collecting adherent peritoneal exudate cells from normal C57B1 mice on collagen, arming them by incubation with SMAF released from spleen cells cultured with the cells of a syngeneic lymphoma (SL2), activating these armed cells by incubating them with tumor-immune lymphoid cells and tumor cells, and then detaching them by incubation with collagenase. A single intraperitoneal injection of 2×10^6 activated armed macrophages 2 hours after intraperitoneal injection of 10^4 SL2 lymphoma cells to C57B1 mice resulted in significantly prolonged survival; after three injections, two out of five mice survived more than 100 days and the other three 23–27 days, whereas mice treated with normal, or armed but not activated, macrophages survived 13 to 15 days. Fidler (1974) cultured C57B1/6 macrophages with supernatants from cultures of a syngeneic melanoma with tumor-immune rat lymphocytes and showed that when these were injected intravenously, but not intraperitoneally, 48 hours after intravenous injection of viable lymphoma cells, the number of tumor nodules which developed in the lungs was significantly reduced.

7.414   NON-SPECIFICALLY STIMULATED CELLS

The tumor inhibitory effect of non-immune lymphoid cells in Winn assays (i.e., mixed with a tumor cell inoculum) may be increased by the addition of interferon (Chernyakhovskaya, Slavina, and Svet-Moldavsky, 1970) or by pretreating the lymphoid cells with methotrexate (Svet-Moldavsky and Kadaghidze, 1968).

It has also been shown (Lundgren and Möller, 1969) that the addition of phytohemagglutinin, streptolysin, or antilymphocyte serum increases the toxicity of non-immune human lymphocytes for allogeneic fibroblasts *in vitro,* but the effect of these agents on the antitumor activity of lymphoid cells *in vivo* does not seem to have been investigated.

Peritoneal exudate cells from some mice, as mentioned previously (5.431), are non-specifically cytotoxic *in vitro* for tumor cells, and injection of such PEC intraperitoneally 2 hours after injection of SL2 lymphoma cells (of DBA/2 origin) to DBA/2 mice resulted in significantly prolonged survival (Den Otter *et al.,* 1977).

7.42 Allogeneic, Semiallogeneic, and Xenogeneic Cells

The effect of transplanted allogeneic or xenogeneic lymphoid cells depends *inter alia* on the capacity of the recipient to reject them. Although this may vary within wide limits, it is convenient to distinguish three situations:

1. The recipient has received radiotherapy or chemotherapy in a dosage which may have caused significant immunosuppression.
2. The recipient is an F1 hybrid of two inbred strains, and the cell donor is a member of one of the parent strains. Transplants of this kind, which will be described as *semiallogeneic (P to F1)*, do not evoke an allograft reaction, in contrast to transplants in the opposite direction, described as *semiallogeneic (F1 to P)*, which are ordinarily rejected in the absence of immunosuppression.
3. The recipient has not received radiotherapy or chemotherapy, and the cells are from an allogeneic or xenogeneic donor.

In the first two cases, cells of donor origin, using this term to include transplanted cells and their descendants, may persist for a long time. This condition, which is termed *chimerism*, may, as we shall see, be associated with severe manifestations of graft-versus-host disease (GVH), particularly if the donor and recipient differ in respect of the major histocompatibility system (H2 in the mouse, HLA in man). In the third case, prolonged chimerism does not occur and GVH usually does not become manifest or takes a mild form; acute GVH may develop, however, after transplantation of a large number of xenogeneic cells from an immunized donor.

7.421 RECIPIENTS SUBJECTED TO RADIOTHERAPY OR CHEMOTHERAPY

In the experiments of Barnes *et al.* (1956), as stated earlier, most of the mice received a supralethal dose (1500 R) of whole body irradiation and were rescued with isogeneic bone marrow. Five mice, however, received allogeneic marrow; three of these developed wasting and diarrhea and died 1–2 months after the treatment, and this was correctly attributed by Barnes *et al.* to "complications of the treatment and not its failure."

The occurrence of this syndrome, which is now often called *secondary disease,* following high-dose irradiation and infusion of allogeneic or xenogeneic bone marrow, was soon confirmed (Congdon, 1957; Congdon and Urso, 1957; van Bekkum and Vos, 1957), and it was observed that an acute form of the disease with a high mortality developed after irradiation and infusion of allogeneic spleen cells (Schwartz, Upton, and Congdon, 1957; Uphoff and Law, 1958; Mathé and Bernard, 1958).

Secondary disease occurs only when the recipient of bone marrow or lymphoid cells possesses histocompatibility antigens which are not present in the cell donor, and for some reason is unable to reject quickly the transplanted cells. It was soon recognized that, with allogeneic donors, secondary disease was likely to be more severe when the donor and recipient differed in respect of the major histocompatibility system (Uphoff and Law, 1958; Mathé, 1960). Like runt disease, which occurs in newborn mice (Billingham and Brent, 1957) and rats (Woodruff and Sparrow, 1957) injected with allogeneic lymphocytes, secondary disease is associated with widespread destruction of lymphoid tissue, and both conditions are manifestations of the GVH reaction.

In many experiments in which animals with transplanted leukemias (DeVries and Vos, 1958; Mathé and Bernard, 1959a) or carcinomas (Woodruff and Symes, 1962c; Woodruff, Symes, and Stuart, 1963) were treated by whole body irradiation followed by infusion of allogeneic, semiallogeneic, or xenogeneic cells, survival has been at best only slightly prolonged, despite evidence in some cases of an inhibitory effect on the tumor, because animals which did not die of the tumor died of secondary disease. Similarly, Mathé, Amiel, and Bernard (1960) found that when mice of a strain (AKR) with a high incidence of spontaneous leukemia were treated by irradiation (750 R) and infusion of allogeneic (C57B1/6 or C3H) bone marrow before they showed signs of leukemia, all the mice died of either leukemia or secondary disease. Mice which received C57B1/6 marrow often died earlier than untreated controls; those which received marrow from C3H mice, which, like AKR, are of haplotype H2k, survived, however, somewhat longer.

Treatment of an allogeneic mouse ascites tumor, the Landschutz carcinoma, by irradiation (400 R) and intraperitoneal injection of spleen cells from normal rats or rats immunized against the tumor, delayed the growth of the tumor and prolonged the survival of the mice; eventually, however, all the animals died of either the tumor or secondary disease (Woodruff, Symes, and Stuart, 1963). Better results were achieved with the same tumor by irradiation and intraperitoneal injection of thoracic duct lymphocytes from immunized rats, and 3 of 23 mice treated in this way survived more than 100 days without evidence of tumor and were then sacrificed; there were, however, many deaths from secondary disease (Woodruff, Symes, and Anderson, 1963). In assessing the significance of these results it must be remembered that allogeneic tumors are easy targets compared with isogeneic or autochthonous tumors; to destroy one is, to borrow Woglom's (1929) graphic phrase, "like shooting a rabbit in its hutch." With isogeneic tumors treatment is often ineffective because, as in the experiments of Gardner et al. (1964), if the treatment is effective in destroying the leukemia the recipients die of GVH.

Much work has been done with the object of finding ways of avoiding this complication (see Nouza, 1968), and the following procedures have been shown under certain conditions to reduce the severity of GVH disease or even prevent it from becoming manifested at all:

1. The use of a fetal donor or a donor compatible with the recipient in respect of the major histocompatibility system.
2. Treatment of the donor with heterologous antilymphocyte serum (Boak and Wilson, 1968).
3. Treatment of the cells prior to infusion:
    (1) Incubation with antilymphocyte globulin or non-cytotoxic Fab derived therefrom (Richie et al., 1975).
    (2) Specific depletion of cells which cause GVH by incubation on monolayers of recipient-type spleen cells (Bonavida and Kedar, 1974).
4. Treatment of the recipient:
    (1) Splenectomy (Biozzi et al., 1964).
    (2) Administration of cytotoxic drugs, of which the most effective appear to have been methotrexate (A-methopterin), cyclophosphamide, and cytosine arabinoside (Nouza, 1968; Floersheim, 1972).

(3) Administration of heterologous antilymphocyte serum (Boak *et al.,* 1968), or alloantiserum raised in the donor strain against recipient strain cells (Silvers and Billingham, 1969).

(4) Administration of lymphoid cells from mature hybrid animals which have not developed fatal GVH following injection of parent-strain lymphoid cells to susceptible (i.e., immature or irradiated) hybrids. The rationale of this procedure, which was devised by McKearn *et al.* (1974), is that mature F1 rats which do not develop severe GVH after injection of parental lymphoid cells have been shown to develop antibody reactive with receptors on donor lymphoid cells for host antigens (ARA); immature or irradiated F1 rats do not develop ARA, and it was predicted that the cells from mature animals, by providing this, would be of therapeutic value.

5. Mixing fetal lymphoid cells with adult cells. This has been shown to reduce local GVH reactions (Skowron-Cendrzak and Ptak, 1976), and the effect has been attributed to suppressor T cells in the fetal cell population.

6. Avoidance of infection by using germ-free animals (Truitt and Pollard, 1976).

The use of these procedures in association with adoptive immunotherapy is, however, restricted by the need to reduce harmful effects of GVH to an acceptable level without either so weakening the antitumor effect as to render the treatment valueless or preventing hematopoietic recovery. This has proved to be a very difficult problem, and only modest progress has been made in the search for a solution.

Irradiation in lethal dosage of mice bearing a transplanted leukemia, followed by infusion of allogeneic fetal liver cells, proved unsuccessful in the hands of Mathé and Bernard (1959a) because, while the animals did not develop GVH, they were not protected against the leukemia. Duplan (1958), however, had some success with this type of procedure in reducing the incidence of a spontaneous murine leukemia.

As already mentioned, Mathé and Bernard (1959b) found that AKR mice reconstituted after lethal irradiation with H2-compatible (C3H) bone marrow survived longer than mice which received H2-incompatible (C57B1/6) marrow. Subsequently Fefer (1969, 1970, 1971, 1973) treated Balb/c mice which had been inoculated with either Moloney sarcoma virus or viable Moloney leukemia cells by chemotherapy with cyclophosphamide and injection of allogeneic H2-compatible (DBA/2) or H2-incompatible (C57B1/6) spleen cells. Many of the mice which received H2-compatible cells from donors immunized with the Moloney virus were cured or showed prolonged survival, but those which received non-immune H2-compatible cells behaved like controls treated with cyclophosphamide only. All mice which received H2-incompatible cells died soon afterwards with secondary disease; at death 15 of 16 mice which had received cells from non-immunized donors, but only 2 of 11 which had received cells from immunized donors, had palpable tumors. On the other hand Bortin *et al.* (1974b) found that all H2-identical cells had little effect.

Woodruff and Symes (1962c) attempted without success to rescue tumor-bearing animals which had been treated with whole body irradiation and allogeneic spleen cells from secondary disease by repeated administration of A-methopterin (methotrexate) starting 2, 4, or 6 days after the first injection of spleen cells. They suggested that injection of isogeneic spleen cells might be more effective, but, in the absence of any other rescue procedures, this did not appear to alter the course of the disease (Woodruff, unpublished).

These lines of attack on the problem were developed further by Boranic (1968), who showed that RF mice with a transplanted isogeneic leukemia treated by 530 R whole body irradiation and infusion of allogeneic (C57B1/Rij) spleen cells and marrow cells died in 2–3 weeks of secondary disease, but if subsequently treated with cyclophosphamide or heterologous antilymphocyte serum they survived 5–8 weeks. The leukemia did not recur, but the state of chimerism persisted, and death was due to a chronic form of secondary disease. Although it appeared from the work of Wallis, Davies, and Koller (1966), who used a chromosomal marker (the T6 translocation), that adoptive immunization was unlikely to be effective in inhibiting the development of radiation leukemia unless chimerism was established, Boranic found that administration of isogeneic bone marrow, blood, splenic, lymph node, and thymic cells after cyclophosphamide often abolished the chimerism without causing recurrence of the leukemia, and 19 out of 36 mice treated in this way were alive and well 5 months later. Many of the mice given cyclophosphamide lost their teeth, and it seems likely that there would have been more long-term survivors if all, instead of only about half, of the mice had been fed on pellets ground with water to form a paste. Subsequently Boranic and Tonkovic (1972) treated RF or (RF × C57B1)F1 mice with the same transplanted myeloid leukemia and A-strain or (A × C57B1)F1 mice with a transplanted A-strain lymphoid leukemia by irradiation in lethal dosage and infusion of allogeneic (C57B1) spleen and bone marrow cells, with or without subsequent attempted rescue from secondary disease with cyclophosphamide alone or cyclophosphamide plus syngeneic bone marrow, blood, splenic, lymph node, and thymic cells. The mice which did not receive cyclophosphamide or syngeneic cells died of secondary disease without evidence of leukemia. Cyclophosphamide alone prevented the manifestation of secondary disease but if given within 3 days of irradiation usually resulted in recurrence of the leukemia. In these experiments, infusion of syngeneic cells given after cyclophosphamide was not well tolerated and shortened survival.

Bortin et al. (1974a) treated AKR mice with tansplanted acute lymphocytic leukemia by 400 R whole body irradiation and intraperitoneal injection of 5 mg cyclophosphamide, followed 4–6 hours later by intravenous injection of allogeneic bone marrow and lymph node cells from H2-incompatible (DBA/2) donors. Six days later the mice were given an intraperitoneal injection of CBA anti-DBA/2 serum and 2 mg cyclophosphamide, followed later that day by an intravenous injection of bone marrow cells from allogeneic but H2-compatible (CBA) mice, and in some animals administration of serum and CBA bone marrow was repeated 7 days later. Thirty-five percent of mice treated in this way survived for over 100 days, and many of these for more than 6 months. The results were less good when the CBA marrow donors had been immunized with DBA/2 tissue, and when the DBA/2 cells were treated with neuraminidase. Intravenously injected neuraminidase-treated lymphocytes are trapped initially in the liver before migrating to lymphoid tissue (Woodruff and Gesner, 1969; Berney and Gesner, 1970), and were tried by Bortin et al. because it had been reported by Im and Simmons (1971) that they caused a less severe GVH reaction than untreated cells in recipients subjected to a moderate degree of immunosuppression.

Merritt et al. (1973) investigated the rescue of non-tumor-bearing rhesus monkeys which had received 900 R whole body irradiation and allogeneic bone marrow. Two animals subsequently treated with cyclophosphamide alone both died of marrow aplasia, and two out of three treated with stored autologous bone marrow alone died of acute GVH disease. Four of nine animals which received cyclophosphamide followed by autologous marrow were rescued; three died of marrow aplasia, one of acute GVH disease, and one of infection. Storb *et al.* (1974) succeeded in rescuing three out of seven dogs which had received 1200 R whole body irradiation and allogeneic bone marrow by a second dose of irradiation (600 R) 14 days later followed by infusion of marrow from a DLA compatible litter mate, but the other four animals died of marrow aplasia or infection.

Truitt and Pollard (1976) treated conventional and germ-free SJL mice with spontaneous reticulum cell sarcomas by whole body irradiation (1000 R for conventional mice and 850 R for germ-free mice) followed 1 day later by intravenous infusion of adult bone marrow cells, using germ-free donors for germ-free recipients and conventional donors for conventional recipients. Conventional tumor-bearing mice which received allogeneic (CBA/H) marrow all died within 30 days with symptoms of severe GVH disease, including weight loss, kyphosis, dermatitis, alopecia, and diarrhea. Seventy percent of germ-free mice which received allogeneic (germ-free CBA/H) marrow survived more than 120 days, and when sacrificed showed no evidence of residual tumor or GVH at autopsy. In contrast 50 percent of germ-free mice which received syngeneic marrow survived 120 days, and all showed evidence of residual tumor.

7.422 SEMIALLOGENEIC (P TO F1) CELLS WITHOUT IMMUNOSUPPRESSION

Transfer of bone marrow or lymphoid cells from inbred parent-strain donors to F1 hybrids clearly has no direct application to the clinical situation, but experiments of this kind have provided important information about the effect of GVH and GVT (graft-versus-tumor) reactions in the absence of irradiation and drug-mediated immunosuppression.

It was reported by Wigzell (1961) that intraperitoneal injection of lymphoid cells from normal members of one parental strain (P1) on day −5, or on day 0 from members of this strain immunized with tissue from the other strain, inhibited growth of lymphoma cells transplanted from the other parent strain (P2) to F1 hybrid recipients on day 0; when similar experiments were performed with two mammary carcinomas and a chemically induced sarcoma, however, only very slight inhibition was observed. The antitumor effect was considered to be mainly specific and directed against histocompatibility antigens, because growth of the lymphoma was inhibited only very slightly by injection of lymphoid cells from the strain of origin of the tumor (P2), which should produce a GVH reaction but not a reaction against histocompatibility antigens represented on the tumor cells. Woodruff and Boak (1965), in experiments which differed from those of Wigzell not only in respect of the strains of mice and tumors used but also in that the lymphoid cell donors were immunized with tumor cells instead of normal cells, found that the growth of an A-strain mammary carcinoma was inhibited by intravenous injection of spleen cells from immunized CBA donors starting 7 days after tumor inoculation. In only 3 out of 60 mice could death be attributed to GVH disease, and it was considered in view of the mildness of the GVH reaction that the antitumor effect was mainly specific.

Rumma and Davies (1975) found that the mortality of F1 hybrid rats inoculated with a parent line tumor was greatly reduced by injection of spleen cells from the strain of origin of the tumor, whereas injection of lymphoid cells from the other strain caused tumor regression but also a high mortality from GVH disease. Injection of lymphoid cells from the strain of origin of the tumor was also moderately effective in preventing metastasis when given as adjuvant therapy after surgical resection of sub-cutaneous tumors which were about 1 cm in diameter.

There is evidence that with other tumor systems tumor inhibition may occur without any specific component as a consequence of the existence of a GVH reaction, and this phenomenon has been termed a "bystander effect" (Johnson and Hersey, 1976). This was first demonstrated by Katz et al. (1972) and Ellman et al. (1972). They found that the survival of adult inbred strain 2 guinea pigs challenged with a le-thal dose of isogeneic leukemia cells (L2C) was markedly prolonged by pretreatment with allogeneic (strain T3) but not with semiallogeneic (F1-P) hybrid (2 × T3)F1 lymphoid cells, and argued that while both categories of cell were liable to rejection only the allogeneic cells had the potential (if not rejected too quickly) to cause a GVH reaction. They showed subsequently that F1 hybrid recipients of the leukemia were protected to an equal extent by lymphoid cells from either parent strain, and argued that this excluded the possibility of the rejection being due to an immune response di-rected against strain 2 histocompatibility antigens presented on the leukemic cells. They thus concluded that the antitumor effect in this system was a consequence of the GVH reaction. More recently, Johnson and Hersey (1976) showed that (PVGe × Wistar)F1 hybrid rats could be protected equally well against a PVGe strain leukemia by lymphoid cells from donors of either parent strain. In each case protection was markedly dependent on the dose and timing of the cell transfer. It should be noted that bystander effects can also occur as the result of local reactions produced in other ways. Thus Bernstein et al. (1971) showed that the growth of a syngeneic guinea pig hepatoma after intradermal inoculation was inhibited if macrophage migration-inhibi-tion factor (MIF), prepared by incubating lymph node cells from guinea pigs immu-nized against killed M. tuberculosis with tuberculin (PPD), was mixed with the tumor inoculum or injected 24 hours before tumor inoculation at the same site.

Treatment with parent line cells may, on the other hand, enhance the growth of tumors in F1 hybrids. This was reported by Palmer and Symes (1974), who found that administration of C57B1 spleen cells to (AKR × C57B1)F1 hybrid mice inoculated with an AKR lymphoma not only caused a strong GVH reaction but also enhanced the growth of the tumor. Injection of AKR spleen cells, on the other hand, caused only a weak GVH reaction and had little effect on tumor growth.

7.423 ALLOGENEIC OR XENOGENEIC CELLS WITHOUT RADIOTHERAPY OR CHEMOTHERAPY

It was found by Woodruff, Symes, and Stuart (1963) that intraperitoneal injec-tion of $8 × 10^8$ normal rat spleen cells to mice 4 days after intraperitoneal inoculation of 10^5 Landschutz ascites tumor cells without any other treatment significantly de-layed the development of the tumor and prolonged the life of the animals. Injection of the same number of cells from rats immunized by repeated injections of Landschutz tumor cells also inhibited the growth of the tumor, but four out of ten mice died with-in 6 to 11 days, and this was thought to be due to acute GVH disease. Similar treat-ment had no beneficial effect on mice inoculated with an isogeneic mammary carcinoma, though Mathé (1966) obtained quite marked inhibition of a syngeneic as-cites tumor with intraperitoneal injection of allogeneic or xenogeneic lymph node cells from immunized donors.

Delorme and Alexander (1964) showed that, in rats with established chemically induced fibrosarcomas, repeated intravenous injection of thoracic duct lymphocytes (total dosage $2 × 10^8$ to $2 × 10^9$ cells) from allogeneic donors immunized 6–10 days previously with irradiated tumor cells obtained by biopsy of the tumor to be treated, caused partial regression in about a third of the animals, and complete regression in one of them. None of the rats developed the usual manifestations of GVH disease, such as weight loss, diarrhea, or lymphoid atrophy, but many died with respiratory failure after the third or fourth injection, and this was attributed to some form of hypersensitivity reaction. Subsequently, Alexander, Delorme, and Hall (1966) used xenogeneic immune lymphoid cells as adjuvant therapy following partial excision of similar rat fibrosarcomas. Sheep were immunized with subcutaneous transplants of tissue from the tumor to be treated, and 3 days later the efferent lymphatic of the draining node was canulated; cells were collected during the next 4 days, washed, and injected intravenously to the rats in a total dosage of 2×10^9 to 5×10^9 cells. Temporary regression of the tumor occurred in 8 out of 18 animals, and none developed symptoms of GVH disease. The effect was clearly specific, since lymph node cells from sheep immunized with tumors other than the one to be treated were ineffective. In preliminary experiments in which goats were used instead of sheep, two tumor-bearing rats were reported to be completely cured.

Alexander and Hall (1970), in discussing these and subsequent experiments, attributed the antitumor effect to cells which they termed *immunoblasts,* which are present in large numbers in lymph collected 4 to 10 days after immunization, but not in lymph collected later or in spleen cells. Since the antitumor effect was not reduced by irradiating the cells in a dosage of 1000 R before they were injected, it was concluded that they do not need to proliferate in the treated animal. It seemed unlikely, moreover, that they survived for more than a very short time, since the recipients were not immunosuppressed, and it was therefore postulated that RNA from the immunoblasts produced a phenotypic transformation in some of the host cells and caused them to acquire immunologically specific antitumor activity (Alexander and Hall, 1970). Experiments bearing on this hypothesis will be discussed later (7.43).

The therapeutic effect in non-immunosuppressed animals of allogeneic spleen cells harvested relatively late from immunized donors, which has been observed mainly in experiments with allogeneic tumors in which the lymphoid and tumor cells were brought into close contact by being injected at the same site (Woodruff, Symes, and Stuart, 1963; Alexander, Connell, and Mikulska, 1966), was attributed by Alexander and Hall to the presence of memory cells which, on contact with antigen, transform into cells with the properties of cytotoxic immunoblasts; it seems unlikely, however, that Jurin's (1972) observation that allogeneic spleen and lymph node cells injected 5–7 days before tumor challenge resulted in a higher TD50 can be explained in this way.

Dullens *et al.* (1974a, 1974b, 1975) observed modest prolongation of survival of mice injected intraperitoneally with a syngeneic lymphoma as the result of a single injection of peritoneal exudate cells from an immunized allogeneic donor 2 hours after injection of the tumor cells. Three or five injections at intervals of 24 hours resulted in even longer survival, but more, or more frequent, injections proved to be less effective. Lymphocytes separated from the PE cells were ineffective; purified macrophages were slightly less effective than unfractionated PE cells.

7.43 Immune RNA

Following the discovery by Fishman (1961) that normal rat lymphoid cells incubated with a cell-free, ribonuclease-sensitive extract prepared from normal rat macrophages exposed to T2 phage acquired the ability to produce anti-T2-phage antibody, it was shown by many investigators (see Fritze *et al.*, 1976a) that normal lymphoid cells treated with RNA prepared from macrophages or lymphoid cells previously sensitized to a variety of antigens acquired the capacity to mediate cellular or humoral reactions both *in vivo* and *in vitro* to the antigen in question. Mannick and Egdahl (1962a, 1962b, 1964) extended this work into the field of transplantation immunology and showed, firstly, that normal rabbit lymphoid cells which had been incubated with RNA from the lymph nodes of rabbits immunized with skin allografts gave a positive transfer reaction (Brent, Brown, and Medawar, 1958) when injected intradermally into the allograft donor, and, secondly, that New Zealand rabbits could be made immune to skin allografts from California rabbits by reinfusion of autologous spleen cells which had been incubated *in vitro* with RNA extracted from the lymph nodes of other New Zealand rabbits which had been immunized with a skin allograft and spleen cells from the same donor. Although these workers did not succeed in transferring immunity to allografts with RNA preparations alone, their findings have stimulated many attempts to transfer tumor immunity with RNA.

Alexander *et al.* (1967) showed that autochthonous chemically induced fibrosarcomas in rats could be made to regress, usually temporarily but occasionally completely, by the injection of material rich in RNA prepared from lymphocytes collected from sheep and allogeneic rats which had been immunized with tissue from the tumor to be treated by canulation of the efferent lymphatic of the prefemoral lymph node and the thoracic duct, respectively. The material was injected into the footpads rather than intravenously because it was thought that intravenously rejected RNA would be degraded by RNAase before it could be taken up by the lymphoid cells of the tumor-bearing animal.

The preparation contained, in addition to RNA, considerable amounts of DNA and some traces of protein, and, although the active principle was thought to be RNA, in subsequent experiments (Alexander *et al.*, 1968) a nucleic acid fraction which consisted of almost pure RNA did not have an antitumor action.

There have been many reports of experiments in which resistance to tumor challenge has been increased specifically by prior administration of syngeneic lymphoid cells incubated with RNA extracted from the lymphoid cells of syngeneic (Rigby, 1969; Deckers and Pilch, 1971a, 1972), allogeneic (Rigby, 1969), or xenogeneic (Ramming and Pilch, 1970, 1971; Pilch and Ramming, 1970) animals immunized against the tumor in question, or of "immune RNA" of allogeneic or xenogeneic origin alone (Londner *et al.*, 1968; Kennedy, Cater, and Hartveit, 1969; Deckers and Pilch, 1971b).

There have also been further reports of inhibition of the growth of established tumors by immune RNA, although only in the experiments of Alexander *et al.* (1967, 1968), which have already been discussed, was an autochthonous tumor used.

Schlager and his colleagues (Schlager and Dray, 1975; Schlager, Paque, and Dray, 1975) injected guinea pig hepatoma cells intradermally at two sites, and 5 days later, when tumor cells had spread to the regional lymph nodes, injected either syngeneic or xenogeneic tumor-immune RNA together with normal syngeneic lymphocytes and tumor-specific antigens to one of the sites. The tumor failed to develop in the treated animals at either site or in the lymph nodes. Pilch *et al.* (1976b) injected xenogeneic (guinea pig) or syngeneic immune RNA as adjuvant therapy in association with excision of syngeneic transplants of a metastasizing mammary carcinoma in Fisher rats. Control animals treated by surgery only all died within 96 days with metastases in the lungs and elsewhere. Additional treatment with xenogeneic immune RNA before and after operation, xenogeneic RNA after operation only, and syngeneic RNA before and after operation resulted in four out of five, six out of nine, and three out of six animals, respectively, being alive and free of tumor after 180 days. Wang, Onikul, and Mannick (1978), in experiments with a transplanted metastasizing C57B1/6 mouse melanoma, found that intraperitoneal injection of normal isogeneic spleen cells which had been incubated *in vitro* with immune RNA from guinea pigs immunized with this tumor, after amputation of the limb bearing the primary transplant, resulted in prolonged survival and some cures. The effect was tumor specific and ribonuclease sensitive.

These findings, together with the discovery that normal lymphoid cells treated with syngeneic (Kern, Drogemuller, and Pilch, 1974) or xenogeneic (Kern and Pilch, 1974) antitumor immune RNA become cytotoxic for the corresponding tumor cells *in vitro,* and that normal tumor-free mice treated with specific xenogeneic immune RNA produce tumor-specific cytotoxic antibody (Fritze *et al.,* 1976a), are of great theoretical interest and offer some encouragement concerning the possible value of immune RNA in the treatment of cancer. One of the attractions of this approach has been the relative freedom from complications, but enhancement of a C3H fibrosarcoma occurred when tumor cells and isogeneic spleen cells treated with immune RNA were mixed together and injected subcutaneously (Pilch and Ramming, 1971), and the possibility that immune RNA alone might cause enhancement should not be ignored.

7.5 NON-SPECIFIC IMMUNOPOTENTIATION

In this section we shall consider agents which stimulate immunological or para-immunological reactions non-specifically, and their effect on tumors when injected systemically or at the tumor site. These will be referred to as *immunopotentiators* or *immunopotentiating agents.* An alternative term proposed by Weiss (1977), which explicitly allows for the possibility of inhibitory as well as stimulatory effects, is *immunomodulator.* The term *immunological adjuvant,* often abbreviated to adjuvant, is also sometimes used to include all agents of this kind, but it seems preferable to use it in its original meaning of something which, when mixed and injected with antigen, results in an augmented immunological response.

Immunopotentiators act in a variety of ways, and these have been reviewed by Weiss (1977). Firstly, they may combine with or modify a weak antigen to make it more immunogenic in normal animals and capable of evoking a response in animals whose immunological responses are generally impaired or which have been made specifically unresponsive to the antigen in question. Secondly, they may create an inflammatory microenvironment which makes for more effective interaction between antigen and cells concerned in the immunological response, or which results in the cells of a tumor or an allograft being damaged as the result of a bystander effect (7.422). Thirdly, they may modify the behavior of lymphocytes, macrophages, and possibly other cells concerned in immunological and para-immunological reactions. The effect on macrophage activity is often particularly striking, and appears to depend on both stimulation of macrophage precursors to differentiate into mature macrophages, and activation of mature cells. These effects have been attributed to increased production of colony-stimulating factor (CSF) and macrophage-stimulating factor (MSF), respectively; it appears from the work of Stanley *et al.* (1976), however, that CSF and MSF assays probably detect the same molecule.

The effect of immunopotentiators on tumor growth *in vivo* depends not only on their effect on immunological and para-immunological responses, but also on the fact that some stimulate the production of interferon, and this may affect the behavior of certain tumors (8.323). The overall therapeutic effect is determined by many factors; these include the particular agent and tumor studied; the dose, route of administration, and time of administration of the agent in relation to chemotherapy (Sansing, Killion, and Kollmorgen, 1977) or other treatment; and the immunological reactivity of the tumor-bearing animal or patient. Insofar as immunological and para-immunological responsiveness may have been impaired by the presence of the tumor, or as the result of treatment, the therapeutic effect will depend on the extent to which the agent can correct this situation (Kerbel, 1974), i.e., on its capacity to achieve what Mathé (1973) has called *immunorestoration*. This may be important in respect of the host's reaction to the tumor and its resistance to infection, both of which may have been seriously impaired.

Various tests, some of which have been discussed by Mathé, Kamel *et al.* (1973), have been used to screen immunopotentiating agents, including their effect on macrophage activity, on immunological activity mediated by T cells, or by T cells in conjunction with B cells, and on the growth of selected animal tumors in normal and T-cell-deficient animals. It is important in applying these tests to use a wide range of doses because, as Bliznakov (1977) has pointed out, the dose–response curve, except over a very limited range, is often non-linear and non-monotonic but W or M shaped with two peaks of relative maximal effect, and agents which inhibit tumor growth at one dose level may stimulate it at another. Although considerable progress has been made in defining the effects of individual agents, it is often still not clear why different tumors respond differently to the same agent, or why a particular tumor responds to some agents but not to others.

When an agent is injected locally, or concentrates selectively in the tumor, the question arises of whether any therapeutic effect which occurs is due, partly or wholly, to direct cytotoxicity. Insofar as this is the case the procedure is only partly immunotherapeutic or even not immunotherapeutic at all. There may be an element of direct cytotoxicity with some of the agents we shall discuss, but it has seemed preferable to err on the side of including too much rather than too little. On the other hand, intralesional injection of some agents has a systemic effect as the result of which the growth of metastases, or other transplants of the same tumor, may be inhibited (Salomon and Lynch, 1976; Salomon *et al.,* 1976).

Immunopotentiating agents will be discussed under the following headings:

1. Bacillus Calmette-Guérin (BCG) and derivatives.
2. *Corynebacterium parvum.*
3. Other bacterial preparations.
4. Viral infection.
5. Polynucleotides.
6. Levamisole.
7. Anticoagulants and fibrinolytic agents.
8. Interferon.
9. Other agents.

7.51 BCG and Derivatives

It was suspected many years ago that the chance of getting cancer was reduced in patients with tuberculosis (see Pearl, 1929), and there was experimental evidence which showed that the growth of allogeneic tumor transplants was inhibited by mixing live *M. tuberculosis* with the tumor inoculum, or even, though to a lesser extent, by injecting the organism at another site (Centanni and Rezzesi, 1926); it was not until

1959, however, that the antitumor effect of Bacillus Calmette-Guérin (BCG) was demonstrated.

This organism was developed by Calmette and Guérin at the Pasteur Institute in Lille by repeatedly culturing *Mycobacterium bovis* in a medium containing ox bile (Guérin, 1957). Although originally intended solely for the prophylaxis of tuberculosis, the adjuvant and immunopotentiating properties of BCG have stimulated experimental and clinical studies of its effect on tumor growth. The original strain has been given to many laboratories throughout the world, and various different substrains have arisen. The preparations used in different studies include living fresh organisms, living organisms which have been frozen or freeze-dried, extracts prepared in various ways, and occasionally killed whole organisms.

Because of strain differences which have arisen, and differences in production and storage, these preparations differ in various ways including their effectiveness as immunopotentiating agents (Mathé, Kamel *et al.,* 1973; Mackaness, Auclair, and Lagrange, 1974; Lagrange *et al.,* 1976; Halle-Pannenko *et al.,* 1976; Turcotte and Quevillon, 1976; Landi *et al.,* 1978; Lagrange, 1978). The main strains available commercially, in alphabetical order (with the city of origin), are Connaught (Ontario), Copenhagen, Glaxo (London), Montreal, Pasteur (Paris), Phipps (Philadelphia), Rio de Janeiro, and Tice (Chicago). Lagrange compared five of these strains which have been widely used clinically (Pasteur, Phipps, Tice, Connaught, and Glaxo), grown and stored in the same way, in respect of immunogenicity, capacity to evoke a lymphoproliferative response *in vivo,* and T-cell-potentiating effect. They found that the first four strains closely resembled each other, Pasteur BCG being the most powerful, whereas Glaxo was much less effective. They also compared fresh and freeze-dried preparations of two strains and found that freeze-dried Pasteur BCG was much less active than its fresh counterpart and also deteriorated on storage, whereas freeze-dried Connaught BCG was nearly as powerful as the fresh preparation. Halle-Pannenko *et al.* (1976) tested nine freeze-dried, five frozen, and one fresh BCG preparation from various strains for their immunopotentiating capacity in mice using three tests: the IgM response to sheep erythrocytes, immunoprophylaxis of the Lewis lung carcinoma, and immunoprophylaxis of the L1210 leukemia. Only fresh Pasteur BCG was effective in all three tests. Two preparations of Glaxo BCG performed very poorly.

In patients (8.242), BCG is commonly given intradermally by scarification or multiple puncture, or intralesionally, though other routes have been used. In animals, BCG may also be given intradermally or intralesionally, but has often been given by other routes, sometimes mixed with tumor cells. Ideally, in both animal experiments and clinical trials, as Baldwin and Pimm (1978) have suggested, the protocol should specify the strain of BCG, the type of preparation (fresh, frozen, freeze-dried, or killed), the dose of organisms expressed as moist weight and/or dry weight, the total number of units (aggregated and single organisms), the number of units containing viable organisms, the number of viable and non-viable organisms, and the route of administration. In practice not all of the information relating to dosage is likely to be available.

The literature concerning the immunological properties and antitumor effect of BCG is large and somewhat repetitive. Useful reviews have been published by Bast *et al.* (1974) and by Baldwin and Pimm (1978). The discussion which follows will be arranged under the following headings:

1. General immunological properties.
2. Systemic treatment of tumors with live BCG.

3. Injection of BCG mixed with the tumor cell inoculum.
4. Intralesional injection of BCG.
5. Treatment with killed BCG and BCG derivatives.

Treatment in which BCG is used together with other immunotherapeutic procedures will be considered later (7.71).

7.511 GENERAL IMMUNOLOGICAL PROPERTIES

Before discussing the effect of BCG on tumors it may be helpful to list some of the observed effects of BCG administration on immunological and para-immunological reactions in general.

Humoral immunity and ADCC.   Humoral responses to both thymus-dependent and thymus-independent antigens may be potentiated (Halpern *et al.,* 1958; Stjernsward, 1966; T.E. Miller, Mackaness, and Lagrange, 1973; Florentin *et al.,* 1976). The effect depends on the dose of BCG and the route of administration. Florentin *et al.* found that, with antigen injected intravenously or intraperitoneally, BCG was effective when given intravenously but not when given subcutaneously. Under certain conditions humoral responses may be decreased; for example, when BCG is administered repeatedly by scarification (Peters *et al.,* 1974).

Antibody-dependent cell-mediated cytotoxicity (ADCC) may be increased (Pollack, 1977).

Cell-mediated immunity.   Cell-mediated responses other than ADCC may be increased (Balner, Old, and Clarke, 1962; T.E. Miller *et al.,* 1973). Sometimes, when a protein–hapten–conjugated antigen is used, hypersensitivity to the carrier may be increased while the antibody response to the hapten is inhibited (Neveu, 1976).

Activity of lymphocytes.   Blast cell transformation of lymphocytes may be increased in lymph nodes draining the site of injection of antigen in animals treated with BCG (Mackaness, Lagrange, and Ishibashi, 1974). It has also been shown that peritoneal exudate cells from mice injected intraperitoneally with BCG followed by tumor cells are very powerfully cytotoxic in Winn assays (5.21), and that this depends on the presence of T cells (Parr, Wheeler, and Alexander, 1977). Lymphocytes cultured *in vitro* with BCG also undergo blast transformation provided there is a critical number of macrophages also present in the culture (Mokyr and Mitchell, 1975; Mitchell, Mokyr, and Kahane, 1975). The response of lymphocytes from BCG-treated animals to a T-cell mitogen, concanavalin A, *in vitro* was reported by Florentin *et al.* (1976) to be markedly depressed, whereas the response to a B-cell mitogen, dextran sulfate, was increased.

Suppressor T-cell activity may be stimulated by high doses of BCG given intravenously. This was reported by Geffard and Orbach-Arbouys (1976), who showed that spleen cells, and also purified T cells prepared by passing spleen cell populations through nylon columns, from mice injected intravenously with 0.75 to 3 mg live Pasteur BCG (whether dry weight or wet weight is not stated) had a markedly lower activity than spleen cells from normal mice, as judged by their capacity to cause a GVH reaction (7.421) *in vivo* and a mixed lymphocyte reaction *in vitro*.

Lymphocyte trapping.   The distribution of lymphocytes in the body may be altered. Florentin *et al.* (1976) found that after intravenous injection of BCG there was an early increase in the trapping of intravenously injected labeled lymphocytes by the spleen, and a long-lasting decrease in trapping by mesenteric lymph nodes and bone marrow. After subcutaneous injection of BCG trapping was increased in the draining lymph nodes and decreased in lymph nodes elsewhere.

Reticuloendothelial system and macrophage function. The production of macrophages by bone marrow precursors may be increased following injection of BCG (B. Fisher *et al.,* 1974b). Macrophage activity may also be increased, as shown by increased phagocytic activity of the reticuloendothelial system (Halpern *et al.,* 1958; Howard *et al.,* 1959), and increased response of macrophages to chemotactic stimuli (Meltzer, Jones, and Boetcher, 1975; Poplack *et al.,* 1976) resulting in increased accumulation of macrophages at inflammatory sites (Perper, Oronsky, and Sanda, 1976); and by evidence of macrophage activation shown *in vitro* by increased metabolic activity, release of lysozomal enzymes, increased phagocytic ability, and increased cytotoxicity for tumor cells (Alexander, 1973; Ferluga, 1973; Hibbs, 1974a, 1974b; Cleveland, Meltzer, and Zbar, 1974; Florentin *et al.,* 1976; Embleton, 1976). The extent to which these manifestations occur may vary to some extent independently; thus, for example, cytotoxicity for tumor cells may be increased while phagocytic activity *in vitro* is decreased (Nathan and Terry, 1977).

NK cells and hemopoietic stem cells. NK-cell activity (5.44) is increased in the peritoneal exudate (Wolfe, Tracey, and Henney, 1976), and in the spleens of normal mice, and to a lesser extent athymic mice (Herberman *et al.,* 1977), after intraperitoneal injection of BCG. The mitotic activity of hemopoietic stem cells has been reported to be increased in mice following intravenous injection of BCG (Pouillart *et al.,* 1975).

Resistance to infection. The resistance to unrelated bacterial infection may be increased by prior injection of BCG (Howard *et al.,* 1959; Blanden *et al.,* 1969).

Shared antigens. There is evidence that BCG and some tumors have antigens in common. Borsos and Rapp (1973) reported that guinea pigs immunized with BCG developed complement-fixing antibodies to a chemically induced guinea pig hepatoma. Subsequently Minden *et al.* (1974a) found that antibody raised in rabbits with BCG sonicates or line-10 guinea pig hepatoma reacted with both of these materials, whereas antiserum raised with a different hepatoma reacted with line-10 hepatoma cells but not with BCG. Faraci *et al.* (1974) reported that, after three injections of BCG, Balb/c mice developed a humoral and cellular immune response to a transplanted melanoma of CBA origin which had been adapted to grow in Balb/c mice; and Minden, Sharpton, and McClatchy (1976) obtained evidence of antigens shared between BCG and human malignant melanoma cells.

BCG derivatives. Many of the immunopotentiating effects of BCG are shown in varying degree by methanol extract residue (MER) (7.515), including the stimulation under defined conditions of humoral (Steinkuller, Krigbaum, and Weiss, 1969; Yashphe and Weiss, 1970; Yashphe, 1972) and cellular (Ben-Ephraim *et al.,* 1973) immune responses to a variety of antigens, including antigens which alone are non-immunogenic (Pass and Yashphe, 1971), and the prevention or correction of states of immunodepression (Weiss, 1972; Kuperman, Feigis and Weiss, 1973). It has also been reported that macrophage activation may be produced by treatment with killed BCG, cell wall skeleton (Kelly, 1976), and cord factor (Yarkoni, Wang and Bekierkunst, 1977b). These materials are described later (7.515).

7.512   SYSTEMIC TREATMENT OF TUMORS WITH LIVE BCG

It was discovered many years ago that resistance to transplanted allogeneic, and also isogeneic, tumors in mice may be increased by prior infection with BCG (Old, Clarke, and Benacerraf, 1959; Biozzi et al., 1959; Halpern et al., 1959; Weiss, Bonhag, and de Ome, 1961). The extent to which this effect is truly systemic has, however, been challenged recently by Parr, Wheeler, and Alexander (1977), who found that with isogeneic transplants of two immunogenic syngeneic mouse sarcomas the heightened resistance which followed injection of BCG was largely restricted to the site at which the BCG was injected.

Intravenous injection of BCG alone 24 hours after subcutaneous inoculation of a murine leukemia (L1210) was reported by Mathé, Pouillart, and Lapeyraque (1969) to cause some inhibition of tumor growth but less than that achieved by active specific immunotherapy with irradiated leukemic cells; Reif and Kim (1971), however, obtained some long-term survivors with BCG alone after investigating the most effective treatment schedule. Baldwin and Pimm (1974) observed a modest reduction in the number of pulmonary metastases in rats with chemically induced primary hepatomas treated with intravenous BCG, though the animals died of the primary tumors in about the same time as untreated controls. Pimm (1976) has also reported a reduction in the number of tumor nodules in the lungs of rats injected intravenously with tumor cells and intrapleurally with BCG; subcutaneous injection of BCG was ineffective in this system, however, so that the effect of intrapleural BCG may have been, once again, local rather than systemic. Administration of BCG via a tube in the esophagus was found by Baldwin, Hopper, and Pimm (1975) to have no effect on the growth of a rat sarcoma following intraperitoneal or intravenous inoculation of the tumor.

BCG has proved more effective when given systemically as adjuvant therapy following surgical excision (Baldwin and Pimm, 1973a; Sparks et al., 1974; Hanna et al., 1976; Economides, Bruley-Rosset, and Mathé, 1976; Owen, 1976) or radiotherapy (Dubois and Serrou, 1976) or transplanted metastasizing solid tumors, or chemotherapy for transplanted leukemia (J.W. Pearson et al., 1972; J.W. Pearson, Chaparas, and Chirigos, 1973; Mathé, Halle-Pannenko, and Bourut, 1974; M. Martin et al., 1975), but the timing may be critical (Amiel and Berardet, 1974). With one exception these findings relate to tumors in experimental animals; Owen (1976), however, treated dogs with spontaneously occurring osteogenic sarcomas by amputation followed by repeated intravenous injection of BCG (Glaxo). Survival ranged from 14 to 76 weeks, with a median survival time of over a year, whereas the usual survival time for dogs treated by amputation only, or amputation and irradiation of one lung, is reported to be 14 weeks. For the most part BCG was injected intravenously, intraperitoneally, or subcutaneously. It was established by M. Martin et al. (1975), however, that Pasteur strain BCG was effective in mice bearing the L1210 leukemia when given intradermally by scarification or with a Heaf gun after suboptimal treatment with cyclophosphamide, whereas administration by gastric tube was ineffective. Administration of BCG by scarification was also investigated by Hanna et al. (1976). They reported temporary inhibition of lymph node metastases in guinea pigs with a subcutaneously transplanted isogeneic hepatoma following excision of the primary transplant and administration of high viability preparations of Phipps and Pasteur strain BCG from the Trudeau Mycobacterial Collection, but commercial freeze-dried preparations of Tice, Pasteur, and Connaught BCG were without effect.

There is evidence that, under certain conditions which are not well defined, systemic administration of BCG may enhance tumor growth. Piessens *et al.* (1970) found that subcutaneous injection of BCG to Sprague-Dawley rats which had developed a single mammary tumor following intragastric administration of dimethylbenzanthracene (DMBA) had no effect on this tumor but resulted in the appearance of more tumors at other sites than occurred in rats which did not receive BCG. Subsequently Piessens *et al.* (1971) found that in rats with DMBA-induced mammary tumors a single injection of BCG 3 weeks after oophorectomy slightly delayed recurrence of the tumor but resulted eventually in the appearance of more new tumors than occurred in rats which did not receive BCG; repeated administration of BCG, however, was beneficial. Vasarevic, Boranic, and Pavelic (1974) found that intradermal administration of BCG prior to transplantation of a C57Bl reticulum-cell sarcoma to (C57Bl ×️ CBA)F1 mice and chemotherapy shortened survival quite markedly.

7.513   LIVE BCG MIXED WITH TUMOR CELL INOCULUM

BCG mixed with a tumor cell inoculum may delay or completely prevent the development of a tumor. This was shown first by Zbar and his colleagues with intradermal inoculation of a syngeneic guinea pig hepatoma (Zbar and Tanaka, 1971; Zbar *et al.,* 1971), and by Baldwin and Pimm (1971) with subcutaneous inoculation of syngeneic chemically induced rat fibrosarcomas. The effect is not due to direct cytotoxicity because tumor cells mixed with similar amounts of BCG grow in tissue culture (Bartlett *et al.,* 1972; M. Moore, Lawrence, and Witherow, 1974).

The inhibitory effect of BCG may be abolished by thymectomy followed by whole body irradiation, or by treatment with antilymphocyte serum and cortisone (Bartlett *et al.,* 1972; Chung *et al.,* 1973; Ray *et al.,* 1977; Tanaka *et al.,* 1977). In the experiments of Bartlett *et al.,* however, both the suppressive effect of admixed BCG in the absence of other treatment, and the abolition of this effect, were demonstrated with two apparently non-immunogenic tumors, suggesting that thymectomy and the other procedures abolished the tumor-inhibitory effect of BCG by modifying the response of the host to the BCG rather than the tumor. M. Moore, Lawrence, and Nisbet (1975, 1976) investigated the matter further by comparing the effect of admixed BCG in normal and T-cell-deficient (thymectomized irradiated) rats, using three different syngeneic rat tumors. With a highly immunogenic, chemically induced osteogenic sarcoma, mixing BCG with the tumor cells virtually prevented growth of the tumor in normal rats and also in T-cell-deficient rats which had been immunized with either BCG or irradiated tumor cells prior to thymectomy, but was somewhat less effective in non-immunized T-cell-deficient rats. It thus appears that there was some degree of T-cell component in the effect of BCG on the growth of this tumor, and this could be attributed to the influence of T cells on the response to either BCG or the tumor. With a weakly immunogenic osteogenic sarcoma induced with radioactive phosphorus, there appeared to be no T-cell component, since admixture of BCG was highly effective in preventing the development of tumor transplants in both normal and T-cell-deficient hosts. With an apparently non-immunogenic fibrosarcoma, which had also been induced with radioactive phosphorus, and which normally metastasized to the lungs after subcutaneous transplantation, admixture of BCG caused modest in-

hibition of primary transplants in both normal and T-cell-deficient hosts, again pointing to the absence of a T-cell component. The incidence of pulmonary metastases,
however, which in the absence of BCG was greater in T-cell-deficient than in normal
rats, was reduced in normal rats when BCG was mixed with the tumor inoculum.
Further evidence that the inhibitory effect of admixed BCG can occur independently
of T cells has been reported by Pimm and Baldwin, who showed that the effect with
isogenic transplants of another rat sarcoma was not weakened by irradiation (450 R)
24–48 hours previously (Pimm and Baldwin, 1976a), and that the growth of rat tumor
xenografts in congenitally athymic mice was totally suppressed by mixing the tumor
cells with BCG (Pimm and Baldwin, 1975a); as might be expected, however, in neither case did the host become resistant to further challenge with tumor cells alone.

The effect does appear to depend on changes in macrophage activity, since it can
be abolished by systemic administration of silica (Chassoux and Salomon, 1975; Hopper et al., 1976) or heterologous antimacrophage serum followed by latex particles
(Tanaka et al., 1977). It has also been reported that there is a positive correlation between the degree of macrophage infiltration of a tumor and its susceptibility to inhibition by mixing BCG with the tumor inoculum (Baldwin, 1976b). Moreover, with
tumor inocula containing relatively few macrophages, addition of peritoneal exudate
(PE) cells increased the susceptibility to admixed BCG, but this did not happen if the
glass-adherent cells were removed from the PE-cell population (Hopper and Pimm,
1977; Pimm, Hopper, and Baldwin, 1978).

7.514 INTRALESIONAL INJECTION OF BCG

Under the heading of intralesional injection of BCG we shall include injection
into a visible tumor; injection at the site of, but subsequent to, tumor inoculation; and
injection into lymph nodes which are possible sites for metastatic tumors.

It was reported by Zbar and Tanaka (1971) that small intradermal transplants of
a syngeneic guinea pig hepatoma often regressed following intralesional injection of
BCG. This treatment, which when successful resulted in the development of humoral
and cell-mediated immunity to the tumor, failed in animals given antilymphocyte serum (Hanna et al., 1973). Regression of various other tumors up to 4 mm in diameter
following intralesional injection of BCG in animals immunized to BCG prior to tumor
transplantation was reported by Bartlett et al. (1972); and Salomon et al. (1976) found
that this form of treatment caused regression both of the tumor injected and of a con-
tralateral transplant of the same, though not of a different, tumor. It has also been
shown that tumor growth after intravenous (Baldwin and Pimm, 1973b), intrapleural
(Pimm and Baldwin, 1975b), and intraperitoneal (Pimm, Hopper, and Baldwin, 1976)
inoculation may be inhibited by intravenous, intrapleural, and intraperitoneal injection of BCG, respectively. The last two cases may clearly be regarded as forms of intralesional treatment; the first case was also claimed to be so by Baldwin and Pimm
(1973b) on the grounds that when radioactively labeled BCG was injected more than
half of it was found in the lungs. On the other hand, negative results following injection of BCG into various tumors have been reported from several laboratories (Baldwin and Pimm, 1971; Simova and Bubenik, 1973; Sparks and Breeding, 1974).

It has also been reported that injection of BCG into the lymph nodes draining the
site of tumor inoculation may prevent, or reduce the incidence of, metastases in these
nodes (Zbar et al., 1972a; Carr and McGinty, 1974; H.G. Smith et al., 1975).

7.515   KILLED BCG AND BCG DERIVATIVES

BCG killed by heating to 65° C for an hour (Zbar, Bernstein, and Rapp, 1971; Chung *et al.,* 1973; M. Moore *et al.,* 1974), or sterilized with gamma radiation (Baldwin *et al.,* 1974a; Ray *et al.,* 1977) has been shown to inhibit the growth of transplanted tumors in varying degree when mixed with the tumor cell inoculum. Zbar *et al.* and Moore *et al.* obtained only a modest degree of inhibition, but Chung *et al.,* using the same material as Zbar *et al.,* found in experiments with a chemically induced mouse fibrosarcoma that it was as effective as live BCG. BCG sterilized by gamma radiation has also been reported to reduce the number of tumors developing in the lungs when injected intravenously following intravenous injection of tumor cells (Baldwin *et al.,* 1974a). It is difficult, however, to make a quantitative comparison of the effectiveness of live and killed BCG because when live organisms are injected they multiply locally or systemically to an extent which is undetermined. According to Muggleton *et al.* (1975), killed organisms when injected intravenously caused more severe granulomatous lesions in the lungs than live organisms.

In the hope of achieving a therapeutic effect without the complications which may result from injecting whole organisms, various extracts of BCG and other mycobacteria have been tested for antitumor activity. These include methanol extract residue (MER); mycobacterial cell wall skeleton, cord factor, and related, chemically defined substances; and a group of water-soluble, lipid-free fractions with reported adjuvant activity.

MER.   It was reported by Weiss, Bonhag, and Leslie (1966) that intraperitoneal injection of a methanol-insoluble residue of phenol-killed acetone-washed BCG, which they referred to as MER, protected mice to a considerable extent against a subcutaneous transplant of a spontaneous isogeneic uterine sarcoma 4 weeks later. Intraperitoneal injection of MER on days 0 and 6 relative to subcutaneous tumor transplantation, and in some case on days 6 and 13, retarded, but did not prevent, growth of the same tumor. Similar findings were obtained with several other isogeneic tumors, but with two tumors growth was stimulated by treatment with MER. Subsequent studies with various tumors have confirmed the antitumor effect of MER when given systemically prior to tumor inoculation (Minden *et al.,* 1974b; Wainberg, Deutsch, and Weiss, 1976) or mixed with the tumor cell inoculum (Hopper, Pimm, and Baldwin, 1975a), and in some experiments when given intralesionally subsequent to tumor inoculation (Weiss, 1972; Wainberg, Margolese, and Weiss, 1977). With systemic administration prior to tumor inoculation, however, the time of administration may be critical; thus Jacobs and Kripke (1974) found that administration several weeks before transplantation of a mouse mammary carcinoma to syngeneic hosts, some of which carried the mouse mammary tumor virus and others of which did not, caused accelerated tumor growth, whereas administration 3 days before tumor inoculation reduced the incidence of tumors. With intralesional injection it has been found in guinea pigs that a marked therapeutic effect may be obtained in one substrain and little effect in another (Wainberg *et al.,* 1977).

Mycobacterial cell wall skeleton and related substances.   BCG cell wall (CW) attached to the surface of oil droplets in aqueous emulsions was found to be as effective as BCG when mixed with the tumor cell inoculum or injected intralesionally to intradermal transplants of a guinea pig hepatoma (Zbar, Rapp, and Ribi, 1972; Zbar, Ribi, and Rapp, 1973).

By treating CW with proteolytic enzymes followed by extraction with organic solvents, Azuma *et al.* (1974) obtained a soluble fraction designated *free lipids* and an insoluble residue designated *cell wall skeleton* (CWS). Subfractions of the free lipids include wax D and cord factor, and Azuma *et al.* prepared from cord factor a chromatographically pure component termed P3, which contained trehalose and mycolic acids. CWS proved to be as effective as CW when mixed with tumor cells but did not cause regression when injected intralesionally to established tumors; CWS mixed with P3, however, was as effective as CW when injected into established tumors (Meyer *et al.*, 1974). Cord factor or P3 alone have been reported to show no antitumor activity (Bekierkunst *et al.*, 1974; Ribi *et al.*, 1975), but Leclerc *et al.* (1976) found that cord factor emulsified in oil and injected intraperitoneally inhibited the growth of intraperitoneally injected L1210 mouse leukemia.

Gray *et al.* (1975) used CW, CWS, and P3 prepared from *M. phlei.* Intralesional injection of mixed CW and CWS caused regression of 60 percent of established guinea pig hepatoma transplants; addition of P3 from *M. phlei,* or of purified trehalose mycolate from a strain of *M. tuberculosis,* to the mixture increased the cure rate to 86 and 90 percent, respectively. Gray *et al.* claimed that *M. phlei* had the advantage of being more easily propagated than BCG, and that CW from this organism could be deproteinized without reducing its antitumor potency. Originally, preparations of CW or killed whole organisms attached to oil droplets were made by prolonged grinding in a tissue homogenizer, but it has been shown by Yarkoni, Rapp, and Zbar (1977) that immunotherapeutically active emulsions can be prepared quickly and reliably by ultrasonication. These authors also showed that an emulsion prepared from *M. smegmatis* by grinding possessed antitumor activity.

Various investigators have studied the effect of chemically defined substances related to material obtained from CW. Gray *et al.* (1975), as mentioned above, mixed purified trehalose, prepared from a strain of *M. tuberculosis,* with CW and CWS from *M. phlei.* Yarkoni and Bekierkunst (1976) found that trehalose dipalmitate had some inhibitory effect when mixed with an inoculum of guinea pig hepatoma cells. Other materials currently being studied are synthetic muramyldipeptide (Audibert *et al.,* 1977; Chedid and Audibert, 1978) and trehalose coupled to bovine or human serum albumin (Gensler and Alam, 1977).

Water-soluble extracts.   Hiu (1972) prepared a lipid-free water-soluble fraction from BCG by removing free lipid with solvents and treating the residue by a process of catalytic hydrogenolysis. He claimed that this material, which he called MAAF (mycobacterial adjuvant and antitumor fraction), was non-toxic and stimulated both cell-mediated and humoral immune responses. He used the material mixed with irradiated tumor cells for combined active immunotherapy (7.711) of the L1210 mouse leukemia.

Other water soluble extracts have been prepared from *M. tuberculosis* by Werner *et al.* (1975) and shown to possess some degree of adjuvant and immunopotentiating activity, but the only one tested for antitumor activity proved negative in this respect.

7.52 "Corynebacterium Parvum" (CP)

Various strains of anaerobic coryneform organisms which have been shown to possess reticuloendothelial stimulating activity have been given the general designation *Corynebacterium parvum* by many authors. It has been suggested (Douglas and Gunter, 1946; Johnson and Cummins, 1972) that all these organisms, and others related to them, should be placed in the genus *Propionibacterium* rather than *Corynebacterium*, but, since the organisms which were formerly called *Propionibacteria* do not possess reticuloendothelial-stimulating activity, McBride *et al.* (1975a) have suggested that the name *Corynebacteria* should be retained. These authors have, however, accepted in all other respects the further subdivision of these organisms, other than the classical *Propionibacteria*, into four main groups, as proposed by Johnson and Cummins (1972) on the basis of serological properties, cell wall composition, and DNA homology: Group 1, *C.* (or *P.*) *acnes* type I; Group II, *C.* (or *P.*) *acnes* type II; Group III, *C.* (or *P.*) *granulosum;* and Group IV, *C.* (or *P.*) *avidum.* Since one or more strains in each group have been, and often still are, referred to as *C. parvum,* usually with a number attached, and since these organisms are administered both experimentally and clinically in the form of heat-killed or formalin-killed suspensions, we shall use the designation "*C. parvum*" (in quotes) or CP as an inclusive label to denote all such suspensions, except when comparing the properties of different organisms.

Stimulation of reticuloendothelial activity by CP was first demonstrated by Halpern *et al.* (1963), who showed that mice injected intravenously or intraperitoneally with a killed suspension of the organism were able to clear intravenously injected colloidal carbon much more rapidly from the bloodstream than untreated mice. This increase in functional activity was associated with an increase in the weight of the liver and spleen. Subsequently Biozzi *et al.* (1965) showed that injection of CP was highly effective in reducing the mortality from graft-versus-host disease caused by injection of parent-line (C57B1.6) spleen cells into (C57B1.6 $\times$ C3H/He)F1 hybrid mice.

In the light of these findings, and the fact that BCG and other agents which stimulate reticuloendothelial activity had been shown to inhibit the growth of some transplanted tumors in mice and rats, Woodruff and Boak (1966) investigated the effect of CP on the growth of experimental tumors and showed that the growth of transplants of two isogeneic murine tumors was inhibited by intravenous injection of CP.

The general immunological properties of CP and its effect on animal and human tumors have subsequently been widely investigated. The subject has been reviewed by Scott (1974d), Oettgen, Pinsky, and Delmonte (1976), and Milas and Scott (1977).

7.521   GENERAL IMMUNOLOGICAL PROPERTIES

Humoral immunity. CP is itself a powerful immunogen, and also modifies the response to other antigens, but the effect depends not only on the dose but also on the route of administration. Since subcutaneous (sc) injection is often ineffective, or much less effective than intravenous (iv) or intraperitoneal (ip) injection, except in the special case when it is mixed with another antigen, the term *systemic injection* will be used in this section to include ip and iv, but not sc, injection.

It was reported by Woodruff, McBride, and Dunbar (1974) that ip injection of CP evoked primary and secondary specific antibody responses to the organism itself in both normal and T-cell-deficient (thymectomized, irradiated, bone marrow reconstituted) mice, whereas sc injection evoked little or no response. A low background level of antibody to CP was regularly observed in untreated mice. The development of an antibody response following systemic injection of CP has been confirmed in mice (Scott and Warner 1976), rabbits (Dawes and McBride, 1975), and man (8.243). Further studies have shown that systemic injection of CP results in an increase in the levels of various immunoglobulin classes and subclasses, especially IgG2b, in normal, and in tumor-bearing but otherwise normal, mice (James *et al.,* 1976); an increase in antibody to CP and in the level of immunoglobulins other than IgG1 in tumor-bearing T-cell-deficient mice (James *et al.,* 1976); and an increase in antibody, and IgG2a and IgM, in athymic nude (nu/nu) mice, though the level of CP antibody was less than in heterozygous (nu/+) littermates (James *et al.,* 1977). It was concluded from the findings in nude mice that CP can act as a partly thymus-independent antigen.

Systemic injection of CP also potentiates the humoral response to other antigens, both thymus dependent (Biozzi *et al.,* 1968; Howard, Scott, and Christie, 1973; James, Ghaffar, and Milne, 1974; Warr and James, 1975; Wiener and Bandieri, 1975) and thymus independent (Howard, Christie, and Scott, 1973; James *et al.,* 1974; Warr and Šljivić, 1974). Pretreatment with CP prevented the development of tolerance to bovine serum albumin in rabbits (Pinckard, Weir, and McBride, 1968), but did not prevent the induction of tolerance by large doses of pneumococcal polysaccharide in mice (Howard, Christie, and Scott, 1973). In the experiments of Warr and James (1975), based on assays of direct and indirect plaque-forming spleen cell responses to sheep erythrocytes using mice of three different strains, the rank order of the potentiating effect of systemic treatment with CP in respect of different antibody classes and subclasses was in general IgG2b > IgG2a > IgM > IgG1, but the findings varied somewhat according to the time of administration of CP in relation to the administration of the sheep erythrocytes. In an experiment with athymic (nu/nu) mice in which both were given on the same day, no potentiation was observed.

Mixing CP with sheep erythrocytes prior to injection into the footpads of mice was found by Bomford (1980a) to increase the number of direct (IgM) plaque-forming cells in the draining popliteal lymph node. It has also been shown that CP has adjuvant activity when injected as a water-in-oil emulsion (O'Neill, Henderson, and White, 1973) or mixed with incomplete Freund's adjuvant (Neveu, Branellec, and Biozzi, 1964).

The discovery that macrophages from CP-treated mice are more effective than normal macrophages in promoting an *in vitro* primary response to sheep erythrocytes by macrophage-depleted spleen cells (Wiener, 1975) but that this difference is abolished if the mice are given an intraperitoneal injection of carageenan two days before CP (Šljivić and Watson, 1977), and that the antibody response to a macrophage independent antigen (DNP-POL) is not affected by CP (Watson and Šljivić, 1976; Šljivić and Watson, 1977), strongly suggests that the potentiation of humoral immunity by CP is mediated by CP-activated macrophages.

Cell-mediated immunity.   Delayed-type hypersensitivity (DTH) to CP has been observed after subcutaneous (footpad) injection of CP (Scott, 1974b, 1976; Tuttle and North, 1975), and also after repeated intravenous injection of CP in low dosage (Scott and Warner, 1976), but intravenous injection of a single large dose actually prevented sensitization by footpad injection of CP 4 days later (Scott, 1974b). The nonspecific inflammatory swelling caused by footpad injection of CP to non-sensitized germ-free mice was the same as in conventional mice, as was DTH following previous CP sensitization (Scott, MacDonald, and Carter, 1978).

Cell-mediated responses to a variety of other antigenic stimuli (Asherson and Allwood, 1971; Allwood and Asherson, 1972; Scott, 1974c), including allogeneic skin grafts (Castro, 1974a; Milas et al., 1975a), may be depressed by prior systemic administration of CP, whereas later treatment may have no such effect. The inhibition of cell-mediated immunity may be due partly to increased trapping of sensitized T cells in the spleen of CP-treated animals (Scott, 1974c), but there is also evidence that macrophages from CP-treated animals may have an inhibitory effect on some T-cell functions. This is suggested by the fact that pretreatment with CP may protect F1 mice injected with parent-line spleen cells from otherwise fatal graft-versus-host disease (Biozzi et al., 1965; Howard et al., 1967), and the more recent discovery that the response of spleen cells from CP-treated mice to phytohemagglutinin and in mixed lymphocyte reactions is impaired (Scott, 1972a) but returns to normal when macrophages are removed from the spleen cell population (Scott, 1972b; Kirchner, Holden, and Herberman, 1975). Further confirmation is provided by the discovery of Kirchner, Glaser, and Herberman (1975) that the capacity of spleen cells from mice immunized with Moloney sarcoma virus (MSV) to mount a secondary cytotoxic response in vitro against an MSV-induced tumor is impaired by injecting the mice with CP after inoculation of the virus, and by mixing the spleen cells from virus-immune mice with spleen cells from syngeneic mice treated with CP.

CP mixed with sheep erythrocytes may potentiate delayed-type hypersensitivity to sheep erythrocytes (Bomford, 1980b). CP mixed with irradiated tumor cells may promote or inhibit the development of immunity to the tumor, depending on the timing and the dose of CP. S.E. Smith and Scott (1972) found with a variety of mouse tumors that intravenous or intraperitoneal injection of 0.7 or 1.4 mg CP 7 days before injection of irradiated tumor cells diminished the immunizing effect. Subsequently Scott (1975b) found that injection of small doses (3.5–175 μg) CP mixed with 1–2×10^7 irradiated mouse mastocytoma cells resulted in the development of strong specific antitumor immunity, whereas injection of irradiated tumor cells alone was ineffective, and the smallest dose of CP (3.5 μg) was the most effective. Woodruff et al. (1976a), in experiments with a strongly immunogenic mouse fibrosarcoma, found that the resistance evoked by injection of 10^6 irradiated tumor cells was impaired by intraperitoneal injection of 1.4 mg CP 5 days before, and virtually abolished by a similar injection 11 days after, the irradiated cells. The effect of subcutaneous injection of 10^6 irradiated cells mixed with CP 14 days before live challenge depended on the dose of CP. With 0.7 mg the development of resistance was largely but not completely abrogated; 0.35 mg resulted in a lesser degree of abrogation; and 0.09 or 0.02 mg had little or no effect. In subsequent experiments (Woodruff and Whitehead, 1977) various possible reasons for the inhibitory effect of a large amount of admixed CP were investigated. There was no evidence of humoral inhibitory factors or an increase in suppressor T cells. The abrogation of immunization could, however, largely be reversed by adoptive immunization and was therefore attributed to the induction of specific immunological tolerance of tumor antigens, probably as the result of prolonged trapping and eventual destruction in the regional lymph nodes of lymphocytes which have responded to tumor antigen.

Lymphocyte trapping.   Frost and Lance (1973) reported that there was a prolonged increase in lymphocyte trapping after intravenous and subcutaneous injection of CP in the spleen and regional nodes, respectively, as measured by the accumulation of intravenously injected ^{51}Cr-labeled syngeneic lymphocytes in these sites. It seems likely that macrophages are concerned in initiating lymphocyte trapping, because this is increased by CP and various other agents which increase phagocytic activity but is not greatly affected by procedures which either selectively or indiscriminately destroy lymphocyte populations (Frost and Lance, 1974; Frost, 1974).

As already mentioned, increased lymphocyte trapping probably contributes to the depression of cellular immunity which may follow administration of CP systemically, intravenously, or mixed with tumor cells.

Activity of lymphocytes.   Systemic injection of CP in high dosage causes atrophy of the thymus (Castro, 1974a; McBride, Jones, and Weir, 1974). There is also evidence, discussed above under the heading of cell-mediated immunity, that the macrophages of CP-treated animals may have an inhibitory effect on some T-cell functions. Nelson (1973) has suggested that this may be due, at least in part, to factors produced by activated macrophages.

Reticuloendothelial system and macrophage function.   As already mentioned (7.52), it was discovered by Halpern *et al.* (1963) that, following systemic injection of CP, mice developed enlargement of the liver and spleen, and increased phagocytic activity as shown by accelerated clearance of intravenously injected colloidal carbon from the bloodstream. These findings have been confirmed in mice by many investigators (see Milas and Scott, 1977); an increase in the weight of the lungs (Adlam and Scott, 1973) and accelerated clearance of aggregated bovine serum albumin (McBride, Jones, and Weir, 1974) and ^{51}Cr-labeled sheep erythrocytes (Warr and Šljivić, 1974), have also been reported. It has also been shown that hepatomegaly and splenomegaly occur after systemic CP injection in rats (Stiffel *et al.,* 1966; Brozovic, Šljivić and Warr, 1975), guinea pigs (Stiffel *et al.,* 1966), and rabbits (Pinckard, Weir, and McBride, 1968). Histologically there is an increase in the number of macrophages of various categories in the liver, spleen, and lungs (Halpern *et al.,* 1963; Collet, 1971; Milas *et al.,* 1974a, 1975a; Brozovic, Šljivić, and Warr, 1975; Šljivić and Warr, 1975), and also marked hematopoietic activity in the spleen involving erythrocyte and granulocyte precursors and megakaryocytes (Halpern *et al.,* 1963; Brozovic *et al.,* 1975; Milas *et al.,* 1975a).

It has also been shown that iv injection of CP results in splenomegaly in germ-free mice and, although the spleens of untreated germ-free mice were smaller than those of conventional mice, the kinetics and magnitude of the increase in the ratio of spleen weight to body weight were similar (Scott, MacDonald, and Carter, 1978).

Subcutaneous injection of CP causes little or no enlargement of the liver and spleen but marked enlargement of the draining lymph node (Scott, 1974b; Tuttle and North, 1975). Cells from the nodes draining the site of subcutaneous injection of CP in non-tumor-bearing mice were found by Fisher, Wolmark, and Coyle (1974) to show no increased cytotoxicity *in vitro* for tumor cells in general; regional lymph node cells from tumor-bearing mice injected subcutaneously with CP at a site between the tumor and the node did, however, show increased cytotoxicity which was specific for the tumor in question.

These effects depend *inter alia* on the strain of animal, the dose of CP, and the strain of organism used. McBride *et al.* (1975a), in a comparative study of nine different organisms, found that antitumor activity correlated rather better with splenomegaly than with an increase in the phagocytic index. The effect on the phagocytic index has, however, been reported to show a strong positive correlation with the capacity of different strains of CP and related organisms to produce a chemotactic factor specific for macrophages (Wilkinson, O'Neill, and Wapshaw, 1973).

CP stimulates production of macrophage precursors in bone marrow, and this has been reported after subcutaneous (Wolmark and Fisher, 1974; Wolmark, Levine, and Fisher, 1974) as well as after systemic (Dimitrov *et al.,* 1975a; Baum and Breese, 1976) injection. In the experiments of Wolmark and Fisher (1974), the effect was greater in tumor-bearing than in normal mice, and it may perhaps be significant that in the tumor-bearing mice the CP was injected into the same limb as the tumor. The increased production of macrophages is accompanied by increased production of granulocytes. Both these effects appear to result from the prompt, sustained elevation of colony-stimulating factor in the serum, which has been shown to occur after CP injection (Foster, MacPherson, and Browdie, 1977).

It has been reported that systemic injection of CP also results in an increase in the number of macrophages which can be harvested from the peritoneal cavity (Basic *et al.,* 1974; Yuhas and Ullrich, 1976) and the pulmonary alveoli (Collet, 1971); Basic *et al.,* however, gave two injections, which caused ascites, and in the writer's experience a single injection has little or no effect on the number of macrophages harvested.

Macrophages from CP-treated animals show more rapid adherence to glass, and increased spreading and vacuolation (Olivotto and Bomford, 1974), increased or modified lysozomal enzyme activity (Wilkinson *et al.,* 1973a; McBride, Jones, and Weir, 1974; Puvion *et al.,* 1976), and cytotoxicity for tumor cells *in vitro.* The cells used in these experiments have been obtained either by peritoneal lavage or from the lungs by lavage via the trachea or expression from minced pulmonary tissue. It would be of interest to compare the effect of unfractionated peritoneal exudate (PE) cells, which contain a considerable number of lymphocytes as well as macrophages, and subpopulations derived from them consisting almost entirely of macrophages. Alternatively, the possible effect of T lymphocytes might be investigated by comparing PE cells from athymic and normal mice, or by studying the effect of a macrophage poison such as trypan blue (Hibbs, 1975).

PE cells from mice treated systemically with CP have been shown to inhibit the growth of a variety of syngeneic tumors *in vitro* (Olivotto and Bomford, 1974; Bomford and Christie, 1975; Christie and Bomford, 1975; Scott, 1974a; Ghaffar *et al.,* 1974; Ghaffar, Cullen, and Woodruff, 1975; Basic *et al.,* 1975; Kirchner, Holden, and Herberman, 1975; Morahan and Kaplan, 1976; Krahenbuhl, Lambert, and Remington, 1976). Intraperitoneal injection of CP was found by Krahenbuhl *et al.* to be somewhat more effective than intravenous injection; subcutaneous injection was ineffective as an initial procedure, but subcutaneous injection 1 week after intravenous injection resulted in increased cytotoxicity. Cytotoxicity for tumor cells *in vitro* has also been observed with pulmonary cells which appeared by both morphological and functional criteria to consist almost entirely of macrophages (Olivotto and Bomford, 1974), and with the glass-adherent fraction, but not the non-adherent fraction, of PE-cell suspensions (Ghaffar *et al.,* 1974; Ghaffar, Cullen, and Woodruff, 1975); it seems reasonable therefore to attribute the effect exclusively to macrophages.

Inhibition of tumor growth may be a manifestation of either cell death or inhibition of cell division. We shall refer to mechanisms which cause cell death as *cytocidal* or *cytolytic,* and those which arrest cell division as *cytostatic.* The term *cytotoxic* is sometimes used as a synonym for cytocidal, but this is redundant and without etymological foundation. We shall use cytotoxic in a broad sense to include both cytocidal and cytostatic effects. The commonly used type of assay, based on measurements of DNA synthesis by the uptake of labeled thymidine or iododeoxyuridine (IUDR) in cultures containing tumor cells and either normal or CP-activated macrophages, however, does not discriminate between cytolysis and cytostasis, since a dead cell is just as incapable of synthesizing DNA as a cell which has been arrested at some point in the cell cycle, and the same problem may arise with assays based on the plating efficiency of a small number of tumor or other cells on macrophage monolayers, as used by Basic *et al.* (1974, 1975). It seems likely that cytostasis is the predominant effect, but there is evidence from morphological studies (Morahan and Kaplan, 1976) that CP-activated macrophages can exert a direct cytocidal effect on tumor cells *in vitro.* The question of whether these mechanisms operate *in vivo* will be discussed later (7.522).

Macrophages activated by a variety of agents including CP may also be cytotoxic for cells transformed *in vitro* (Basic *et al.,* 1974) and to a lesser extent for embryonic fibroblasts (Kaplan, Morahan, and Baird, 1976), but not for normal syngeneic or allogeneic adult cells (Hibbs, Lambert, and Remington, 1972a, 1972b; Hibbs, 1973; Basic *et al.,* 1975). Milas and Scott (1977) have suggested that this discrimination may be related to the membrane properties of macrophages and tumor cells facilitating close contact, and this is consistent with the findings of Puvion, Fray, and Halpern (1976) that contact between intact or dead tumor cells and peritoneal macrophages was demonstrable by electron microscopy with PE cells from CP-treated, but not from untreated, mice. An alternative explanation has been put forward by Currie and his colleagues (Currie, 1978; Currie and Basham, 1978), who have shown that macrophages activated with bacterial lipopolysaccharide or CP (Currie, Gyure, and Cifuentes, 1979) liberate large amounts of arginase, and have claimed that this exerts a deleterious effect on tumor cells both *in vitro* and *in vivo* (Currie, Gyure, and Cifuentes, 1979) because they require more L-arginine than normal cells and the amount available to them when grown in tissue culture with macrophages, or at the microenvironmental level in animals treated with CP or other macrophage-activating agents is depleted by the action of the enzyme. There is also evidence (Kung *et al.,* 1977) that suppression of T-cell function by macrophages *in vitro* may be brought about in the same way, and it seems plausible to postulate that this is true also of the inhibition of T-cell function by CP *in vivo.*

The discovery that macrophages become cytotoxic for tumor cells after incubation *in vitro* with a mixture of CP and spleen cells from CP-immune mice, or with CP mixed with supernatants from cultures of CP-immune spleen cells, but not by incubation with CP alone or with CP and CP-immune spleen cells treated with anti-Thy 1 serum and complement (Christie and Bomford, 1975; Bomford and Christie, 1975), suggests that activation is due to soluble factors released from CP-sensitized T cells on contact with CP; and the further observation that macrophage activation occurs more rapidly in mice immunized with CP 60 or 130 days previously (Bomford and Christie, 1975) suggests that the same mechanism may operate also *in vivo*. Since macrophage activation also occurs in thymectomized, irradiated, bone-marrow-reconstituted (TIR) mice (Bomford and Christie, 1975) and athymic mice (Ghaffar, Cullen, and Woodruff, 1975); however, there must be an alternative T-cell-independent mechanism of activation. It has been suggested that this may be mediated by complement cleavage products, since CP incubated with serum has been shown to activate complement. In human scrum, which normally has a background titer of antibody to CP, this activation can occur via the classical pathway. Activation by the alternative pathway has also been shown to occur, however, both in human serum after absorption with CP and in guinea pig serum which contained no detectable antibody (McBride *et al.,* 1975c), and this generates the cleavage product C3b, attachment of which to mouse macrophages in culture leads to the release of lysozomal enzymes (Schorlemmer, Davies, and Allison, 1976) and has been reported (Allison, 1977b) to render the macrophages cytotoxic for tumor cells *in vitro*.

The effect of irradiation on the activation of macrophages *in vivo* by CP has been investigated by Woodruff, Ghaffar, and Whitehead (1976). The increase in phagocytic activity, as judged by accelerated clearance of intravenously injected colloidal carbon, which normally follows intravenous or intraperitoneal injection of CP, was reduced but not abolished in mice given 350–500 rad whole body irradiation 4 days before CP injection, whereas irradiation of up to 1000 rad 4 days after CP injection had no such effect. The antitumor cytotoxicity of PE and spleen cells from CP-treated mice for tumor cells *in vitro* was abolished by irradiation of the cell donor (400–800 rad) 4 days before CP injection but was not reduced by irradiation (800 rad) of the cell donor 4 days after CP injection, or by irradiation of the effector cells *in vitro*. These findings provide further evidence that systemic injection of CP stimulates macrophage precursors to differentiate into mature cells; they show in addition that these cells then become activated, and strongly suggest that this is the main pathway for the production of cytotoxic macrophages. The fact that the stimulating effect of CP on phagocytic activity was only partly reduced by prior irradiation points to the conclusion that this effect of CP is due partly to stimulation and activation of macrophage precursors and partly to activation of a population of mature non-dividing phagocytic cells in the liver and spleen.

It was reported by Watson and Šljivić (1976) that splenic macrophages from CP-treated mice enhanced the primary antibody response to sheep erythrocytes *in vitro*. In subsequent experiments (Šljivić and Watson, 1977) it was found that macrophages with this property appeared in the spleen and peritoneal exudate of irradiated mice reconstituted with purified T lymphocytes, but not in T-cell-deficient mice. It was therefore postulated that activated macrophages capable of enhancing antibody responses to sheep erythrocytes (and other T-cell-dependent antigens) are generated by the action of CP on a non-dividing population of cells, resident in the spleen and peritoneal exudate, but that this only occurs in the presence of T cells.

If all these findings are confirmed it would then appear that systemic administration of CP (1) stimulates macrophage precursors in bone marrow to differentiate into cytotoxic and phagocytic mature macrophages; (2) stimulates non-dividing macrophages in the liver and spleen to become increasingly phagocytic; and (3) stimulates non-dividing macrophages in the spleen and peritoneal exudate so that they are able to enhance antibody responses to T-cell-dependent antigens. The first effect depends, *inter alia,* on increased production of colony-stimulating factor, and does not require the presence of T cells. The second effect also does not require T cells, but the third effect is T-cell dependent.

NK-cell activity.   As stated earlier (5.441), intraperitoneal administration of CP results in increased NK-cell activity in the spleens of normal, and also, to a smaller extent, athymic, Balb/c mice (Herberman *et al.,* 1977; Ojo *et al.,* 1978a, 1978b), whereas intravenous injection decreases NK-cell activity. Intraperitoneal injection of CP has also been reported to increase NK-cell activity in the peritoneal exudate cells of rats of strains W/Fu and BN, and in the spleen cells of strain W/Fu (Oehler *et al.,* 1978b). A smaller increase in activity was observed in the spleen cells of BN rats, which normally show a low level of NK-cell activity.

Hematopoiesis.   In mice there is a transient leukopenia involving lymphocytes (Woodruff and Dunbar, 1973; Brozovic, Šljivić, and Warr, 1975; Milas *et al.,* 1975a) and polymorphs (Woodruff and Dunbar, 1973) following injection of CP. Subsequently anemia may develop (Halpern and Fray, 1969; McCracken, McBride, and Weir, 1971). This is associated with hemolytic autoantibody (McCracken *et al.,* 1971; McBride, Jones, and Weir, 1974) and increased phagocytosis of red cells (McBride *et al.,* 1974). It has been suggested by Cox and Keast (1974) that the antibody reacts with antigens from CP adsorbed by erythrocytes.

The anemia is associated, as already mentioned, with increased hematopoiesis in the spleen. There is also an increase in the number of colony-forming units in the spleen and bone marrow (Toujas, Dazord, and Guelfi, 1975), associated with increased production of colony-stimulating factor (CSF) (Foster, MacPherson, and Browdie, 1977).

Resistance to infection.   Systemic injection of CP may protect both normal (Fauve and Hevin, 1971; Adlam, Broughton, and Scott, 1972; Halpern *et al.,* 1973a; Collins and Scott, 1974; Swartzberg *et al.,* 1975; Ruitenberg and van Noorle Jansen, 1975) and athymic (Ruitenberg and van Noorle Jansen, 1975) mice against infection with a variety of bacteria, and has also been shown to protect normal mice against some viral (Cerutti, 1975) and protozoal infections (Nussenzweig, 1967; Clark, Cox, and Allison, 1977). On the other hand, intravenous injection of CP appeared to reduce the resistance of rats to a helminth (*Trichinella spiralis*) infection (Ruitenberg and Steerenberg, 1973).

The increased resistance to bacterial infection appears to be due to increased destruction of bacteria by activated macrophages in the liver and spleen (Fauve and Hevin, 1971, 1974; Collins and Scott, 1974; Fauve, 1975). Collins and Scott (1974) found that administration of CP after bacterial infection was not protective.

Sensitivity to endotoxin, histamine, and intravenous anesthetics.   Systemic injection of CP may make mice sensitive to endotoxin (Howard, 1969), histamine (Adlam, Broughton, and Scott, 1972; Adlam, 1973), and pentobarbitone and tribromethanol (Mosedale and Smith, 1975). Sensitivity to endotoxin and histamine has been attributed to release of lysozomal enzymes from CP-activated macrophages, and sensitivity to intravenous anesthetics to impaired destruction of the drug by microsomal enzymes in the liver (Milas and Scott, 1977).

Distribution of injected CP.   Scott and Milas (1977) labeled killed CP with either fluorescein isothiocyanate or ^{125}I and, after showing that both preparations retained lymphoreticular stimulatory and antitumor activity, used them to study the distribution of injected CP by fluorescence microscopy and by gamma counting of samples of tissue and blood. Large amounts of intravenously injected CP were found in the liver, spleen, and lungs, and less in bone marrow and lymph nodes. Much of the label disappeared from the lungs within 24 hours, but label remained much longer in the other tissues. It was observed that an inactive strain of CP was destroyed in the liver more rapidly than the active strain. Clearance of labeled CP from the blood was more rapid in tumor-bearing mice than in normal mice, and the absolute amount (though not the amount per unit weight of the organ) in the liver and draining lymph node was increased. Labeled CP was found in established solid tumors, but the amount was unrelated to the response of the tumor to treatment with CP. After subcutaneous or intralesional injection the bulk of the inoculum was retained at the site of injection and in the regional lymph node (see also Scott, 1978).

Very similar results were obtained by Sadler, Cramp, and Castro (1977, 1978) with a formol-killed vaccine of CP which had been labeled by growing the organism in the presence of ^{3}H-thymidine, with the additional observation that a moderate amount of label was found in the small bowel. Barth and Singla (1978) also reported similar findings with technetium (^{99}Tc)-labeled CP, except that with the particular tumor they used (the B16 melanoma in C57Bl/6 mice) there was a very high concentration of label in the tumor (39 percent of the recoverable activity) at 24 hours.

More recently Scott and Decker (1978) have studied the distribution of fluorescein- or ^{125}I-labeled CP after intrapleural injection. Cells harvested by pleural lavage, which consisted mainly of activated macrophages, were found to have become heavily labeled, as were the mediastinal lymph nodes, but very little label was found in the lung. There was less CP taken up by the liver and spleen than after iv injection, and the spleen was less enlarged.

7.522   SYSTEMIC TREATMENT OF TUMORS WITH CP

It was reported by Woodruff and Boak (1966) that intravenous injection of CP either 2 days before or 8–12 days after subcutaneous inoculation of 10^5 or 10^4 viable cells of a syngeneic mouse mammary carcinoma significantly delayed the development of tumors, which appeared at about the same time in CP-treated mice which received 10^5 tumor cells as in untreated mice which received 10^4 cells. Once the tumor had become palpable, however, the rate of growth was much the same in treated and untreated animals. Injection of CP also delayed the appearance of a palpable tumor following subcutaneous inoculation of 10^5 or 10^4 viable sarcoma cells, but the effect was less marked than with the mammary tumor.

Some months after this work was published, Halpern *et al.* (1966) reported inhibition of the growth of an allogeneic mouse sarcoma by intravenous or intraperitoneal injection of CP, the maximal effect being obtained when the CP was injected 2 days prior to tumor inoculation. The mortality following intraperitoneal inoculation of another allogeneic tumor, the Ehrlich ascites tumor, was markedly reduced by intraperitoneal injection of CP on the day of inoculation of the tumor, whereas intravenous injection was ineffective.

There have been many subsequent reports of protection of mice in various degrees against subcutaneously inoculated syngeneic solid tumors of many different kinds, including mammary carcinomas (Woodruff and Inchley, 1971b; Milas et al., 1974a, 1974b), chemically induced (Woodruff, Inchley, and Dunbar, 1972; Woodruff and Dunbar, 1973; J.C. Fisher, Grace, and Mannick, 1974; Milas et al., 1974a, 1974b, 1974c, 1974d; Castro, 1974b; Bomford, 1975; McBride, Tuach, and Marmion, 1975; Suit et al., 1975, 1976b) and other (S.E. Smith and Scott, 1972) fibrosarcomas, osteosarcoma (van Putten et al., 1975), mastocytoma (Scott, 1974a), plasmacytoma (Woodruff and Warner, 1977), and Lewis lung carcinoma (Mathé, Kamel et al., 1973; Sadler and Castro, 1976a), by intravenous or intraperitoneal injection shortly before, on the day of, or up to a few days after tumor inoculation. Subcutaneous injection of CP at a site remote from that of tumor inoculation has as a rule been ineffective or much less effective (Woodruff and Inchley, 1971b; Milas et al., 1974a), but an exception to this rule was reported by Fisher, Grace, and Mannick (1970). Oral administration of CP proved completely ineffective in mice inoculated with the Lewis lung carcinoma (Sadler and Castro, 1975).

Protection against intravenously inoculated fibrosarcoma cells has been observed in mice given systemic injections of CP (Milas and Mujagic, 1972; Milas et al., 1974a, 1974d; Bomford and Olivotto, 1974). Subcutaneous injection of CP was also reported to be effective by Fisher, Grace, and Mannick (1970), though not by Bomford and Olivotto (1974).

With ascitic or other tumors inoculated intraperitoneally, intraperitoneal injection of CP has proved highly effective (S.E. Smith and Scott, 1972; Halpern et al., 1973b; Castro, 1974b), but this should perhaps be regarded as local rather than systemic treatment.

Protection has also been achieved against transplanted leukemias and lymphomas (Lamensans et al., 1968; Amiel, Litwin, and Berardet, 1969; Stiffel, Mouton, and Biozzi, 1971; S.E. Smith and Scott, 1972; Mathé, Kamel et al., 1973; Kouznetzova et al., 1974; Halpern, Crepin, and Rabourdin, 1975; Roumiantzeff et al., 1978), but this has usually been less marked than with other types of tumor except when both the leukemia and the CP were injected intraperitoneally (Lamensans et al., 1968; Halpern, Crepin, and Rabourdin, 1975).

Yuhas and Ullrich (1976) treated spontaneous mammary tumors which developed in old, previously irradiated mice with three weekly intraperitoneal injections of CP, and obtained temporary remissions.

In rats, Pimm and Baldwin (1977b) found that intravenous injection of CP on the day of subcutaneous inoculation of a strongly immunogenic sarcoma or a moderately immunogenic hepatoma caused enhanced growth, whereas subcutaneous injection of CP either had no effect or slightly delayed the appearance of tumors. In these experiments the dose of CP was only 0.7 mg, i.e., the same amount as is commonly given to mice. This may have been suboptimal, since Likhite (1977) found that weekly injection of 1.5 mg CP, divided equally between the intraperitoneal and intravenous routes, prolonged the survival of rats inoculated subcutaneously with a metastasizing mammary carcinoma when treatment was begun as late as 20 days after tumor inoculation.

The therapeutic response to systemic administration of CP depends on many factors, including the schedule of treatment, the site of inoculation of the tumor, the bulk of the tumor at the start of treatment, characteristics of the tumor, and host factors which may be modified by various experimental procedures.

Schedule of treatment. In mice the optimal single dose of CP appears to be in the range 0.35 to 0.7 mg. Above 0.7 mg toxic symptoms begin to develop, and below 0.35 mg there may be a gradual decline in the therapeutic effect (Scott, 1974a; Suit *et al.,* 1976b). In rats doses of 0.7 to 1.4 mg have been used, but further studies are required to determine the optimal level. The comparative effectiveness of different routes of administration has been discussed already. Repeated treatment using small or moderate doses may be advantageous (Suit *et al.,* 1976b; Likhite, 1977), but repeated large doses have usually not resulted in an increased antitumor effect (Scott, 1974b; Suit *et al.,* 1976b) and may cause increased toxicity.

In view of the fact that in man intravenous injection of CP may cause severe pyrexial reactions, and that endotoxin fever is mediated by E prostaglandins (Feldberg, 1974), the possibility of controlling pyrexia due to CP by administration of antipyretics like aspirin and indomethacin which block prostaglandin synthesis (Vane, 1971) merits consideration. Such treatment would be pointless if these agents also abrogated the antitumor effect of CP, but this seems unlikely in view of the observation of Lynch and Salomon (1979) that, under conditions in which systemic treatment with CP alone failed to induce regression of a mouse sarcoma, administration of CP followed by continued treatment with indomethacin caused complete regression of the tumor in 75 percent of mice, and that indomethacin alone also inhibited tumor growth though it did not cause any complete regressions.

Tumor site. It was reported by Suit *et al.* (1976b) that CP was more effective after intradermal and subcutaneous inoculation of a murine fibrosarcoma than after intramuscular inoculation. The response to CP after intravenous and intraperitoneal inoculation of various tumors has already been discussed. It was reported by Woodruff, Hitchcock, and Whitehead (1977) that intravenous or intraperitoneal injection of CP before intracerebral inoculation of a murine fibrosarcoma prolonged survival though the tumor grew in most of the mice, whereas similar treatment three days after tumor inoculation has little or no effect.

Bulk of the tumor. Within limits, systemic treatment with CP appears to be more effective when the initial tumor inoculum is relatively small and treatment is begun at the latest a few days after tumor inoculation (see Milas and Scott, 1977). There is, however, evidence that when the inoculum is very small—for example, in the region of the TD50 (1.22) or less—administration of CP may increase the number of tumors which develop (Peters *et al.,* 1978).

With larger tumors which do not respond to CP alone, it may be therapeutically advantageous to combine administration of CP with other procedures which reduce the bulk of the tumor.

The potentiation of the response to chemotherapy by CP was first demonstrated by Currie and Bagshawe (1970), who reported that subcutaneous transplants of an isogeneic fibrosarcoma which regressed only temporarily when treated with cyclophosphamide, regressed completely in 70 percent of mice treated with an intraperitoneal injection of cyclophosphamide followed 12 days later by an intradermal injection of

CP. Injection of CP 6 or 16 days after cyclophosphamide also had some effect, but injection of CP on the day of, or before, injection of cyclophosphamide had no antitumor effect and was highly toxic. Subsequently, intraperitoneal or intravenous, and in some cases intradermal, injection of CP has been shown to potentiate the therapeutic effect of cyclophosphamide (Woodruff and Dunbar, 1973; J.W. Pearson et al., 1975; B. Fisher et al., 1975b, 1975c; Woodruff, Whitehead, and Speedy, 1978; Scott, 1979a) and other chemotherapeutic agents (Amiel and Berardet, 1970; J.W. Pearson et al., 1972, 1974; Houchens and Gaston, 1976; B. Fisher et al., 1976a; Scott, 1979a) in mice with a variety of transplanted tumors, including fibrosarcomas, mammary carcinomas, and leukemias. It has been widely accepted that when single doses of each agent are used, CP should follow the chemotherapeutic drug, and the optimal interval was found by Scott (1979a, 1979b), in experiments with a mouse fibrosarcoma, to be 4 days. Scott showed, however, that potentiation also occurred when CP was given 15–18 days, and to a lesser extent 1–4 days, before cyclophosphamide, but not when CP was given 8 days or 12 days before cyclophosphamide. Various regimens have also been devised in which repeated doses of a chemotherapeutic drug and CP were given alternately (B. Fisher et al., 1975b, 1975c; Woodruff, Whitehead, and Speedy, 1978).

Systemic injection of CP has been shown to reduce the dose of irradiation needed to cause regression of an immunogenic fibrosarcoma (Milas et al., 1975c) and to increase the cure rate after fractionated irradiation (Suit et al., 1975, 1976b; Milas et al., 1978). CP given 2 to 4 days before irradiation was more effective than CP 2 days after irradiation, and the adjuvant effect was much greater with relatively small doses of irradiation. Repeated intraperitoneal injection prior to irradiation has also been shown to potentiate the local effect of irradiation on transplants of a non-metastasizing rat fibrosarcoma (Moroson and Schechter, 1976). Administration of CP prior to irradiation of a transplanted, weakly immunogenic, metastasizing mammary carcinoma reduced the incidence of pulmonary metastases (Milas, Mason, and Withers, 1976); CP also caused further slowing of the growth of this tumor when combined with fractionated irradiation, but did not significantly increase the cure rate (Milas et al., 1978). Administration of CP also reduced the incidence of pulmonary metastases when given 7–14 days after surgical excision of a subcutaneously transplanted rat hepatoma (Proctor, Rudenstam, and Alexander, 1973a), or prior to excision of transplants of a metastasizing mammary carcinoma (Milas, Mason, and Withers, 1976) or the Lewis lung carcinoma (Sadler and Castro, 1976a).

Properties of the tumor.   The extent to which the response of tumors to systemic treatment with CP correlates with their immunogenicity in syngeneic or autochthonous hosts is controversial. Milas et al. (1975b) observed only occasional temporary remission of transplants of a weakly immunogenic mammary carcinoma in mice treated with CP alone; Suit et al. (1976a) found that CP given as adjuvant therapy in conjunction with irradiation had at most a feeble effect; and Hewitt and Blake (1978), in experiments with transplants of two spontaneous mouse adenocarcinomas, found that a single intravenous or intraperitoneal injection of CP 4 days before excision of a transplant had no effect on the number or distribution of metastases in viscera or lymph nodes. Woodruff, Whitehead, and Speedy (1978), on the other hand, working with transplants of a spontaneous murine adenocarcinoma which on thorough investigation appeared to be virtually non-immunogenic, found that systemic injection of CP 3 days after tumor inoculation significantly delayed the appearance of tumors. Moreover, when used as adjuvant therapy in conjunction with administration of cyclophosphamide for the treatment of established tumors, the effect of CP was comparable to that observed in similar experiments with transplants of a highly immunogenic tumor. The reasons for these discrepancies have not been established, but a plausible hypothesis is that the response of a non-immunogenic tumor to CP depends on its susceptibility to attack by activated macrophages.

Host factors.   Systemic treatment with CP has been shown to exert an inhibitory effect on primary syngeneic tumor transplants in thymectomized, irradiated, bone-marrow-reconstituted (TIR) mice (Woodruff, Dunbar, and Ghaffar, 1973; Scott, 1974a), congenitally athymic mice (Woodruff and Warner, 1977), mice treated with antilymphocyte serum (Hattori and Mori, 1973; Castro, 1974b), and mice with defective humoral immune responses due to genetic causes (Biozzi *et al.*, 1972) or splenectomy (Castro, 1974b; Mazurek *et al.*, 1976); on the other hand, antilymphocyte serum was found by Sadler and Castro (1976b) to abrogate the antimetastic effect of CP on the Lewis lung carcinoma. In both TIR and athymic mice the response to CP was usually similar to that seen with CP-sensitive tumors in normal mice. Among the tumors studied by Woodruff and Warner (1977), two lymphomas, which regressed spontaneously in untreated normal mice but grew progressively in untreated athymic mice, grew progressively in normal mice given systemic CP, though their growth was slowed in similarly treated athymic mice.

It is more difficult to determine the effect of macrophage deficiency because of the difficulty of establishing, and even more of maintaining, a state of macrophage deficiency uncomplicated by other changes which may influence tumor behavior, but some important data have been obtained by studying the effect of whole body irradiation, and administration of cortisone and macrophage poisons such as silica and gold salts.

As already mentioned (7.521), both the increase in phagocytic index and the development of macrophages in the spleen and peritoneal exudate which are cytotoxic for tumor cells *in vitro,* which normally follow systemic injection of CP, may be inhibited by whole body irradiation (350–500 rad) 4 days before, but not after, CP injection (Woodruff, Ghaffar, and Whitehead, 1976), and it was concluded from this that injection of CP promotes the proliferation of macrophage precursors and their development into activated mature macrophages. Evidence that this process may be important in relation to the effect of CP on tumor growth *in vivo* is provided by the observation of Bomford and Olivotto (1974) that the protective effect of intravenous CP administration 1 day before intravenous inoculation of syngeneic murine fibrosarcoma cells was abolished by irradiation (800 rad) 1 day before, but not by irradiation on the day of or 1 day after, CP administration. It was found, on the other hand, by Woodruff, Ghaffar, and Whitehead (1976) that the response of subcutaneous fibrosarcoma transplants to intraperitoneal injection of CP was impaired by whole body irradiation (350–500 rad) irrespective of whether this was given 4 days before or 4 days after CP injection. To account for this apparently anomalous result, it was suggested that, in this system, the antitumor effect of CP *in vivo* was dependent on the recruitment and differentiation of new effector cells over a fairly long time.

Olivotto and Bomford (1974) found that the effect of an intravenous injection of CP in reducing the number of tumors which developed in the lungs after intravenous injection of tumor cells 1 day after the CP was not altered by injection of silica between 6 days before and 4 days after CP injection. Injection of silica did, however, reduce the splenonegaly in CP-treated mice, and also the number of lung tumors in mice injected with tumors but not with CP. No reason was suggested for this apparently protective effect of silica, but it may well be related to the failure of silica to interfere with the protective effect of CP. McBride, Tuach, and Marmion (1975) found that injection of the anti-inflammatory agent sodium aurothiomalate, which inhibits lysozomal enzyme activity in phagocytic cells (Persellin and Ziff, 1966), probably by sulfydryl bonding (Ennis, Granda, and Posner, 1968), also failed to reduce the protective effect of CP against intravenous injection of tumor cells; in contrast to the findings of Olivotto and Bomford (1974) with silica, however, one or more injections of gold salt in the absence of CP increased the number of tumors which developed in the lungs after intravenous injection of tumor cells; and repeated injection of gold salt also inhibited the antitumor effect of systemic administration on CP or subcutaneously inoculated tumors.

Injection of cortisone may also inhibit the antitumor effect of CP. Scott (1975a), in reporting this, suggested that cortisone might prevent exocytosis of lysozomal enzymes by stabilizing the macrophage membrane.

7.523   CP MIXED WITH TUMOR CELL INOCULUM

It was reported by Likhite and Halpern (1973, 1974) that if CP is mixed and injected subcutaneously with viable cells of a syngeneic mouse mammary carcinoma, tumors fail to develop and the mice become highly resistant to subsequent live challenge with the same tumor. This phenomenon has been demonstrated with other syngeneic tumors in rats (Pimm and Baldwin, 1977b) as well as mice, and also with an allogeneic rat tumor (Likhite and Halpern, 1973).

The development of isogeneic tumors after subcutaneous inoculation in T-cell-deficient mice and intracerebral inoculation in normal mice (Woodruff, Hitchcock, and Whitehead, 1977), and of rat tumors in congenitally athymic mice (Pimm and Baldwin, 1976b), is also inhibited by mixing CP with the tumor inoculum. It seems clear therefore that, as in the case of BCG (7.513), when the tumor inoculum is mixed with the immunopotentiating agent, inhibition of growth of the primary transplant, as distinct from the development of immunity, is not T-cell dependent.

7.524   LOCAL INJECTION OF CP

The term *local injection* will be used to denote (1) *intralesional injection*, i.e., injection subsequent to, but at the site of, tumor inoculation, or into a manifest tumor; and (2) *neighborhood injection*, i.e., injection at a site near to the site of tumor inoculation or a manifest tumor, and in the same area of lymphatic drainage.

Intralesional injection of CP has been shown to cause marked inhibition, and often complete regression, of a variety of animal tumors including mouse (Likhite and Halpern, 1974) and rat (Likhite, 1974) mammary carcinomas, mouse mastocytoma (Scott, 1974b, 1976), mouse fibrosarcomas (Woodruff and Dunbar, 1975; Milas *et al.,* 1975b; Tuttle and North, 1975; Morahan *et al.,* 1976; Suit *et al.,* 1976b), and hamster melanoma (Paslin, Dimitrov, and Heaton, 1974). In some cases metastases have regressed as well as the injected tumor (Likhite, 1974), but Boak and Tebbutt (1977) found that intralesional injection of CP, which strongly inhibited subcutaneous transplants of a mouse fibrosarcoma, had no effect on artificial metastases made by injecting tumor cells into the femoral condyle 14 days after the initial inoculation. Neighborhood injection has proved somewhat less effective than intralesional injection, but may nevertheless cause marked inhibition (Likhite and Halpern, 1974; Scott, 1974b, 1975b), whereas subcutaneous injection at a remote site, as already mentioned (7.522), is ineffective. An important control was introduced by Woodruff and Dunbar (1975), who showed that *C. diphtheriae* and *C. granulosum* (NTC 10387), both of which failed to inhibit tumor growth when given systemically, were also ineffective when given intralesionally.

The antitumor effect of intralesional injection of CP is completely T cell dependent, since it does not occur in either thymectomized, irradiated, bone marrow reconstituted mice (Scott, 1974b; Woodruff and Dunbar, 1975) or congenitally athymic mice (Woodruff and Warner, 1977). Moreover, in experiments with a virtually non-immunogenic tumor (Woodruff, Whitehead, and Speedy, 1978), intralesional injection of CP as early as 3 days after tumor inoculation was completely ineffective, although, as mentioned earlier (7.522, 7.523), growth was inhibited by systemic treatment or by mixing CP with the tumor inoculum.

The optimal dose of CP is lower when given intralesionally than when given systemically, and in mice Scott (1974b) found that it was in the region of 0.07 mg for a mastocytoma; doses of 0.7 mg, though probably well above the optimal level, nevertheless cause marked inhibition of a fibrosarcoma (Woodruff and Dunbar, 1975).

7.525 MECHANISMS UNDERLYING THE THERAPEUTIC EFFECT OF CP

As we have seen, systemic injection of CP results in widespread activation of macrophages, but may inhibit some T-cell functions (7.521), including the expression of cell-mediated immunity to tumor antigens, and there is evidence that this last effect may be due to trapping of antitumor effector cells in the spleen, or in the lymph nodes draining the site of subcutaneous CP injection (Bomford, 1977a; Woodruff and Whitehead, 1977). It is also clear that systemic injection of CP can inhibit tumor growth *in vivo* independently of T cells (7.522). It seems likely therefore that the therapeutic effect of this form of treatment is mediated, at least partly and perhaps mainly, by activated macrophages. This is consistent with the finding of McBride, Tuach, and Marmion (1975) that gold salts can abrogate the antitumor effect of systemic injection of CP, though there is no obvious explanation of the failure of Jones and Castro (1977) to achieve similar abrogation with silica or trypan blue. It seems likely, though direct evidence is lacking, that CP-activated macrophages exert a cytotoxic effect on tumor cells *in vivo* as they have been shown to do *in vitro* (7.521); in addition, as Milas and Scott (1977) have suggested, they may expedite the removal or destruction of tumor-protective blocking factors in the form of antigen–antibody complexes.

There is evidence, however, that although systemic injection of CP may inhibit T-cell function it may also, under conditions which are not yet clearly defined, potentiate the development of specific immunity to a tumor. It was reported by Yuhas, Toya, and Wagner (1975) that specific immunity to a mouse carcinoma developed after intraperitoneal injection of irradiated tumor cells and intravenous injection of CP, but not after either of these procedures alone. Milas *et al.* (1975d) found that T cells were required to induce optimal resistance to pulmonary metastases of a mouse fibrosarcoma, and, as mentioned earlier, Sadler and Castro (1976b) found that repeated subcutaneous injection of antilymphocyte serum (ALS) abolished the inhibitory effect of intravenous injection of CP on metastasis of the Lewis lung tumor. In discussing their experiments Sadler and Castro (1976b) considered that the effect could not be attributed to a cytoxic effect of ALS on macrophages, and suggested that the action of CP on metastases is dependent on a population of long-lived circulating T cells.

The tumor inhibitory effect of intralesional injection of CP subsequent to tumor inoculation, as we have seen, is T cell dependent, whereas when CP is mixed with the inoculum, growth of a tumor may be prevented in the absence of T cells.

Successful CP treatment is typically associated with the development of specific antitumor immunity; the response to intralesional injection of CP may, however, depend also to some extent on a specific local reaction to CP, since, in the experiments of Tuttle and North (1975), regression of a mouse fibrosarcoma occurred only in mice which had been previously sensitized to CP and which were treated by intralesional injection when delayed-type hypersensitivity to CP was maximal.

7.526 CP DERIVATIVES

Various cell wall (CW) preparations of anaerobic corynebacteria and related organisms have been shown to possess reticuloendothelial-stimulating activity (Kouznetzova et al., 1974), to act as adjuvants in promoting antibody production and delayed-type hypersensitivity (Kouznetzova et al., 1974; Azuma et al., 1975), and to manifest some degree of antitumor activity (Kouznetzova et al., 1974; McBride, Dawes, and Tuach, 1976). Lipid material, which lies on the surface of the cell, is a chemoattractant for macrophages (R.J. Russell et al., 1976), and in the experiments of McBride et al. the observed antitumor activity, which was feeble but could be increased by adsorbing the material onto latex particles, was found in the lipid component of the CW extract. Lipid-free extracts, which contain peptidoglycan and carbohydrate, possess reticuloendothelial-stimulating and adjuvant activity (Adlam, Reid, and Torkington, 1975; Jolles et al., 1975), but antitumor activity has not been found or has been demonstrated only with an allogeneic tumor (Adlam, Reid, and Torkington, 1975) or, with a syngeneic tumor, by mixing the material with the tumor inoculum, and in the latter case the animal did not become resistant to subsequent challenge with the same tumor (Riveros-Moreno, Bomford, and Scott (1978).

It was concluded by Riveros-Moreno et al. (1978) that, since the only derivative of CP that had been shown to retain full antitumor activity consisted of phenol-treated unbroken cells and contained CW as well as an undefined amount of non-CW components, complete antitumor activity is not associated with a single molecular component capable of being isolated in pure form; in other words, "synergism between, or molecular assocation of, CW and non-CW components may be required." A month or two after this paper was accepted for publication, however, Millman, Scott, and Halbherr (1977) reported that intralesional injection of a cytoplasmic fraction of CP (P. acnes) pelleted by high-speed centrifugation inhibited the growth of a mouse mastocytoma inoculated into one footpad 7 days previously as fully as whole cells injected in one-fifth of the dose (in terms of nitrogen content) and, unlike whole cells, inhibited the growth of an uninjected second tumor in the opposite footpad. The possibility of developing therapeutically effective extracts of CP should therefore be regarded as still open.

7.53 Other Bacterial Preparations

Bacterial lipopolysaccharide from *Salmonellae* and other gram-negative bacilli and polysaccharide-free lipid derived from it have been reported to render macrophages cytotoxic for tumor cells *in vitro* (Alexander and Evans, 1971) and also to inhibit tumor growth *in vivo* (Mizuno et al., 1968; Parr, Wheeler, and Alexander, 1973).

Heat- and formalin-killed *Brucella abortus* injected intraperitoneally 3 days after inoculation of the Ehrlich ascites tumor was found by Pilet and Sabolovic (1970) to have a more powerful tumor-inhibitor effect than injection of CP. In later experiments (Toujas et al., 1972) injection of the same material inhibited the growth of a syngeneic mouse leukemia provided it was given not less than 20 days before tumor inoculation.

Spleen and peritoneal exudate cells from mice immunized with viable *Listeria monocytogenes* have been reported to be cytotoxic for tumor cells *in vitro* (Youdim and Sharman, 1976).

On the other hand, Mathé, Pouillart, and Laperaque (1969) observed no prolongation of survival of mice which received a single injection of killed *Bordetella pertussis* vaccine 1 day after tumor inoculation, or five injections at 4 day intervals; and Hirano et al. (1967) found that administration of *B. pertussis* augmented the growth of an allogeneic mouse leukemia.

Parker et al. (1947) observed marked oncolysis after injection of *Clostridium histolyticum* intralesionally to sarcoma transplants in mice. Treatment with penicillin and antitoxin enabled some treated mice to survive longer than the controls. Malmgren and Flanigan (1955) found that the presence of a tumor protected mice from tetanus after injection of spores of *Cl. tetani* in a dosage which caused death of non-tumor-bearing mice in 48 hours. Möse and Möse (1959) observed that when *Cl. tetani* spores were injected intravenously to mice bearing solid transplants of the Ehrlich ascites tumor, there was selective rapid germination of the spores in the tumor and extensive destruction of tumor tissue, but this was followed invariably by death of the animals.

These findings encouraged Möse and Möse to search for clostridia which were non-pathogenic and whose spores would germinate selectively in tumor tissue, and it has been shown subsequently that a strain of *Cl. butyricum* known as M55 which fulfils these criteria, or material extracted therefrom, has a powerful antitumor effect against a variety of animal tumors (Engelbart and Gericke, 1964; Gericke and Engelbart, 1964; Gericke, 1971; Thiele et al., 1964; Möse et al., 1967; Heppner, 1967; Fredette and Plante, 1970, 1972; Fredette et al., 1971).

The antitumor capacity of another *Clostridium* was discovered by Mohr et al. (1968, 1972a, 1972b). They found that an extract of pig skin, whose inhibitory effect on tumors in hamsters and mice was originally attributed to epidermal or melanocyte chalones (4.22), was contaminated with the spores of a previously unidentified *Clostridium*, and that these were responsible for the tumor inhibition. They showed further that sterile filtrates of cultures of this organism had a similar therapeutic effect.

It seems clear from Fredette's (1973) studies that clostridial spores and extracts may be cytotoxic for tumor cells *in vitro*, and it seems likely that the antitumor effect *in vivo* is due at least in part to direct cytotoxicity. It is an open question, however, whether this is the only factor concerned. Most of the experiments have been performed in outbred animals, or with tumors like the Ehrlich mouse ascites carcinoma and the Walker rat carcinoma. It would be of interest to repeat them with isogeneic tumors, both immunogenic and non-immunogenic, in inbred animals, to determine whether immunological factors are involved.

7.54   Viral Infection

Occasional reports of regression of human cancer following a viral infection (8.245) have stimulated interest in the possibility of treating tumors by inoculation of live virus. Webb and Gordon Smith (1970) have suggested three ways in which this procedure might cause tumor regression: (1) by direct cytolysis, the virus being preferentially destructive for tumor cells; (2) by making the tumor cells more immunogenic; and (3) by interfering with an oncogenic virus directly or by stimulating production of interferon. For the procedure to be feasible, however, the virus must be adapted to grow in the tumor, and the host must not be killed by the virus. These conditions have proved difficult to fulfil, but some success has been achieved, mainly with transplanted allogeneic tumors.

Many years ago Sharpless, Davies, and Cox (1950) showed that a transplanted lymphoid tumor of chickens could be caused to regress, without any apparent damage to the host, by inoculation of Russian Spring-Summer, West Nile, Japanese B encephalitis, St. Louis encephalities, or louping-ill virus, and chickens cured in this way became resistant to rechallenge with the same tumor. Later, A.E. Moore (1953) showed that sarcoma 180 could be destroyed in a strain of mice resistant to Russian encephalitis virus by inoculating the tumor with this virus, and experiments with other allogeneic mouse tumors, in particular the Ehrlich ascites tumor, have been reported by various authors (Koprowski, Love, and Koprowska, 1957; Lindenmann, 1962, 1963, 1964, 1973, 1974; Lindenmann and Klein, 1967a, 1967b; Cassel and Garrett, 1966). Initially Lindenmann used human influenza virus, but he subsequently found a strain of avian influenza virus which was much more easily adapted to grow in mouse tumor tissue. Various other viruses have been used experimentally or suggested as possible candidates. Lindenmann (1974) has also suggested that instead of inoculating the tumor-bearing host with live virus a therapeutic effect might be achieved by injecting what he called *viral oncolysate,* prepared by homogenizing tumor tissue infected in another animal or *in vitro* with virus, and then inactivating the virus with formalin or, preferably, ultraviolet light.

There have been a few studies of the immunogenicity of virus-infected syngeneic tumors, which open the way to further experiments of a therapeutic kind. Boone *et al.* (1974) made the interesting observation that injection of homogenates of a transplantable SV40-transformed Balb/c fibrosarcoma failed to immunize mice against subsequent challenge with live tumor cells, whereas intact tumor cells, and homogenate infected with mouse-adapted influenza virus or vesicular stomatitis virus, were more or less equally immunogenic by this criterion; uninfected tumor homogenate was however able to elicit a delayed type hypersensitivity reaction. They attributed the effect of the virus to a helper antigen mechanism. Kobayashi *et al.* (1970) showed that rat tumors, after being infected with Friend leukemia virus, lost their ability to grow progressively in rats and were able to immunize rats against the original uninfected tumor. Lindenmann (1974), in commenting on these experiments of Kobayashi, says they show features of both heterogenization (7.63) by Friend antigens, which prevented the infected tumor from growing, and adjuvanticity, which enabled the virus-infected tumor to behave as a more potent immunogen with respect to the weak tumor-specific antigens of the original tumor. Lindenmann (1973, 1974) has suggested also that a carrier-hapten type of association is achieved by the viral antigens becoming incorporated in the membrane of tumor cells, or alternatively by cellular antigens becoming incorporated in the viral envelope.

7.55   Polynucleotides

The possible use of nucleotides in the treatment of cancer is suggested by two considerations. In the first place, certain categories of nucleotide have been shown to stimulate humoral and cell-mediated immunity, macrophage activity, and the production of interferon. Secondly, deoxyribonucleotides have been shown under certain conditions to be cytotoxic for tumor cells.

Before reviewing the results of immunotherapeutic experiments it may be helpful to examine these properties in more detail.

7.551   IMMUNOPOTENTIATION AND MACROPHAGE ACTIVATION

It was shown by Braun and his colleagues that oligodeoxyribonucleotides produced by enzymatic partial degradation of DNA stimulate DNA synthesis and cell multiplication in bacteria (Braun and Whallon, 1954; Braun, Firshein, and Whallon, 1957) and also in mammalian cells (Braun, 1958). In subsequent investigations the stimulatory effect of oligonucleotides on cells concerned in immunological responses, including macrophages, and/or their precursors has been manifested in the following ways:

1. An increase in the number of hemolysin-forming cells in the spleens of mice immunized with sheep erythrocytes (Braun, 1965; Braun and Nakano, 1965, 1967a). Studies of the distribution of these cells in the spleen suggest that the number of antibody-forming clones does not increase but that the absolute number of antibody-forming cells in each clone does; it would seem therefore that stimulation affects committed cells rather than stem cells.
2. An increase in the titer of antibody in the sera of mice immunized with bovine gamma globulin (Merritt and Johnson, 1965).
3. Partial restoration of immunological responsiveness in mice exposed to x-irradiation (Taliaferro and Jaroslow, 1960) or treated with 6-mercaptopurine (Feldman, Globerson, and Nachtigel, 1963). Further work (Jaroslow, 1968; Simic and Kanazir, 1968) suggests that four processes are involved, namely, restoration of the capacity of cells to respond to antigen, repair of reproductive potential, stimulation of proliferation, and enhancement of spontaneous DNA repair.

Braun and his colleagues reported that only oligonucleotides obtained from DNA gave positive results in studies of the immunological response to sheep erythrocytes. This is difficult to understand in view of subsequent work with polyribonucleotides (*vide infra*), and is clearly not a general rule, since others (Taliaferro and Jaroslow, 1960; Merritt and Johnson, 1965) have reported that oligodeoxyribonucleotides and oligoribonucleotides were both effective in their systems.

The observation of Nakano and Braun (1967) that a stimulating fraction rich in oligodeoxyribonucleotides is released by spleen cells from immunized mice when exposed *in vitro* to the relevant antigen raises the possibility that release of oligonucleotides may play a role in secondary immunological responses *in vivo.* It would seem that oligonucleotides are broken down or cleared from the bloodstream fairly slowly, since, according to Braun and Nakano (1967b), stimulatory activity is still demonstrable in the serum of mice 48 hours after injection of a stimulating dose of oligodeoxyribonucleotides, though not after 72 hours. These data are similar to those relating to the passive transfer of activity elicited by Freund's adjuvant (Dawe, Segre, and Myers, 1965).

Variations in the activity of enzyme digests prompted similar studies with polynucleotides, on the assumption that these would go through a stage of partial depolymerization *in vivo,* and it has been shown that administration of double-stranded (ds) synthetic polyribonucleotides or dsRNA of natural origin can elicit or potentiate the following types of response:

1.   Blast transformation and uptake of ^{3}H-thymidine *in vitro* by spleen cells from normal mice of certain strains (Dean *et al.,* 1972), and from cortisone-treated and congenitally athymic mice (Ruhl *et al.,* 1974), and also by human spleen cells (Dean *et al.,* 1972).
2.   Activation of mouse macrophages *in vitro* so that they become cytotoxic for other mouse cells (Alexander and Evans, 1971; H.G. Johnson and A.G. Johnson, 1971).
3.   Activation of macrophages *in vivo,* manifested by accelerated clearance of intravenously injected colloidal carbon (Freedman and Braun, 1965), increased macrophage antibacterial activity (Braun, Ishizuka *et al.,* 1971; Fauve, 1971), and increased resistance of both normal and athymic mice to infection with *Listeria monocytogenes* (Remington and Merigan, 1970) and *Brucella abortus* (Cheers and Cone, 1974).
4.   The primary antibody response *in vitro* of spleen cells from normal but not athymic mice to sheep erythrocytes (Ishizuka *et al.,* 1971; Cone and Marchalonis, 1972).
5.   The secondary antibody response *in vitro* of (1) mouse spleen cells primed with human gamma globulin (Stout and Johnson, 1972) and (2) hapten-primed mouse B cells to a hapten-heterologous carrier conjugate through the activation of nonprimed T cells (Yamashita and Kitagawa, 1974).
6.   The primary antibody response of mice to thymus-dependent antigens such as sheep erythrocytes when the polynucleotide is given with or soon after, but not before, the antigen (Braun and Nakano, 1967b; Braun, Nakano *et al.,* 1968; Braun, Ishizuka *et al.,* 1971; Turner *et al.,* 1970; Cone and Johnson, 1971, 1972; Schmidtke and Johnson, 1971; Cone and Marchalonis, 1972; Collavo *et al.,* 1972; Hamaoka and Katz, 1973), but not to thymus-independent antigens (Renoux *et al.,* 1972). Even 4-day-old mice, which normally show only a very feeble antibody response to sheep erythrocytes, respond well when treated with Poly A: Poly U (Braun, 1970). The poor response of aged mice, which Braun, Ishizuka *et al.* (1971) suggest may be due to lack of the adjuvant effect of endogenous nucleic acid resulting from the presence in aged mice of antibody to nucleic acid (Friou and Teague, 1964), can be similarly boosted (Winchurch and Braun, 1969).
7.   The antibody response of a low responder strain of mice to a synthetic polypeptide antigen (Mozes *et al.,* 1971).

8. Antibody production in mice injected with peritoneal exudate cells which have been exposed to antigen *in vitro* (H.G. Johnson and A.G. Johnson, 1968).
9. The secondary antihapten antibody response *in vivo,* especially when the polynucleotide is given with the second antigen (Yamashita and Kitagawa, 1974).
10. Cell-mediated immunity *in vivo,* exemplified by the graft-versus-host reaction (Cantor *et al.,* 1970), and the response of guinea pigs to tuberculin (Braun, Ishizuka *et al.,* 1971).
11. NK-cell activity. Herberman *et al.* (1977) found that the NK-cell cytotoxic activity of spleen cells, peritoneal exudate (PE) cells, and peripheral blood leukocytes harvested from BN rats 24 hours after intraperitoneal injection of 1 mg Poly I: Poly C was significantly increased. The activity of spleen cells and blood lymphocytes had returned almost to normal by 48 hours, but that of PE cells was still high after 72 hours. The NK-cell activity of spleen cells was also studied after injection of Poly I, Poly C, Poly CI, cytidylyl cytidine (CpC), Poly I + CpC, and PolyA:Poly U, but was not found to be consistently elevated.

In large dosage polynucleotides cause toxic effects very similar to those caused by bacterial endotoxin (Alexander and Evans, 1971), and even small doses of both agents may be lethal if actinomycin D is given at the same time (Pieroni *et al.,* 1971). Long continued repeated administration of polynucleotides causes thymic atrophy, splenic hypoplasia and lymphopenia (Leonard, Eccleston, and Jones, 1969), and immunosuppression manifested by prolonged survival of skin allografts (J.C. Fisher, Cooperband, and Mannick, 1972).

These findings suggest that the polynucleotides in non-toxic doses stimulate macrophages and T lymphocytes, but have no direct effect on B lymphocytes. At first sight this is at variance with the stimulation of spleen cells from cortisone-treated and congenitally athymic (nude) mice which Ruhl *et al.* (1974) attributed to a direct effect on B cells; the nude mouse spleen is, however, particularly rich in NK cells, and it seems likely that it was these cells which responded to the polynucleotide. It is uncertain whether the T-cell response is due primarily to increased proliferation of T cells in response to antigen or to increased activity of individual T cells, but Yamashita and Kitagawa (1974) claim that their observations on the antihapten response favor the second of these possibilities.

A clue to the mechanism underlying some at least of these stimulatory effects is provided by the discovery of Firshein and his colleagues that treatment of Type III pneumococci with Poly rC, and to a lesser extent Poly rA, or oligonucleotides derived therefrom, induces the formation of nucleotide kinases, in particular deoxycytidylate (d CMP) kinase and deoxyguanylate (d GMP) kinase, which are concerned with the step from nucleoside monophosphates to di- and triphosphates in the synthesis of DNA (Firshein *et al.,* 1967; Firshein and Benson, 1968). Firshein and Benson suggested that much the same mechanism is involved in mammalian cells, and Braun, Nakano *et al.* (1968) have produced evidence in support of this hypothesis. In the bacterial model study of oligonucleotides of different chain length prepared by chromatography showed that tetramers and larger molecules were equally active; tri- and dinucleotides were, respectively, three-quarters and one-quarter as effective as tetramers, and mononucleotides were inactive. When the organisms were treated with polyribonucleotides only single-stranded molecules were effective, whereas, as already mentioned, double-stranded molecules are required for *in vivo* stimulation in mammals, but this difference probably merely reflects different rates of degradation of the polymers in the two systems; it may well be, as Firshein and Benson point out, that in the bacterial assay, which lasts 25 minutes, ds polynucleotides are not broken down to active oligomers, whereas in the mammal ss polynucleotides are broken down too quickly to be effective. The lack of activity of Poly U and Poly I in the bacterial model suggests that the stimulatory effects are not due simply to the addition of polyanions but depend on the particular bases present in the polymer (Firshein and Benson, 1968); studies of the effect of chromatographic fractions of DNA digests on the stimulation of antibody to bovine gamma globulin in mice, on the other hand, led A.G. Johnson, et al. (1968) to conclude that the effect was independent of the base composition of the oligonucleotides.

Stimulation of the antibody response of mouse spleen cells to sheep erythrocytes by PolyA:PolyU is prevented if kinetin riboside is injected with the nucleotide, but this substance does not interfere with the normal unstimulated response to the same antigen (Braun, Nakano et al., 1968). It would seem therefore that stimulation by the nucleotide recruits a different population of cells, and experiments in which spleen cells were separated on density gradients have provided some confirmation of this suggestion. Since oligonucleotides and PolyA:PolyU do not cause any change in the background number of spleen cells forming antibodies to various antigens when given alone, but do increase the number of such cells if given with chlorpromazine, phenoxybenzamine, streptolysin C, or low concentrations of cortisone, all of which are permeability-altering agents, Braun, Nakano et al. (1968) suggest that stimulatory oligonucleotides cannot ordinarily get into lymphocytes, but can do so when cell permeability is altered by these agents or by administration of an antigen at about the same time. On the other hand, neither antigen nor a non-specific modifier of cell permeability seems to be necessary for the stimulation pf phagocytic activity (Freedman and Braun, 1965).

It has been suggested by Herberman et al. (1977) that stimulation of NK-cell activity is due to interferon induction (7.552) on the ground that Poly I, Poly I + CpC, and PolyA:Poly U, which did not stimulate NK activity in their experiments, cause interferon induction only when given in much higher dosage (Field et al., 1967).

7.552 INTERFERON INDUCTION

It has been shown that ds RNA of both synthetic and natural origin stimulates the production of interferon in animals (Lampson et al., 1967; Field et al., 1967; Vilcek et al., 1968; Leonard et al., 1969; Colby and Chamberlain, 1969; De Clercq and Merigan, 1969; Hilleman, 1970; Baron et al., 1970; Colby et al., 1971) and man (Hilleman et al., 1971), and also by mouse kidney cells in tissue culture (Hilleman et al., 1971). It is of interest that ds RNAs containing IC or GC base pairs appear to be more active than those containing AU base pairs, and this property seems to be associated with somewhat greater toxicity and pyrogenicity (Braun, Ishizuka et al., 1971).

The mechanism of interferon induction has not been fully elucidated, but studies with isotope-labeled synthetic ds RNA have shown that although some of this material gains entry to cells, and some of the degradation products are incorporated in the cellular DNA, the bulk of the material is still on the cell surface at the time the commitment to interferon production is made (Merigan et al., 1971). Whatever the mechanism, it seems a plausible hypothesis that polynucleotides are, as Merigan et al. suggest, the critical interferon stimulating factors during the process of natural virus infection.

7.553 CYTOTOXICITY FOR TUMOR CELLS

It was reported by Glick and Goldberg (1965, 1966) that DNA from the thymus of BDF_1 or DBA/2 mice, when mixed with L1210 mouse leukemia cells, inhibited the growth of tumors after subcutaneous inoculation, whereas tumor cells alone grew well in both strains. DNA from the tumor alone, from the thymus of Swiss mice, and from *E. coli* had no such effect. They also found that DNA from one human cell line was toxic to cells of a second human cell line but not to a third. The phenomenon appears to depend on loss of cell viability, since tumor cells incubated first with the appropriate DNA and subsequently in DNA-free medium show progressive loss of viability.

Glick (1968) has postulated that the mechanism involves entry of some of the foreign DNA into the cell, leading to synthesis of the corresponding RNA; and this in turn leads to the synthesis of a protein which is cytotoxic. In support of this hypothesis he has advanced the following evidence:

1. Only high molecular weight helical DNA is effective.
2. Studies with labeled DNA *in vitro* show that DNA enters cells rapidly; in the experiments described about 50 percent of the DNA to enter the cell did so within 5 minutes.
3. Isotope studies *in vitro* show that DNA synthesis followed by RNA synthesis does occur within the target cells. Moreover, the cytotoxic effect is lost if DNA synthesis is blocked with 5-fluorodeoxyuridine (FUDR), or DNA-dependent RNA synthesis is blocked with actinomycin D, but is not lost if the target cells are exposed to actinomycin D and then washed before being exposed to DNA.
4. Exposure to appropriate DNA stimulates protein synthesis by L1210 leukemia cells *in vitro* as shown by increased uptake of ^{14}C-lysine, and the cytotoxic effect is blocked if protein synthesis by DNA-treated cells is blocked with puromycin.

According to Glick (1968), however, the proportion of cells destroyed by treatment with appropriate DNA "is much too large to be explained on the basis of genetic transformation for a specific genetic marker." He has therefore suggested that any one of a number of genetic sites present in BDF_1 or DBA/2 DNA is capable of directing the formation of a cytotoxic foreign protein within L1210 cells, and that a cell will be destroyed if one or more of these lethal genetic sites gains entry to it.

7.554 EFFECT ON TUMOR GROWTH *IN VIVO*

As discussed earlier (2.2) ds RNA prepared synthetically or of natural origin may inhibit chemical, radiation, and viral carcinogenesis.

Systemic (intravenous or intraperitoneal) administration of these agents has been shown to inhibit the growth of subcutaneous transplants of many tumors, including tumors induced with polyoma virus (J.C. Fisher, Cooperband, and Mannick, 1972), chemically induced fibrosarcomas (Fisher *et al.*, 1972; Parr, Wheeler, and Alexander, 1973) and lymphomas (H.B. Levy, Law, and Rabson, 1969; Zelerznick and Bhuyan, 1969; Mathé, Hayat, Sakouhi, and Choay, 1970), the B16 melanoma (Bart and Kopf, 1969; Bart, Kopf, and Silagi, 1971; Kreider and Benjamin, 1972), the Lewis lung carcinoma (Heyes *et al.*, 1974), and a reticulum cell sarcoma, a fibrosarcoma, and a lymphoma of spontaneous origin (H.B. Levy *et al.*, 1971) in mice; and a variety of rat tumors of both viral and non-viral origin (Kreider and Benjamin, 1972). In the experiments of Fisher *et al.* (1972) primary transplants up to 3 mm diameter were made to regress; this effect was usually only temporary, but in a few mice transplants of poly-oma-induced tumors regressed completely. Complete regression of many subcutane-ous and intradermal transplants of chemically induced lymphomas and fibrosarcomas was reported by Parr *et al.* (1973), and reduced metastasis of the Lewis lung tumor by Heyes *et al.* (1974). On the other hand, Meier, Myers, and Huebner (1970) reported that Poly I:Poly C had little or no effect on transplants of chemically induced fibrosar-comas in mice, and Pimm, Embleton, and Baldwin (1976) found that systemic injec-tion of a ds RNA of fungal viral origin was equally ineffective in rats with transplants of chemically induced and spontaneous tumors.

Lacour *et al.* (1972) used repeated intravenous injection of Poly A:Poly U as ad-juvant therapy after surgical excision of spontaneous mammary adenocarcinomas in C3H mice and transplants of a metastastizing melanoma in hamsters. In both cases the incidence of metastases was reduced and survival of the animals prolonged, but mice treated by administration of PolyA:Poly U without surgery did not survive long-er than untreated animals.

Double-stranded RNA has also been shown to inhibit the growth of subcutane-ous (Parr *et al.*, 1973; Heyes *et al.*, 1974) and intraperitoneal (H.B. Levy, Law, and Rabson, 1969; Ball and McCarter, 1971; Svec *et al.*, 1972; Pimm and Baldwin, 1976d) tumor transplants in mice and rats when injected at the site of tumor inoculation, and also when mixed with a suspension of tumor cells and injected subcutaneously (Pimm, Embleton, and Baldwin, 1976). In some experiments the therapeutic effect was strik-ing but may have been due in part to a direct cytoxic effect of the ds RNA on the tu-mor cells, since the agent used was cytotoxic for cultured tumor cells *in vitro,* but Pimm *et al.* suggest that this is not the complete explanation because regression *in vivo* was sometimes preceded by temporary growth of the tumor.

Whatever the explanation of the antitumor effect of local treatment, it seems like-ly that the effect of systemic treatment depends on increased host reactivity of some kind, though the possibility of some direct effect on tumor cells cannot be excluded on the evidence available (Kreider and Benjamin, 1972). The observation of Kreider and Benjamin (1972) that treatment with Poly I:Poly C retarded tumor growth in thymec-tomized ALS-treated rats and ALS-treated mice but did not restore the ability of these animals to reject skin allografts suggests that stimulation of T lymphocytes is not an essential factor, but experiments in athymic mice with a variety of immunogenic and non-immunogenic tumors are required to delineate precisely the role, if any, of T-cell stimulation. It seems likely that activation of macrophages is important, but NK cells may also be involved. In the case of tumors of viral origin, and tumors induced by chemical carcinogens and irradiation in which activation of latent oncogenic virus is involved, interferon induction may play a key role.

It is surprising, in view of its possible therapeutic importance, that Glick's work (7.553) on the cytotoxicity of DNA has not been followed by detailed study of the ef-fect of DNA from various sources on tumor growth *in vivo.*

7.56 Levamisole

An antihelminthic drug, tetramisole, was introduced for veterinary use in 1965 and for human use one year later. It consists of a mixture of two optical isomers, of which the levorotatory isomer, L-2,3,5,6-tetrahydro-6-phenylimidazole [2,1-b]thiazole hydrochloride, termed *levamisole*, is the more potent antihelminthic and has been found to have immunopotentiating properties (Willoughby and Wood, 1977).

Levamisole has been shown to potentiate various manifestations of T-cell-mediated immunity including delayed-type hypersensitivity (Renoux *et al.*, 1976), the graft-versus-host reaction (Renoux and Renoux, 1972b), the rejection of skin grafts across an HY barrier (i.e., from males to females) in C57B1 mice (Chirigos, Pearson, and Pryor, 1973), and the IgG response to sheep erythrocytes (Renoux *et al.*, 1976). It has also been shown to restore the capacity of aged mice to respond immunologically to sheep erythrocytes (Renoux and Renoux, 1972a), and to increase the phagocytic activity of macrophages (Hoebeke and Franchi, 1973; Verhaegen *et al.*, 1973).

Levamisole has been reported to inhibit the growth of subcutaneous transplants and pulmonary metastases of the Lewis lung tumor in C57B1 mice (Renoux and Renoux, 1972c), to protect newborn hamsters against a virus-induced sarcoma (Thiry *et al.*, 1977), and to inhibit metastasis by cells transformed by herpes simplex virus (Sadowski and Rapp, 1975). Levamisole has also been reported to potentiate the effect of chemotherapy in Balb/c mice with Moloney-virus-induced leukemia (Chirigos *et al.*, 1973, 1975). On the other hand, it has failed to inhibit the growth of isogeneic transplants of a variety of other tumors in mice and rats when administered systemically (Potter *et al.*, 1974; Hopper, Pimm, and Baldwin, 1975b) or admixed with tumor cells (Hopper, Pimm, and Baldwin, 1975b).

7.57   Anticoagulants and Fibrinolytic Agents

Platelet aggregation and fibrin formation are commonly seen around tumors, and it has been reported that anticoagulants and fibrinolytic agents may reduce the number of tumors which develop after intravenous injection of tumor cells (Terranova and Chiossone, 1952; Cliffton, 1966; Back, Shields, and Ambrus, 1966; Gasic, Gasic, and Stewart, 1968) and also inhibit spontaneous metastasis from a variety of experimental tumors (Retik *et al.*, 1962; Back *et al.*, 1966; Hagmar, 1968, 1970; Hagmar and Boeryd, 1968; Ryan, Ketcham, and Wexler, 1968b; J.M. Brown, 1973; Berkarda, d'Souza, and Bakemeier, 1974). Warfarin and other coumarin derivatives may have an antimetastatic effect when heparin does not (Hagmar, 1968; Berkarda *et al.*, 1974), and appear to inhibit the growth not only of metastases but of some primary tumors, but the diverse pharmacological actions of these agents make interpretation of the experimental results difficult (Hilgard and Thornes, 1976).

The chemical combination of alkylating agents with heparin has been reported to increase their effectiveness against tumors in animals (Csaba *et al.*, 1964) but, again, interpretation is difficult.

7.58   Interferon

The discovery of interferon (Isaacs and Lindemann, 1957; Isaacs *et al.*, 1957) arose out of the study of the phenomenon of viral interference, i.e., the capacity of a cell exposed to one virus, which may be inactivated, to resist infection by another live virus. It is now known, however, that cells exposed to virus may produce a range of biologically active glycoproteins, referred to collectively as interferons, which not only inhibit viral replication but may also inhibit the growth of both normal and tumor cells *in vitro* and of tumors *in vivo* (see Tan, 1976).

The effect of interferons on mouse tumors has been studied particularly by Gresser and his colleagues. Their findings and conclusions may be summarized as follows:

1. Repeated injection of mouse interferon delayed the development of leukemia in mice previously inoculated with Friend or Rauscher virus (Gresser *et al.,* 1968). It was thought likely that this was due to inhibition of virus replication, but a direct effect on the proliferation of virus-infected cells was not excluded.
2. Repeated administration of mouse, but not human or rabbit, interferon inhibited the growth of a variety of transplanted syngeneic mouse tumors and also the allogeneic Ehrlich ascites tumor, and prolonged the survival of the recipients (Gresser *et al.,* 1969, 1970a; Gresser and Bourali, 1970; Gresser, 1972). Two of the syngeneically transplanted tumors studied, the RC19 Balb/c ascites tumor and the E ♂ G2 DBA/2 tumor, had been induced originally with Rauscher virus and Gross virus, respectively; two others, the EL4 and L1210 ascites tumor, had been induced chemically, but both exhibited A-type particles on electron microscopy.
3. Mouse interferon preparations inhibited the multiplication of L1210 and Ehrlich ascites cells *in vitro,* but prolonged exposure of L1210 cells to interferon resulted in the development of a cell subline resistant to the inhibitory effect of interferon on cell multiplication (Gresser *et al.,* 1970b).
4. Treatment with interferon increased the survival of mice inoculated with the interferon-resistant subline of the L1210 tumor (Gresser, Maury, and Brouty-Boyé, 1972). It was concluded that interferon can act not only on virus and virus-transformed cells, but can also render the host more resistant to tumor growth. It was found subsequently that the antitumor effect of interferon on both the interferon-sensitive and the interferon-resistant lines of L1210 was unaffected by pretreating the mice with antilymphocyte serum, and reduced but not abolished by pretreatment with silica (Gresser and Bourali-Maury, 1973). It was concluded that the effect is mediated at least in part by mechanisms which do not involve T lymphocytes and macrophages. In the light of subsequent developments it would seem likely that NK cells (5.44) are involved.

7.59 Other Agents

A variety of glucans, including glucan prepared from yeast cell walls, and lentinan prepared from mushrooms (Maeda and Chihara, 1971), have been reported to possess antitumor activity (Maeda *et al.,* 1971, 1973, 1975; Maeda and Chihara, 1973). Bomford and Moreno (1978) found, however, that none of the glucans they tested, including lentinan, reproducibly potentiated immunization when mixed with irradiated tumor cells, nor did they inhibit the growth of subcutaneous syngeneic tumor transplants when injected intravenously or intralesionally.

Some new immunopotentiating agents which have become available recently, but whose effect on tumor growth has not yet been evaluated, are discussed in the next chapter (8.322). Hyperthermia will also be considered later [8.24(11)] because most of the data concerning its effect on tumors have come from clinical studies.

7.6   SPECIFIC ACTIVE IMMUNIZATION

In this section we shall consider treatment with unmodified, irradiated, enzyme-treated, and "xenogenized" tumor cells, selected subpopulations of tumor cells, and tumor cell extracts, without the use of immunopotentiating agents. Administration of tumor cells or extracts combined with systemic or local administration of immunopotentiating agents will be discussed later (7.71).

7.61   Unmodified and Irradiated Cells. Cell Extracts

It was stated by Jensen in 1903 that it is possible not only to produce immunity against a tumor in normal mice but also to inhibit and destroy an existing tumor by treatment with separated tumor cells. To quote his words: ". . . es nicht nur möglich ist, bei gesunden Mäusen eine aktive Immunität den Geschwulstzellen gegenüber hervorzurufen, sondern dass es auch möglich ist, bei einer bereits von einem Tumor angegriffenen Maus eine aktive Immunität durch Behandlung mit losgetrennten Geschwulstzellen zu erzeugen, so dass das fortgesetzte Wachstum der Geschwulst verhindert und das Geschwulstgewebe nach und nach getötet und resorbiert wird."*

Half a century later Cohen and Cohen, in a series of experiments extending from 1956 to 1960 (summarized by A. Cohen, 1964), showed that the radiosensitivity of mammary adenocarcinomas in C3H mice could be increased by inoculating the animal with autochthonous tumor tissue which had been excised and irradiated *in vitro,* and somewhat similar results were obtained by Haddow and Alexander (1964) with chemically induced primary fibrosarcomas in rats.

More direct confirmation of Jensen's claim has been provided by the demonstration that the growth of various experimental tumors, including transplanted Shope virus-induced tumors (C.A. Evans *et al.,* 1962a), transplanted syngeneic mouse leukemia (Mathé, Schwartzenberg *et al.,* 1967; Mathé, 1968) and mouse fibrosarcomas (Vanwijck *et al.,* 1971), and autochthonous bladder tumors induced in rats by dietary (vitamin B₆) restriction and administration of acetylaminofluorene (Fingerhut and Veenema, 1975) may be inhibited by treatment with irradiated or unmodified tumor tissue. The results with the rat bladder tumors were striking; 15 out of 33 regressed completely following autotransplantation of a small fragment of tumor to the peritoneal cavity, and 12 others showed histological evidence of regression with marked round cell infiltration. Regression of the leukemia occurred, however, only if the tumor inoculum was small or the tumor burden was reduced by chemotherapy; and with the fibrosarcomas the immunotherapy, which was preceded by surgical excision of the primary transplant, suppressed or stimulated metastasis depending on the number of cells injected. Subcutaneous injection of irradiated mouse fibrosarcoma cells was found by Woodruff, Hitchcock, and Whitehead (1977) to prolong the survival of mice inoculated intracerebrally with viable tumor cells on the same day, though most

---

*It is not only possible to induce active immunity against tumor cells in healthy mice, but it is also possible to generate active immunity in a mouse already bearing a tumor graft by treatment with free tumor cells so that established growth of the tumor is inhibited and tumor tissue is killed and absorbed.

of the animals developed tumors and died eventually; the same treatment 3 days after tumor inoculation was ineffective.

Aptekman and Lewis (1951) treated rats bearing syngeneically transplanted methylcholanthrene-induced fibrosarcomas by repeated injection of an alcoholic extract of tumor tissue starting 6 days after transplantation. All the tumors regressed and the animals became resistant to rechallenge; injection of distilled water, or alcohol diluted with water, however, was completely ineffective. More recently Morton *et al.* (1971b) have reported that injection of cell-free tumor antigenic extracts from methylcholanthrene-induced guinea pig sarcomas at a site remote from the tumor caused inhibition of growth when given before, at the time of, or even after tumor inoculation. Forni and Comoglio (1974), however, found that repeated injection of solubilized tumor cell membrane antigen starting 24 hours before tumor inoculation was of no benefit in mice inoculated with either a syngeneic IgA plasmacytoma or a spontaneous adenocarcinoma, although the material used was shown to induce, and react with, specific antibody.

While the pattern of immunological response depends *inter alia* on the route of administration and dose of antigen (Lagrange, Mackannes, and Miller, 1974), it does not seem surprising that not very much has been achieved by injecting antigen which is likely to be available, perhaps in excessive amounts, from the tumor. The possibility of modifying the antigenic stimulus would seem to be of greater interest, and this we shall now consider.

7.62   Neuraminidase-treated Tumor Cells

Incubation with the enzyme neuraminidase derived from *Vibrio cholerae* (VCN) has been shown to increase the immunogenicity of a variety of mouse tumors, both non-strain-specific (Currie, 1967; Currie and Bagshawe, 1968a, 1968b; Sanford, 1967; Lindenmann and Klein, 1967b), and strain-specific (Bagshawe and Currie, 1968; Currie and Bagshawe, 1969; Bekesi, St. Arneault, and Holland, 1971; Sethi and Brandis, 1973), as indicated by failure of the tumor to grow after inoculation of enough cells to yield tumors if they had not been treated, induction of resistance to subsequent challenge with untreated cells, and in some cases the demonstration of antibody (Currie and Bagshawe, 1968a, 1968b) or sensitized lymphocytes (Faraci, Marrone, and Ketcham, 1975) specifically cytotoxic for the tumor cells. A similar but weaker effect was demonstrated by Currie and Bagshawe (1968b) with neuraminidase from *Clostridium perfringens* but not with neuraminidase prepared from influenza virus. It has also been shown (Simmons, Rios, and Ray, 1971) that normal lymphoid cells treated with VCN become more immunogenic, in the sense that they are more effective than normal lymphoid cells in eliciting allograft immunity when transplanted across a major histocompatibility barrier.

To explain the effect of neuraminidase on immunogenicity, Currie and Bagshawe (1967a, 1968a, 1968b) postulated that sialomucin on the cell surface prevents antigen-sensitive cells from making contact with some cell surface antigens, either by steric hindrance or electrostatic repulsion, and that these antigens may become accessible when the cell is treated with the enzyme by a process which they called unmasking. Sanford (1967) suggested originally that major histocompatibility antigens might be masked by sialic acid and unmasked by neuraminidase. Subsequently Sanford and

Codington (1971) revised this hypothesis in the light of their finding that cells of a non-strain-specific mouse ascites tumor became susceptible to lysis by naturally occurring antibodies in normal guinea pig serum, and in the sera of some mouse strains, but did not show increased binding of antibodies directed against H2 antigens; and they suggested that, while some new antigenic sites might be exposed by cleavage of neuraminozyl groups at the cell surface by neuraminidase, altered molecular conformation resulting from a decreased negative surface charge might also contribute to the antigenic change. The biological significance of cell surface sialic acids, and the mechanism underlying the effect of neuraminidase on cell interactions, have been reviewed by L. Weiss (1973).

The discovery of the effect of exposure to neuraminidase on the immunogenicity of tumor cells prompted investigation of the therapeutic value of injecting neuraminidase-treated autochthonous or syngeneic tumor cells to tumor-bearing animals.

It was reported by Simmons et al. (1971a) that a single injection of 10^6 VCN-treated mouse fibrosarcoma cells 20–30 days after subcutaneous inoculation of the same tumor, by which time the tumors were 5–10 mm diameter, caused permanent regression of the smaller tumors and temporary cessation of growth of the remainder, and that the successfully treated animals became resistant to rechallenge; treatment with cells which had been incubated with inactivated VCN, or with VCN in the presence of excess sialic acid, or with VCN-treated cells from a different fibrosarcoma, however, was ineffective. Simmons and Rios confirmed and extended these experiments, using tumor cells which had been treated with mitomycin to prevent further division, or killed by freezing and thawing, besides being incubated with VCN (Simmons and Rios, 1971a, 1971b, 1972b, 1974; Rios and Simmons, 1974a); they showed also that with fibrosarcoma transplants more than 10 mm diameter, treatment by subtotal excision and injection of VCN-treated cells was more effective than either of these procedures alone (Rios and Simmons, 1974b). In contrast, Spence, Simon, and Baker (1978) reported that treatment with VCN-treated cells was ineffective in mice with established fibrosarcomas; Simmons and Rios (1973a) found that chemotherapy plus administration of VCN-treated cells was less effective than either procedure alone; and Godrick et al. (1972), in a study of the incidence of pulmonary metastases after treatment of primary mouse fibrosarcoma transplants by amputation, found that if therapeutically optimal doses were used, injection of unmodified viable tumor cells was as effective as injection of VCN-treated cells.

Studies with other types of tumor, using cells treated with VCN and mitomycin, or with VCN and irradiation, have also yielded discordant results. With mouse leukemias, administration of VCN-treated cells combined with chemotherapy has been found beneficial in some experiments (Holland, St. Arneault, and Bekesi, 1972; Bekesi and Holland, 1974; Bekesi, Roboz, and Holland, 1977; Le Fever, Killion, and Kollmorgen, 1976) but not in others (Dore et al., 1973; Ghose et al., 1977). With a transplanted mouse melanoma, Rios and Simmons (1974b) reported inhibition of growth, and in one animal complete remission, following injection of VCN-treated cells; others, however, working with similar tumors, have reported no benefit (Jamieson, 1974) or enhanced tumor growth (Froese, Berczi, and Sehon, 1974), and in the experiments of Rios and Simmons (1974b) administration of VCN-treated cells combined with surgical enucleation of the tumor was no more effective than either procedure alone. In rats with intraperitoneal transplants of an ascitic form of a chemically induced colon carcinoma, Enker and Jacobitz (1976) reported cures in 70 percent of animals which received repeated subcutaneous injections of VCN-treated tumor cells starting 24 hours after tumor inoculation, whereas all the untreated animals died. In mice with transplanted mammary carcinomas, Simmons and Rios (1973b, 1976), and Rios and Simmons (1974b), reported that injection of VCN-treated cells resulted in temporary inhibition of growth of small tumors, and reduced incidence of recurrence when combined with incomplete surgical excision of large tumors; in rats, however, Pimm, Cook, and Baldwin (1978) found that administration of VCN-treated cells had no effect on syngeneic mammary tumor transplants, and in dogs with spontaneous mammary tumors, Sedlacek, Meesman, and Seiler (1975) found that administration of VCN-treated tumor cells caused tumor regression in some animals and enhanced growth in others.

Attempts to treat tumors by intralesional injection of neuraminidase have also been reported to cause regression in some experiments (Simmons and Rios, 1972a; Simmons, Rios, and Kersey, 1972; Sparks and Breeding, 1974; Alley and Snodgrass, 1977), and no change or enhanced tumor growth in others (Binder et al., 1975). It was found moreover by Simmons et al. that mice with spontaneous mammary tumors which regressed following intralesional injection of VCN, developed new tumors of similar histological type, possibly, they suggested, because the animals developed immunity to weak specific antigens of the treated tumor but not to antigens of the mouse mammary tumor virus.

A clue to the explanation of the lack of uniformity in the therapeutic response to injection of neuraminidase-treated cells is provided by the discovery that the response depends not only on such factors as the type of tumor and the immunological status of the host, but also on the concentration of VCN used to treat the cells, which has differed greatly in different experiments, and which, if it exceeds a certain level, may cause little or no increase in immunogenicity of the treated cells (Simmons et al., 1971a, 1971c; Bekesi et al., 1972; Sethi and Brandis, 1973). It is difficult to account for this relationship on the assumption that the effect of VCN depends solely on the splitting of cell-surface sialic acid. It has been shown, however, with radio-actively labeled material (Lüben, Sedlacek, and Seiler, 1976) that when tumor cells are incubated with VCN some active enzyme becomes bound to the surface of the cells, the amount depending on the concentration to which the cells are exposed. This bound enzyme is able to split off sialic acid from lymphocytes and other cells with which the tumor cells come in contact in vivo (Petitou, Rosenfeld, and Sinay, 1977), to stimulate macrophages and lymphocytes, and to act as an immunological adjuvant; moreover, the adjuvant effect of VCN follows a dose–response curve similar to the V-shaped dose–response curve for VCN-treated tumor cells in tumor immunotherapy (Sedlacek and Seiler, 1978).

Bekesi and Holland (1977, 1978) have suggested that the number of VCN-treated cells causing the strongest local delayed-type hypersensitivity (DTH) reaction might be the optimal dose for immunotherapy, and have set up a prospective study to investigate this in patients with acute myeloid leukemia. Seiler and Sedlacek (1978) have carried this approach a stage further, and have designed a procedure called *chessboard vaccination,* in which various numbers of tumor cells combined with various amounts of VCN are injected intradermally at different sites, to determine which combination causes the strongest DTH reaction. In dogs with a small residual tumor burden after surgical removal of mammary tumors, the greatest effect was produced by either a small number of tumor cells combined with a relatively large amount of VCN, or a large number of cells combined with a small amount of VCN (Sedlacek et al., 1979); in dogs with a large tumor burden, no amount of VCN caused a clear increase in the DTH reaction.

7.63 Modified Tumor Cells and Cross-reacting Antigen

Administration of conjugated (Nachtigal and Feldman, 1964; Nachtigal, Eschel-Zussman, and Feldman, 1965; Weigle, 1964, 1965) and cross-reacting (Scales and Cruse, 1970) antigen has been reported to abolish tolerance to various soluble antigens. This suggests that it might be of therapeutic value to immunize tumor-bearing hosts with what have since been called *xenogenized* (Kobayashi, Kodama, and Gotohda, 1977) or *heterogenized* tumor cells, i.e., cells modified in such a way that they acquire antigens which they do not normally possess. Various possible procedures have been discussed by Prager (1973).

The use of chemically xenogenized cells was pioneered by Czajkowski et al. (1966), who treated C3H mice bearing spontaneous mammary adenocarcinomas and methylcholanthrene-induced squamous cell carcinomas by repeated injection of tumor cells prepared from excised tumor tissue and coupled to human IgG by means of *bis*-diazobenzidine. None of the tumors decreased in size, but growth was retarded, and histological sections showed increased necrosis, lymphocytic infiltration, and fibrosis in tumors from the treated mice as compared with tumors from untreated controls.

Fixation with glutaraldehyde or formaldehyde may selectively impair cell antigenicity, and the question arises of whether this phenomenon could be turned to therapeutic account. Dennert and Tucker (1972) showed that erythrocytes treated with these agents retained their immunogenicity towards T cells but were unable to evoke a humoral response as judged by plaque-forming assays, and suggested that tumor cells treated in the same way might retain their capacity to stimulate CMI but not the production of antibody. It was shown subsequently by others that cells of methylcholanthrene-induced mouse sarcomas which had been treated with glutaraldehyde were able to protect animals against subsequent live challenge with the same tumor (Sanderson and Frost, 1974), and that the cells of a MLV-induced lymphoma lost the capacity to evoke an antibody response after treatment with either formaldehyde or glutaraldehyde (Gatti, Ostborn, and Fagraeus, 1974). It would seem important to develop this approach further, and to assess the effect of glutaraldehyde and formalin fixation on the capacity of cells from a variety of tumors to evoke cell-mediated and humoral immunity, and on their therapeutic effectiveness when used to treat tumor-bearing animals.

Erythrocytes may also lose the capacity to evoke a humoral response while retaining the capacity to induce DTH following partial digestion by macrophages in vitro (Pearson and Raffel, 1971), and it would be of interest to study the effect of this procedure on tumor cell immunogenicity.

The use of neuraminidase-treated cells has been considered in a separate section because it was originally thought that treatment with this enzyme did no more than unmask hidden antigens. As we have seen (7.62), however, some neuraminidase becomes firmly attached to the cell surface, and, in so far as it is immunogenic, the process of xenogenization is involved. Another way in which xenogenization occurs is by virus infection; non-specific immunopotentiation may also occur, however, and the use of viral infection in experimental immunotherapy also was discussed in an earlier section (7.54).

Watkins and Chen (1969) immunized mice against the Ehrlich ascites tumor with a hamster-Ehrlich ascites tumor hybrid cell line. It would be of interest to undertake similar experiments with isogeneic tumors using hybrids of the tumor and normal allogeneic or xenogeneic cells, and to investigate the therapeutic possibilities of the procedure.

Immunization with fetal antigens which cross-react with tumor antigens may afford some protection against subsequent challenge with live tumor cells (Hanna *et al.*, 1971), but it seems unlikely that fetal cells would be more effective than tumor cells, or even as effective, when used for active immunotherapy. The existence of oncofetal antigens does however raise the possibility, which was discussed earlier (2.2), of immunoprophylaxis against some forms of carcinogenesis.

7.64   Selected Subpopulations of Tumor Cells

It was found by Killion and Kollmorgen (1976) that when cells of the L1210 mouse leukemia were fractionated on cell-affinity columns prepared by coupling concanavalin A to nylon fibers with glutaraldehyde, the fractions differed greatly in their therapeutic effectiveness when injected to mice bearing the L1210 tumor following reduction of the tumor burden by chemotherapy; furthermore, the relative effectiveness of different fractions was altered by treating the cells with neuraminidase. They concluded that the immunogenicity of the various subpopulations was related to the expression of cell surface carbohydrates, and they postulated that specific immunotherapy following chemotherapy might fail because of antigenic differences between metastatic and drug-resistant residual tumor cells and the cells forming the bulk of the primary tumors which were used for immunization. They suggested therefore that attempts should be made to identify, and expand for therapeutic use, subpopulations of cells which matched antigenically the residual tumor.

This approach has been taken a stage further by Killion (1978), using columns coated with concanavalin A, fucose-binding protein, ricin-communis agglutinin, or PHA to collect tumor cells and eluting with phosphate-buffered saline or solutions of carbohydrate-competitors of lectins such as α-D-galactose and L-fucose. Immunotherapy with L1210 cells eluted from fucose-specific columns following chemotherapy proved beneficial, whereas administration of cells eluted from galactose-specific columns was deleterious. It will be interesting to see whether similar results can be obtained with other tumors.

7.7   COMBINED IMMUNOTHERAPEUTIC PROCEDURES

The general problem of determining whether two or more therapeutic agents have a synergistic effect has been discussed by Berenbaum (1977). When studying combinations of immunotherapeutic procedures the kind of analysis which might be undertaken with combinations of therapeutic drugs has not been attempted, and the question—whether explicit or implicit—which seems to have prompted most investigations is whether it is possible by using two procedures to produce a therapeutic effect greater than that produced by either alone when given in an optimal way, with no greater harmful effects. Since combinations of treatment which are advantageous for one tumor model may not be for another, it is important to define classes of tumors for which particular combinations seem favorable, and then try to discover why this should be so.

7.71 Combined Active Specific and Non- Specific Immunotherapy

7.711 IMMUNOPOTENTIATING AGENTS MIXED WITH TUMOR CELLS OR ANTIGEN

Repeated subcutaneous and intravenous injection of tumor homogenate mixed with hyaluronidase and *Bordetella pertussis* vaccine, starting 14 days after tumor inoculation, was reported by Wissler *et al.* (1968) to inhibit the growth of subcutaneous isogeneic transplants of a rat hepatoma, whereas treatment 9 days before tumor inoculation resulted in enhanced tumor growth.

Injection of BCG mixed with tumor cells has been reported to delay or entirely prevent the development of tumors in animals inoculated at the same time, but at a different site, with viable cells of the same isogeneic tumor. The greatest effect has been observed with strongly immunogenic tumors, including chemically induced guinea pig (Bartlett and Zbar, 1972) and rat (Embleton, 1976) hepatomas and rat fibrosarcomas (Baldwin and Pimm, 1971, 1973c). With such tumors a sufficient number of viable tumor cells may be given with BCG with little risk of tumor development at the site of treatment, but irradiated and mitomycin-treated cells, which eliminate this risk completely, are also effective (Bartlett and Zbar, 1972; Bekierkunst, 1975), and some effect has been obtained with lyophilized cells and BCG (Yarkoni, Zbar and Rapp, 1977). With weakly immunogenic tumors, however, it may not be possible to achieve anything like the same effect, either with the maximum number of viable tumor cells that can be given with BCG, or with a mixture of BCG and irradiated or mitomycin-treated cells. It is therefore not surprising that these procedures have proved ineffective in irradiated and athymic animals (Pimm and Baldwin, 1976a, 1976b).

Similar treatment subsequent to tumor challenge has given more variable results even with immunogenic tumors. Bartlett and Zbar (1972) obtained complete regression of subcutaneous guinea pig hepatoma transplants up to 1.5 cm diameter, and Baldwin and Pimm (1973b) prevented the development of tumors in the lungs by subcutaneous injection of tumor cells mixed with BCG up to 10 days after intravenous injection of rat sarcoma cells; on the other hand, this treatment has had little or no effect on subcutaneously transplanted rat fibrosarcomas (Baldwin and Pimm, 1973c; Thomson, 1975; Salomon *et al.*, 1976). When used as adjuvant therapy following surgical excision of metastasizing rat mammary carcinomas, subcutaneous injection of mixed BCG and tumor cells was found by Sparks and Breeding (1974) to prolong survival, but in similar experiments with rat fibrosarcoma transplants Baldwin and Pimm (1973a) found that the adjuvant therapy had no significant effect.

When administration of BCG mixed with tumor cells is effective it may be associated with increased lymphocytic infiltration of the tumor (Hopper, Robins, and Baldwin, 1978), a tumor-specific antibody response and disappearance from the circulation of tumor antigen (Thomson, 1975; Embleton, 1976), and a fall in the amount of antigen–antibody complex in the serum (Jennette and Feldman, 1977; Hoffken *et al.*, 1978).

In most of the experiments cited, live BCG has been used, but MER (7.515) and other derivatives have been used with tumor cells in immunization experiments and will no doubt also be tried therapeutically. The possibility of using soluble tumor antigen adsorbed on BCG is raised by the observation of Crum and McGregor (1977) that this material is highly immunogenic. Another material which has been shown to be highly immunogenic, and which will no doubt be tried in therapeutic experiments, was prepared by Lachmann and Sikora (1978) by coupling PPD (7.515) to concanavalin A with glutaraldehyde, and then binding this complex to tumor cells.

As an alternative to injecting BCG mixed with VCN-treated tumor cells, Simmons, Rios, and Kersey (1972) injected VCN and BCG intralesionally in C3H mice with spontaneous mammary tumors. Injection of either agent alone slowed the growth of the tumors. Injection of both together resulted in total regression of the tumors and prolonged survival, but other mammary tumors developed subsequently; it was postulated therefore that immunity was induced to weak antigens of the treated tumor but not to the mammary tumor virus.

Treatment with CP mixed with irradiated tumor cells has been shown in a variety of experiments to inhibit the growth of isogeneically transplanted mouse fibrosarcomas, but the dose of CP and the time at which the treatment is given are critical. Bomford (1975) found that footpad injection of 5–120 μg CP mixed with not less than 50,000 irradiated (10,000 rad) tumor cells prevented the development of tumors when given 2 or 6 days, but not when given 10 days, after dorsal subcutaneous injection of the same number of viable tumor cells, and also when given two days before intravenous injection of viable cells. Treatment with isogeneic fetal cells, or allogeneic* tumor cells, and CP was ineffective. Treatment was also ineffective in T-cell-deficient mice, though Woodruff, Hitchcock, and Whitehead (1977) observed moderate inhibition of mouse fibrosarcoma transplants in an immunologically privileged site when a mixture of irradiated tumor cells and CP was injected either subcutaneously or intralesionally 3 days after intracerebral tumor inoculation.

The optimal dose of CP when mixed with tumor cells in Bomford's experiments was much below the optimal dose of CP when given alone by intravenous injection, and a similar difference was observed by Scott (1974b) in experiments with a mouse mastocytoma. As mentioned previously (7.521), there is support for the hypothesis that the abrogation of immunization by subcutaneous injection of large doses of CP mixed with irradiated tumor cells is due to prolonged trapping and eventual destruction of lymphocytes which have responded to tumor antigen in the lymph nodes draining the site of injection (Woodruff and Whitehead, 1977).

It was found by Proctor, Rudenstam, and Alexander (1973a) that injection of irradiated tumor cells prior to surgical excision of transplants of a metastasizing rat hepatoma resulted in either inhibition or enhancement of tumor growth depending on the dose of irradiated cells; if CP (or BCG) was mixed with the cells, however, enhancement did not occur. Scott (1979a, 1979b) found that injection of a mixture of irradiated cells and CP added to the antitumor effect of cyclophosphamide in mice with established fibrosarcoma transplants if the immunotherapy was given after the chemotherapy, an interval of 14 days giving the best results; injection of CP and irradiated cells before cyclophosphamide, however, was ineffective.

Likhite (1976) observed a reduced incidence of spontaneous mammary carcinomas in DBA/2 mice following injection of a mixture of CP and syngeneic mammary carcinoma cells.

---

*Referred to by Bomford as *heterologous*.

7.712 SEPARATE ADMINISTRATION OF SPECIFIC AND NON-SPECIFIC AGENTS

Injection of BCG or CP at one site and tumor cells at another has also been found in some experiments to be more effective than either treatment alone. This was shown by Mathé, Pouillart, and Laperaque (1969) with mice bearing the L1210 leukemia which received a single subcutaneous injection of irradiated tumor cells 24 hours after tumor inoculation, repeated intravenous injection of BCG starting 24 hours after tumor inoculation, or both forms of treatment; and by Simmons and Rios (1971b) with mice bearing established fibrosarcoma transplants which received a subcutaneous injection of tumor cells treated with mitomycin and neuraminidase, or a subcutaneous injection of BCG, or subcutaneous injections of both these materials at different sites.

Similar results have been obtained with *Corynebacterium parvum* and cells treated with mitomycin and neuraminidase or by irradiation in mice with transplanted fibrosarcomas (Woodruff and Dunbar, 1973) and other tumors (Yuhas, Toya, and Wagner, 1975).

7.72 Combined Active and Passive Immunotherapy

There have been a few reports of experiments in which active and passive immunotherapeutic procedures were combined.

In experiments with an A-strain mouse mammary carcinoma and a CBA fibrosarcoma (Woodruff and Inchley, 1971b; Woodruff, Inchley, and Dunbar, 1972), intravenous administration of heterospecific antitumor globulin failed to potentiate the effect of treatment with CP. Since preincubation of the tumor cells with ATG in the absence of complement prior to inoculation, combined with administration of CP, had a greater inhibitory effect than either procedure alone, it was concluded that when ATG was given intravenously the amount reaching the tumor cells was insufficient to have an effect.

In rats treated a few hours after inoculation of a syngeneic fibrosarcoma by active immunization with Friend-virus-infected tumor cells, adoptive immunization with lymphoid cells from mice immunized with a Friend virus-induced tumor, or chemotherapy, Gotohda *et al.* (1974) found that the survival rate ranged from 17 to 19 percent. Active immunization and chemotherapy combined gave 56 percent survival, and all three forms of treatment 85 percent survival. It seems pertinent to ask, however, whether the same or better survival could have been obtained by chemotherapy alone in optimal dosage.

7.8 PROCEDURES TO ELIMINATE BLOCKING FACTORS AND SUPPRESSOR CELLS

7.81 Thoracic Duct Drainage and Plasmapheresis

It was reported by Noonan *et al.* (1974) that tumor-specific blocking factors could be detected by the macrophage migration inhibition test in thoracic duct lymph collected 14–48 hours after inoculation of two chemically induced isogeneic mouse fibrosarcomas. Drainage of lymph during this period, with replacement of the cells, inhibited subsequent tumor growth. With mice inoculated with a third fibrosarcoma, blocking factor was not demonstrated and growth of this tumor was not affected by thoracic duct drainage. These findings are consistent with the observation of Rose (1973) that tumors induced in splenectomized rats with mouse sarcoma virus regressed after drainage of thoracic duct lymph and replacement of the lymphocytes; other workers (Proctor, Rudenstam, and Alexander, 1973; Thomson, Eccles, and Alexander, 1973a), however, have reported that thoracic duct drainage and cell replacement in rats bearing methylcholanthrene-induced sarcomas results in an increase in pulmonary metastases, and have suggested that there is a factor in the serum of sarcoma-bearing rats which inhibits metastases.

Another possible way of eliminating blocking factors is *plasmapheresis,* i.e., removal of blood plasma and replacement with solutions containing electrolytes and possibly also albumin and other substances. This procedure appears to have been used first in patients and will be considered in the next chapter (8.27).

7.82   Administration of Antibody

The use of specific antitumor serum or Ig has already been discussed (7.21). Here we shall consider various other kinds of antibody which have been suggested, and in some cases investigated, as possible therapeutic agents.

7.821   UNBLOCKING SERUM

It was discovered by I. Hellström and K. Hellström (1970) that the serum of mice in which MSV-induced sarcomas had regressed spontaneously was able to neutralize the blocking activity of serum from tumor-bearing animals. Unblocking activity was subsequently demonstrated in the serum of rats after surgical excision of transplanted polyoma virus-induced tumors (Bansal and Sjögren, 1971) and also in the sera of rats and rabbits which received an intraperitoneal injection of BCG followed 8–12 days later by an injection of polyoma virus-induced tumor cells which had been treated with neuraminidase and mitomycin (Bansal and Sjögren, 1972). The unblocking factor appears to be an immunoglobulin, and Sjögren (1974) has suggested that it may be free antibody which acts by removing tumor antigen from lymphocyte receptor sites.

Repeated injection of unblocking serum combined with splenectomy caused marked inhibition of polyoma-induced tumors in rats associated with the disappearance of blocking activity from the serum of the treated animals (Bansal and Sjögren, 1972).

7.822   ANTI-PLASMA-CELL AND ANTI-IMMUNOGLOBULIN SERA

N.S. Harris *et al.* (1972) prepared anti-plasma-cell serum by immunizing rabbits with mouse myeloma cells and showed that this greatly reduced the number of IgM plaque-forming cells when administered to mice 1, 2, and 3 days after immunization with sheep erythrocytes. They suggested that this might be of therapeutic value in animals bearing antigenic tumors by reducing or preventing the production of blocking antibody.

Anti-immunoglobulin sera prepared by immunizing rabbits with mouse immunoglobulin or their component heavy or light chains may inhibit antibody production by mouse spleen cells *in vitro;* they have also been shown to inhibit antibody formation by newborn mice and to modify the humoral responses of adult mice, but not to affect the survival of skin allografts (Manning and Jutila, 1972a, 1972b, 1972c). It might be of interest to study the effect of such sera on levels of blocking factor and survival in tumor-bearing mice.

7.823 ANTI-I-J ALLOSERUM

As discussed earlier (5.521), suppressor T cells generate products which are capable of suppressing antibody responses and contact sensitivity, and also of enhancing the growth of various tumors. Since, in the mouse, both the cells and their products bear determinants coded for by the I-J subregion of the H2 complex, it was predicted that anti-I-J antisera would possess antisuppressor properties, and this was confirmed by Pierres et al. (1977), using sheep erythrocytes as antigen. Furthermore, since progressively growing syngeneic methylcholanthrene-induced sarcomas in the mouse stimulate the development of suppressor T cells capable of preventing rejection of the tumor (Fujimoto, Greene, and Sehon, 1976a, 1976b), it was predicted, and subsequently confirmed, by M.I. Greene et al. (1977) that the growth of such tumors might be inhibited by treatment of the host with an anti-I-J alloantiserum. Daily administration of as little as $2\mu l$ of the serum, starting on the day of tumor inoculation, markedly suppressed the growth of the two tumors studied in A/J mice for as long as the serum was administered (15 days), and the effect was clearly specific because no inhibition occurred if the appropriate I-J specificity (in this case I-J^k) was absorbed.

7.824 ANTI-IDIOTYPE ANTIBODY

Administration of anti-idiotype antibody usually causes unresponsiveness to the corresponding antigen, but under certain conditions a small dose of anti-idiotype antibody may potentiate both T-cell and B-cell responses (Eichmann, 1974; Eichmann and Rajewsky, 1975). The possibility of raising antibody to a tumor, preparing the corresponding anti-idiotype antibody, and using this to treat tumor-bearing hosts therefore merits investigation.

7.83 Other Procedures

Immunization with xenogenized cells and cross-reacting antigens has been discussed in Section 7.63.

The extent to which immunotherapy fails because sensitized cells, antibody, and complement fail to gain access to tumor cells has not been thoroughly investigated. If, however, as seems quite likely, this is an important factor, a search for pharmacological methods of improving such access might prove rewarding.

8

Immunotherapy of Human Cancer

8.1 INTRODUCTION

In recent years the search for immunotherapeutic procedures, using this term in the broad sense defined earlier (7.1), which could be used effectively in patients with cancer, has been greatly intensified. This is illustrated by the reviews and reports of symposia published during the last two decades (Southam, 1961; Koldovsky, 1966b; World Health Organization Scientific Group Report, 1966; Sophocles and Nadler, 1971; Motta, 1971; Currie, 1972; Baker and Taub, 1973a; Mathé, Schwarzenberg *et al.*, 1974b; Thomas, Storb, Clift *et al.*, 1975; Mathé, 1976a; National Cancer Institute Radiation Oncology Committee, 1976; MacGregor and Falk, 1976; Nathanson, 1977; Rosenberg and Terry, 1977; Gutterman, 1977; Griffith and Regamey, 1978; Terry and Windhorst, 1978; Woodruff, 1979).

The impetus for this work has a threefold origin: firstly, growing awareness of the limitations of conventional methods of treatment (6.3); secondly, the discovery of tumor-associated antigens and other less well defined markers which distinguish many tumor cells from normal cells (5.2), and which might conceivably provide a *point d'appui* for immunotherapeutic attack; and, thirdly, the encouraging results obtained in some studies of the response of animal tumors to immunological and para-immunological manipulations (Chapter 7). The optimism which these results engendered, despite warnings of possible limitations (Koldovsky, 1966b), has been succeeded by a mood of pessimism which often appears to be equally uncritical. A balanced view of the situation has been published by D.W. Weiss (1977).

It has been argued by Hewitt, Blake, and Walder (1976) that tumors induced experimentally in animals are completely inappropriate as models of human cancer, and therefore of no value as guides for planning clinical trials, but, for reasons discussed earlier (1.23), this seems altogether too extreme a view. As we have seen, environmental carcinogens play a role in the etiology of many human tumors, and there is no obvious reason why such tumors should not possess antigens of the kind which, following Klein and Oettgen (1969), we have designated TSARIPAH (5.2), such

234

same extent as one finds in animal tumors induced experimentally with similar agents. In animals, para-immunological manipulations may be therapeutically effective in the absence of such antigens (7.522), and it seems reasonable to postulate that the same will be true of some human tumors. Indeed, even in the absence of all markers characteristic of tumor cells, the possibility of immunotherapeutic attack is not necessarily excluded (Woodruff, 1964) because the agent concerned may be injected into the tumor or may conceivably be induced to localize there preferentially by prior local treatment of a non-immunological kind, for example, radiotherapy.

8.2 CLINICAL TRIALS

The immunotherapeutic procedures used clincially may be classified under the same general headings as the experimental procedures discussed in Chapter 7, viz.:

1. Passive immunotherapy.
    (1) Passive immunization with serum, plasma, or immunoglobulin.
    (2) Immunochemotherapy (i.e., the use of antibodies as carriers for chemotherapeutic agents).
    (3) Passive immunization, with cells and cell products (sometimes termed adoptive immunotherapy).
    (4) Passive immunization with both antibody and cells.
2. Active immunotherapy.
    (1) Non-specific immunopotentiation.
    (2) Specific immunization.
    (3) Combined non-specific and specific procedures.
3. Combined passive and active immunotherapy.
4. Removal of blocking factors, and procedures to increase access of cells, antibody, and complement to a tumor.

It should be noted that the immunological reaction to a tumor may also be stimulated unknowingly, either specifically as a consequence of partial destruction of the tumor (Strauss, Saphir, and Appel, 1956) by procedures such as electrocoagulation or other forms of heating [8.24(11)] and conceivably also by ligation of the blood supply to the tumor (Mori, Masuda, and Miyanga, 1966; McDermott and Hensle, 1974) and radiotherapy; or non-specifically as the result of infection (Nauts, 1969, 1973, 1977; Ruckdeschel et al., 1972). In either case this may be of therapeutic importance.

Immunotherapy has been used as the sole method of treatment, particularly in Phase I trials (1.113), in patients with locally advanced or disseminated disease. It has also been used extensively as adjuvant therapy in patients whose tumor mass has been reduced to undetectable levels by surgical excision or chemotherapy.

However thorough the experimental studies preceding a clinical trial, it is impossible to eliminate all risk. The hazards which may be encountered are of three kinds. Firstly, the therapeutic agent used may cause toxic effects, irrespective of the presence or absence of a tumor. Secondly, the procedure may enhance rather than inhibit tumor growth. Thirdly, successful destruction of a tumor may give rise to hemorrhage, and in the case of intracerebral tumors, whether primary or metastatic, this may be rapidly fatal. A major objective of Phase I studies (1.113) is to assess each type of risk, and to establish regimens of treatment which, at the very least, do not enhance tumor growth, and for which the severity and frequency of complications have been reduced to acceptably low levels.

In Phase II and Phase III trials (1.113) the crucial questions are the extent to which the treatment has inhibited growth and spread of the tumor, and whether it has been of benefit to the patient. As discussed earlier (1.112, 1.113), length of survival is an important criterion, but other precisely defined criteria may also be used, such as disease-free interval if complete regression has been achieved, and rate of progression of the tumor based on surface measurement, serial radiographs, or biochemical investigations. The quality of life enjoyed by the patient, though it does not lend itself to measurement, is also important.

A subsidiary objective in all trials should be to monitor throughout the course of treatment the patient's immunological response to his tumor, and to the therapeutic agent employed if this happens to be antigenic, and his capacity to respond to unrelated antigens. Such studies are important because they may reveal why a particular treatment has succeeded or has failed, and so provide a rational basis for planning future trials. The methods which have been used include the following:

1. Assessment of the patient's response to his tumor.
    (1) *In vitro* tests for humoral immunity (5.224), ADCC 5.225), and lymphocyte-mediated cytotoxicity (5.226), using as targets the patient's tumor cells or established cell lines derived from similar tumors.
    (2) Migration inhibition and adherence inhibition assays (5.227).
    (3) Mixed lymphocyte–tumor cell culture (5.228).
    (4) Tests for skin hypersensitivity to tumor extracts (5.229).
    (5) Special tests for OFA (5.23) where appropriate.
    (6) Tests for blocking factors (5.521).
2. Assessment of the response to immunopotentiating agents which happen to be immunogenic.
    (1) Intradermal skin test with old tuberculin or PPD in patients treated with BCG.
    (2) Lymphocyte transformation by PPD in patients treated with BCG.
    (3) Titer of antibody to CP in patients treated with this organism.
3. Assessment of general immunological competence by methods discussed previously (4.42).

In most of the earlier trials, and in many recent Phase I trials, patients with a variety of tumors have been included. Other trials have been concerned with a single type of cancer, notably acute lymphatic leukemia (ALL), acute myeloblastic leukemia (AML), Hodgkin's disease and other lymphomas, melanoma, osteogenic sarcoma, and carcinomas of the lung, breast, stomach, colon, rectum, kidney, bladder, ovary, and skin.

Many of the more recent trials reviewed below were reported at a conference held in October 1976, a report of which has now been published (Terry and Windhorst, 1978); and a list of trials in progress, with a summary of each protocol, is published at intervals by the International Registry of Tumor Immunotherapy. As we shall see, some trials have been well designed in accordance with the principles discussed earlier (1.123). In many others, however, changes of protocol, assessment based on clinical impressions rather than on length of survival or precisely defined criteria of tumor regression and recurrence, and the absence of randomized controls cast serious doubt on the validity of the conclusions reported. In others again, there does not appear to have been any firm biological basis for the trial, so that, in the words of Bernard Fisher (1978), "What is judged as a therapeutic failure may in reality never have been a therapeutic contest." This is exemplified by trials in which an agent which is effective in animals only when given by certain routes is given to patients by some other route.

8.21   Passive Immunotherapy with Serum, Plasma, or Immunoglobulin

Many patients have been treated with serum, plasma, or Ig of human or animal origin.

8.211   ALLOGENEIC SERUM OR PLASMA

The human serum or plasma used in trials of immunotherapy has been obtained from three sources: (1) normal donors; (2) donors immunized with normal or neoplastic cells; and (3) patients in remission. The results have been uniformly disappointing.

It was reported by G.E. Moore, Sandberg, and Amos (1957) that normal human Ig had no beneficial effect in 13 patients with a variety of disseminated tumors, and Albo, Krivit, and Hartmann (1968) found, in a controlled study, that normal plasma, whether from the patients' parents or unrelated donors, was ineffective as adjuvant therapy in children with acute leukemia in whom a remission had been induced by chemotherapy.

Following the discovery (I. Hellström et al., 1973; K.E. Hellström and I. Hellström, 1974) that the plasma of North American blacks often showed "unblocking effects" (5.521) when tested with melanoma cells in vitro, a trial was set up to study the effect of normal human plasma from black and white donors in patients with Stage II and Stage III (disseminated) melanoma (Wright et al., 1976, 1978). All patients received conventional treatment in the form of surgery or chemotherapy; some received in addition BCG and plasma from black or white donors. The use of BCG complicates the situation, but when last reported there was no significant effect attributable to the immunotherapy.

Plasma or serum from volunteers immunized with normal (Laszlo, Buckley, and Amos, 1968) or leukemic (Brittingham and Chaplin, 1960; Izawa et al., 1966; Sakurai, 1966) leukocytes was reported to be of no benefit in patients with leukemia, though many showed a transient fall in the blood leukocyte count.

Administration of plasma from patients in remission was followed by temporary remission in two patients with Burkitt's lymphoma treated by Ngu (1967). In one case the tumor disappeared completely, but it later recurred and killed the patient. No benefit was observed in five cases similarly treated (Fass et al., 1970c), and in two others treatment was followed by marked and rapid growth of the tumor (Clifford, Singh et al., 1967), although in both these studies the material was shown to react in vitro with Burkitt tumor cells.

Horn and Horn (1971) treated a patient who had had a nephrectomy for carcinoma of the kidney, and subsequently a left upper lobectomy for pulmonary metastases, with repeated infusions of plasma from his uncle, who had been successfully treated surgically for a similar tumor. At the time of the lobectomy some lymph nodes were removed, but others which were also thought to be invaded by tumor were left in situ. The patient was still in remission 15 months later, and this was regarded by Horn and

Horn as evidence of the effectiveness of the plasma infusions; 5 months later however, the patient was found to have cerebral metastases, and he died 26 months after his first infusion of plasma (Wright, Hellström *et al.,* 1976). It seems doubtful whether the immunotherapy had any beneficial effect.

Treatment with whole blood, or with plasma plus leukocytes, will be considered later (8.23).

8.212   XENOGENEIC SERUM

Xenogeneic serum used in trials of immunotherapy has been obtained from animals immunized with (1) pooled tissue or tissue extracts from a variety of human tumors; (2) pooled tissue or tissue extracts from tumors of the same kind as the patient's; (3) normal human leukocytes; and (4) tissue or tissue extracts from the patient's own tumor. Various animal species have been used, including rabbits, sheep, goats, pigs, dogs, horses, and monkeys.

It is not always clear in the earlier papers whether the antigenic material used was of type (1) or type (2). This might not matter very much if, firstly, as Björklund and his colleagues have claimed (5.223), the cells of many different human tumors possess a common surface antigen as a result of which they are subject to lysis *in vitro* by antibody which reacts with this antigen, and, secondly, this antibody is also effectively cytolytic *in vivo.* As we have seen, however, Björklund's conclusion has not found general acceptance, and there is no convincing evidence in support of the second proviso.

Héricourt and Richet (1895) published a brief account of some 50 patients with advanced cancer who had been treated with serum from dogs and monkeys immunized with pooled human tumor tissue. They reported various beneficial effects including diminution of pain, healing of ulcers, temporary slowing of tumor growth and in some cases partial regression, and improvement in general health, but sooner or later the tumor began once again to progress. Side effects consisted of mild urticaria and erythema, and in four cases syncopal attacks of brief duration. Symptomatic improvement in many patients treated with xenogeneic antitumor serum, and dramatic but temporary regression in a few patients was subsequently reported by Vidal (1911) and Berkeley (1914). Héricourt and Richet suggested that better results might be obtained by combining their treatment with surgical excision of the tumor. This was tried in 39 patients by Berkeley (1914) but does not seem to have been particularly effective.

More recently Murray (1958, 1965) has reported improvement, sometimes of a dramatic kind, in many patients with advanced, and often terminal, cancer who were treated with serum from horses immunized with pooled human tumor tissue. This work, which was based initially on a study of 233 patients, has been strongly criticized because of lack of detail in the case reports and undue reliance on symptomatic improvement, and also because no immunological studies were undertaken in the patients (Currie, 1972; Rosenberg and Terry, 1977). In general, this criticism seems justified, but Murray does cite instances of objective improvement, for example, decrease in the size of some primary tumors or improvement in anaemia, and the disappearance of cranial nerve palsies in a patient with cerebral metastases, which it seems not unreasonable to attribute to the treatment.

De Carvalho (1963) prepared antigenic extracts from (1) a mixture of solid human tumors of many different kinds; (2) a mixture of splenic tissue from patients with various types of leukemia; and (3) a mixture of various normal human tissues. Extracts of types (1) and (2) were absorbed with IgG from horses which had previously been immunized with extract (3), with the object of removing normal tissue antigens, and one or the other of these absorbed preparations was then used to immunize other horses and donkeys. IgG from these latter animals was used therapeutically in patients with solid tumors and leukemia, respectively.

De Carvalho reported remissions lasting from 1 to 29 months in 13 to 15 patients with leukemia, alleviation of pain in virtually all patients with solid tumors, and objective evidence of temporary regression of skin nodules in one patient with breast cancer and of supraclavicular nodes in another such patient. In one patient with a recurrent retroperitoneal fibrosarcoma the tumor ceased to be palpable on vaginal examination after treatment with IgG, and no trace of it was seen when a hysterectomy was performed 14 months later on account of uterine fibroids. De Carvalho reported only mild side effects in the form of local inflammatory reactions at the injection site and slight pyrexia; on the other hand, one patient reported earlier by De La Pava et al. (1962), who was given whole horse serum, developed fatal nephritis.

De Carvalho's work has also been strongly criticized because the improvement in his patients was mainly subjective, but his cases are described in reasonable detail and, as he said, his report was preliminary and "definitive evaluation of the clinical value [of his method] may require . . . homogeneous cancer patient groups, double-blind and double-check studies by several groups, and time." In the absence of further work along these lines no firm conclusions can be drawn, though it seems unlikely that the use of antigenic extracts of such a heterogeneous kind to prepare immune globulin is the best way to tackle the problem.

Reports concerning the effect of sera raised in animals with normal and leukemic human leukocytes in patients with leukemia are conflicting. Lindstrom (1927) reported remissions in patients with acute myeloid leukemia treated by radiotherapy and administration of serum, but his results, which were not confirmed by Hueper and Russell (1932), may have been due solely to the radiotherapy. More recent studies of this kind in patients with lymphatic leukemia (Sekla et al., 1967; Tsirimbas et al., 1968) have also yielded mainly negative results. Administration of serum from animals immunized with human melanomas (Parks, Smith et al., 1975) or cerebral gliomas (Mahaley, 1965) has proved similarly ineffective in patients with these tumors.

A few of the patients treated by Berkeley (1914) received serum from animals immunized with their own individual tumor, and this has encouraged other attempts of a similar kind despite the logistic difficulties involved.

McCredie, Brown, and Cole (1959) treated two patients with advanced breast cancer with immunoglobulin from sheep immunized in this way, but with no effect apart from some decrease in size of the supraclavicular lymph nodes.

In the light of earlier experimental studies (Levi, Schechtman et al., 1959; Garb et al., 1962), Sekla et al., (1967) immunized sheep and pigs which had been pretreated within 3 weeks of birth with normal human blood, with tissue from four patients with leukemia and one with osteosarcoma. Each animal received tissue from a single patient, and immunoglobulin prepared from its serum was used to treat only this patient. The cases were regarded as "beyond any hope of cure or improvement" and "no real therapeutic effects were expected," but one of the leukemic patients had a further remission of 1 year after administration of immunoglobulin.

Newman et al. (1977) immunized goats with five weekly injections of cell suspensions prepared from the individual tumors of patients with operable lung cancer treated by lobectomy or pneumonectomy. Each goat was bled 1 week after the last injection. The serum was absorbed with allogeneic spleen cells until it showed no complement-dependent cytotoxictiy against cultured human lymphoblasts, and then fractionated and sterilized by filtration. Following operation, 37 patients were given two courses of chemotherapy, during the second of which they received also four intravenous injections of antitumor Ig. Thirty-four other patients received chemotherapy only. The assignment of patients to these two treatment groups was not strictly random; instead, alternate cases in each of a series of prognostic groups were allocated to different treatment groups. There were fewer recurrences and deaths in the group receiving both immunotherapy and chemotherapy, but the difference was said to be not statistically significant.

Stevenson and his colleagues raised anti-idiotype antibody against surface immunoglobulin on human neoplastic lymphocytes (Hough, Eady, Hamblin, Stevenson, and Stevenson, 1976), and have used this in a few patients with lymphocytic leukemia. The results so far have been described as encouraging but not conclusive (Stevenson, Elliott, and Stevenson, 1977).

8.22 Immunochemotherapy

The use of antibody as a carrier for cytotoxic or radioactive agents is an attractive idea and, as we have seen, has had some success in animal experiments. There have been a few trials in patients with melanoma and neuroblastoma.

Nungester, Bierwaltes, and Knorpp (1952) treated a patient with disseminated malignant melanoma with serum raised in rabbits with tissue from the patient's tumor and subsequently tagged with ^{131}I. They reported that the tumor regressed completely and the patient died 8 years later of myocardial infarction. At autopsy (exclusive of the head) there was no evidence of tumor. As a result of this report, Vial and Callahan (1957) treated an unspecified number of melanoma patients with ^{131}I-tagged serum raised in rabbits by injection of cell suspensions, cell fractions, or melanin from the patient's tumor or other melanomas. No tumor regression was observed, however, and in only one patient was there any evidence of selective uptake of the label in tumor tissue.

Ghose and his colleagues (Ghose et al., 1972, 1975a, 1975b) treated two patients with disseminated malignant melanoma with intravenous and intralesional injections of antimelanoma antibody conjugated with chlorambucil. The antibody was raised in goats by repeated injections of human melanoma tissue and was absorbed with normal human tissue. Some subcutaneous metastatic nodules regressed temporarily in both patients. Oon et al. (1974) treated a patient with malignant melanoma by active immunization followed by injection of autochthonous antibody conjugated with chlorambucil, and three children with neuroblastomas with parental immunoglobulin conjugated with the same drug. Only minor therapeutic effects were observed.

These disappointing results may conceivably be due to the antibody being insufficiently specific or of low affinity, or to the tumors not being sufficiently sensitive to the drug to which the antibody was coupled.

8.23 Passive Immunization with Cells and Cell Products

The agents used in this form of treatment, which is sometimes termed adoptive immunotherapy, comprise non-immune bone marrow and lymphoid cells, immune and non-specifically stimulated lymphoid cells, transfer factor, and RNA. As in the previous chapter, the term lymphoid cells is used simply as a convenient generic term to include lymphocytes obtained from the spleen, lymph nodes, peripheral blood, or thoracic duct lymph, but not lymphocytes in bone marrow or thymus.

In discussing the use of cells from immunized donors we shall, as a matter of convenience, include studies in which patients have received whole blood, or cells plus serum or plasma, as well as those in which the patients received only cells.

8.231 BONE MARROW

Bone marrow has been infused in cancer patients with two aims: to promote hemopoietic recovery following damage caused by chemotherapy or radiotherapy, and as adoptive immunotherapy to cause cytotoxic damage to the tumor. Insofar as the treatment has been followed by tumor regression, however, it is difficult if not impossible to determine the extent to which this has been due to the chemotherapy.

The development of satisfactory methods for storing living cells made it possible to remove bone marrow prior to whole body or wide field irradiation, or immunotherapy, and replace it afterwards as an autograft. There have been many reports of cases of advanced cancer treated in this way (Kurnick et al., 1958; Kurnick, 1962; Newton et al., 1959; Westbury et al., 1959; McFarland et al., 1959; Woodruff, 1961). Good hemopoietic recovery has been observed frequently, but in no case does there appear to have been more than temporary regression.

Transplantation of isogeneic bone marrow from a healthy monozygotic twin to patients with acute leukemia following treatment by chemotherapy and/or whole body irradiation has been reported by Atkinson et al. (1959) and by E.D. Thomas and his colleagues (Thomas, Lochte et al., 1959; Thomas, Herman et al., 1961; Thomas, Rudolph et al., 1971b; Thomas, Buckner et al., 1978; Rudolph et al., 1973; Fefer et al., 1973, 1974). Hemopoietic recovery was satisfactory, but the leukemia recurred in the case of Atkinson et al. in 7 weeks, and in the first five cases of Thomas et al., who received no other form of immunotherapy, in 2–12 weeks. Later patients, who received also specific active immunotherapy in the form of killed leukemic cells plus donor lymphocytes (Fefer et al., 1974; Thomas, Buckner et al., 1978), fared, however, much better. Complete remission occurred in about 90 percent of these cases, and there were survivors 7 years after treatment for acute lymphatic leukemia and 5 years after treatment for acute myeloid leukemia. These results are impressive because almost all the patients had had extensive prior chemotherapy and were in relapse at the time of irradiation and marrow infusion.

Allogeneic bone marrow infusion following whole body irradiation was first used for the treatment of leukemia by E.D. Thomas and his colleagues (Thomas, Lochte et al., 1957). Since then there have been many further reports of cases in which allogeneic marrow was given, in association with irradiation or chemotherapy, for the treatment of leukemia by Thomas and his colleagues (Thomas, Buckner et al., 1971a, 1973, 1978; Thomas, Storb et al., 1975; Storb et al., 1973), Mathé and his colleagues (Mathé, Bernard et al., 1959, 1960b; Mathé, Amiel et al., 1963, 1965; Mathé, Schwarzenberg, et al., 1967, 1974b), and others (van Bekkum and de Vries, 1967; Santos et al., 1969, 1971; Graw and Santos, 1971; Graw, Yankee et al., 1972). There has also been a report of similar treatment in patients with Hodgkin's disease (Santos et al., 1971). The aim in these cases was to ensure that the transplanted marrow survived either indefinitely or sufficiently long to permit recovery of the patient's marrow, and to achieve an effective graft-versus-tumor (GVT) reaction without causing serious graft-versus-host (GVH) disease. Until recently there appeared to have been little progress towards this goal (Bortin, 1970). The suggestion (Mathé, Amiel *et al.*, 1963) that it might be advantageous to use several donors for each recipient was not confirmed. The use of an HLA-identical sibling donor in one case was of little or no benefit, and treatment of the recipient with antilymphocyte serum before marrow transplantation, while successful in preventing GVH, was followed by rejection of the marrow graft and death from recurrent leukemia (Mathé, Amiel *et al.*, 1970a). There is now evidence, however, that the incidence of serious GVH can be reduced by using an HLA-compatible sibling donor and treating the recipient with methotrexate for up to 100 days after grafting, and it is beginning to look as if the risk of recurrence of the leukemia can be reduced by giving chemotherapy as well as irradiation prior to marrow transplantation. In a review of 120 cases, comprising 52 with acute lymphatic leukemia, 58 with acute myeloid leukemia, and 10 with chronic myeloid leukemia in a state of blast crisis, treated along these lines from 1969 to 1975, E.D. Thomas *et al.* (1978) reported that during the first 4 months after grafting there was a considerable mortality due to the poor state of the patient at the time, recurrent leukemia, and GVH. During the next 16 months deaths occurred due to recurrent leukemia, but the survival curve then flattened and no more relapses occurred. Seventeen patients were alive in mid-1977, and the longest survivor had been grafted 7 years previously.

Some investigators have used chemotherapy only before marrow grafting (Graw *et al.*, 1972, 1974; Santos *et al.*, 1976), but the incidence of recurrent leukemia has been extremely high.

It is of interest that among the patients treated by Thomas *et al.* there were two females with acute lymphatic leukemia, who had received marrow from an HLA-identical brother, in whom leukemia recurred and cytogenetic studies showed that the leukemic cells contained a Y chromosome (Fialkow *et al.*, 1971b; E.D. Thomas *et al.*, 1978). It seems likely therefore that malignant transformation had occurred in donor cells, though Thomas *et al.* considered, as a possible alternative explanation, that there had been "a transfer of a Y chromosome to a surviving remnant of the original leukemic cell population following a cell fusion event."

The question of whether or not allogeneic marrow has an antileukemic effect in man remains unresolved. It has been argued that the effect is not great because relapse of leukemia has occurred in patients who have had severe but not fatal GVH, but this is far from conclusive.

Hattori *et al.* (1972) compared the survival of patients with cancer of the stomach following gastrectomy alone, gastrectomy plus chemotherapy, and gastrectomy plus chemotherapy plus infusion of allogeneic bone marrow. The marrow did not have a statistically significant effect (at the $p = 0.05$ level), but most patients received less than 2×10^9 marrow cells.

8.232 NON-IMMUNE UNSTIMULATED LYMPHOID CELLS

Woodruff and Nolan (1961) removed the spleen in three patients with advanced cancer, prepared and stored a cell suspension from each spleen, and administered this intravenously after treatment with cytotoxic drugs. The aim was to promote hemopoietic recovery and in particular recovery of lymphoid tissue following the damage caused by the chemotherapy, and it was considered that spleen cell suspensions were less likely than bone marrow suspensions to contain viable tumor cells. The infusions were well tolerated, and the blood lymphocyte count rose satisfactorily, but the extent to which this was due to the spleen cells is open to question.

In the light of this experience and studies in animals, Woodruff and Nolan (1963) subsequently treated eight patients with advanced cancer by intravenous or intraperitoneal injection of allogeneic spleen cell suspensions after preparatory treatment with a cytotoxic drug or prednisone designed to delay rejection of the cells. No attempt was made to produce the maximal antitumor effect because it was thought that this would entail the risk of severe graft-versus-host disease, but in every case some change occurred in either the patient's symptoms, the physical signs, or the findings on serial biopsy. Some of these changes were probably due to the chemotherapy or other treatment which the patient received in addition to spleen cell infusion, and others may have been fortuitous. In four patients, however, changes occurred which are difficult to account for except as a consequence of the infusion. One of these patients had multiple subcutaneous melanomatous deposits, and a local hyperemic reaction developed at the site of each nodule within a few hours of intravenous spleen cell infusion. This was associated with an initial rise in skin temperature of 5° C, and 3 weeks after the infusion the skin temperature over the nodule was still 2° C higher than the temperature of normal skin in the corresponding region on the opposite limb. The other three patients had ovarian cancer associated with malignant ascites, and the ascites cleared completely after spleen cell infusion. This was given in one case intravenously and in the other cases intraperitoneally, and none of the patients received any other treatment by the intraperitoneal route.

Israel et al. (1966, 1967a) treated 25 patients with advanced cancer by repeated intravenous infusion of allogeneic spleen cells or blood lymphocytes preceded, unless there was marked lymphopenia as a result of earlier chemotherapy, by administration of cytotoxic drugs. Some temporary objective improvement occurred in nine cases. In one patient with malignant ascites who received an intraperitoneal infusion of spleen cells, the ascites disappeared completely, but in three patients with malignant pleural effusions infusion of lymphocytes into the pleural cavity was ineffective.

Four patients with advanced malignant melanoma were treated by Symes et al. (1968) with a small dose of phenylalanine mustard, followed by intravenous infusion of allogeneic spleen cells. Temporary regression was observed in three patients, and in each of these there was a significant increase in skin temperature over the tumors following the infusion.

Yonemoto and Terasaki (1972) tackled the problem of early rejection of the transplanted cells by using HLA-matched donors, but some of their patients also received preliminary chemotherapy. No benefit was observed in patients given one pint of whole blood or $1-3 \times 10^9$ blood leukocytes, but temporary regression occurred in two patients who received $20-70 \times 10^9$ thoracic duct cells, and this lasted in one case for 6 months. Two patients who did not respond to thoracic duct cells nevertheless showed evidence of chimerism 2–6 weeks after the infusion.

Schwarzenberg, Mathé et al. (1966) treated 21 patients with acute leukemia with infusions of $60-120 \times 10^{10}$ allogeneic blood leukocytes from patients with chronic myeloid leukemia. All except one of these patients were resistant to available forms of chemotherapy or could not be treated conventionally on account of marked neutropenia. There were six complete and three partial remissions, but these were of short duration (1–3 weeks only in seven patients; 80 days and 4 months in the other two). A patient treated in this way by Graw et al. (1970) developed severe GVH and died from septicemia.

George Moore and his colleagues pioneered the large-scale cultivation of human lymphocytes (Moore, Gerner, and Franklin, 1967) and treated 31 patients with advanced cancer with autochthonous or allogeneic cultured lymphocytes (Moore and Moore, 1969; Moore and Gerner, 1970). None of the patients who received allogeneic cells, in total amounts up to 236 g, responded, nor did patients who received up to 100 g of autologous cells. Significant but temporary remission did, however, occur in two of three patients who received more than 300 g of autologous cells. No severe reactions occurred. Subsequently Douglass *et al.* (1975) treated four patients with osteogenic sarcoma with pulmonary metastases by infusing cultured lymphocytes; the dose of cells is not stated, but no benefit resulted. Moore and Gerner (1970) suggested that their treatment should be tried as what we have termed adjuvant therapy in patients with a small residual tumor burden.

8.233 IMMUNE AND NON-SPECIFICALLY STIMULATED LYMPHOID CELLS

Skurkovich *et al.* (1969b) treated nine patients with acute leukemia in remission with autologous leukocytes and plasma taken from the same patient 1–2 weeks previously, and reported remissions of 491 days or more as compared with 171 days in patients who did not receive immunotherapy. The difference appears considerable, but its significance cannot be assessed because the controls were historical and the patients in the two groups may have differed in various ways. The same authors also teated 12 patients with acute leukemia in relapse with autologous leukocytes and plasma obtained during previous remission. They reported some improvement, but this was mainly subjective, and the evidence of a definite therapeutic effect is not very convincing. The procedure would however seem to merit further study, and, if this appeared promising, a properly controlled trial.

Frenster and Rogoway (1968) reinfused autologous lymphocytes which had been stimulated *in vitro* with PHA in five patients with disseminated cancer and observed temporary partial regression in three of them. Cheema and Hersh (1972) injected PHA-stimulated autologous lymphocytes locally into subcutaneous secondary melanomatous deposits, and observed total disappearance of a few nodules and decrease in size of many others, but the treatment does not appear to have altered the general course of the disease. Schlosser and Benes (1971) injected PHA-stimulated lymphocytes intravenously, subcutaneously, and intraperitoneally in ten patients with advanced cancer and reported partial regression in three of them. It is not clear whether these cells were autologous or allogeneic. Attempts have also been made, though so far without much success, to treat cancer patients with autologous lymphocytes which had been exposed *in vitro* to autochthonous tumor cells. McKhann and Jagarlamoody (1972) treated four patients with metastatic malignant melanoma and one with metastatic liposarcoma, which were refractory to chemotherapy, in this way over periods ranging from 2 weeks to 5 months. In one of the patients with malignant melanoma some large tumor masses regressed completely; at no time, however, was the patient clinically free of tumor, and he relapsed after a year and died a few months later. The other four patients did not benefit from the treatment and died of cerebral or pulmonary metastases. As Rosenberg and Terry (1977) have pointed out, there is a risk that these procedures may cause autoimmune disease, and also, when specific immunization is attempted *in vitro,* that suppressor cells may be generated.

Studies with presumptively immune allogeneic cells have taken various forms.

Sumner and Foraker (1960) treated two patients with malignant melanoma with whole blood from another patient in whom a melanoma had regressed spontaneously

4 years previously. In the first patient, who had multiple metastases, the tumor disappeared completely between 16 and 24 weeks after transfusion; in the other patient the treatment had no apparent effect. Teimourian and McCune (1963) treated a further four patients with disseminated melanoma with blood from a patient who had been treated surgically 10 years previously for a melanoma of the back with bilateral axillary lymph node metastases and whose tumor had not recurred. In one case pulmonary metastases almost disappeared, but the patient developed cerebral metastases and died a year later; in the other patients the treatment had no apparent effect. Complete regression of disseminated melanoma, with no evidence of recurrence after 5 years, was reported by McPeak (1971), however, in a patient who received intralymphatic infusions of leukocytes from two patients who had been treated surgically for melanomas 4 and 18 years previously and who showed no evidence of recurrence.

Nadler and Moore (1966, 1969) chose pairs of patients with disseminated cancer and immunized each member of the pair by subcutaneous transplantation of tissue of the other's tumor. They then interchanged blood leukocytes over a period of 3 weeks starting 5–15 days after the tumor transplantation. The immunization technique was varied in some cases by using Freund's adjuvant and transplanting tumor tissue repeatedly, and some patients received leukocytes not only from their partner but also from various other donors. In all, 118 patients were treated, of whom 86 had malignant melanoma. Complete remission, with disappearance of all detectable tumor tissue, occurred in two patients with malignant melanoma. Complete regression was also reported in a patient in whom, following above-knee amputation for osteogenic sarcoma, radiological diagnosis of bilateral lymphangetic pulmonary metastases was made, but in the absence of other evidence the diagnosis cannot be regarded as definitely established. In 20 other patients decrease in tumor size or other evidence of partial regression was reported. Many patients experienced chills and fever, but apart from this the treatment was well tolerated. In two patients the tumor transplants grew but fortunately did not recur after excision. Much the same procedure, involving cross-immunization with tumor tissue or homogenates, or cultured tumor cells, and subsequent infusion of leukocytes and plasma, has been used by other investigators, mainly in patients with disseminated malignant melanoma (Humphrey et al., 1968, 1971a, 1971b: Krementz et al., 1971, 1974; Mansell et al., 1975). Partial regression has been reported in about one-sixth of the cases. In three patients treated by Krementz et al., and one treated by Humphrey et al., all the visible metastases disappeared completely, but one of Krementz's patients died 14 months after treatment, probably with recurrent tumor.

Krementz et al. (1974) used the same procedure as adjuvant therapy in two patients with Stage II melanoma following radical surgery, and in another patient following excision of a recurrence of melanoma in the neck. Although these patients were all apparently tumor-free 15–29 months later, it is impossible to say whether the immunotherapy contributed to this result.

A feature of the treatment just described, which might conceivably affect the results, is that each patient was exposed to histocompatibility antigens of the donor from whom he subsequently received leukocytes as a result of the tumor graft. To avoid this, Enneking and his colleagues (Marsh et al., 1972; Neff and Enneking, 1975) studied the effect of sensitized allogeneic leukocytes in patients with osteogenic sarcoma whose tumors had been used to immunize the leukocyte donors but who had not themselves been immunized in the reverse direction. A similar protocol was used by

Oon *et al.* (1974), with the difference that the tumor cells used for immunization were irradiated. Andrews *et al.* (1967) treated one patient with acute leukemia and one with melanoma with thoracic duct lymphocytes from a healthy relative who had been immunized with the patient's tumor. No therapeutic effect was observed in three patients with frank metastases from osteogenic sarcoma by Marsh *et al.* (1972), in five patients with melanoma and two with neuroblastoma treated by Oon *el al.* (1974), or in the two patients treated by Andrews *et al.* (1967); and the death of one of Andrews's patients 9 days after the infusion with diarrhea and other symptoms consistent with GVH suggests that infusion of lymphoid cells to cancer patients may be dangerous even in the absence of treatment with immunosuppressive agents. The survival of 32 patients who, following amputation, appeared to be clinically free of tumor but who nevertheless received sensitized leukocytes as adjuvant therapy was not significantly longer than that of comparable historical controls who were treated by amputation only (Neff and Enneking, 1975), but the dose of cells ranged from 1.7×10^9 to 10.6×10^9, and Rosenberg and Terry (1977) have pointed out that patients who received more than 3.9×10^9 cells seemed to do better than those who received fewer cells. Further study of this procedure in patients with a high probability of having occult residual disease (3.34), but using higher cell doses, might therefore be rewarding.

Instead of infusing cells, Starzl *et al.* (1965) transplanted a whole spleen by vascular anastomosis to four patients with advanced cancer. Each patient was first immunized with tumor tissue from another member of the group and each subsequently donated a spleen to the patient against whose tumor he had been immunized. No benefit was observed, and in one patient the progress of the disease appears to have been accelerated.

Symes and his colleagues have pioneered the therapeutic use of immune xenogeneic lymphocytes for the treatment of bladder cancer (Symes and Riddell, 1973; Symes *et al.,* 1973; Feneley *et al.,* 1974). They immunized pigs by transplanting tumor tissue to the ileal mesentry, harvested mesenteric lymph node cells 7 days later, and injected these into the arterial blood supply of the tumor. In 7 out of 25 patients with transitional cell carcinoma of the bladder, infusion of pig cells was the only treatment; in 7 others pig cells were given following radiotherapy for the treatment of tumor recurrence, and in 11 patients pig cell infusion was followed 4–8 weeks later by an attenuated course of radiotherapy. In these three treatment groups, 5, 3, and 9 patients, respectively, obtained clinical benefit as shown by cessation of hematuria and increased tumor necrosis in biopsy specimens. A controlled trial designed to compare the effect of treating matched pairs of patients by radical radiotherapy (5500 rad in 25 daily fractions over a period of 5 weeks) only, or by pig cell infusion followed by radiotherapy 6 weeks later, has shown no significant difference in remission rates or survival times in the two groups, but it is of interest that 6 of the 15 patients who received pig cells showed evidence of remission before radiotherapy was given (Symes *et al.,* 1978a). The results were in fact not as good as those seen in six patients who had been treated previously with pig cells followed by a smaller dose (4000 rad) of irradiation. Symes *et al.* have postulated therefore that the higher dose of irradiation somehow interferes with the action of the pig cells and have suggested setting up another trial to test this hypothesis. Meanwhile, they had studied the effect of intra-arterial infusion of tumor-immune pig lymphocytes in 24 patients with invasive transitional cell carcinoma of the bladder which recurred following radiotherapy (Symes *et al.,* 1978b). In 11 patients there was a remission, and three patients were alive and showed no evidence of residual tumor over a year after treatment (Symes *et al.,* 1978b).

8.234 TRANSFER FACTOR

The discovery by Lawrence (1955) that, in man, delayed type hypersensitivity (DTH) can be transferred from one individual to another with leukocyte extracts as readily as with viable leukocytes suggested a possible new method of immunotherapy, and interest in this approach has been stimulated as the result of further investigations (Lawrence, 1974). The material responsible, to which Lawrence gave the general name *transfer factor* (TF), is effective despite histoincompatibility between donor and recipient (Rapaport *et al.,* 1965) and does not evoke a graft-versus-host reaction (Lawrence, 1974). Activity persists in dialysates, and material so treated has been named TF_D. TF_D has a molecular weight below 10,000 Daltons, is non-immunogenic, and is unaffected by DNase and RNase. According to Lawrence it is immunologically specific (Lawrence, 1969, 1974), but there is some evidence that it may also stimulate the immune system non-specifically as shown by increased response of lymphocytes to mitogens (Griscelli *et al.,* 1973) and in mixed lymphocyte cultures (Dupont *et al.,* 1974), and increased macrophage chemotaxis (Gallin and Kirkpatrick, 1974). It has been shown that patients with disseminated cancer, even if anergic—i.e., unresponsive to antigenic stimulation—may respond to TF from normal donors sensitized to a variety of microbial antigens (Solowey *et al.,* 1967; Lawrence, 1974); moreover, cell-mediated immunity may be augmented in this way without at the same time boosting production of antibody.

Transfer factor used to treat cancer patients has been prepared from cells derived from either (1) untreated individuals chosen because it was thought, for one of the reasons discussed below, that they might be capable of mounting a cell-mediated reaction against the patient's tumor, or (2) other cancer patients deliberately immunized with the tumor of the patient to be treated.

Untreated donors. Oettgen *et al.* (1971, 1974) prepared TF_D from blood leukocytes of healthy women over 45 years of age, and used this to treat five women with advanced breast cancer. They argued that, if the hypothesis of immunological surveillance is correct (5.51), "mature women who are free of breast cancer may have been exposed to and raised a specific TF verus neoplastic breast cells from puberty onwards." Each patient received daily or thrice-weekly subcutaneous injections of TF_D for periods ranging from 21 to 310 days, and the total amount given was equivalent to 17×10^9 to 217×10^9 cells. Although reactivity to PPD or streptokinase–streptodornase was shown to be transmitted to three of the patients, a therapeutic effect was observed in only one. This took the form of partial regression of the tumor which was sustained for 6 months. When relapse occurred the patient was treated with TF_D from a different pool but failed to respond. No harmful side effects were observed.

Goldenberg and Brandes (1972) prepared TF_D from EB-virus-positive young adults who had recovered from infectious mononucleosis and administered it to two patients with nasopharyngeal carcinoma refractory to conventional treatment. In both patients there was temporary tumor regression; in one case this was associated with intense lymphocyte infiltration of the tumor, transfer of reactivity to PPD and *T. rubrum,* and a fall in antibody titer to viral capsid antigen of the EB virus.

Patients with malignant melanoma (Spitler *et al.,* 1973; Price *et al.,* 1974), soft-tissue and osteogenic sarcomas (LoBuglio *et al.,* 1973; Neidhart and LoBuglio, 1974; Levin *et al.,* 1975), leukemia (Neidhart and LoBuglio, 1974), and other tumors (Vetto *et al.,* 1976) have been treated with TF obtained from cells donated by members of the same family as the patient and living in the same household. In some cases the donors were chosen because their lymphocytes reacted against the patient's or a similar tumor *in vitro*, as shown by a MIF (macrophage-inhibition factor) assay or by direct cytotoxicity (LoBuglio *et al.*, 1973; Spitler *et al.*, 1973; Neidhart and LoBuglio, 1974; Levin *et al.*, 1975); Vetto *et al.*, however, used family member cohabitants without preliminary *in vitro* testing. Price *et al.* (1974) also treated melanoma patients with TF prepared from leukocytes from patients who had been cured of melanoma and from healthy Black donors. In most of the patients with advanced cancer little if any therapeutic effect was observed, but Vetto *et al.* (1976) reported six partial and three complete remissions among 35 patients treated.

In five patients in whom TF was given as adjuvant therapy after amputation for osteogenic sarcoma, Levin *et al.* (1975) reported tumor-free survival times ranging from 12 to 24 months; and in another similar series LoBuglio and Neidhart (1976) reported that two patients developed recurrences after 4 months and 12 months, respectively, but that the other three were alive and clinically tumor-free 7, 8, and 17 months after treatment. Ivins and his colleagues (Ivins *et al.*, 1976; Ritts *et al.*, 1978) compared the effect of adjuvant immunotherapy in the form of injection of TF, and adjuvant chemotherapy, following amputation for osteogenic sarcoma. The TF was prepared from leukocytes from donors who had themselves had an amputation for osteogenic sarcoma and had survived for longer than 5 years, and who showed a marked recall microbial DTH skin reaction. The trial is described as randomized, but five patients in whom transfer of DTH did not occur after administration of TF were transferred to the chemotherapy group. Neither form of adjuvant therapy seems to have been of benefit; comparison with historical controls treated by amputation only is difficult, however, because of differences in survival between patients treated by surgery only at different times or in different institutions.

Immunized donors. Brandes, Galton, and Wiltshaw (1971) performed reciprocal immunization in two patients with disseminated malignant melanoma, and subsequently treated each one with a leukocyte extract presumed to contain TF from the other patient. The extract was injected thrice weekly subcutaneously; in addition, later in the course of therapy, intralesional injections were given into two subcutaneous metastases. In one patient the locally injected nodules became intensely inflamed and were removed for histological examination, and the other nodules showed an overall regression of 20–25 percent. Death occurred suddenly from cerebral hemorrhage, however, 17 days after the first injection, and autopsy revealed widespread disease with hemorrhage into a cerebral metastasis. The other patient was not fully reported, but apparently no tumor regression was observed.

Further reports of the local or systemic use of TF prepared from the cells of other patients immunized with the tumor of the patient to be treated have been published by Thompson (1971), G.V. Smith, Morse, and Deraps (1973), and Krementz *et al.* (1974). Thompson reported that 7 of 19 patients with advanced cancer showed "a greater than 50 percent regression in measurable tumor with clinical improvement of up to 17 months". Smith *et al.* also reported some partial regressions, and instances of "complete regression of some lesions," in patients with advanced cancer, but there is not sufficient information to evaluate the results critically. The same problem arises with the series of 21 patients with minimal or non-detectable residual disease reported by Thompson in which TF was given as adjuvant therapy.

Attention has already been drawn to the danger to which recipients of viable tumor grafts are exposed (1.112). A further matter to be considered is the possible danger of repeated leukapheresis when the cell donor is himself a cancer patient, although in practice this seems so far to have been well tolerated.

8.235   IMMUNE RNA

In the light of evidence that human lymphocytes treated *in vitro* with xenogeneic RNA extracted from the lymphoid organs of sheep immunized with human tumors become specifically cytotoxic for human tumor target cells (Pilch, Veltman, and Kern, 1974; Pilch *et al.*, 1976c; Kern *et al.*, 1976a, 1976b, 1977) and preliminary animal studies (7.43), Pilch *et al.* (1976a, 1976b, 1978) instituted Phase I clinical trials of xenogeneic immune RNA in patients with advanced cancer, and also in patients without detectable tumors but in whom the probability of occult residual disease was considered to be greater than 50 percent.

Cell suspensions prepared from fresh or frozen tumor tissue removed at operations were emulsified with complete Freund's adjuvant and injected intradermally to sheep on three occasions at weekly intervals. Ten days after the last injection the animals were killed and RNA was extracted from their spleens and lymph nodes, and purified. This material, suspended in physiological saline, was injected intradermally to patients at weekly intervals. Administration was discontinued after 8 weeks if progression of the disease had occurred. Whenever possible patients received RNA from animals immunized with their own tumors; failing this RNA from animals immunized with tumors of similar type was used.

Symptoms of toxicity were minimal and consisted of transient malaise and occasional pyrexia. No anaphylactic reactions occurred. No claims of therapeutic benefit were made in respect of the patients with advanced cancer. The results in patients suspected of having occult residual disease after surgical treatment for melanoma, colorectal cancer, or hypernephroma are described as encouraging, but the follow-up period at the time of the last report ranged from only 2 to 25 months. Pilch *et al.* have drawn attention to the desirability of giving RNase inhibitors to delay destruction of the immune RNA. They have used sodium dextran sulfate for this purpose in animals but state that they know of no RNase inhibitor suitable for use in patients.

8.24   Non-specific Immunopotentiation

In this section we shall examine the use of agents which have been reported to stimulate immunological or para-immunological responses non-specifically, in the absence of other forms of immunotherapy. Combined non-specific and active specific procedures will be considered later (8.26).

The agents will be discussed under the following headings:

1.   Coley's bacterial toxins.
2.   Bacillus Calmette-Guérin (BCG) and derivatives.
3.   *"Corynebacterium parvum."*
4.   Other bacterial preparations.
5.   Viral infection.
6.   Polynucleotides.
7.   Levamisole.

8. Anticoagulants and fibrinolytic agents.
9. Phytohemogglutinin (PHA), polysaccharides, thymosin.
10. Substances used to evoke a local hypersensitivity reaction.
11. Hyperthermia.

8.241   COLEY'S BACTERIAL TOXINS

Investigation of the effect of bacterial toxins on human tumors, which was initiated by W.B. Coley, was prompted by reports, reviewed fairly recently by Nauts (1969, 1973), that prolonged tumor regression sometimes followed episodes of infection of various kinds. Coley used mixed toxins derived from *Streptococcus pyogenes* and *Serratia marcescens* (formerly called *Bacillus prodigiosus*), but at least 15 variations in formulae have been used by Coley and other investigators. Nauts and her colleagues, in a series of papers and monographs, have reviewed a total of 894 cases of cancer treated with this material between 1893 and 1973 (Nauts, Swift, and Coley, 1946; Nauts and Fowler, 1969; T.R. Miller and Nicholson, 1974; Nauts, 1973, 1974, 1975a, 1975b, 1975c, 1976a, 1976b, 1978). During the first half of this period many of the cases were treated and reported by Coley himself (Coley, 1893, 1894, 1898, 1901, 1906, 1910, 1929); since his papers tend to overlap and are listed by Nauts, we have cited only a few leading references.

Coley's toxins have been administered both systemically (intravenously, intramuscularly, subcutaneously, and intradermally) and intralesionally.

The 5 year survival figures for treated patients reported by Nauts (1978) are shown in Table 1, and more detailed information can be found in the reviews cited earlier. Cases listed as operable received bacterial toxin as an adjuvant to surgery.

Table 8-1
Nauts' (1978) 5 Year Survival Figures

Type of Tumor	Inoperable Cases		Operable Cases	
	Total No.	No. Surviving 5 Years	Total No.	No. Surviving 5 Years
Ewing's tumor of bone	52	11	62	18
Osteogenic sarcoma	23	3	139	43
Reticulum cell sarcoma of bone	49	9	23	13
Multiple myelomas	8	4	4	2
Giant cell tumor of bone	19	15	38	33
Lymphosarcomas	86	42		
Other soft tissue sarcomas	137	77	49	35
Hodgkin's disease	15	10		
Cancer of breast	20	13	13	13
Cancer of ovary	15	10	1	1
Cancer of cervix	3	2		
Sarcoma of uterus	11	8		
Malignant tumor of testes	43*	14	21	15
Malignant melanoma	17	10	14	10
Colorectal cancer	11	5	2	2
Renal cancer in adults	7	3	1	1
Wilms' tumor			3	1
Neuroblastoma	6	1	3	2

*Including 16 terminal cases.
From *Dev Biol Stand 38.* (Reprinted with permission of S. Karger, A.G. Basel, and H.C. Nauts.)

Conservative operations were performed in preference to amputation in many patients with giant cell tumors and soft tissue sarcomas, and in some patients with osteogenic sarcoma, involving the extremities. This conservative approach was an innovation in Coley's day but is now commonly adopted in treating giant cell tumors and soft tissue sarcomas, and it is open to question whether similar results might have been obtained by surgery alone or combined with radiotherapy. It is also difficult to assess the extent to which treatment with toxins affected the course of the disease in the inoperable cases, though it may well have contributed to the prolonged relief of pain and improvement in general condition which occurred in many patients. The important question is whether a *prima facie* case has been made which is strong enough to justify setting up controlled clinical trials of bacterial toxins, particularly as adjuvant therapy in conditions like osteogenic sarcoma where the prognosis with conventional treatment is still so poor.

8.242   BCG AND DERIVATIVES

As we have seen (7.51) there are now many different strains and preparations of BCG, and these differ considerably in their effect on immunological responses. BCG is commonly given intradermally by scarification or multiple puncture with an instrument such as the Heaf gun fitted with a number of tines, but it has been given as a single intradermal injection, and also intravenously orally, intraperitoneally, intrapleurally, intralymphatically, intralesionally, and as an aerosol. BCG derivatives have been given intradermally and intralesionally.

We shall begin by considering intradermal administration of living BCG in patients with a variety of neoplastic conditions.

Intradermal BCG in leukemias and lymphomas. The use of BCG for the treatment of cancer patients was introduced by Georges Mathé, who in 1963 started a randomized clinical trial in patients with acute lymphatic leukemia (ALL). He chose ALL because, at that time, it was one of the rare diseases in which it was possible to maintain long remission with chemotherapy, and it was thought that it might be possible to reduce the number of leukemic cells by chemotherapy sufficiently for the residual cells to be susceptible to immunotherapeutic attack (Mathé, Olsson *et al.,* 1980). There were 40 patients in the trial, aged between 3 and 50 years, and in all of them a remission had been induced and maintained for up to 2 years by chemotherapy. They were divided at random into four groups. Group I consisted of ten patients who received no further treatment after cessation of chemotherapy. Group II consisted of eight patients who were treated with the Pasteur Institute strain of BCG by cutaneous scarification, initially every fourth day and later every eighth day. Each of the scratches was 5 cm long and they were arranged in a square; into this scarified area was placed 2 ml of a suspension containing 75 mg of living bacteria per ml. Group III consisted of five patients who received intradermal and subcutaneous injection of formalin-treated or irradiated allogeneic leukemic cells and Group IV of seven patients who received both BCG and cells.

Progress reports of this trial have been published from time to time (Mathé, Amiel *et al.,* 1968, 1969a, 1977a; Mathé, Schwarzenberg *et al.,* 1978). At the time of the first report, all the patients in Group I had relapsed within 130 days of stopping chemotherapy, whereas in Groups II, III, and IV there were five, three, and four patients, respectively, who were still in remission. In subsequent reports the patients in the three groups who received immunotherapy have been pooled so that it is not possible to assess the effect of BCG alone. The results will therefore be considered later, together with those of many other trials in which BCG has been used in conjunction with other immunotherapeutic procedures (8.26).

In the light of Mathé's work a trial of BCG in ALL was started in the United Kingdom under the auspices of the Medical Research Council (MRC), and reports of this have been published by the MRC Working Party on Leukemia in Childhood (1971) and by Kay (1978). After induction of remission and consolidation by chemotherapy, the patients were divided randomly into three groups. Those in the first group received no further treatment, those in the second were treated with methotrexate, and those in the third group received weekly intradermal treatment with the Glaxo strain of BCG administered with a Heaf gun. Prolonged remission occurred in patients treated with methotrexate but not in those treated with BCG. In another randomized trial in which 502 children with ALL received either no further treatment, or chemotherapy or BCG, after induction of remission and consolidation, there were again no prolonged remissions in the group treated with BCG, nor, in this trial, in those given chemotherapy (Heyn et al., 1975, 1978). A freeze-dried preparation of the Pasteur strain of BCG grown in Chicago was given repeatedly by the tine technique. No benefit from BCG following induction of remission with chemotherapy and prophylactic irradiation of the central nervous system was also reported by Ekert et al. (1978) in a small non-randomized trial in which Pasteur-strain BCG grown at the Commonwealth Serum Laboratories in Melbourne was used.

Benefit in the form of prolonged remission was reported by Gutterman, Hersh et al. (1974a) in adult patients with acute myeloblastic leukemia (AML) who, after remission induction and consolidation with a three drug chemotherapy regimen, were given Pasteur-strain BCG by scarification three times per month in addition to maintenance chemotherapy. This conclusion was based on comparison with historical controls and has been strongly criticized by Peto and Galton (1975). Moreover, in a later report of this trial (Gutterman, Rodriguez et al., 1978c), there was no significant prolongation of remission duration, although survival was longer in the patients who received BCG in comparison with historical controls, and the difference was said to be just significant at the $p=0.05$ level; and in a randomized trial from the same hospital (Hewlett et al., 1978), the addition of administration of lyophilized Pasteur-strain BCG to maintenance chemotherapy in adult acute leukemias had no significant effect on either duration of remission or survival. Gutterman, Mavligit et al. (1976b) have also reported prolongation of the disease-free interval in adults with acute leukemia who received BCG only after remission induction and consolidation with chemotherapy, as compared with those who received no further treatment or chemotherapy; once again, however, the trial was non-randomized.

Two other trials of BCG in AML, both of which were randomized, have yielded conflicting results. In one (Vogler and Chan, 1974; Vogler et al., 1978), in which maintenance with chemotherapy alone was compared with maintenance with chemotherapy plus administration of Tice-strain BCG given twice weekly for 4 weeks by the tine technique, remission duration but not survival was reported to be significantly prolonged. In the other (Whittaker and Slater, 1978), in which lyophilized Glaxo-strain BCG was used, patients maintained with chemotherapy plus BCG were reported to survive longer than those maintained with chemotherapy alone, but remission duration was the same in the two groups.

Sokal, Aungst, and Snyderman (1974), in a randomized trial, compared the effect of giving BCG or no further treatment to patients with malignant lymphoma who were in remission following chemotherapy. There were 50 patients in the trial, of whom 32 had Hodgkin's disease. Freeze-dried Tice BCG was given by intradermal injection in a dose of 0.8×10^6 viable bacilli. Ten patients received only a single dose; 13 received two doses, and 5 received three or more doses, the principal reason for repeating the dose being that the patient had failed to become tuberculin positive. During the 6–8 years follow-up, 16 out of 22 controls relapsed, the mean time to the first new lesion being 10.6 months. Of the 28 treated patients, 17 relapsed, with a mean time to the first new lesion of 25.9 months. The differences on detailed analysis were reported to be statistically significant ($p=0.01$), but the authors pointed out that, by the time the studies were published, better results could be obtained without immunotherapy.

In more recent trials in which BCG was given repeatedly, there was no significant beneficial effect, as judged by duration of remission and survival, in Hodgkin's disease (Hoerni et al., 1976; Bakemeir et al., 1978) and Burkitt's lymphoma (Magrath and Ziegler, 1976), and at most a very slight effect in other types of lymphoma (J.W. Thomas et al., 1975, 1976; S.E. Jones et al., 1978).

Intradermal BCG for solid non-lymphoid tumors.   Following reports by Bluming et al. (1972, 1974) of delayed reappearance of melanoma after surgical excision in African patients treated with Pasteur BCG by scarification, though not in those given intradermal injections of Glaxo BCG, there have been many trials of BCG as an adjuvant to chemotherapy in patients with disseminated melanoma, and as an adjuvant to surgery in operable cases. Gutterman et al. (1974b, 1978a) reported longer remissions in patients with disseminated melanoma who received Pasteur BCG by scarification plus dimethyltriazenoimidazole carboxamide (DTIC) than in historical controls treated with DTIC only, but only a few patients remained in remission. Costanzi (1978) and Simmons et al. (1978), in randomized trials in patients with disseminated disease, found that the addition of BCG to chemotherapy conferred no significant benefit.

Reports on the value of BCG as an adjuvant to surgery are conflicting. Gutterman et al. (1976b, 1978b) reported that patients with melanoma on the trunk, but not in other sites, given Pasteur BCG by scarification following surgical excision, survived longer than historical controls treated by surgery alone. Morton and his colleagues (Eilber et al., 1976; Morton et al., 1976, 1978) have also reported a lower recurrence rate in patients treated with BCG after surgical excision of melanomas and the related lymph nodes, especially when tumor was found in only one node, but the fact that the trial was non-randomized again makes interpretation uncertain. In trials with randomized controls, postoperative treatment with Tice or Pasteur BCG made little or no difference (Cunningham et al., 1978; Pinsky et al., 1978b; Beretta et al., 1978).

Mavligit et al. (1975, 1976, 1978) gave intradermal BCG alone, or intradermal BCG plus oral 5-fluorouracil (5FU) as adjuvant therapy after operation for colorectal cancer of grade C in Dukes' classification. They reported that, in terms of disease-free interval and length of survival, these two groups behaved similarly but fared significantly better than historical controls treated by surgery only. The use of historical controls and the validity of this conclusion have been strongly criticized by P.R.M. Thomas et al. (1976), Moertel (1978), and others. A trial by Engstrom et al. (1978) of Glaxo BCG, or BCG plus chemotherapy with 5FU, in patients with advanced or recurrent colorectal cancer, showed no significant differences between the two groups in respect of objective responses or survival.

In patients with advanced breast cancer, the addition of repeated treatment with Tice or Pasteur BCG to chemotherapy has been reported to result in the same remission rate but somewhat longer survival of responders (Gutterman, Cardenas *et al.,* 1976a; Hortobagyi *et al.,* 1978). Once again, however, the conclusion is based on historical controls, and the evidence is unconvincing. In contrast, Pines (1976), in a randomized trial comparing patients with advanced squamous cell carcinoma of the lung treated by radiotherapy alone or radiotherapy plus repeated treatment with Glaxo BCG administered with a Heaf gun, found that survival during the first year of observation was longer, and the incidence of peripheral metastases less, in the patients who received BCG.

Oral, intravenous, and intralymphatic administration of BCG. It was originally suggested by Calmette that BCG should be given orally, but, with the dose recommended, sensitization to tuberculin did not always occur. Later, however, it was found that large doses were effective by mouth in children, though not always in adults.

Oral administration of BCG for the treatment of cancer seems to have been initiated by J.W. Thomas (1972), who observed prolonged remission of metastatic melanoma, found at laparotomy to be limited to the small bowel, in a patient who was given a blood transfusion from another patient who was sensitized to both BCG and vaccinia virus, followed by repeated administration of BCG by mouth and vaccinia virus by subcutaneous injection. Encouraged by this result, Thomas and his colleagues (Clements *et al.,* 1976) conducted a small pilot study followed by a randomized trial in patients with non-Hodgkin's malignant lymphoma. Patients in Stages I and II in whom a remission had been induced with chemotherapy received either no further treatment or repeated administration of BCG both orally and by scarification; patients in Stages III and IV in whom a remission was induced received either oral cyclophosphamide or BCG both orally and by scarification. The treatment was well tolerated but the trial, when reported, had not been running long enough to give any clear indication of whether or not it was beneficial. MacGregor *et al.* (1975) gave BCG by mouth as an adjuvant to conventional treatment in 47 patients with all stages of malignant melanoma. They considered that the treatment delayed recurrence and metastasis, and increased survival in patients with disseminated melanoma except in the case of intracerebral metastases, or hepatic metastases from a primary ocular melanoma. The evidence, however, is far from convincing, and some of the patients received intralesional injections of BCG and other forms of immunotherapy in addition to BCG by mouth. Ambus *et al.* (1978) found that a single intraperitoneal injection of BCG followed by repeated oral administration, given in addition to administration of 5FU, was of no significant benefit in patients with various forms of cancer of the gastrointestinal tract. In a randomized trial of oral BCG as adjuvant therapy following surgical resection for operable colorectal cancer (Dukes' stages B and C) Ambus *et al.* claimed that the combined treatment was clearly more favorable, but it is not clear whether the difference in survival was statistically significant.

Whittaker *et al.* (1973) administered reconstituted freeze-dried Glaxo BCG intravenously to three patients with AML in whom a remission had been induced with chemotherapy. Dilutions of 1 in 10^6, 1 in 10^5, 1 in 10^4, and so on up to full strength were prepared, and an injection of 0.1 ml was given daily, starting with the most dilute suspension and following this with the next in the series unless the pyrexia, which typically developed 2 hours after injection, persisted. The course of treatment, which was well tolerated, was repeated monthly. The results were considered sufficiently encouraging to justify setting up a randomized trial, and this is in progress. It has been reported, however, by Mathé (1976b) that BCG injected intravenously may cause immunosuppression and possibly enhance tumor growth in allergic patients.

Cascinelli et al. (1977) gave a single injection of BCG, ranging in amount from 0.2 to 80 mg, into a lymphatic vessel on the dorsum of the foot in 20 patients with visceral metastases from malignant melanoma. After 21 days, when none of the patients showed any evidence of therapeutic benefit, they were given chemotherapy.

Intralesional and regional administration of BCG.   It was reported by Morton *et al.* (1970), and subsequently confirmed by others (Krementz, 1971; Nathanson, 1972; Pinsky *et al.*, 1973; G. V. Smith *et al.*, 1973), that subcutaneous melanoma metastases often regressed after intralesional injection of BCG. In a later paper (Morton *et al.*, 1974) it was reported that melanoma nodules distant from the one injected with BCG also regressed in 15–20 percent of patients who were immunologically competent as judged by their ability to be sensitized to dinitrochlorobenzene or to respond to tuberculin after BCG administration. Some of the patients treated by Pinsky *et al.* and Morton *et al.* became apparently disease-free, and remained so during follow-up periods of several years.

McKneally, Maver, and Kausel (1976, 1978), in a randomized trial to which 95 patients were admitted, studied the effect of intrapleural injection of BCG (Tice strain) 4–6 days after pulmonary resection for operable lung cancer (other than small cell undifferentiated tumors), followed by isoniazid. Control patients received only isoniazid after their operation. The incidence of recurrence and the length of the disease-free interval were significantly improved in patients whose tumor was not more than 3 cm in diameter, irrespective of whether the hilar lymph nodes were involved or not, and in patients with larger tumors without involvement of adjacent structures or hilar nodes, but not in patients with more advanced disease. This clear-cut result in a properly controlled trial should certainly stimulate further study of this form of treatment. It has also been reported that intrapleural injection of BCG sterilized by γ-radiation (Pimm and Baldwin, 1976c), or BCG cell wall skeleton attached to oil droplets (Yamamura *et al.*, 1976a, 1976b; Yasumoto *et al.*, 1976), may reduce the rate of accumulation of malignant pleural effusions and prolong survival. The use of these materials avoids the need for subsequent administration of isoniazid.

Falk *et al.* (1976) administered BCG intraperitoneally to 35 patients with advanced cancer of the stomach, pancreas, biliary tract, or colon. Subsequently the patients were given BCG orally and also chemotherapy. A brisk febrile reaction occurred in most patients within 2 to 5 days of the intraperitoneal injection. Some patients experienced more prolonged low grade fever and malaise, but this responded well to treatment with isoniazid. Progression of the tumor was reported to be arrested or retarded in patients with all types of tumor, most notably in those with hepatic metastases from cancer of the colon, but it is impossible to say to what extent this was due to BCG.

Garner *et al.* (1975) administered BCG repeatedly in the form of an aerosol to 15 patients with metastatic cancer involving the lungs. The procedure resulted in malaise and fever, beginning 4–8 hours after completion of the administration and lasting usually for 24–36 hours, but was otherwise well tolerated; progression of the tumor occurred, however, in all cases.

Morales, Eidinger, and Bruce (1976, 1978) administered BCG intradermally by Heaf gun, and also by instillation of a saline suspension of the organisms into the urinary bladder, in 16 patients in whom a superficial bladder cancer had recurred after surgical treatment and who had subsequently been treated by endoscopic resection or fulguration and intralesional instillation of thiotepa. They claimed that the immunotherapy reduced the incidence of further recurrence, but the evidence does not seem sufficient to justify this conclusion.

BCG derivatives.   Moertel *et al.* (1975, 1978) used the methanol extraction residue fraction (MER) of BCG as an adjuvant to chemotherapy in patients with advanced colorectal cancer, but observed no significant advantage in respect of completeness or duration of response, or survival, as compared with patients treated by chemotherapy only. It has been suggested, however, that the dose of MER, namely, 2 mg on days 1, 7, 21, 36, and then every 2 weeks (or without the first two doses in some cases), was excessive. Weiss *et al.* (1975), in a randomized trial, treated patients with AML in whom complete or partial remission had been induced by chemotherapy, with either chemotherapy alone or chemotherapy plus MER (1–2 mg monthly by intradermal injection divided between five to ten sites). Analysis of the first 28 patients showed significant prolongation of both duration of remission and survival, but the authors wisely refrained from drawing firm conclusions at this stage. Cuttner *et al.* (1978), in another randomized trial, used either chemotherapy for 7 days, or chemotherapy for 7 days plus 1.0 mg MER by intradermal injection divided between five sites on the first day of treatment, to induce remission in AML. In patients under the age of 60 there were 22 complete remissions in 33 patients who received MER as compared with 67 complete remissions in 132 patients treated by chemotherapy only. Patients in whom remission was induced with chemotherapy only were later subdivided randomly into two groups; members of one group were maintained by chemotherapy, the others by chemotherapy plus MER. When reported, the trial had not been running long enough to allow a firm conclusion to be drawn, but there was a suggestion that administration of MER was beneficial.

Yamamura (1978) gave BCG cell wall skeleton intralesionally or intradermally weekly for 30 weeks, and then monthly, as an adjuvant to surgery, chemotherapy, or irradiation in patients with all stages of lung cancer. It was suggested that survival in advanced cases was prolonged as compared with historical controls.

Complications of BCG therapy.   Transient malaise and low grade fever are common sequelae of BCG administration. Local pruritis is also common. Local pain and ulceration is fairly common after intradermal injection of either BCG (Bakemeier *et al.,* 1978) or MER (Cuttner *et al.,* 1978), but not after administration of BCG by scarification (Schwarzenberg *et al.,* 1976). Severe or prolonged fever, nausea, and vomiting occur occasionally, particularly, according to Serrou and Domas (1978), after intralesional injection of BCG. Intralesional injection may also be followed by persistent sinuses and lymphadenopathy (Morton *et al.,* 1976). Serrou *et al.* (1975) have reported one case of granulomatous hepatitis following treatment of a malignant melanoma by intralesional injection of BCG. After intravenous injection of BCG all the patients treated by Whittaker and Slater (1978) developed fever within 6–12 hours and this lasted for 12–72 hours. Some patients experienced headaches and muscle pains, and two had non-fatal anaphylactic reactions. Two patients developed splenomegaly and transient jaundice, and at autopsy granulomas were found in the spleen, liver, and lungs (Whittaker *et al.*, 1976).

Fatal generalized BCG infection has been described in two patients by Šicević (1972), but both were said to have a severe pre-existing deficiency of cellular immunity.

Effect on immunological responses. Administration of BCG by scarification to cancer patients promotes the conversion of tuberculin (PPD)-negative patients to tuberculin positive (Cochran *et al.*, 1978; Richardson *et al.*, 1978), and may lead to an increased response by the patient's leukocytes to PPD *in vitro*, as shown in the leukocyte migration-inhibition assay (Richardson *et al.*, 1978), but has been reported to have no effect on the response of the patient's lymphocytes to tumor antigens *in vitro* (Cochran *et al.*, 1978). Patients treated in this way have also been reported to have a higher proportion of T cells (indicated by their capacity to form E rosettes with sheep erythrocytes) as compared with similar patients not given BCG (Anthony *et al.*, 1975b; Kerman and Stefani, 1978), and to show a greater response to PHA (Kerman and Stefani, 1978; Thatcher and Crowther, 1978). The effect on the patient's response to recall antigens appears to depend on the dose of BCG and the immunological state of the patient. Thus Mathé and his colleagues (Mathé, 1976a; Simmler, Schwarzenberg, and Mathé, 1976) found that application of 75 mg fresh living Pasteur BCG to four scarified areas increased responses in allergic patients and depressed responses in those who were anergic, whereas application to a single area had the opposite effect.

Oral administration of BCG to cancer patients may fail to promote conversion to tuberculin positivity, or to stimulate the response to PHA (Mankiewicz *et al.*, 1977). It has also been reported that oral BCG leads to unresponsiveness to cytoplasmic melanoma antigens, but does not inhibit the response to membrane antigens evoked by administration of irradiated autologous tumor cells (M.G. Lewis *et al.*, 1976b).

Wybran *et al.* (1976) studied variations in the number of T cells in the blood of six patients with melanomas treated by intralesional BCG. They used two techniques for detecting cells which formed rosettes with sheep erythrocytes: the "active T-rosette test," in which the sheep erythrocytes were incubated for only a very short time with the patient's lymphocytes, and the "total T-rosette test," in which incubation was more prolonged. Four of the patients showed a good therapeutic response with regression of some or all the skin nodules; all of these patients showed an increase in active rosette-forming cells (T-Ea), and two showed also an increase in total rosette-forming cells (T-Et). The other two patients did not respond to the treatment. One of these showed an increase in T-Ea cells only; the other showed no increase in either type of cell. It was suggested from these findings, and from other immunological studies in the same patients (Lieberman *et al.*, 1975), that intralesional BCG may bind to melanoma antigens, and that this complex, or a product released from the melanoma cells, activates T cells.

Prophylaxis of cancer with BCG. It was reported by Davignon *et al.* (1970) that death from leukemia was only half as common among BCG-vaccinated as among non-vaccinated individuals less than 15 years of age in the Province of Quebec, Canada, for each of the years 1960–1963. The table published in this report erroneously showed the population at risk as one-tenth of the true figure, but this did not affect the ratio

Table 2

Distribution of Children of 0–14 Years of Age Who Died of Leukemia,
by Year and According to BCG Vaccination Status

Group	1960	1961	1962	1963
Non-vaccinated				
Population (0–14 years)	887,500	868,000	838,500	824,600
Number of leukemia deaths	52	46	44	49
Rate per 100,000	5.8	5.2	5.2	5.9
Vaccinated				
Population (0–14 years)	938,400	995,300	1,052,900	1,092,400
Number of leukemia deaths	20	22	33	21
Rate per 100,000	2.1	2.2	3.1	1.9

Table 3

Distribution of Children of 0–4 Years of Age Who Died of Leukemia,
by Year and According to BCG Vaccination Status

Group	1960	1961	1962	1963
Non-vaccinated				
Population (0–4 years)	361,300	354,600	347,700	344,700
Number of leukemia deaths	22	29	30	22
Rate per 100,000	6.0	8.1	8.6	6.3
Vaccinated				
Population (0–4 years)	302,100	316,600	325,000	327,300
Number of leukemia deaths	8	13	16	9
Rate per 100,000	2.6	4.1	4.9	2.7

From Davignon *et al.,* 1971a. (Reprinted with permission of the *Lancet* and L. Frappier Davignon.)

between vaccinated and non-vaccinated groups. The correct figures, which are shown here in Table 2, and some further information (Table 3) were published in a later paper (Davignon *et al.,* 1971a). The Central Record System, from which these figures were obtained, was started when the first Canadian was vaccinated with BCG in 1926, and all vaccinations were performed by specially trained teams and recorded at the time; it would seem therefore that the data can be accepted as accurate. In the 0–14 years group the proportion of children who were vaccinated at birth is not given, but, in the 0–4 years group, 90 percent of the children vaccinated were vaccinated at birth. It seems clear that there is a significant difference in mortality due to leukemia between the two groups. Whether this difference is due to BCG or some other cause, as Divignon *et al.* (1971b) point out, can only be determined by further study, and, in particular, by some form of cohort analysis. Studies undertaken in the United Kingdom are also difficult to interpret. If it is assumed that, in the absence of BCG vaccination, the leukemia mortality rate would have continued to increase at the same rate as it did during the first half of this century, the data collected by Hems and Stuart (1971) would seem to indicate that BCG-vaccinated children have approximately half the risk of dying from leukemia as unvaccinated children, but Hems and Stuart suggest that other changes occurring before about 1955 may have been responsible for the difference.

8.243 *"C. PARVUM"* (CP)

As in the previous chapter (7.52), *"C. parvum"* (in quotation marks) or CP will be used to denote heat-killed or formalin-killed suspensions of a variety of organisms classified as *Corynebacteria* or *Propionibacteria* which stimulate lymphoreticuloendothelial activity and have been shown under certain conditions to inhibit the growth of tumors in experimental animals.

The organisms which have been used clinically included the following:

1. The Pasteur strain numbered 936B, prepared by Prévot, which was used in the original experiments with animal tumors by Woodruff and Boak (1966) and Halpern *et al.* (1966). This strain is no longer available and remains an unknown entity.
2. An organism grown at the Pasteur Institute, Paris, by Raynaud and referred to as *C. granulosum.*
3. An organism from the Institut Merieux designated IMI585, identified by Roumiantzeff *et al.* (1975) as *P. avidum.*
4. An organism from the Wellcome Foundation in the United Kingdom, and from Burroughs Wellcome Laboratories in the United States, designated CN6134, which has been identified as a *P. acnes* Type I (Milas and Scott, 1977), or, in the terminology of McBride *et al.* (1975a), *C. acnes* Type I. This organism was originally obtained from Raynaud and is serologically identical with the organism referred to by the Pasteur Institute as *C. granulosum* (Adlam and Reid, 1978).

Therapeutic effects. CP was first used clinically by Israel (Halpern and Israel, 1971; Israel and Halpern, 1972) in a randomized trial in which 41 patients with disseminated cancer received either chemotherapy with five drugs, or the same chemotherapy plus weekly subcutaneous injections of CP (2 mg to each arm). The patients were tested for sensitivity to tuberculin before treatment was begun and subsequently and were stratified retrospectively according to whether they were initially tuberculin positive or negative. A comparison was then made of the length of survival from the start of treatment in the resulting four groups. The group mean value ranged from 13 months in patients who were tuberculin positive and received CP to 3.6 months in tuberculin-negative patients who received only chemotherapy. CP treatment significantly prolonged survival in both tuberculin-positive and tuberculin-negative patients, and the survival of tuberculin-negative patients who received CP was not significantly different from that of tuberculin-positive patients who received only chemotherapy.

Further reports have been published of the beneficial effect of subcutaneous injection of CP as an adjuvant to chemotherapy in patients with advanced cancer of various kinds, including carcinomas of the lung, breast, and ovary, melanomas, and sarcomas (Israel and Edelstein, 1975; Israel, 1975; Ochoa *et al.,* 1976; Mayr *et al.,* 1978a). In the experience of Israel and his colleagues, the administration of CP counteracted to a considerable extent the damaging effect of chemotherapy on the hemopoietic tissues. De Jager and his colleagues, on the other hand, found no significant differences in response rate or survival in patients with advanced breast cancer who received weekly subcutaneous injections of CP (4 mg) plus chemotherapy with cyclophosphamide, adriamycin, methotrexate, and 5FU as compared with those who received chemotherapy alone (De Jager *et al.,* 1976; Pinsky *et al.,* 1978a); and Dimitrov *et al.* (1978) found that the addition of repeated subcutaneous and intradermal injection of CP to chemotherapy did not influence tumor progression or survival in patients with lung cancer, though the incidence of leukopenia was less in the patients who received CP. Slight increase in survival was reported by Mahé et al. (1975) in patients with head and neck cancer who received subcutaneous injections of CP; and Ishmael et al. (1976), in a small trial (28 patients) comparing adjuvant therapy with BCG and with subcutaneous injections of CP after surgical treatment for melanoma, observed four relapses in patients who received BCG but none, at the time of the report, in those given CP.

In the studies described above, Israel used Pasteur-strain 936B vaccine until 1967, Raynaud's C. granulosum vaccine from 1967 to 1973, and thereafter Mérieux vaccine IM1585. Wellcome vaccine 6134 was used in the other trials.

Intravenous injection of CP was first used by Woodruff et al. (1974a, 1975) in 20 patients with advanced inoperable cancer in a Phase I trial which began in 1973 when Wellcome vaccine (Coparvax) became available for clinical use. The intravenous route was chosen because it had been found in experiments extending over many years that subcutaneous administration of CP (excluding intralesional injection) had far less effect on the growth of tumors in animals, and also on phagocytic activity and antibody response to CP, than intraperitoneal or intravenous administration, and appeared to be well tolerated in mice in a dosage of 35–70 mg/kg body weight. The first 12 patients received a single intravenous infusion of a saline dilution of CP. It was intended to give 1 mg/kg body weight in 500 ml saline over a period of 3–4 hours, but the infusions had to be stopped on account of febrile reactions when a total dose ranging from 15 to 48 mg had been given. The other patients received 20 mg CP in 100 ml saline intravenously, followed by 2 mg weekly by intramuscular injeciton. No spectacular regressions were observed in this small group of patients, but arrest of tumor growth for over a year in a patient with a metastasis in the opposite lung after pulmonary resection for bronchogenic carcinoma, and for 7 months in a patient with an extensive ulcerating cancer of the breast, was considered sufficiently encouraging to justify starting a randomized trial of CP as adjuvant therapy following pulmonary resection for operable bronchogenic cancer. The results of this trial will be discussed later.

Many other Phase I trials of intravenous infusion of CP as an adjuvant to chemotherapy in patients with advanced cancer have now been reported (Israel, 1975; Israel et al., 1975; Band et al., 1975; Harvey et al., 1976; Reed et al., 1975; Hirshaut et al., 1975; Ossorio et al., 1975; B. Fisher et al., 1976b; Minton et al., 1976; Takita and Moayeri, 1976; Valdivieso et al., 1976; Cheng et al., 1976; Humphrey et al., 1976; Haskell el al., 1976; Osborn and Castro, 1977; Mitcheson and Castro, 1978; Gordon, 1978; Chare et al., 1978; Presant et al., 1978). Many authors have employed a dose of 5 mg/m², weekly or every 2 weeks for varying times (Harvey et al., 1976; B. Fisher et al., 1976; Presant et al., 1978), or as a single dose (Minton et al., 1976; Takita and Moayeri, 1976; Valdivieso et al., 1976). Band et al. (1975) gave 0.5 to 6 mg/m² daily for 10 days, Israel (1975) 4 mg daily 5 days per week for 4–16 weeks, Mitcheson and Castro (1978) 10 mg/m² monthly, and Chare et al. (1978) either a single dose of 15 mg or five daily injections of 4 mg. Objective remissions were reported in 4 out of 20 patients by Band et al. and Harvey et al., in 8 out of 20 patients by Israel et al., and in 3 out of 21 patients with locally advanced breast cancer by Chare et al. Minton et al. (1976) reported that of six patients with disseminated breast cancer who had received a single injection of CP 10–11 months previously, two showed no evidence of tumor and in two the condition was stationary. One patient had a recurrence in her mastectomy scar and one had had a hypophysectomy following only temporary improvement. Takita and Moayeri, and Valdivieso et al., found that a single injection of CP made the patient more tolerant of chemotherapy, but this was not the experience of Haskell et al. (1976).

In another pilot study Israel (1975) treated nine patients with ocular melanomas, after removal of the eye, with a combination of subcutaneous injections of CP (4 mg weekly) and intradermal injection of Pasteur BCG. Eight of the patients were reported to be alive and without clinical evidence of disease 6 to 50 months later.

Trials of CP as an adjuvant to surgery in more favorable cases are in progress. Results in the author's randomized trial of a single intravenous infusion of 20 mg CP 2 weeks after pulmonary resection for operable lung cancer, entry to which was closed in 1976, are summarized in Table 4 (Woodruff, McCormack, and Walbaum, unpublished). Although in this small study the differences are not statistically significant at the $p = 0.05$ level, the number of long-term survivors among the patients given CP, especially among those with undifferentiated tumors, would seem to justify setting up a larger trial of the same kind. In view of the febrile reactions which many patients experienced despite the fact that they were given a single dose of aspirin prior to the CP infusion, it is suggested that the dose of CP should be reduced to about 7 mg and that repeated doses of aspirin or indomethacin should be given. The reasons for this last suggestion are discussed later (8.322).

Intratumor injection of CP was used by Israel (1975) and Cunningham-Rundles et al. (1975) in patients with cutaneous metastases, mostly of malignant melanoma. Both groups reported complete regression of some of the injected nodules (11 out of 12 and 3 out of 14, respectively), but there was no effect on the growth of the nodules that were not injected. Dykes and Trejdosiewicz (1978) injected CP into carcinomas of the stomach using a gastroscope. Each patient received two doses of between 1.5 and 8 mg CP, and operation was performed 2 weeks after the last injection. Various immunological parameters were studied (vide infra), but no information is given about the subsequent behavior of the patients. In a similar kind of study Boak (1978) injected CP into mammary carcinomas in seven patients 10–14 days before simple mastectomy, and observed enlargement of the ipsilateral axillary lymph nodes associated with marked sinus histiocytosis.

Table 4

Effect of a Single Intravenous Injection of C. Parvum on Survival
After Pulmonary Resection for Lung Cancer

Category	Controls (Pulmonary Resection Only)			Adjuvant Therapy Group (Pulmonary Resection + CP)		
	No. of Patients	No. Alive 3 Years Postop.	No. Alive November 1, 1979	No. of Patients	No. Alive 3 Years Postop.	No. Alive November 1, 1979
All Patients	24	10	7	25	13	13
Patients with undifferentiated tumors	8	2	1	12	5	5

Log rank test for entire table: $x^2 = 1.67$, $p < 0.2$
Data of Woodruff, McCormack, and Walbaum (unpublished).

Webb *et al.* (1978) treated six patients with malignant effusions, five from carcinomas and one from a melanoma, with one or more intrapleural or intraperitoneal injections of CP (Wellcome strain) in a dosage ranging from 3.5 to 14 mg dry weight of organisms. The patients survived for periods ranging from a week to just under a year. The treatment was symptomatically beneficial, however, in that the effusions diminished or disappeared completely. More recently the Ludwig Lung Cancer Study Group (1978) injected CP intrapleurally, or both intrapleurally and intravenously, in 62 patients prior to lobectomy or pneumonectomy for bronchogenic cancer. This was essentially a feasibility trial, and a randomized study has been started to investigate the therapeutic effect of this procedure.

The use of CP in combination with active specific immunotherapy will be considered later (8.26).

Complications of CP therapy.   A fairly clear picture of the complications of CP therapy has begun to emerge from the investigations already cited and other studies (Palmer *et al.*, 1978; Mayr *et al.*, 1978b), and the subject has been reviewed by Milas and Scott (1977) and Whisnant (1978).

For a period of about half an hour to 2 hours after the start of an intravenous infusion of CP there are usually no untoward symptoms. The patient then begins to feel cold and usually shivery and may experience quite severe rigors, lasting from half an hour to an hour, and associated with peripheral vasospasm and tachycardia. The temperature rises, sometimes to as much as 105°F, and the patient may experience nausea, vomiting, and headache. The pyrexia usually subsides within a few hours but may persist for several days. With succeeding injections the reactions become less severe. The severity of the initial reaction may be reduced by administration of hydrocortisone (B. Fisher *et al.*, 1976b), aspirin (Woodruff, unpublished), or promethazine (Osborn and Castro, 1977), but the question arises as to whether these agents may reduce the therapeutic effect of the CP (7.522). In a few patients more severe complications have developed, including angina associated with hypertension (Band *et al.*, 1975), generalized Schwartzman reaction with acute azotemia and severe thrombocytopenia, which did not clear for 10 days (Reed et al., 1975), and transient jaundice with biochemical evidence of hepatocellular damage (Woodruff *et al.*, 1975). After subcutaneous injection of CP the symptoms are usually milder, and consist mainly of local soreness, erythema, and induration, together with mild fever and headache, but local abscess formation has occurred in some cases (Sexauer *et al.*, 1976). To counteract the local pain Israel and Halpern (1972) mixed local anesthetic with the CP. Intratumor injection is associated with the same symptoms as subcutaneous injection. After intrapleural injection about half the patients experienced dyspnea, chest pain, chills, or nausea (Ludwig Lung Cancer Study Group, 1978).

Effect of CP on immunological responses.   Blood lymphocyte, T-cell, and monocyte counts in patients given intravenous infusions of CP vary considerably, but are often temporarily depressed (Israel, 1975; Reed *et al.*, 1975; Ossorio *et al.*, 1975; Woodruff *et al.*, 1975; Cheng *et al.*, 1976; Minton *et al.*, 1976; Ochoa *et al.*, 1976; Gill *et al.*, 1978). There is a very transient fall in the polymorphonuclear leukocyte count, which returns to normal within 24 hours (Gill *et al.*, 1978). Several authors have been unable to find any consistent pattern in sequential studies of the response of the patient's lymphocytes to PHA and other mitogens (Woodruff *et al.*, 1975; R.A. Fisher *et al.*, 1978; Webster *et al.*, 1978), but others have reported a transient depression for a few days (Reed *et al.*, 1975; Minton *et al.*, 1976; Gill *et al.*, 1978), followed by increased reactivity to PHA and concanavalin A 1 to 2 months later in patients who received multiple injecitons (Reed *et al.*, 1975). Transient depression of antibody-dependent and PHA-dependent cell-mediated cytotoxicity has also been reported (Gill *et al.*, 1978).

Increased skin sensitivity to recall antigens and DNCB has been reported in some patients, but no very consistent pattern has emerged (Reed *et al.*, 1975; Hirshaut *et al.*, 1975; Cheng *et al.*, 1976; Webster *et al.*, 1978).

A consistent increase in the levels of IgG, especially of the IgG_{2b} subclass, the development of antibodies to CP, and the transient appearance of "rheumatoid-factor-like" substances in the serum of patients who received repeated small doses of CP (the first intravenously) were reported by James *et al.* (1975). Similar changes in IgG and antibody to CP were reported subsequently by Osborn and Castro (1977) in patients who received repeated intravenous infusions of CP. In later studies James *et al.* (1978) observed changes similar to those they had previously described, but less marked, in patients with advanced bronchogenic cancer treated with cyclophosphamide and CP. In one out of seven of these patients, and in three out of seven patients with malignant cerebral gliomas* who received intralesional CP, there was a transient appearance of antinuclear factor (James *et al.*, 1978).

Depression of serum levels of the third (C3) and fourth (C4) components of complement has been observed in patients given CP intravenously (Dimitrov, Israel, and Peltier, 1975; Biran *et al.*, 1975), and there is evidence that CP activates complement, via both the classical pathway and the alternative pathway, when natural or induced antibodies to CP are present (McBride *et al.*, 1975c; Biran *et al.*, 1975).

8.244   OTHER BACTERIAL PREPARATIONS

Bordetella pertussis.   Guyer and Crowther (1969) studied the effect of weekly or twice weekly intramuscular injections of *B. pertussis* vaccine in eight patients with acute lymphoblastic leukemia who had been brought into remission by chemotherapy. The median time to relapse was 186 days, as compared with 112 days in a matched group of patients who received no further treatment after a similar course of chemotherapy, but there were no long-term remissions in either group.

Pseudomonas aeruginosa.   It was observed in a trial designed to see whether the incidence of infectious complications in patients with acute non-lymphoblastic leukemia could be reduced by the administration of *Ps. aeruginosa* vaccine, that a number of long remissions occured in the vaccine-treated patients (Young *et al.*, 1973; Clarkson *et al.*, 1975). A randomized trial was therefore set up in patients with this form of leukemia to compare the effect of chemotherapy alone and chemotherapy combined with repeated intramuscular injections of a lipopolysaccharide preparation derived from *Ps. aeruginosa* (Gee *et al.*, 1978). If a remission occurred treatment was continued throughout the consolidation period. In addition, 4 of 12 patients in whom a complete remission had been achieved with chemotherapy only, were treated with the lipopolysaccharide.

No significant difference was observed in the proportion of patients in each group

---

*Under the care of Mr. E. R. Hitchcock, at the Western General Hospital, Edinburgh.

who went into remission or in the length of remission, but when reported there were only 29 patients in the randomized trial.

Clostridia.   Spores of *C. butyricum* (strain M55) were injected intralesionally or intravenously to patients with advanced tumors by Möse *et al.* (1967). This evoked a pyrexial reaction, which was sometimes marked and persistent. There was reported to be evidence of oncolysis in some patients. Subsequently, Carey *et al.* (1967) treated five patients with advanced, and for the most part unusual, tumors, with an intravenous infusion containing 10^{10} spores of *C. butyricum,* together with penicillin and polymyxin. The patients survived for 10 days, 22 days, 54 days, 4 months, and 13 months. Some oncolysis was observed, but in general the tumors continued to progress. Carey *et al.* suggest that the procedure is likely to have only a limited place in treatment; their paper, however, leaves the reader with the feeling that it is unlikely to have any.

8.245   VIRAL INFECTION

De Pace (1912) reported regression of carcinoma of the cervix in a woman undergoing Pasteur's treatment for rabies. More recently, natural infection with measles has been reported to have had a beneficial effect in children with acute lymphoblastic leukemia (Starr and Berkovich, 1964; Smithwick and Berkovich, 1966), and to have been followed by complete regression of Burkitt's lymphoma in an untreated African child who contracted measles shortly after biopsy of the tumor (Bluming and Ziegler, 1971).

Attempts to treat solid tumors and leukemias by inoculation of live virus have on the whole been discouraging (Pack, 1950; Southam and Moore, 1952; Newman and Southam, 1954; R.S. Smith *et al.,* 1956; Webb *et al.,* 1966), apart from intralesional injection of melanomas with vaccinia virus. This last procedure was used initially in patients with disseminated disease (Burdick, 1960; Belisario and Milton, 1961; Burdick and Hank, 1964; Milton, 1963; Milton and Lane Brown, 1966; Hunter-Craig *et al.,* 1970) who had received various other forms of treatment previously. It has been the general experience that intradermal metastases injected with vaccinia often regress completely. Hunter-Craig *et al.* emphasized that subcutaneous metastases and lymph nodes which were injected never disappeared completely, though some showed partial regression; and they observed no regression of uninjected lesions. Milton and his colleagues, however, observed regression in some cases at sites other than those injected, and among 30 patients treated there were 4 in whom it was considered that survival had been prolonged by the treatment. One of these patients was alive and clinically free of tumor 5 years after treatment of widespread recurrence by intralesional injection together with radiotherapy to the inguinal region but not extending to lesions in the flank. The treatment of primary melanomas by injection of vaccine virus was initiated by Dent *et al.* (1972), and subsequently Everall *et al.* (1975) conducted a non-randomized trial in which 23 patients with primary malignant melanoma were treated by injection of the lesion with vaccinia virus followed 14 days later by wide local excision, and 25 patients were treated by wide local excision only. It is noteworthy that all but three of the vaccinia-treated patients had previously been vaccinated. The preliminary results reported were interpreted as suggesting that "intralesional vaccinia may delay or possibly prevent the onset of metastases from a primary melanoma," but the evidence is insufficient to allow a firm conclusion to be drawn.

Opinions have differed as to whether previous vaccination of a patient affects the response of his tumor to treatment with vaccinia. Milton and Lane Brown (1966) concluded that a worthwhile remission could only be achieved if the patient was not immune to the virus. If this is correct the fact that Hunter-Craig *et al.* (1970) deliberately vaccinated or revaccinated some of their patients before intralesional injection may account for their failure to obtain any regression except in the lesions injected. It also suggests that the results obtained by Everall *et al.* (1975) might have been more decisive if more of their patients had been previously unvaccinated.

As an alternative to injecting live virus into tumors *in situ,* Lindenmann (1973, 1974) suggested preparing a "viral oncolysate" by growing a suitably adapted virus in excised tumor tissue, and injecting this back into the patient. The original intention was to render the virus innocuous either by inactivating it or by preimmunizing the patient, but in the first case reported (Sauter *et al.*, 1972) the virus used, an avian influenza virus, was thought to be non-pathogenic for man and was not inactivated. This patient was suffering from acute myelogenous leukemia, and a remission was achieved comparable with those obtained by chemotherapy. A randomized trial was set up later in which patients with AML were brought into remission with chemotherapy and then maintained either with chemotherapy alone or with chemotherapy plus monthly intradermal and subcutaneous injections of formalin-inactivated viral oncolysate prepared from allogeneic leukemic myeloblasts infacted with an avian myxovirus, given on the 15th day of the chemotherapy cycle (Sauter *et al.*, 1978). When reported there was no significant difference between the two groups. It was proposed to undertake a further study with oncolysate from autologous cells, possibly using ultraviolet light rather than formalin to inactivate the virus.

Possible mechanisms of viral oncolysis were discussed in the previous chapter (7.54). Evidence in support of the hypothesis that inoculation with vaccinia virus may activate cell-mediated immunity against melanoma cells has been reported by Roenigk *et al.* (1974).

8.246   POLYNUCLEOTIDES

Phase I studies of Poly I:Poly C in patients with large tumor burdens have defined safe levels of dosage but have not revealed any significant antitumor effect (De Vita *et al.*, 1970; Young, 1971; Hilleman *et al.*, 1971; Robinson *et al.*, 1976). The study by Robinson *et al.* included 7 patients with acute lymphatic leukemia, 2 with acute myeloid leukemia, 2 with chronic myeloid leukemia in blast crisis, and 26 with advanced solid tumors of various kinds which had proved refractory to conventional treatment. No objective remissions were observed following intravenous administration of Poly I:Poly C in three dose schedules: 0.3–75 mg/m^2 on day 0 and then daily for up to 35 days; 12–37.5 mg/m^2 every second day for 6–9 doses; 4–50 mg/m^2 daily for 28 days. Moreover, progression of the disease during the treatment was observed in all the patients with leukemia and in 17 of those with solid tumors. Four patients were given Poly I:Poly C by intramuscular injection, and two by inhalation, without benefit. Mathé *et al.* (1970b) reported five complete remissions in 15 patients with ALL whose bone marrow contained less than 50 percent of blast cells treated with Poly I:Poly C in a dosage of 1 mg/m^2 per day for 8–16 days, but treatment of patients with AML who were in remission following chemotherapy with Poly I:Poly C has been ineffective, or at most marginally effective (McIntyre *et al.*, 1978; Sodomann *et al.*, 1972).

A possible reason for the ineffectiveness of Poly I:Poly C in man is that it appears to be rapidly broken down by an enzyme present in human serum (Nordlund *et al.*, 1970). H.B. Levy *et al.* (1975) have therefore started a trial of a stabilized Poly I:Poly C-Poly-L-lysine compound which is resistant to the action of this enzyme.

Toxicity. Mathé *et al.* (1970b), using the dose stated above, observed no evidence of toxicity. Robinson *et al.* (1976) reported fever in 29 of 44 separate trials conducted in their 26 patients, lasting usually for 24–36 hours, with a mean peak elevation of temperature of 1.5°C occurring 6–12 hours after administration of Poly I:Poly C. In 26 trials there was a slight increase in the thrombin time and in the serum level of fibrin degradation products, and in 11 trials transient elevation of serum glutamic-oxaloacetic transaminase (SGOT) and glutamic-pyruvic transaminase (SGPT), but the level of these enzymes appeared to be unrelated to the dose of Poly I:Poly C. One patient receiving a dose of 2.5 mg/m^2 developed laboratory evidence of disseminated intravascular coagulation, and two patients developed moderately severe hypersensitivity reactions characterized by bronchospasm, chest and flank pain, and pedaledema after doses of 2.5 and 35 mg/m^2. Cornell *et al.* (1976) reported a flu-like illness, characterized by fever, occasional chills, myalgia, and nausea, in nearly all patients receiving Poly I:Poly C in a dosage greater than 1 mg/kg and a transient increase of SGOT in 4 of 13 patients receiving doses greater than 6 mg/kg.* The degree of fever correlated with the dose and was associated with an increase in the absolute granulocyte count. There was laboratory evidence of intravascular coagulation in one patient who received a dose of 10 mg/kg. McIntyre *et al.* (1978) observed fever, sometimes with chills, nausea, and vomiting, in patients receiving doses of 300 mg/m^2, and in one patient vasomotor collapse and wheezing which responded to antihistamines and adrenalin.

Effect on immunological activity and interferon production. Mathé *et al.* (1970b) reported that three of their 15 patients developed sensitivity to recall antigens, and three showed an increased lymphocyte response to PHA *in vitro.*

Although, as already mentioned, Poly I:Poly C appears to be rapidly destroyed by an enzyme in human plasma (Nordlund *et al.*, (1970), its administration in acceptable dosage may induce the formation of small but measurable amounts of interferon in patients (Robinson *et al.*, 1976; Cornell *et al.*, 1976; McIntyre *et al.*, 1978), first detectable after 6–8 hours and reaching its peak after 15–24 hours. The response to different doses of Poly I:Poly C has, however, varied widely. Robinson *et al.* found no measurable response with doses below 1 mg/m^2; thereafter the response increased in a rather erratic way and then declined sharply with doses of 50 mg/m^2 or more. Cornell *et al.* found that doses of 1–10 mg/kg evoked the same response, whereas with doses below 1 mg/kg there was no response. McIntyre *et al.* observed a response in 28 out of 33 patients who received 300 mg/m^2.

8.247 LEVAMISOLE

A multicenter randomized double-blind study of levamisole as an adjuvant to pulmonary resection in patients with operable cancer has been undertaken by the

---

*It may be helpful to remember that in human adults ranging in height from 1.5 to 1.8 m (5 to 6 feet), and weighing between 50 and 110 kg (110 to 240 pounds), a dose of 1 mg/kg corresponds to somewhere between 35 and 50 mg/m^2.

Study Group for Bronchogenic Cancer (1975), and more recent reports of this study have been published by the chairman of the Group (Amery, 1976, 1978). The patients received either a placebo or levamisole by mouth in a dosage of 50 mg three times per day for 3 days prior to operation, and this course was repeated every 2 weeks thereafter. The results show that, in patients weighing 70 kg or less, there were fewer recurrences in those who received levamisole, and when recurrence did occur it was confined to the chest except in one patient, though the number of deaths attributed to cancer was not significantly different in the treated and control (placebo) groups. In patients weighing over 70 kg, of whom there were 77 out of a total of 147 in the trial, there was no significant difference in the number of recurrences in the two groups, and it was concluded that the dose per kg received by these patients was too small. The validity of conclusions based on the retrospective separation of patients into two groups according to their weight has been challenged, and it has been suggested that a new trial should be undertaken using weight-related doses of the drug.

Rojas et al. (1976, 1978) investigated the effect of administering levamisole in a dose of 150 mg orally three times a week in alternate weeks to patients with locally advanced inoperable breast cancer who were said to have been rendered clinically disease-free by radiotherapy to the breast, supraclavicular region, and axilla. Twenty patients treated in this way were compared with alternate patients who received the same radiotherapy but no levamisole. There was reported to be significant prolongation of the median disease-free interval (25 months as against 9 months) and of survival (90 percent alive at 30 months as against 35 percent of the controls). It is of interest, however, in relation to the suggestion that levamisole is particularly effective in preventing distant metastases from developing (Amery, 1976), that the incidence and distribution of metastases was not significantly different in the levamisole-treated and control patients, except that lung metastases were actually more frequent in those who received levamisole (8 out of 20 as compared with 4 out of 23), possibly because the treated patients survived longer.

Spitler et al. (1978), in a randomized study, investigated the effect of levamisole, again in a dosage of 150 mg on three occasions every second week, as an adjuvant to surgical excision of all known tumor, in patients with various stages of melanoma. No significant benefit was observed.

Toxicity.   In most cases there has been no evidence of serious toxicity in the dosage employed. Some patients have complained of nausea, vomiting, diarrhea, tiredness, headache, bitter taste, itchy erythematous rashes, and insomnia. These symptoms have in general not been severe or of long duration (Oettgen et al., 1976; Rojas et al., 1976), but Thornes (1978a) has reported severe nausea, vomiting and skin rashes which made it necessary to stop administration of levamisole.

Effect on immune responses.   Tripodi et al. (1973) reported that 14 out of 20 cancer patients who were anergic to DNCB or tuberculin or both, and who received 150 mg levamisole daily by mouth, showed increased responses, whereas 14 control patients who did not receive levamisole remained anergic. Increased responses to DNCB was also observed by Rojas et al. (1976) in patients with advanced breast cancer who remained clinically free of disease 30 months after radiotherapy and commencement of treatment with levamisole, whereas patients who developed recurrence before 20 months showed no significant increase in reactivity. Hirshaut et al. (1973), however, in a randomized study of patients with advanced cancer, failed to demonstrate a clear effect of levamisole on reactivity to DNCB; in another study, while prolonged treatment boosted reactivity to DNCB in some patients it failed to restore reactivity in any patient who was initially unresponsive to 200 μg DNCB (Verhaegen *et al.,* 1973), in contrast to the findings of Tripodi *et al.* Conflicting results have also been reported concerning the *in vitro* response of lymphocytes from patients treated with levamisole to PHA (Verhaegen *et al.,* 1973; Renoux, Renoux, and Palat, 1975; Oettgen, Pinsky, and Delmonte, 1976). In Hodgkin's disease the number of T cells as estimated by their capacity to form E rosettes *in vitro* is increased by levamisole administration (Biniaminov and Ramot, 1975), and the chemotactic response of human monocytes may be increased by incubation with levamisole *in vitro* (Pike and Snyderman, 1976b). Resistance to infection of various kinds may also be increased by administration of levamisole.

8.248   ANTICOAGULANTS AND FIBRINOLYTIC AGENTS

Michaels (1964) reviewed the histories of 540 patients on oral anticoagulant therapy for thromboembolic disease who had been observed for a total of 1569 patient years, and found a total of 22 cancers in 19 patients, in contrast to 8 predicted. This report has stimulated interest in the possible use of anticoagulants and fibrinolytic agents in the treatment of cancer.

Thornes (1969) reported 100 patients with advanced or recurrent cancer who were given conventional chemotherapy together with warfarin or some other coumarin derivative in sufficient dosage to keep the prothrombin time at about twice the normal level. Fifteen patients showed objective responses, characterized by partial regression of the tumor, maintenance of the hemoglobin level, and a return to active status in the community for more than 2 years; 14 others showed subjective improvement. A second trial was therefore undertaken (Thornes, 1972a, 1975) in which alternate patients with recurrent tumors of particular types, including lymphosarcoma, carcinoma of the ovary, and carcinoma of the breast, were given warfarin in addition to standard chemotherapy. This increased the 2 year survival, though the difference was significant only in the patients with cancer of the breast. Thornes (1972b) has also reported that, in a small group of patients on maintenance therapy for lymphoma or chronic leukemia, sensitivity to cytotoxic drugs was restored in 21 patients out of 30 by the addition of warfarin to the treatment schedule. In another trial patients with Stage IV breast cancer are being treated with either chemotherapy alone or chemotherapy plus levamisole, BCG, and warfarin (Thornes, 1978a). When reported there were fewer deaths in the group receiving immunotherapy and these patients appeared to tolerate their chemotherapy better, but further time is required to see whether these trends are maintained.

Hoover *et al.* (1978) used warfarin as an adjuvant to amputation in patients with osteosarcomas. Survival was better than in another group of patients treated by amputation only, but this was not a randomized trial and it is not possible to assess the significance of the findings.

A fibrinolytic agent, streptokinase, has been tried as an adjuvant to surgery in the treatment of operable colorectal cancer (Thornes, 1975, 1978b). The patients were randomly subdivided into two groups; those in one group were given an infusion of streptokinase in the operating room immediately after resection of the tumor, while those in the other group received an infusion of saline instead. When last analyzed

(Thornes, 1978b), the 3 year and 5 year survival rates were greater in the patients who received streptokinase, but the differences were not statistically significant. The dose of streptokinase required to achieve effective fibrinolysis was titrated just prior to infusion, and if the dose predicted exceeded 500,000 units the patient was not admitted to the trial. This precaution, combined with careful hemostasis, sufficed to avoid serious bleeding.

The suggestion that the antitumor effects we have been discussing depend, at least in part, on immunological mechanisms gains support from the observation that, in patients anergic to a variety of antigens, sensitivity may be restored by administration of streptokinase, or of brinase—a proteolytic enzyme from *Aspergillus oryzal* which lowers antiplasmin levels in man and promotes the appearance of antilymphocytic and antileukemic antibodies in patients with leukemia (Thornes, 1974; Thornes *et al.*, 1974).

8.249 PHYTOHEMAGGLUTININ, POLYSACCHARIDES, THYMOSIN

E. Robinson (1966) treated five patients with generalized carcinomatosis with PHA, and observed clear-cut but temporary improvement in each case. No information concerning dosage was given. Chretien *et al.* (1978) have reported that the survival of patients with oat cell carcinoma of the lung treated by chemotherapy, and who showed evidence of immunosuppression, was increased if they were given thymosin (see Goldstein, 1978; G.D. Marshall, 1978).

Trials are in progress or about to start with a variety of other substances, including a naturally occurring polysaccharide from a species of mushroom and the synthetic polysaccharide glucan (Muggia, 1977).

8.24(10) SUBSTANCES TO EVOKE A LOCAL HYPERSENSITIVITY REACTION

E. Klein and her colleagues treated skin tumors by repeated application of DNCB, or other substances which also evoke skin hypersensitivity reactions. This caused a more intense reaction in the tumor than in the surrounding normal skin, and by daily application of an appropriate dose it was possible to achieve complete and permanent regression of some tumors, including basal cell carcinomas and squamous cell carcinomas *in situ,* at the cost of only a minimal reaction in normal skin (Helm and Klein, 1965; E. Klein, 1968a, 1968b, 1969). The same procedure has been used in patients with mycosis fungoides and basal cell carcinomas by Ratner, Waldorf, and Scott (1968) and Stjernsward and Levin (1971), with complete or partial regression in many cases; Stjernsward and Levin also observed regression of metastases in the skin from lymphoma and carcinoma of the breast. Castermans-Elias *et al.* (1977) applied DNCB to primary melanomas on three occasions at weekly intervals, and then performed wide local excision of the tumors without lymphadenectomy. DNCB was applied subsequently to the site of operation every 3 months for a year and then every 6 months. All patients (23 in number) whose tumors had not been biopsied prior to the start of treatment, and 10 out of 14 whose tumors had been biopsied, showed no evidence of recurrence after 3 years. The authors concluded modestly that the treatment had not worsened the prognosis in the patients not previously subjected to biopsy.

Guthrie and Way (1975) treated six patients who had previously had a hysterectomy and in whom three or more vaginal smears had been positive for malignant cells, but who were free of symptoms, by application of DNCB to the arm or leg, followed by an application to the vagina 3 weeks later. Before the vaginal application skin tests were done, and a dose was chosen which only just produced a reaction in the skin. When reported the patients had been followed up for 2, 13, 17, 24, 27, and 35 months, and the smears had remained negative throughout.

8.24(11) HYPERTHERMIA

There have been many studies of the sensitivity of tumor cells to hyperthermia *in vitro* and *in vivo*. The methods of heating used *in vivo* include *whole body hyperthermia* by immersion in hot water (Kirsch and Schmidt, 1966; Von Ardenne, 1971) or by covering the body with molten wax combined in some cases with inhalation of heated gases (Henderson and Pettigrew, 1971; Pettigrew *et al.,* 1974a, 1974b); and *local hyperthermia* by limb perfusion, sometimes with solutions containing cytotoxic drugs (Woodhall *et al.,* 1960; Cavaliere *et al.,* 1967, 1976; Stehlin *et al.,* 1975; Stehlin, 1976), immersion of the part in a hot bath (Crile, 1961a, 1962; Hartman and Crile, 1968; Dickson and Muckle, 1972; Dickson and Ellis, 1976), local irrigation (Hall *et al.,* 1974), application of a heat pipe (Dickson and Shah, 1977), short-wave diathermy (Westermark, 1927; Hartman and Crile, 1968), electrocoagulation (Strauss *et al.,* 1962, 1965; Strauss, 1969; Crile and Turnbull, 1972), and radio frequency heating (Le Veen *et al.,* 1976; Dickson and Shah, 1977).

Temperatures in the vicinity of 42°C, though in general well tolerated by normal cells, are lethal to some, though by no means all, tumor cells (Selawry, Goldstein, and McCormick, 1957; Mondovi *et al.,* 1969; Dickson and Suzanger, 1976; Mondovi, 1976; Dickson, 1977). Raising the body temperature to this level has been shown to cause regression or partial regression of some animal tumors (Westermark, 1927; Crile, 1961a, 1962) and partial regression of some human tumors (Cavaliere *et al.,* 1967; Hartman and Crile, 1968; Pettigrew *et al.,* 1974a). Radio frequency heating has been used to raise the intratumor temperature to between 45°C and 50°C; by this means animal tumors resistant to lower temperatures have been made to regress without destruction of normal tissues (Le Veen *et al.,* 1976; Dickson and Shah, 1977), and substantial partial regression has been achieved with some human tumors (Le Veen *et al.,* 1976). Hyperthermia may also potentiate the effect of radiotherapy (Rohdenburg and Prime, 1921; Warren, 1935; Selawry, Carlson, and Moore, 1958; Crile, 1962; Brenner and Yerushalmi, 1975) and of cytotoxic drugs given systemically (Pettigrew *et al.,* 1974a) or by regional perfusion (Woodhall *et al.,* 1960; Stehlin, 1976). This may be related to the fact that, in an animal tumor, hyperthermia has been shown to bring non-cycling cells back into cycle (Dickson and Calderwood, 1976). Cavaliere *et al.* (1976) have used hyperthermic perfusion prior to amputation for osteogenic sarcoma and recurrent melanoma. Six out of twelve patients with osteogenic sarcoma were alive with no evidence of disease 3 to 8½ years after the perfusion. Both Stehlin and Cavaliere *et al.* have reported the disappearance of metastases in patients treated by hyperthermic perfusion, and have suggested that this is due to stimulation of the host immune reaction as a result of destruction of the tumor.

On the other hand, it has been shown in animal systems that hyperthermia may cause increased dissemination of a transplanted tumor (Dickson and Ellis, 1974) and impair the functional activity of cytotoxic T lymphocytes (McDonald, 1977). The effect on T cells requires further investigation, however, and Thornes *et al.* (1978) have preliminary evidence that radio frequency heating of the thymus may, under certain conditions, increase the proportion of T cells in the circulation.

As already mentioned (8.2), the question arises as to whether destruction of a tumor by hyperthermia or other means stimulates immunological defence mechanisms. Conversely, it has been suggested (Norman, 1975; Muggia, 1977) that the antitumor effect of agents like BCG, CP, viruses, and polynucleotides, which evoke a marked febrile reaction, may be due, at least in part, to the rise in temperature within the tumor. The general body temperature, which rarely exceeds 40.5°C (105°F) and is commonly not more than 39.5°C (103°F), is below the temperature at which tumor cells are likely to be destroyed. The important parameter, however, is the temperature within the tumor, and the observation by Gough and Furnival (1978) that 24 hours after intralesional injection of *C. parvum* the temperature in the center of the tumor was 44°C, while the sublingual temperature was 39.5°C, suggests that hyperthermia may play a part in this form of therapy. It may be thought unlikely that intratumor temperatures of this order would occur in patients treated by systemic administration of any of the non-specific immunopotentiating agents we have been discussing, but pending further investigation the question should be regarded as *sub judice*. The matter is of practical as well as theoretical importance because many investigators have refrained from attempting to control the pyrexial reactions for fear that, if successful, this might weaken the antitumor effect.

8.25   Active Specific Immunization

8.251   EARLY INVESTIGATIONS

The treatment of cancer patients with material derived from tumors was initiated by von Leyden and Blumenthal (1902), who injected three patients with advanced cancer with fluid expressed from their own tumors. During the next 50 years or so material prepared from autologous or allogeneic tumor tissue was widely used in an empirical way, mainly in patients with advanced cancer but also, in some patients, prior to surgical excision of an operable tumor. Some of these preparations were fresh and undoubtedly contained viable tumor cells; others had been treated with alcohol, formalin, or phenol, or frozen and thawed. Kellock, Chambers, and Russ (1922) used irradiated autologous tumor tissue, but the dose of irradiation was so small that it would seem to be of no significance. Many of the reports relate to only a few cases, but quite large series were published by Coca, Dorrance, and Lebredo (1912) (87 cases), Vaughan (1914) (over 200 cases), Kellock *et al.* (1922) (30 cases), and Witebsky, Rose, and Shulman (1956) (20 cases). This work has been reviewed by Southam (1961), and subsequently by others (Currie, 1972; Baker and Taub, 1973a). Some objective remissions were reported, and Vaughan (1914) made the perhaps prophetic comment that "the best results are obtained in cases in which the amount of tumor tissue is small, and in which the differential leucocyte count of the patient shows a decided reaction following administration of the cancer protein." The evidence, however, does not stand up well to critical examination, and Southam's (1961) conclusion that there is no proof that this treatment, or other forms of immunotherapy attempted during the same period, had any influence on the behavior of the tumour, seems fully justified. Southam added, however, and the comments seem reasonable, that "unless we could prove that the occasional clinical responses which were observed were unrelated to the treatment used, these rare instances cannot be considered biologically insignificant," and that "if any one of these reported responses was in fact a result of some immunological reaction we cannot say that it is inconsequential."

8.252   UNMODIFIED OR IRRADIATED TUMOR CELLS
WITH OR WITHOUT ADJUVANTS

A more rational approach to active immunization was introduced by Graham
and Graham (1959, 1962), who based their trials on a previous investigation (Graham
and Graham, 1955) in which they had demonstrated complement fixation when sera
from 12 of 48 patients studied who had recently been treated by surgery or radiotherapy for gynecologic cancers were incubated with water-soluble extracts of autologous
tumor tissue. Graham and Graham (1959, 1962) treated in all 232 patients, most of
them suffering from advanced or recurrent cancer of the cervix, body of the uterus,
and ovary, with intradermal and intramuscular injections of autologous whole tumor
cells, cell fragments, or tumor extracts in Freund-type adjuvant. The procedure was
shown to be safe, and there was some suggestion that when patients in whom the bulk
of the tumor had been surgically removed were treated in this way the residual disease
was more responsive to radiotherapy. Apart from this it was concluded that the treatment failed to alter the course of the disease with sufficient regularity to justify its use.
Taylor and Odili (1972) also injected tumor homogenate in Freund's adjuvant in 12
patients with advanced tumors and observed some partial regression associated with
histological changes suggestive of delayed type hypersensitivity. Finney, Byers, and
Wilson (1960) treated three patients with secondary subcutaneous melanomas by intralesional injection of antibody containing globulin prepared from the patient's plasma after active immunization with frozen–thawed autologous tumor tissue in
Freund's adjuvant. The injected lesions were reported to decrease in size and showed
extensive necrosis on histological examination.

Treatment with irradiated autologous cells in patients with melanoma may evoke
both cytotoxic antibody (Ikonopisov et al., 1970) and specific lymphocyte cytotoxicity
(Currie, Lejeune, and Fairley, 1971), but despite this it appears to have had little or no
beneficial effect (van den Brenk, 1969; Ikonopisov et al., 1970; Currie et al., 1971; Krementz et al., 1971), apart from one remarkable case reported by Krementz et al. of a
patient given immunotherapy for recurrence of a melanoma after hindquarter amputation in whom the tumor regressed completely and who died 4 years later, reportedly
from a heart attack. In osteogenic sarcoma, although the initial report of Marcove et
al. (1973) appeared moderately encouraging, subsequent reports (Douglass et al.,
1975; Miké and Marcove, 1978) have not revealed any clear beneficial effect from active immunization procedures. In cancer of the breast, Gorodilova et al. (1965) reported "better survival" in 32 patients with Stage II and Stage III lesions who received
autologous tumor vaccine than in other patients who did not. Anderson et al. (1974,
1978) injected irradiated autologous tumor cells, subcutaneously and intradermally,
a few hours after mastectomy to 12 patients with Stage II and 4 with Stage III breast
cancer. All the patients were subsequently given radiotherapy. Forty to 66 months later these patients' leukocytes showed significantly increased reactivity to allogeneic
mammary cancer cells in leukocyte migration-inhibition tests. The survival of the 16
patients given autologous tumor cells was compared with that of 139 patients with
Stage II breast cancer treated in the same hospital by surgery and radiotherapy alone.
Ten of the 16 patients were alive after 6 years as compared with 41 of the 139 who did
not receive immunotherapy, and more detailed analysis of the two survival curves was
reported to show a significant difference. It was suggested in the discussion of this paper that the differences in the leukocyte migration tests were not as significant as they

appeared, and that a randomized study should be undertaken to see if this would confirm the reported prolongation of survival in the patients given immunotherapy.

Nadler and Moore (1970) treated 173 patients with advanced cancer with either irradiated or non-irradiated allogeneic cultured tumor cells, but without beneficial effect except in one patient with an osteogenic sarcoma who also received chemotherapy.

As mentioned previously (8.242), in Mathé's first trial of immunotherapy for acute lymphoblastic leukemia, there were five patients who, after remission induction by chemotherapy, received only intradermal and subcutaneous injections of formalin-treated or irradiated allogeneic leukemic cells; three of these were still in remission at the time of the first report, but in later reports the three groups of patients who received different forms of immunotherapy were pooled. Skurkovich et al. (1969a) treated pairs of children with various forms of acute leukemia by repeated intravenous and intramuscular injections of blood leukocytes and bone marrow from the other member of the pair. They observed a fall in the blood leukocyte count, a decrease in the size of the lymph nodes, spleen, and liver, and improvement in the general condition in 8 out of 12 patients. Eight to 15 days after the last injection plasma and peripheral blood leukocytes were interchanged between members of each pair, and this resulted in a further fall in the blood leukocyte count. Powles et al. (1971), as a preliminary to a trial of combined specific and non-specific immunotherapy (8.26) in AML, studied the response of patients in remission to injection of irradiated autologous leukemic cells. They found that injection of 1×10^9 cells was required to increase transiently the reactivity of the patient's blood lymphocytes to autologous lymphocytes which had been collected and stored before induction of a remission by chemotherapy, as judged by transformation in mixed cultures. This observation was confirmed by Gutterman et al. (1973).

8.253 ENZYME-TREATED TUMOR CELLS

Wilson et al. (1963) treated 25 patients with advanced solid tumors by injecting autologous tumor cells mixed with Freund's adjuvant and hyaluronidase. Temporary regression was observed in some patients.

Bekesi et al. (Bekesi, Roboz, and Holland, 1977; Holland and Bekesi, 1978), in a randomized trial, found that patients with acute myeloid leukemia in whom a remission had been induced with chemotherapy remained in remission significantly longer if given maintenance chemotherapy plus intradermal injections of neuraminidase-treated allogeneic myeloblasts than if given maintenance chemotherapy only. The cell dose was considerable: 2×10^8 cells at each of 48 sites monthly, midway between chemotherapy courses.

The use of neuraminidase-treated cells in conjunction with BCG will be considered later (8.26).

8.254 ANTIGENIC TUMOR EXTRACTS

Hughes, Kearney, and Tully (1970) treated 20 patients with advanced tumors with a vaccine consisting of microsomal and mitochondrial fractions of autologous tumor cells mixed with adjuvants of various kinds. Ten of the patients developed delayed-type hypersensitivity to autologous tumor antigens. Seven showed temporary regression but no long-term benefit.

Humphrey et al. (1971a, 1971b), in the course of studying the effect of interchange of plasma and lymphocytes between pairs of patients with advanced cancer reciprocally immunized with a crude tumor homogenate of each other's tumor (8.233), observed an objective response in four patients before completion of the exchange of plasma and leukocytes, and suggested that this might be due to the active immunization. Subsequently (Humphrey *et al.,* 1972) they observed partial remission in the form of a decrease in size of superficial or pulmonary tumors in 42 of 181 patients with advanced cancer following injection of the same type of allogeneic tumor homogenate, or a concentrated cell-free preparation derived from this.

Stewart *et al.* (1978), in a trial in which there were some randomized and some historical controls, compared the effect of adjuvant chemotherapy with methotrexate, and adjuvant therapy with methotrexate plus monthly injections of a soluble extract of allogeneic lung cancer tissue in Freund's adjuvant, following pulmonary resection for operable lung cancer. The disease-free interval was reported to be shorter in patients with Stage I tumors in the immunotherapy group, but the significance of this is uncertain because the number of patients was small, and the chemotherapy was not entirely uniform.

8.255 XENOGENIZED TUMOR CELLS

The term xenogenization has, as we have seen (7.63), been used to denote the process of altering tumor cells in such a way that they acquire foreign antigens, i.e., antigens which they do not normally possess (Kobayashi, Kodama, and Gotohda, 1977).

Xenogenized tumor cells were first used clinically by Czajkowski *et al.* (1967) in 14 patients with advanced cancer. A cell suspension was prepared from excised autologous tumor tissue and the cells were coupled to rabbit gamma globulin (Cohn fraction II) with *bis*-diazobenzidine, washed, and resuspended. The final suspension was emulsified with incomplete Freund's adjuvant and injected intradermally and intramuscularly every 2–3 weeks. Two patients were alive and clinically tumor-free 4 years after the beginning of immunization. One of these had been given two courses of immunotherapy for an inoperable squamous cell carcinoma invading the mandible; the other, one course of treatment for a carcinoma of the breast which had recurred after operation. Neither of these patients received any other treatment after the start of the immunotherapy, apart from plastic surgery to repair the tissue defect in the first patient. Three other patients showed stabilization or slow progression of the tumor, and nine died 9 weeks to 18 months after treatment was begun. Of the 14 patients, 13 showed precipitating antibody in their serum to a fluorocarbon extract of their own tumor and also to pooled tumor antigen, and frozen sections of tumors from 11 of the patients showed specific immunofluorescence when treated with posttreatment serum and fluorescein-labeled antihuman globulin. Eight of ten patients tested were found to have developed skin sensitivity to extracts of their own tumors. Other reports of similar treatment are conflicting. Takita and Brugarolas (1972) reported prolongation of survival in patients with residual mediastinal lymph node metastases after pulmonary resection for lung cancer, whereas Cunningham *et al.* (1969) observed only one objective remission attributable to the immunotherapy in 41 patients with a variety of tumors treated with autologous tumor cells coupled to rabbit globulin.

Ayre (1969) treated seven patients with carcinoma of the cervix *in situ* by intralesional injection of protein material derived from a wide variety of cancers and coupled to rabbit gamma globulin with *bis*-diazobenzidine. In two patients the lesion regressed completely, and in another only minimal dysplasia was observed after the treatment.

Two other patients showed moderate regression and were treated and cured surgically, and two were under observation at the time of the report. It is difficult to assess the significance of these results. The patients were under very close supervision, but despite this the trial of new procedures in a condition so readily curable but so potentially dangerous as carcinoma-in-situ of the cervix uteri raises difficult ethical questions.

The use of viral oncolysate has been discussed earlier (8.245).

8.256 PATERNAL CELLS OR TISSUE IN CHORIONCARCINOMA

In the special case of postgestational chorioncarcinoma the possibility exists of evoking an antitumor reaction by immunizing the patient with cells or tissue grafts from the father of the fetus, because the tumor arises from tissue which is of fetal origin.

This was first attempted by Doniach, Crookston, and Cope (1958), who treated one patient by injection of leukocytes and transplantation of skin from her husband. She remained symptom-free for a year but then developed metastases. Hackett and Beech (1961) treated another patient by intradermal, subcutaneous, and intravenous injection of her husband's leukocytes, followed by skin grafts from her husband and an independent donor, which were rejected after 8 days and 28 days, respectively. The patient was then given chemotherapy in the form of 6-mercaptopurine, but the tumor did not regress and she died soon afterwards.

Cinader *et al.* (1961) and Jakoubkova *et al.* (1965) each reported one successful case, but both patients received chemotherapy and both were examples of early disease following hydatidiform mole, a form of the disease which, according to Bagshawe (1966), not infrequently regresses spontaneously. Both received active immunotherapy with paternal cells, and Cinader's patient received in addition passive immunotherapy in the form of serum from rabbits immunized with the husband's seminal fluid.

Bagshawe and Golding (1970) observed a remission in 8 out of 21 patients who received intradermal injections of BCG and skin grafts from the husband, but in only one case was this attributed to the immunotherapy.

Commenting some years ago on the outlook for immunotherapy, the British Medical Journal (1966) suggested that unless it could be shown that chorioncarcinoma was susceptible to immunological attack, the case for using this against other tumors was weak. As Bagshawe (1966) pointed out in reply, however, even normal trophoblast seems remarkably non-susceptible to immunological attack, and there is no obvious reason why neoplastic trophoblast should be any more susceptible.

8.26 Combined Non-specific and Active Specific Immunotherapy

There have been many trials in which patients received both BCG and tumor cells, and a few in which *C. parvum* and other immunopotentiating agents were used instead of, or in addition to, BCG.

In Mathé's original trial of immunotherapy in patients with ALL, as we have seen (8.242, 8.252), seven patients, after induction of a remission by chemotherapy, were treated with BCG plus irradiated allogeneic cells. Except in the first progress report (Mathé, Amiel *et al.*, 1968, 1969a), these patients were pooled with others who received either BCG or irradiated leukemic cells but not both. Seven of the patients in this combined group, but none of the ten patients who did not receive immunotherapy, were alive and in complete remission 10–13 years later (Mathé, Schwarzenberg *et al.*, 1978), and no one else today has any long-term survivors from the chemotherapy available in 1963. Although this trial has been strongly criticized by Peto (1978b) and others, notably on the ground that the patients who did not receive immunotherapy fared unexpectedly badly even by 1963 standards, the results were considered by Mathé to be so decisive that in subsequent trials, undertaken to compare different therapeutic regimens which included new drugs as they became available, all patients received active immunotherapy in the form of BCG or BCG plus CP, together with irradiated frozen or cultured allogeneic leukemic cells (Mathé, Amiel *et al.*, 1971; Mathé, DeVassal *et al.*, 1976, 1977b; Mathé, Schwarzenberg *et al.*, 1978). The addition of CP did not make any significant difference to the results, and it was not established whether cultured cells were more or less effective than frozen cells. Mathé *et al.* concluded that there were fewer late relapses and more second remissions in their patients than in patients treated elsewhere by chemotherapy only. Moreover, there were no lethal complications attributable to immunotherapy, whereas there were 4–28 percent of deaths occurring during remission in patients submitted to maintenance chemotherapy. The prognosis in patients given immunotherapy could be assessed by cytological typing and estimates of the tumor volume, and it was claimed that in the good prognosis category one particular protocol gave an 80 percent cure expectancy (Mathé, De Vassal *et al.*, 1977).

In another trial (Mathé, Belpomme *et al.*, 1975a) 42 patients suffering from terminal leukemic lymphosarcoma were treated as acute lymphoid leukemia patients. Twenty-six entered apparently complete remission. They were then submitted to complementary cell reducing treatment in the form of systemic and intrathecal chemotherapy, and radiotherapy of the CNS and the lymphosarcomatous masses that had been detected at the beginning of leukemic conversion. Eight patients relapsed during this treatment, and 18 were still in complete remission at the end of it. Nine of the patients in remission were submitted to active immunotherapy (BCG plus CP plus irradiated allogeneic leukemic lymphosarcoma cells), and five of these were reported to have remained free of disease for 13 to 66 months; the other nine served as controls, and all except two had died from leukemic manifestations when the report was published.

Trials of combined active immunotherapy in ALL from other centers have been less encouraging than those of Mathé. Andrien *et al.* (1978) conducted a randomized trial with 167 patients. If a remission was induced the patients received one of two chemotherapeutic regimes for consolidation, and if still in complete remission after 1 year they were randomized to receive either maintenance chemotherapy, or immunotherapy in the form of BCG (Pasteur strain) by scarification twice weekly for 6 months and then weekly, together with 4×10^7 frozen allogeneic non-irradiated leukemic blast cells from untreated patients weekly for 3 months and then monthly. Treatment was stopped after 4 years. No difference was observed in relapse rate or survival between the groups, and it seemed doubtful if either had added to the effectiveness of the consolidation therapy. Poplack *et al.* (1978) gave consolidation chemotherapy plus CNS irradiation to patients under 20 years of age with ALL in whom a remission had been induced, followed, if the patient remained in remission, by maintenance chemotherapy alone or in combination with administration of BCG (Pasteur strain) with a Heaf gun plus intradermal injection of allogeneic leukemic cells. There was no significant difference in relapse rate or duration of remission. Some of the patients given

BCG developed positive skin reactions to tuberculin, but there was no other evidence of immunostimulation; indeed both groups showed a decrease in the response of their lymphocytes to PHA *in vitro* (Leventhal *et al.,* 1976).

The use of BCG and allogeneic leukemic cells in AML was initiated by Powles *et al.,* and reports of the first trial were published at an early stage, and 2½ years after entry of the last patient (Powles *et al.,* 1973b, 1977). Prior to any treatment patients were aloocated on an alternate basis to determine what treatment they would receive subsequently if they achieved remission. Of 60 patients who did achieve remission on chemotherapy, 22 were maintained on chemotherapy alone and 38 were given the same chemotherapy together with immunotherapy in the form of weekly administration of BCG (Glaxo strain) with a Heaf gun and weekly intradermal and subcutaneous injections of irradiated allogeneic myeloblasts leukemia cells (total weekly dose 10^9 cells). The cells were collected with a blood cell separator and preserved in a viable state at —179°C in the presence of DMSO (Powles *et al.,* 1973a, 1974). The median survival times were 270 days, and after relapse 75 days, for the patients who received chemotherapy only; 510 days, and after relapse 165 days, for those who received both immunotherapy and chemotherapy. It was concluded that the immunotherapy resulted in both prolongation of the first remission and prolongation of survival after the first relapse, but the difference was statistically significant at the 5 percent level only with respect to survival after the first relapse. It was thought that this might be due to stimulation of the bone marrow, enabling patients who had relapsed after immunotherapy to tolerate the high doses of chemotherapy necessary to constrain the disease. Freeman *et al.* (1973), in an uncontrolled trial using the same immunotherapy protocol, also reported a long period of survival after relapse, and commented on the high proportion of patients in whom they were able to induce a second remission. Similar findings were reported by Fennely, McBride, and O'Connell (1975) following an uncontrolled trial in six patients.

In view of the encouraging early results of the first trial, Powles and his colleagues undertook a second (non-randomized) trial to compare the effectiveness of irradiated and non-irradiated allogeneic leukemic cells, when used in combination with BCG, as maintenance therapy in AML, but observed no difference in either duration of remission or survival (Powles, 1974; Russell, Chapuis, and Powles, 1976). Some of the patients in this study who had received BCG and irradiated cells (to different sites) were subsequently given intradermal injections of a mixture of BCG and cells, but this addition had no effect on either duration of remission or survival (Russell *et al.,* 1976).

Mathé *et al.* (1975b) treated 18 patients with AML in remission with BCG (Pasteur strain) by scarification and injection of irradiated allogeneic frozen AML cells and reported longer duration of complete remission and survival than in historical controls. They considered that the results were disappointing because the remission duration and survival after remission curves both declined steadily, and were not broken to form a "cure expectancy plateau" such as they had observed in patients with ALL given immunotherapy.

Reizenstein *et al.* (1978), in a small randomized trial involving 30 patients with acute non-lymphatic leukemia, reported longer survival in those given immunotherapy in the form of BCG plus non-irradiated leukemic cells injected to the same limb.

Peto (1978a), reporting a randomized trial organized by the British Medical Research Council which compared chemotherapy alone with chemotherapy plus immunotherapy in the form of BCG and irradiated allogeneic leukemic blast cells for maintenance of patients with AML in remission, stated that there was no substantial difference between the two groups, but added a note in proof stating that as the trial progressed it had become apparent that survival after the first relapse was prolonged in the patients given immunotherapy, as reported by others in the papers discussed above.

Oliver (1977), in a randomized trial, compared maintenance of patients with AML in remission by monthly chemotherapy plus weekly BCG, with monthly chemotherapy plus weekly BCG and irradiated allogeneic leukemic blast cells. When reported, there was little difference between the two groups. A similar kind of comparison was made by Bekesi et al. (Bekesi, Roboz, and Holland, 1977; Holland and Bekesi, 1978), who in another randomized trial compared maintenance by monthly intradermal injections of neuraminidase-treated allogeneic leukemic blast cells with injections of cells and MER (8.242). Treatment with allogeneic cells, as mentioned earlier (8.253), significantly prolonged the duration of remission, but the addition of MER was of no benefit.

Seigler et al. (1972, 1973) treated 142 patients with malignant melanoma who had previously undergone combinations of surgical treatment, irradiation, cytotoxic limb perfusion, and chemotherapy, and had subsequently developed recurrent disease, with a staged immunotherapeutic procedure. The first two stages were non-specific and consisted of sensitization with BCG followed by intralesional injection of BCG. In the third stage, autologous lymphocytes were harvested, incubated in vitro with neuraminidase-treated autochthonous tumor cells, and readministered to the patient by subcutaneous or intralesional injection. In the fourth stage the patient was challenged with a subcutaneous injection of irradiated neuraminidase-treated autochthonous tumor cells plus BCG. There was an interval of 6–8 weeks between stages, and various immunological parameters were measured before treatment and after each successive stage. When reported the follow-up period ranged from 3 to 39 months. Forty-eight patients (34 percent) had died "of causes secondary to the melanoma," 61 (43 percent) were alive but had detectable disease, and 33 (23 percent) were clinically free of tumor. Thirty-one of the first 70 patients completing the treatment developed detectable tumor-specific antibody. Forty-three of the first 62 patients developed evidence of cell-mediated immunity to the tumor as shown by in vitro cytotoxicity tests, but the serum of 27 of these patients contained blocking factors which interfered with this test. The 19 patients who failed to develop evidence of cell-mediated immunity all died with progressive disease.

In the discussion of this paper the question was raised as to whether equally good results might have been obtained with BCG alone; clearly, however, the only way to tackle this question is to undertake a randomized prospective trial.

In another uncontrolled trial (R.M. Grant et al., 1974) three patients with metastatic or locally recurrent melanoma were treated with BCG (Glaxo) and irradiated autochthonous tumor cells; in one of them 70 cutaneous metastases disappeared prior to the patient's death 5 months after immunotherapy was begun. One patient who had local recurrence of a nasal melanoma received radiotherapy plus BCG plus irradiated autochthonous tumor cells plus heterologous antitumor antibody coupled to chlorambucil. This multifactorial attack was followed by complete regression of the recurrence, and 16 months later the patient was well and clinically free of tumor. In another patient, who received the same immunotherapeutic cocktail but no radiotherapy, pulmonary metastases decreased in size over 4 months but death occurred from melanoma 6 months after the first administration of BCG.

BCG combined with specific active immunization has been used in randomized trials as an adjuvant to chemotherapy with a variety of drugs in patients with disseminated melanoma (Newlands *et al.,* 1976; Simmons *et al.,* 1978; Mastrangelo *et al.,* 1978), and as an adjuvant to radical surgery (wide local excision and excision of regional lymph nodes) in patients with operable lesions (McIllmurray *et al.,* 1977; Simmons *et al.* 1978), but in none of the papers cited above was any significant benefit attributable to the immunotherapy observed. Indeed, the trial of McIllmurray *et al.* was stopped after a year when four out of eight patients who received immunotherapy had died of widespread recurrence whereas the seven controls were all alive, although in three of them the tumor had recurred. The immunotherapy varied considerably. Newlands *et al.* initially injected BCG (Glaxo) mixed with irradiated allogeneic melanoma cells intradermally, but in view of severe local reactions they modified the protocol and gave BCG alone with the first two courses of chemotherapy and cells alone with subsequent courses. Mastrangelo *et al.,* who also used BCG mixed with irradiated allogeneic cells, continued to inject this material on five occasions at intervals of 2 weeks in every 8 week course of chemotherapy. McIllmurray *et al.* injected a mixture of BCG (Glaxo) and irradiated autologous cells to multiple sites on a single occasion on the 14th postoperative day. Simmons *et al.* administered BCG (Tice strain) with a Heaf gun and injected irradiated, neuraminidase-treated frozen autochthonous tumor cells intradermally to the same arm.

Mankiewicz *et al.* (1977) reported that, whereas routine radiotherapy was of no benefit in patients with inoperable lung cancer, survival was prolonged by immunotherapy in the form of BCG plus irradiated autochthonous tumor cells. Patients with advanced lung cancer treated by radical but non-curative pulmonary resection have also been reported to benefit from additional treatment in the form of repeated intradermal injection of non-irradiated neuraminidase-treated autochthonous tumor cells every 2 weeks plus weekly intradermal injections of BCG (Takita *et al.,* 1978), but the number of patients was small and twice as many pneumonectomies (and correspondingly fewer lobectomies) were performed in the patients who received immunotherapy as in those who did not.

Hudson *et al.* (1976) treated ten patients with advanced or recurrent ovarian cancer with chemotherapy plus repeated intradermal injection of irradiated allogeneic frozen tumor cells mixed with BCG. The duration of disease stasis and survival were reported to be longer than in a retrospective matched group of historical controls treated by chemotherapy only. In patients with disseminated osteogenic sarcoma it was found by Eilber, Townsend, and Morton (1978) that immunotherapy in the form of repeated intradermal injection of cultured allogeneic osteogenic sarcoma cells plus repeated administration of BCG at a separate site by the tine technique was of no benefit as an adjuvant to radical surgery including resection of pulmonary metastases. The authors suggested that this negative result might have been due to the large residual tumor burden in these patients, and felt in retrospect that chemotherapy should have been given after operation but before the immunotherapy.

Clifford *et al.* (1967) combined injection of irradiated autochthonous tumor cells and of a variety of immunopotentiating agents, including oleic acid and triple (diphtheria, pertussis, and tetanus) vaccine, in patients with Burkitt's lymphoma, but were unable to evaluate accurately the effect of the immunotherapy because different forms of chemotherapy were used to treat those who received immunotherapy and those who did not.

Mathé *et al.* (1978) found that giving CP in addition to BCG and irradiated allogeneic leukemic cells to patients with ALL in remission did not improve the results.

Reed (1976) gave CP intravenously and irradiated cultured melanoma cells subcutaneously as an adjuvant to chemotherapy with DTIC in patients with disseminated malignant melanoma. Seven of eleven patients treated in this way showed objective regression of liver metastases as compared with 2 out of 13 patients who received chemotherapy only, and the median survival time was 7.5 months in the immunotherapy group as compared with 4 months in patients who received chemotherapy only.

8.27 Plasmapheresis

Attempts have been made to remove blocking factors by plasmapheresis. This approach was initiated by Hersey *et al.* (1976b), who treated four patients with multiple subcutaneous melanoma metastases but no detectable visceral metastases, by repeated plasmapheresis with a continuous-flow blood cell separator. The procedure was performed twice weekly in alternate weeks for the first four exchanges and thereafter once every 2 weeks. About 4 liters of plasma were removed on each occasion and replaced with various fluids, including physiological saline, Hartmann's solution, heat-treated stable plasma protein solution, human serum albumin, and Haemacel (Hochst). Each procedure was concluded with the infusion of at least two units of fresh–frozen plasma. Chromium-release assays, performed with a melanoma cell line, and effector cells and serum from the patient showed that cell-mediated toxicity was inhibited by pretreatment serum but increased by posttreatment serum or IgG. At least two exchanges were required before the serum increased cell-mediated toxicity. It was concluded that plasmapheresis removed a blocking factor from the serum. The nature of the blocking agent was not determined, but it was thought to be different from the non-specific blocking activity which is manifested by inhibition of the mitogenic effect of PHA, since there was little correlation between the removal of PHA-blocking activity and the increased cell-mediated cytotoxicity to melanoma cells. The increased cytotoxicity in the presence of later posttreatment serum was attributed to the presence of leukocyte-dependent cytotoxic antibody. The treatment was well tolerated, and although no therapeutic benefit was claimed it was considered that further studies of plasmapheresis should be undertaken.

Israel *et al.* (1976) treated 26 patients with disseminated tumors, including seven with malignant melanoma and five with breast cancer, by twice weekly plasmapheresis, and washed the patients' leukocytes before they were replaced. Partial regression of the tumor was observed in eight patients. Six patients developed an increased response to recall antigens, but this did not correlate with the antitumor effect. Unlike Hersey *et al.* (*vide supra*), Israel *et al.* suggested that the main effect of the plasmapheresis was to remove *non-specific* blocking factors. It was proposed to give further treatment in the form of non-specific immunotherapy with CP.

8.3 PRESENT POSITION AND FUTURE PROSPECTS

8.31 The Present Position

It is interesting to compare immunotherapy for cancer in 1979 with organ transplantation in 1960. At that time (Woodruff, 1960) much had been learned about the behavior of allografts and the mechanism by which they are rejected. Means had been found of preventing rejection under certain conditions in experimental animals, but the problem of making allografts survive indefinitely, or even for long enough to be of some real clinical benefit to the patient, appeared difficult—indeed, to many people working in the field, including some who had made major contributions to it, insoluble. Yet within 2 years the situation was transformed by the introduction into clinical practice of the immunosuppressive drug azathioprine. Previously, when whole body irradiation was the main method of immunosuppression, the results, with the notable exception of one patient who received a transplant in 1960 (Merrill *et al.,* 1960) and was alive and well 18 years later, can only be described as dismal. With azathioprine, worthwhile benefit to patients began to be achieved; indeed, the first patient treated with azathioprine by the writer following renal transplantation from his father in 1962 was still alive 18 years later.

Today much is known about tumor immunology, and it has been shown that the growth of various tumors in experimental animals may be inhibited by immunotherapeutic procedures; opinions differ, however, regarding the present status and future prospects of immunotherapy in man.

It has been suggested that immunotherapy already has a place, albeit a limited one, in the management of some forms of cancer, notably acute leukemia and malignant melanoma when the tumor burden has been reduced to a low level by other methods of treatment. Many clinicians and tumor biologists consider, however, that the evidence is insufficient to justify this conclusion. They are unimpressed by trials not based on randomized controls unless the effects demonstrated are striking, and point out that with so many trials in progress—according to Peto (1978c) there were, for example, 68 trials of immunotherapy for melanoma running in 1975, and many more have begun since then—one would expect a few to show differences which were significant at the $p=0.05$ level, even if the randomization procedure was impeccable and the treatment was of no value whatsoever. Some who take this view, like the present author, are optimistic concerning the future prospects for immunotherapy but feel that to introduce it into clinical practice now would probably do patients on the whole more harm than good, and might discredit the subject so much as to prejudice future developments. Others, however, see no future for immunotherapy and regard the whole approach as unsound. Since this view is quite widely held it merits critical examination.

Among clinicians, the main reason for skepticism seems to be disappointment that the high hopes raised by the discovery of tumor-associated antigens, and the striking response of some tumors in experimental animals to immunotherapeutic procedures, have not been fulfilled. Slow progress, however, does not imply that the problem is insoluble; it can be explained by the fact that the problem is intrinsically difficult, by the ethical and other factors which necessarily limit clinical research (1.12), and by the fact that, within these limits, the problem has often not been tackled in an effective way. It is not only that trials have often been poorly controlled. What is worse is that many, as we have seen, have not had a firm biological basis, or have involved such a multiplicity of agents that if a therapeutic effect occurred it was impossible to be sure what caused it. Moreover, although many interesting observations have been made by monitoring the immunological reaction of a patient to his tumor, and his capacity to respond to unrelated antigens at various times during the course of treatment, no clear picture has yet emerged of the factors which determine why particular forms of treatment sometimes appear to succeed but often fail.

In the case of biologists there appear to be five main grounds for skepticism:

1. Rejection of the hypothesis of immunological surveillance (5.5).
2. The phenomenon of immunostimulation (5.522).
3. The assumption that tumors induced in experimental animals are of necessity inappropriate models for human cancer (1.21, 1.23).

4. The failure of immunotherapy in the special case of postgestational chorioncarcinoma, which possesses antigens foreign to the patient which are the product of paternal genes (8.256).

5. The lability of tumor cell populations, as a result of which a particular form of attack may cease to be effective (3.114, 5.521).

The first four grounds have been discussed in the sections indicated, and reasons given for not regarding any of them as decisive. The last, to which we shall return later, is not so much a reason for abandoning the search for immunotherapeutic weapons as a factor to be taken into consideration in deciding in what direction to look.

8.32 The Way Ahead

If immunotherapy is going to play an important role in the treatment of cancer, what is this likely to be, and where will the way ahead be found?

It is widely accepted that the answer to the first question is, "for the treatment of residual disease after the mass of the tumor has been reduced to a small and perhaps undetectable amount by surgery, chemotherapy, or radiotherapy." The available evidence is consistent with this view, although opinions may differ concerning the maximum number of tumor cells in the face of which immunotherapeutic procedures are likely to be of value. It seems possible that this number might be substantially increased by using plasmapheresis as an initial step to reduce the amount of circulating tumor antigen or antigen–antibody complex.

The answer to the second question is a matter of conjecture, and any such conjecture must be subject to revision in the light of new data. The following suggestions represent the personal views of the author at the time of writing.

8.321 PASSIVE IMMUNIZATION

Infusion of allogeneic bone marrow from a normal HLA-identical sibling donor seems likely to continue to have a place in association with chemotherapy in the treatment of leukemia, although, as we have seen, it is not clear whether this has any antileukemic effect or whether the clinical benefit is due to its effect in promoting hemopoietic recovery.

It seems unlikely that immunization of healthy volunteers or other cancer patients to provide antibody, sensitized cells, or transfer factor for passive immunotherapy will find a definitive place in treatment. The use of such agents from patients who have been treated unsuccessfully for cancer cannot be expected to be effective unless the tumors of patient and donor have virus associated, oncofetal or other TAA in common, and even when this condition is fulfilled the possible risk to the donor may be a decisive limiting factor. In the special case of Burkitt's lymphoma the possibility exists of specific immunotherapy with Ig from patients who have recovered from infectious mononucleosis, since the Epstein-Barr virus is associated with both conditions, and this would seem to merit further investigation.

The use of Ig from rabbits, goats, and other animals immunized with the patient's tumor presents some logistic problems but has been shown to be feasible. Although somewhat discredited by unconvincing claims based on some of the earlier studies, Ig raised in this way, or with other tumors having TAA in common with the patient's tumor, might have much to offer if it were of sufficiently high specificity since even if it was not cytotoxic it could be coupled to a cytotoxic chemical or to radioactive material. Attempts to increase specificity by absorption procedures, or by raising sera in animals previously made specifically tolerant of normal human tissue, offer little prospect but the scope of passive immunotherapy and immunochemotherapy may be dramatically altered as a result of the development by Kohler and Milstein (1976) of a technique for making monoclonal antibody in which lymphocytes from immunized animals are hybridized with the cells of a plasmacytoma cell line and antibody-producing cells of appropriate specificity are selected. The rapidity of technological advance in this field raises the possibility that monoclonal antibodies will be used in clinical trials in cancer patients within the next few years.

Three other procedures which would seem to merit further study are removal of autologous lymphocytes and replacement after immunization with autochthonous tumor cells *in vitro;* treatment with transfer factor from allogeneic lymphocytes immunized *in vitro;* and treatment with RNA from the lymphocytes of animals immunized *in vivo.* With the first of these procedures steps may have to be taken to eliminate suppressor cells, and autoimmune disease is a possible complication. If RNA is to be of value, means will have to be found of preventing it from being rapidly destroyed by RNase in the patient's serum.

8.322 ACTIVE IMMUNOTHERAPY

The value of the non-specific immunopotentiating agents which have already been used in clinical trials cannot as yet be fully assessed. In the case of BCG there are important differences between strains, and although the optimal dosage has been studied in various animal models the optimal dose for systemic administration in man is open to question. It seems likely that in many trials too much has been given rather than too little. Moreover, there is still much to be learned concerning the extent to which BCG stimulates suppressor cell activity in man, and how this effect may best be overcome. Trials of CP and other agents now in progress in patients with minimal residual cancer may yield important information. One pertinent question is whether the severe pyrexial reactions evoked by CP and other agents may be prevented by administration of aspirin and indomethacin and other drugs which inhibit prostaglandin synthesis (Vane, 1971; Feldberg, 1975), without weakening the antitumor effect. Intralesional injection of CP and other agents some time before excision of the tumor, with or without the regional lymph nodes, would seem to merit further study.

It seems likely, however, that the agents which have been tried will be replaced by new agents, which Mathé *et al.* (1980) have suggested should fulfill the following conditions: (1) they will be well defined chemical compounds, or at least quantifiable agents; (2) their action will be limited to stimulation of one or few populations of cells; (3) they will not induce suppressor cells; and (4) their side effects will be minimal. Among agents suggested for study by Mathé *et al.* are thymosin (8.249), and an antibiotic, bestatin, isolated from actinomycetes (Umezawa *et al.,* 1976a, 1976b), which appear to stimulate mainly T cells, although bestatin also stimulates macrophages to some extent; an azaridine derivative, BM12 531 (Boehringer, Mannheim) (Bicker *et al.,* 1977; Schulz *et al.,* 1978), which stimulates T cells and possibly also hemopoietic stem cells and macrophages to some extent; glucan (β-1-3 polyglucose), extracted from yeast cell wall, and tuftsine, a basic tetrapeptide synthesized by Martinez *et al.* (1978), which seem to be particularly effective macrophage activators; and muramyl dipeptide (MDP), which appears to be particularly effective for stimulating K cells (Chedid, Audibert, and Johnson, 1978; Kiger *et al.*, 1978). With all the agents discussed, both old and new, data are needed concerning the response to repeated as well as to single doses.

Specific active immunization seems likely to be effective only when the endogenous tumor antigen in the circulation has fallen to a low level, or if the antigen can be presented in a form which makes it more effective than endogenous antigen. It seems likely therefore that developments in this area will be concerned with the use of antigen in association with adjuvants, or "xenogenized antigen," after the bulk of a tumor has been excised or eliminated in other ways. Much work remains to be done with animal models as a basis for future clinical trials.

8.323 ADMINISTRATION OF INTERFERON

As we have seen, many non-specific immunopotentiating agents are interferon inducers. It is pertinent to ask, therefore, whether the interferon system, which until quite recently was widely believed to have evolved solely as a protection against virus infections but is now known to influence a wide range of biological phenomena (see Gresser, 1979), may be concerned in surveillance against neoplasia, and whether administration of interferon may be a useful therapeutic procedure in patients with cancer. A trial of human leukocyte interferon in patients with osteosarcoma has been in progress in Stockholm since 1971 (Adamson *et al.*, 1980) and has engendered much optimism, but may be difficult to assess because there were no control patients (i.e. patients who did not receive interferon) in the same hospital; encouraging results have also been reported in pilot studies of interferon therapy in patients with multiple myeloma (Mellstedt *et al.*, 1979) and non-Hodgkin's lymphoma (Merigan *et al.*, 1978). A major limitation has been the cost of producing sufficient interferon; despite this, however, work in this field is expanding rapidly, due in large measure to the initiative of Cantell in Helsinki, and it seems likely that some answers to the questions posed above will be found during the next few years.

8.324 OTHER PROCEDURES

The possible value of plasmapheresis, when the residual tumor burden is so great that immunotherapy would otherwise be ineffective, has already been mentioned.

Another procedure, which does not appear to have been tried in cancer patients, is to administer anti-ideotype antibody which reacts with the ideotypic determinant by which the patient's lymphocytes recognize the cells of his tumor. As we have seen (7.824), the rationale of this procedure is that anti-ideotype antibody, if administered in small quantity, may stimulate rather than suppress cells bearing the ideotype in question.

8.325 COMBINED IMMUNOTHERAPY

Since tumor cell populations are heterogeneous, and also highly labile, it seems likely that for optimal benefit more than one form of immunotherapy will be required. Criticism earlier in this chapter of therapeutic trials in which a multiplicity of agents was used is not incompatible with this assertion. So far the combinations mainly studied have consisted of specific active immunotherapy together with administration of one or more non-specific immunopotentiating agents. Other possibilities which would seem to merit consideraiton include passive immunization with antibody combined with administration of an agent, such as CP, which activates complement; passive immunization with antibody combined with passive immunization with immune lymphocytes, transfer factor, or RNA; and combinations of non-specific agents which act principally on different cell populations. Combinations, however, must be designed rationally in the light of previous studies with single agents, and information concerning the tumor and the reaction of the host, the mode of action of each agent, and the stage of the cell cycle at which its effect on tumor cells, directly or indirectly, is likely to be greatest. When a combination has been chosen further decisions have to be made about the timing of the immunotherapy in relation to other forms of treatment, and the efficiency of the combination has to be assessed in clinical trials which incorporate all necessary—though, of course, not all possible—controls. Clearly, wherever the way ahead may lie, the going will not be easy, but the prospect is exciting.

References

The references are arranged in alphabetical order except that *Mc* and *Mac* are both treated as *Mac,* indexed separately before *M.* Names beginning *De, de, D,* or *d'* are treated as beginning with *D;* those beginning *Van, van, Von,* or *von* as beginning with *V.* The letters a, b, c, etc., are used to distinguish publications in the same year with the same first author. In the text these letters are included when the reference takes the form of the first author followed by et al.; when sufficient names are given in the text to define the reference uniquely the letters a, b, c are, as a rule, omitted.

A

Abbey Smith, R. Cure of lung cancer—From incomplete surgical resection. Br Med J *2*, 563–565, 1971

Abdou, N. I., and Abdou, N. L. The monoclonal nature of lymphocytes in multiple myeloma: Effects of therapy. Ann Intern Med *83*, 42–45, 1975

Abelev, G. I. Study of the antigenic structure of tumors. Acta Unio Int Contra Cancrum *19*, 80–82, 1963

Abelev, G. I. Alpha-fetoprotein in ontogenesis and its association with malignant tumors. Adv Cancer Res *14*, 295–358, 1971

Abelev, G. I., Perova, S. D., Khramkova, N. I., Postnikova, Z. A., and Irlin, I. S. Production of embryonal α-globulin by transplantable mouse hepatomas. Transplantation *1*, 174–180, 1963

Abercrombie, M., and Ambrose, E. J. The surface properties of cancer cells: A review. Cancer Res *22*, 525–548, 1962

Abercrombie, M., Heaysman, J. E. M., and Karthauser,H. M. Social behaviour of cells in tissue culture. III. Mutual influence of sarcoma cells and fibroblasts. Exp Cell Res *13*, 276–291, 1957

Ablashi, D. V., Easton, J. M., and Guegan, J. H. Herpesviruses and cancer in man and subhuman primates. Biomedicine *24*, 286–305, 1976

Ablashi, D. V., Glaser, R., Easton, J. M., Nonoyama, M., and Armstrong, G. R. Athymic nude mice: Induction of tumors containing Ep-

stein-Barr virus using Burkitt's-related cell lines. Exp Hematol *6*, 365–374, 1978

Ablashi, D. V., Loeb, W. F., Valerio, M. G., Adamson, R. H., Armstrong, G. R., Bennett, D. G., and Heine, U. Malignant lymphoma with lymphocytic leukemia induced in owl monkeys by Herpesvirus saimizi. J Natl Cancer Inst *47*, 837–846, 1971

Achong, B. G., Trumper, P. A., and Giovanella, B. C. C-type virus particles in human tumours transplanted into nude mice. Br J Cancer *34*, 203–206, 1976

Ackerman, N. R. The blood supply of experimental liver metastases. IV. Changes in vascularity with increasing tumor growth. Surgery *75*, 589–596, 1974

Adams, G. E., Dische, S., Fowler, J. F., and Thomlinson, R. H. Hypoxic cell sensitisers in radiotherapy. Lancet *1*, 186–188, 1976

Adams, J. B., and Wong, M. S. F. Paraendocrine behaviour of the human breast carcinoma: In vitro transformation of steroids to physiologically active hormones. J Endocrinol *41*, 41–52, 1968

Adamson, U., Aparisi, T., Broström, L. A., Cantell, K., Einhorn, S., Hall, K., Inyimarrson, S., Nilsonne, U., Strander, H. and Södeberg, G. In: The Role of Non-Specific Immunity in the Prevention and Treatment of Cancer. Vatican City: Pontifical Academy of Sciences, 1980

Adlam, C. Studies on the histamine sensitisation produced in mice by Corynebacterium parvum. J Med Microbiol *6*, 527–536, 1973

Adlam, C. Broughton, E. S., and Scott, M. T. Enhanced resistance of mice to infection with bacteria following pre-treatment with Coryne-

289

bacterium parvum. Nature New Biol *235*, 219–220, 1972

Adlam, C., and Reid, D. E. Comparative studies on the cell wall composition of some anaerobic coryneforms of varying lympho-reticular stimulatory activity. Dev Biol Stand *38*, 115–120, 1978

Adlam, C., Reid, D. E., and Torkington, P. The nature of the active principle of C. parvum, pp 33–39, In Halpern, B. (Ed): Corynebacterium Parvum and Its Application in Experimental and Clinical Oncology. New York: Plenum Press, 1975

Adlam, C., and Scott, M. T. Lympho-reticular stimulatory properties of Corynebacterium parvum and related bacteria. J Med Microbiol *6*, 261–273, 1973

Adler, W. H., Takiguchi, T., and Smith, R. T. Phytohemagglutinin unresponsiveness in mouse spleen cells induced by methylcholanthrene sarcomas. Cancer Res *31*, 864–867, 1971

Aherne, W. A., Camplejohn, R. S., and Wright, N. A. An Introduction to Cell Population Kinetics. London: Edward Arnold, 1977

Aisenberg, A. C. Studies of lymphocyte transfer reaction in Hodgkin's disease. J Clin Invest *44*, 555–564, 1965

Aisenberg, A. C. Immunologic status of Hodgkin's disease. Cancer *19*, 385–394, 1966

Aisenberg, A. C., Bloch, K. J., and Long, J. C. Cell-surface immunoglobulins in chronic lymphocytic leukemia and allied disorders. Am J Med *55*, 184–191, 1973

Aisenberg, A. C., and Leskowitz, S. Antibody formation in Hodgkin's disease. N Engl J Med *268*, 1269–1272, 1963

Albertini, R. J., and DeMars, R. Somatic cell mutation. Detection and quantification of x-ray induced mutation in cultured, diploid human fibroblasts. Mutat Res *18*, 199–224, 1973

Albo, V., Krivit, W., and Hartmann, J. Fresh plasma as an adjuvant to the chemotherapy of acute lymphatic leukemia in children. Proc Am Assoc Cancer Res *9*, 2, 1968

Alexander, J. W., and Altemeier, W. A. Susceptibility of injured tissues to hematogenous metastases: An experimental study. Ann Surg *159*, 933–944, 1964

Alexander, J. W., Braunstein, H., and Altemeier, W. A. Transplantation studies of the venereal sarcoma of dogs. J Surg Res *4*, 151–159, 1964

Alexander, P. Immunotherapy of leukemia: The use of different classes of immune lymphocytes. Cancer Res *27*, 2521–2526, 1967

Alexander, P. Foetal "antigens" in cancer. Nature *235*, 137–140, 1972

Alexander, P. Activated macrophages and the anti-

tumour action of BCG. Natl Cancer Inst Monogr *39*, 127–133, 1973

Alexander, P. Personal communication, 1974

Alexander, P., Connell, D. I., Mikulska, Z. B. Treatment of a murine leukemia with spleen cells or sera from allogeneic mice immunized against the tumor. Cancer Res *26*, 1508–1515, 1966

Alexander, P., Delorme, E. J., and Hall, J. G. The effect of lymphoid cells from the lymph of specifically immunised sheep on the growth of primary sarcomata in rats. Lancet *1*, 1186–1189, 1966

Alexander, P., Delorme, E. J., Hamilton, L. D. G., and Hall, J. G. Effect of nucleic acids from immune lymphocytes on rat sarcomata. Nature *213*, 569–572, 1967

Alexander, P., Delorme, E. J., Hamilton, L. D. G., and Hall, J. G. Stimulation of anti-tumor activity of the host with RNA from immune lymphocytes, pp 527–534, In Plescia, O. J., and Braun, W. (Eds): Nucleic Acids in Immunology. New York: Springer-Verlag, 1968

Alexander, P., Eccles, S. A., and Gauci, C. L. L. The significance of macrophages in human and experimental tumors. Ann NY Acad Sci *276*, 124–133, 1976

Alexander, P., and Evans, R. Endotoxin and double stranded RNA render macrophages cytotoxic. Nature New Biol *232*, 76–78, 1971

Alexander, P., Evans, R., and Mikulska, Z. B. The relationship between concomitant immunity and metastasis. The role of macrophages in concomitant immunity involving the peritoneal cavity. In Garattini, S., and Franchi, G. (Eds): Dissemination and Metastasis. New York: Raven Press, pp 177–185, 1973

Alexander, P., and Hall, J. G. The role of immunoblasts in host resistance and immunotherapy of primary sarcomata. Adv Cancer Res *13*, 1–37, 1970

Alexander, P., and Horning, E. S. Observations on the Oppenheimer method of inducing tumours by subcutaneous implantation of plastic films, pp 12–25, In Wolstenholme, G. E. W., and O'Connor, M. (Eds): CIBA Fdn Symp on Carcinogenesis: Mechanisms of Action. Boston: Little, Brown, 1959

Alexander, R. F., and Spriggs, A. I. The differential diagnosis of tumor cells in circulating blood. J Clin Pathol *13*, 414–424, 1960

Alford, C., Hollinshead, A., and Herberman, R. E. Delayed cutaneous hypersensitivity reactions to extracts of malignant and normal human breast cells. Ann Surg *178*, 20–24, 1973

Algire, G. H., and Chalkley, H. W. Vascular reactions of normal and malignant tissues in vivo. I. Vascular reactions of mice to wounds and to normal and neoplastic implants. J Natl Cancer Inst 6, 73–85, 1945

Allen, E. P. Malignant melanoma: Spontaneous regression after pregnancy. Br Med J 2, 1067, 1955

Alley, C. D., and Snodgrass, M. J. Effectiveness of neuraminidase in experimental immunotherapy of two murine pulmonary carcinomas. Cancer Res 37, 95–101, 1977

Allison, A. C. Immunological surveillance of tumours. Cancer Immunol Immunother 2, 151–155, 1977a

Allison, A. C. Cited as personal communication by Milas and Scott (1977), 1977b

Allison, A. C. Mechanisms by which activated macrophages inhibit lymphocyte responses. Immunol Rev 40, 5–32, 1978

Allison, A. C., Berman, L. D., and Levey, R. H. Increased tumor induction by adenovirus type 12 in thymectomized mice and mice treated with anti-lymphocytic serum. Nature 215, 185–187, 1967

Allison, A. C., and Law, L. W. Effects of antilymphocyte serum on virus oncogenesis. Proc Soc Exp Biol Med 127, 207–212, 1968

Allison, A. C., Monga, J. N., and Hammond, V. Increased susceptibility to virus oncogenesis of congenitally thymus-deprived nude mice. Nature 252, 746–747, 1974

Allison, A. C., and Taylor, R. B. Observations on thymectomy and carcinogenesis. Cancer Res 27, 703–707, 1967

Allwood, G. G., and Asherson, G. L. Depression of delayed hypersensitivity by pretreatment with Freund-type adjuvants. III. Depressed arrival of lymphoid cells at recently immunized lymph nodes in mice pretreated with adjuvants. Clin Exp Immunol 11, 579–584, 1972

Alpert, E., Hershberg, R., Schur, P., and Isselbacher, K. J. α-Fetoptotein in human hepatoma: Improved detection in serum, and quantitative studies using a new sensitive technique. Gastroenterology 61, 137–143, 1971a

Alpert, E., Pinn, V. W., and Isselbacher, K. J. Alpha-fetoprotein in a patient with gastric carcinoma metastatic to the liver. N Engl J Med 285, 1058–1059, 1971b

Al-Sarraf, M., Sardesai, S., and Vaitkevisius, V. K. Clinical immunologic responsiveness in malignant disease. II. In vitro lymphocyte response to phytohemagglutinin and the effect of cytotoxic drugs. Oncology 26, 357–368, 1972

Al-Sarraf, M., Wong, P., Sardesai, S., and Vaitkevisius, V. K. Clinical immunologic responsiveness in malignant disease. I. Delayed hypersensitivity reaction and the effect of cytotoxic drugs. Cancer 26, 262–268, 1970

Amaral, L., and Werthamer, S. Identification of breast cancer transcortin and its inhibitory role in cell-mediated immunity. Nature 262, 589–590, 1976

Ambrose, E. J., Batzdorf, U., Osborn, J. S., and Stuart, P. R. Sub-surface structures in normal and malignant cells. Nature 227, 397–398, 1970

Ambus, U., Falk, R. E., Landi, S., Bugala, R., and Langer, B. Randomized trial of chemoimmunotherapy for resectable and non-resectable gastrointestinal cancer. Dev Biol Stand 38, 541–545, 1978

Amery, W. K. Double-blind trial with levamisole in resectable lung cancer. Ann NY Acad Sci 277, 260–268, 1976

Amery, W. K. A placebo-controlled levamisole study in resectable lung cancer, pp 191–200, In Terry, W. D., and Windhorst, D. (Eds): Immunotherapy of Cancer: Present Status of Trials in Man. New York: Raven Press, 1978

Ames, B. N., Durston, W. E., Yamasaki, E., and Lee, F. D. Carcinogens are mutagens: A simple test system combining liver homogenates for activation and bacteria for detection. Proc Natl Acad Sci USA 70, 2281–2285, 1973

Amiel, J. L., and Berardet, M. An experimental model of active immunotherapy preceded by cytoreductive chemotherapy. Eur J Cancer 6, 557–559, 1970

Amiel, J. L., and Berardet, M. Factor time for active immunotherapy after cytoreductive chemotherapy. Eur J Cancer 10, 89–91, 1974

Amiel, J. L., Litwin, J., and Berardet, M. Attempts at active nonspecific immunotherapy using formolized Corynebacterium parvum. Rev Fr Etudes Clin Biol 14, 909–912, 1969

Amino, N., and Degroot, L. J. A sensitive microassay system for lymphocyte-mediated cytotoxicity induced by PHA and PPD. J Immunol 111, 464–471, 1973

Amos, D. B., and Day, D. Passive immunity against four mouse leukoses by means of isoimmune sera. Ann NY Acad Sci 64, 851–858, 1957

Amos, D. B., Hattler, B. G., and Shingleton, W. W. Prolonged survival of skin-grafts from cancer patients on normal recipients. Lancet 1, 414–415, 1965

Anastassiades, O. T., and Pryce, D. M. Immunological significance of the morphological changes in lymph nodes draining breast cancer. Br J Cancer 20, 239–249, 1966

Andersen, V., Bendixen, G., and Schrodt, T. An in vitro demonstration of cellular immunity against autologous mammary carcinoma in man. Acta Med Scand 186, 101–103, 1969

Andersen, V., Bjerrum, O., Bendixen, G., Schrodt, T., and Dissing, I. Effect of autologous mammary tumour extracts on human leukocyte migration in vitro. Int J Cancer *5*, 357–363, 1970

Anderson, D. E. Some characteristics of familial breast cancer. Cancer *28*, 1500–1504, 1971

Anderson, D. E. A genetic study of human breast cancer. J Natl Cancer Inst *48*, 1029–1034, 1972

Anderson, D. E., and Skinner, P. E. Studies on bovine ocular squamous carcinoma ('cancer eye'). XI. Effects of sunlight. J Anim Sci *20*, 474–477, 1961

Anderson, E. E., and Glenn, J. F. Cushing's syndrome associated with anaplastic carcinoma of the thyroid gland. J Urol *95*, 1–4, 1966

Anderson, J. M., Kelly, F., and Gettinby, G. Stimulatory immunotherapy with autografts of mammary cancers. Dev Biol Stand *38*, 433–440, 1978

Anderson, J. M., Kelly, F., Wood, S. E., and Halnan, K. E. Stimulatory immunotherapy in mammary cancer. Br J Surg *61*, 778–784, 1974

Andreassen, M., and Dahl-Iversen, E. Recherches sur les métastases microscopiques des ganglions lymphatiques sus-claviculaires dans le cancer du sein. J Internat Chir *9*, 27–40, 1949

Andreini, P., Drasher, M. L., and Mitchison, N. A. Studies on the immunological response to foreign tumor transplants in the mouse. III. Changes in weight and content of nucleic acids and protein of host lymphoid tissues. J Exp Med *102*, 199–204, 1955

Andrews, G. A., Congdon, C. C., Edwards, C. L., Gengozian, N., Nelson, B., and Vodopick, H. Preliminary trials of clinical immunotherapy. Cancer Res *27*, 2535–2541, 1967

Adrien, J. M., Beumer-Jockmans, M. P., Bury, J., Cauchie, C., *et al.* Immunotherapy versus chemotherapy as maintenance treatment of acute lymphoblastic leukemia, pp 471–480, In Terry, W. D., and Windhorst, D. (Eds): Immunotherapy of Cancer: Present Status of Trials in Man. New York: Raven Press, 1978

Anthony, H. M., Kirk, J. A., Madsen, K. E., Mason, M. K., and Templeman, G. H. E and EAC rosetting lymphocytes in patients with carcinoma of bronchus. I. Some parameters of the test and of its prognostic significance. Clin Exp Immunol *20*, 29–40, 1975a

Anthony, H. M., Kirk, J. A., Madsen, K. E., Mason, M. K., and Templeman, G. H. E and EAC rosetting lymphocytes in patients with carcinoma of bronchus. II. A sequential study of thirty patients: Effect of BCG: Clin Exp Immunol *20*, 41–54, 1975b

Anthony, H. M., and Parsons, M. Globulin on cells of cancer patients. Nature *206*, 275–276, 1965

Aoki, T. Murine type-C RNA viruses: A proposed reclassification, other possible pathogenicities

and a new immunologic function. J Natl Cancer Inst *52*, 1029–1034, 1974

Aoki, T., Boyse, E. A., and Old, L. J. Occurrence of natural antibody to the G (Gross) leukemia antigen in mice. Cancer Res *26*, 1415–1419, 1966

Aoki, T., Boyse, E. A., Old, L. J., Harven, E. de, Hammerling, U., and Wood, H. A. G (Gross) and H-2 cell-surface antigens: Location on gross leukemia cells by electron microscopy with visually labeled antibody. Proc Natl Acad Sci USA *65*, 569–576, 1970

Aoki, T., Huebner, R. J., Chang, K. S. S., Sturm, M. M., and Lui, M. Diversity of envelope antigens on murine type-C RNA viruses. J Natl Cancer Inst *52*, 1189–1197, 1974

Aoki, T., and Takahashi, T. Viral and cellular surface antigens of murine leukemias and myelomas. Serological analysis by immunoelectron microscopy. J Exp Med *135*, 443–457, 1972

Aptekman, P. M., and Lewis, M. R. Evidence of resistance to tumor graft in early stages of induced oncolysis. J Immunol *66*, 361–364, 1951

Arcomano, J. P., Barnett, J. C., and Bottone, J. J. Spontaneous disappearance of pulmonary metastases following nephrectomy for hypernephroma. Am J Surg *96*, 703–704, 1958

Ariel, I. M. The use of lymphangiography in melanoma. Surgery *76*, 654–665, 1974

Armitage, P., and Doll, R. The age distribution of cancer and a multistage theory of carcinogenesis. Br J Cancer *8*, 1–12, 1954

Armitage, P., and Doll, R. A two-stage theory of carcinogenesis in relation to the age distribution of human cancer. Br J Cancer *11*, 161–169, 1957

Armstrong, B., Skegg, D., White, G., and Doll, R. Rauwolfia derivatives and breast cancer in hypersensitive women. Lancet *2*, 8–12, 1976

Armstrong, B., Stevens, N., and Doll, R. Retrospective study of the association between use of rauwolfia derivatives and breast cancer in English women. Lancet *2*, 672–675, 1974

Armstrong, D., Henle, G., and Henle, W. Complement fixation tests with cell lines derived from Burkitt's lymphoma and acute leukemias. J Bacteriol *91*, 1257–1262, 1966

Armstrong, M. Y. K., Ruddle, N. H., Lipman, M. B., and Richards, F. F. Tumor induction by immunologically activated murine leukemia virus. J Exp Med *137*, 1163–1179, 1973

Aschoff, K. A. L. Lectures on Pathology. New York: Hoeber, 1924

Asherson, G. L., and Allwood, G. G. Depression of delayed hypersensitivity by pretreatment with Freund-type adjuvants. I. Description of the phenomenon. Clin Exp Immunol *9*, 249–258, 1971

Ashikawa, K., Inoue, K., Shimizu, T., and Ishibashi, Y. An increase of serum alpha-globulin in tumor-bearing hosts and its immunological significance. Jpn J Exp Med *41*, 339–355, 1971

Ashikawa, K., Motoya, K., Sekiguchi, M., and Ishibashi, Y. Immune response in tumor-bearing patients and animals. II. Incidence of tuberculin anergy in cancer patients. Gann *58*, 565–573, 1967

Ashley, D. J. B. The two 'hit' and multiple 'hit' theories of carcinogenesis. Br J Cancer *23*, 313–328, 1969

Ashworth, T. R. A case of cancer in which cells similar to those of the tumor were seen in the blood after death (1869). [*Cited by W. K. Hughes.*] Med J Aust *14*, 146–147, 1909

Atkinson, J. B., Mahoney, F. J., Schwartz, I. R., and Hesch, J. A. Therapy of acute leukemia by whole-body irradiation and bone marrow transplantation from an identical normal twin. Blood *14*, 228–234, 1959

Attia, M. A. M., DeOme, K. B., and Weiss, D. W. Immunology of spontaneous mammary carcinomas in mice. II. Resistance to a rapidly and slowly developing tumor. Cancer Res *25*, 451–457, 1965

Attia, M. A. M., and Weiss, D. W. Immunology of spontaneous mammary carcinomas in mice. V. Acquired tumor resistance and enhancement in strain A mice infected with mammary tumor virus. Cancer Res *26*, 1787–1800, 1966

Aub, J. C., Tieslau, C., and Lankester, A. Reactions of normal and tumor cell surfaces to enzymes. I. Wheat-germ lipase and associated mucopolysaccharides. Proc Natl Acad Sci USA *50*, 613–619, 1963

Audibert, F., Chedid, L., Lefrancier, P., Choay, J., and Lederer, E. Relationship between chemical structure and adjuvant activity of some synthetic analogues of N-acetyl-muramyl-L-alanyl-D-isoglutamine (MDP). Ann Immunol (Paris) *128C*, 653–661, 1977

Auerbach, R., Arensman, R., Kubai, L., and Folkman, J. Tumor-induced angiogenesis: Lack of inhibition by irradiation. Int J Cancer *15*, 241–245, 1975

Aurelian, L., Royston, I., and Davis, H. J. Antibody to genital herpes simplex virus: Association with cervical atypia and carcinoma in situ. J Natl Cancer Inst *45*, 455–464, 1970

Auster, L. S. The role of trauma in oncogenesis: A judicial consideration. JAMA *175*, 946–950, 1961

Avis, F., Avis, I., Cole, A. T., Fried, F., and Haughton, G. Antigenic cross-reactivity between benign prostatic hyperplasia and adeno-carcinoma of the prostate. Urology *5*, 122–130, 1975

Avis, F., Avis, I., Newsome, J. F., and Haughton, G. Antigenic cross-reactivity between adenocarcinoma of the breast and fibrocystic disease of the breast. J Natl Cancer Inst *56*, 17–25, 1976

Avis, F., Mosonov, I., and Haughton, G. Antigenic-reactivity between benign and malignant neoplasms of the human breast. J Natl Cancer Inst *52*, 1041–1049, 1974

Avis, P., and Lewis, M. G. Tumor-associated fetal antigens in human tumors. J Natl Cancer Inst *51*, 1063–1066, 1973

Axel, R., Gulati, S. C., and Spiegelman, S. Particles containing RNA-instructed DNA polymerase and virus-related RNA in human breast cancer. Proc Natl Acad Sci USA *69*, 3133–3137, 1972

Axel, R., Schlom, J., and Spiegelman, S. Presence in human breast cancer of RNA homologous to mouse mammary tumour virus RNA. Nature *235*, 32–36, 1972a

Axel, R., Schlom, J., and Spiegelman, S. Evidence for translation of viral-specific RNA in cells of a mouse mammary carcinoma. Proc Natl Acad Sci USA *69*, 535–538, 1972b

Axelrad, A. A. Changes in resistance to the proliferation of iso-transplanted Gross virus-induced lymphoma cells, as measured with a spleen colony assay. Nature *199*, 80–83, 1963

Ayre, J. E. Studies of an immuno-active coupled tumor protein antigen. Cyto-immunology of carcinoma in situ. Oncology, *23*, 177–200, 1969

Azuma, I., Ribi, E. E., Meyer, T. J., and Zbar, B. Biologically active components from mycobacterial cell walls. I. Isolation and composition of cell wall skeleton and component P3. J Natl Cancer Inst *52*, 95–102, 1974

Azuma, I., Sugimura, K., Taniyama, T., Aladin, A., and Yamamura, Y. Chemical and immunological studies on the cell walls of P. acnes strain C7 and C. parvum ATCC 11829. Jpn J Microbiol *19*, 265–275, 1975

Azzarone, B., Pedulla, D., and Romanzi, C. A. Spontaneous transformation of human skin fibroblasts derived from neoplastic patients. Nature *262*, 74–75, 1976

B

Bach, M. L., Bach, F. H., and Joo, P. Leukemia associated antigens in the mixed leukocyte culture test. Science *166*, 1520–1522, 1969

Back, N., Shields, R. R., and Ambrus, J. L. Role
of the fibrinolysin system in the metastatic distribution of spontaneously metastasizing and
intravenously injected rodent tumor cells. Proc
Am Assoc Cancer Res 7, 4, 1966

Bagshawe, K. D. Immunotherapy of cancer. Br
Med J 2, 463, 1966

Bagshawe, K. D. Choriocarcinoma. The Clinical
Biology of Trophoblast and its Tumours. London: Edward Arnold, 1969

Bagshawe, K. D. Tumour-associated antigens. Br
Med Bull 30, 68–73, 1974

Bagshawe, K. D., and Currie, G. A. Immunogenicity of L1210 murine leukemia cells after
treatment with neuraminidase. Nature 218,
1254–1255, 1968

Bagshawe, K. D., and Golding. P. R. Immunology
of trophoblastic tumors. Effect of specific and
nonspecific immunization procedures on rejection of husband skin graft and course of the
disease in patients with choriocarcinoma, pp
1–273, In Severi, L. (Ed): Immunity and Tolerance in Oncogenesis. Perugia: Pub Div Cancer Res, 1970

Bagshawe, K. D., and Harland, S. Detection of
intracranial tumours with special reference to
immunodiagnosis. Proc R Soc Med 69, 51–
53, 1976

Baird, D. T., Uno, A., and Melby, J. C. Adrenal
secretion of androgens and oestrogens. J Endocrinol 45, 135–136, 1969

Bakemeir, R. F., Costello, W., Horton, J., and De-
Vita, V. T. BCG immunotherapy following
chemotherapy-induced remission of stage III
and IV Hodgkin's disease, pp 513–517, In Terry, W. D., and Windhorst, D.(Eds): Immunotherapy of Cancer: Present Status of Trials
in Man. New York: Raven Press, 1978

Baker, M. A., and Taub, R. N. Immunotherapy
of human cancer. Prog Allergy 17, 227–299,
1973a

Baker, M. A., and Taub, R. N. Production of antiserum in mice to human leukaemia-associated
antigens. Nature New Biol 241, 93–94, 1973b

Baker, P. J. Homeostatic control of antibody responses: A model based on the recognition of
cell-associated antibody by regulatory T cells.
Transplant Rev 26, 3–20, 1975

Baldwin, R. W. Tumour-specific immunity against
spontaneous rat tumours. Int J Cancer 1, 257–
264, 1966

Baldwin, R. W. Immunological aspects of chemical
carcinogenesis. Adv Cancer Res 18, 1–76, 1973

Baldwin, R. W. Relevant animal models for tumor
immunotherapy. Cancer Immunol Immunother 1, 197–198, 1976a

Baldwin, R. W. Role of immunosurveillance against

chemically induced rat tumors. Transplant Rev
28, 62–74, 1976b

Baldwin, R. W., and Barker, C. R. Antigen deletions in carcinogen-induced rat hepatomata.
Nature 214, 292–293, 1967a

Baldwin, R. W., and Barker, C. R. Antigenic composition of transplanted rat hepatomas originally induced by 4-dimethylaminoazobenzene.
Br J Cancer 21, 338–345, 1967b

Baldwin, R. W., and Barker, C. R. Tumour-specific
antigenicity of aminoazo-dye-induced rat hepatomas. Int J Cancer 2, 335–364, 1967c

Baldwin, R. W., and Barker, C. R. Demonstration
of tumour-specific humoral antibody against
aminoazo-dye-induced rat hepatomata. Br J
Cancer 21, 793–800, 1967d

Baldwin, R. W., Bowen, J. G., and Price, M. R.
Detection of circulating hepatoma D23 antigen
and immune complexes in tumour bearer serum. Br J Cancer 28, 16–24, 1973

Baldwin, R. W., Cook, A. J., Hopper, D. G., and
Pimm, M. V. Radiation-killed BCG in the
treatment of transplanted rat tumours. Int J
Cancer 13, 743–750, 1974a

Baldwin, R. W., and Embleton, M. J. Immunology
of 2-acetylaminofluorine-induced rat mammary adenocarcinomas. Int J Cancer 4, 47–53,
1969a

Baldwin, R. W., and Embleton, M. J. Immunology
of spontaneously arising rat mammary adenocarcinomas. Int J Cancer 4, 430–439, 1969b

Baldwin, R. W., and Embleton, M. J. Detection
and isolation of tumour-specific antigen associated with a spontaneously arising rat mammary carcinoma. Int J Cancer 6, 372–382,
1970

Baldwin, R. W., and Embleton, M. J. Demonstration by colony-inhibition methods of cellular
and humoral immune reactions to tumour-specific antigens associated with aminoazo-dye-
induced rat hepatomas. Int J Cancer 7, 17–
25, 1971

Baldwin, R. W., and Glaves, D. Solubilization of
tumour-specific antigen from plasma membrane of an aminoazo-dye-induced rat hepatoma. Clin Exp Med 11, 51–56, 1972

Baldwin, R. W., Glaves, D., and Pimm, M. V.
Tumor-associated antigens as expressions of
chemically induced neoplasia and their involvement in tumor-host interaction, pp 907–
920, In Amos, B. (Ed): Progress in Immunology. New York: Academic Press, 1971

Baldwin, R. W., Glaves, O., Pimm, M. V., and
Vose, B. M. Tumour specific and embryonic
antigen expression on chemically induced rat
tumours. Ann Inst Pasteur 122, 715–728,
1972a

Baldwin, R. W., Glaves, D., and Vose, B. M. Embryonic antigen expression in chemically induced rat hepatomas and sarcomas. Int J Cancer 10, 233–243, 1972b

Baldwin, R. W., Glaves, D., and Vose, B. M. Immunogenicity of embryonic antigens associated with chemically induced rat tumours. Int J Cancer 13, 135–142, 1974

Baldwin, R. W., Harris, J. R., and Price, M. R. Fractionation of plasma membrane-associated tumour specific antigen from an aminoazo dye-induced rat hepatoma. Int J Cancer 11, 385–397, 1973

Baldwin, R. W., Hopper, D. G., and Pimm, M. V. Influence of orally administered BCG on growth of transplanted rat tumours. Br J Cancer 31, 124–128, 1975

Baldwin, R. W., and Moore, M. Isolation of membrane-associated tumour-specific antigen from an aminoazo-dye-induced rat hepatoma. Int J Cancer 4, 753–760, 1969

Baldwin, R. W., and Pimm, M. V. Influence of BCG infection on growth of 3-methylcholanthrene-induced rat sarcomas. Rev Eur Etudes Clin Biol 16, 875–881, 1971

Baldwin, R. W., and Pimm, M. V. BCG immunotherapy of local subcutaneous growths and post-surgical pulmonary metastases of a transplanted rat epithelioma of spontaneous origin. Int J Cancer 12, 420–427, 1973a

Baldwin, R. W., and Pimm, M. V. BCG immunotherapy of pulmonary growths from intravenously transferred rat tumor cells. Br J Cancer 27, 48–54, 1973b

Baldwin, R. W., and Pimm, M. V. BCG immunotherapy of a rat sarcoma. Br J Cancer 28, 281–287, 1973c

Baldwin, R. W., and Pimm, M. V. BCG suppression of pulmonary metastases from primary rat hepatomata. Br J Cancer 30, 473–476, 1974

Baldwin, R. W., and Pimm, M. V. BCG in tumor immunotherapy. Adv Cancer Res 28, 91–147, 1978

Baldwin, R. W., and Vose, B. M. Embryonic antigen expression on 2-acetylamino-fluorene induced and spontaneously arising rat tumours. Br J Cancer 30, 209–214, 1974

Ball, J. K., and McCarter, J. A. Effect of polyinosinic-polycytidylic acid on induction of primary or transplanted tumors by chemical carcinogen or irradiation. J Natl Cancer Inst 46, 1009–1014, 1971

Balme, H. W. Metastatic carcinoma of the thyroid successfully treated with thyroxine. Lancet 1, 812–813, 1954

Balner, H., and Dersjant, H. Neonatal thymectomy and tumor induction with methylcholanthrene in mice. J Natl Cancer Inst 36, 513–521, 1966

Balner, H., and Dersjant, H. Increased oncogenic effect of methylcholanthrene after treatment with anti-lymphocyte serum. Nature 224, 376–378, 1969

Balner, H., Old, L. J., and Clarke, D. A. Accelerated rejection of male skin isograft by female C57B1 mice injected with bacillus Calmette-Guérin (BCG). Proc Soc Exp Biol Med 109, 58–62, 1962

Baltimore, D. RNA-dependent DNA polymerase in virions of RNA tumour viruses. Nature 226, 1209–1211, 1970

Band, P. R., Jao-King, C., Urtasun, R., and Haraphongse, M. A phase I study of intravenous Corynebacterium parvum in solid tumors. Proc Am Assoc Cancer Res 16, 9, 1975

Bansal, S. C., Hargreaves, R., and Sjögren, H. O. Facilitation of polyoma tumor growth in rats by blocking sera and tumor eluate. Int J Cancer 9, 97–108, 1972

Bansal, S. C., and Sjögren, H. O. "Unblocking" serum activity in vitro in the polyoma system may correlate with antitumour effects of antiserum in vivo. Nature New Biol 233, 76–78, 1971

Bansal, S. C., and Sjögren, H. O. Counteraction of the blocking of cell-mediated tumor immunity by inoculation of unblocking sera and splenectomy: Immunotherapeutic effects on primary polyoma tumors in rats. Int J Cancer 9, 490–509, 1972

Bansal, S. C., and Sjögren, H. O. Correlation between changes in antitumor immune parameters and tumor growth in vivo in rats. Fed Proc 32, 165–172, 1973

Bar, R. S., DeLor, C. J., Clausen, K. P., Hurtubise, P., Henle, W., and Hewetson, J. F. Fatal infectious mononucleosis in a family. N Engl J Med 290, 363–367, 1974

Barker, H. R., Sommers, S. C., Snyder, R., and Kwon, T. H. Histologic and nuclear grading and stromal reactions as indices for prognosis in ovarian cancer. Am J Obstet Gynecol 121, 795–804, 1975

Barnes, D. W. H., Corp, M. Y., Loutit, J. F., and Neal, F. E. Tratment of murine leukaemia with x rays and homologous bone marrow. Preliminary communication. Br Med J 2, 626–627, 1956

Barnes, D. W. H., and Loutit, J. F. Treatment of murine leukaemia with x-rays and homologous bone-marrow. Br J Haematol 3, 241–252, 1957

Baron, S., de Buy, H., Buckler, C. E., Johnson, M. L., Park, J., Billiau, A., Sarma, P., and

Huebner, R. J. Induction of interferon and viral resistance in animals by polynucleotides. Ann NY Acad Sci *173*, 568–581, 1970

Barr, M., and Fairley, G. H. Circulating antibodies in reticuloses. Lancet *1*, 1305–1310, 1961

Barr, R. D., and Fialkow, P. J. Clonal origin of chronic myelocytic leukemia. N Engl J Med *289*, 307–309, 1973

Barrett, A., DeSouza, I., Morgan, L., Tovey, F., and Hobbs, J. R. A breast carcinoma dependent on human placental lactogen. Lancet *1*, 1347, 1975

Barrett, M. K. The influence of genetic constitution upon the induction of resistance to transplantable mouse tumors. J Natl Cancer Inst *1*, 387–393, 1940

Barrett, M. K. The nature of tumor immunity. Reprinted by U.S. Dept. Health, Education and Welfare, U.S. Public Health Service, with permission from Origins of Resistance to Toxic Agents—New York, Academic Press, 1955

Barrett, M. K., and Deringer, M. K. Induced adaptation in transplantable tumor of mice. J Natl Cancer Inst *11*, 51–59, 1950

Barrett, M. K., and Deringer, M. K. Induced adaptation in a tumor: Permanence of the change. J Natl Cancer Inst *12*, 1011–1017, 1952

Barrett, M. K., Deringer, M. K., and Hansen, W. H. Induced adaptation in a tumor: Specificity of the change. J Natl Cancer Inst *14*, 381–394, 1953

Barski, G., and Cornefert, F. Characteristics of "hybrid"-type clonal cell lines obtained from mixed cultures in vivo. J Natl Cancer Inst *28*, 801–821, 1962

Bart, R. S., and Kopf, A. W. Inhibition of the growth of murine malignant melanoma with synthetic double-stranded ribonucleic acid. Nature *224*, 372–373, 1969

Bart, R. S., Kopf, A. W., and Silagi, S. Inhibition of the growth of murine malignant melanoma by polyinosinic-polycytidylic acid. J Invest Dermatol *56*, 33–37, 1971

Barth, R. F., and Singla, O. Distribution of technetium-99m labeled Corynebacterium parvum in normal and tumor bearing mice. Dev Biol Stand *38*, 129–135, 1978

Bartlett, G. Effect of host immunity on the antigenic strength of primary tumors. J Natl Cancer Inst *49*, 493–504, 1972

Bartlett, G. L., and Zbar, B. Tumor-specific vaccine containing Mycobacterium bovis and tumor cells: Safety and efficacy. J Natl Cancer Inst *48*, 1709–1726, 1972

Bartlett, G. L., Zbar, B., and Rapp, H. J. Suppression of murine tumor growth by immune reaction to the bacillus Calmette-Guérin strain

of Mycobacterium bovis. J Natl Cancer Inst *48*, 245–257, 1972

Bartsch, H. Predictive value of mutagenicity tests in chemical carcinogenesis. Mutat Res *38*, 177–190, 1976

Bashford, E. F., Murray, J. A., and Haaland, M. Resistance and susceptibility to inoculated cancer. London, Third Sci Rep Imp Cancer Res Fund, pp 359–397, 1908a

Bashford, E. F., Murray, J. A., Haaland, M., and Bowen, W. H. General results of propagation of malignant new growths. London, Third Sci Rep Imp Cancer Res Fund, pp 262–292, 1908b

Basic, I., Milas, L., Grdina, D. J., and Withers, H. R. Destruction of hamster ovarian cell cultures by peritoneal macrophages from mice treated with Corynebacterium granulosum. J Natl Cancer Inst *52*, 1839–1842, 1974

Basic, I., Milas, L., Grdina, D. J., and Withers, H. R. In vitro destruction of tumor cells by macrophages from mice treated with Corynebacterium granulosum. J Natl Cancer Inst *55*, 589–596, 1975

Basombrio, M. A. Search for common antigenicities among twenty-five sarcomas induced by methylcholanthrene. Cancer Res *30*, 2458–2462, 1970

Bast, R. C., Zbar, B., Borsos, T., and Rapp, H. J. BCG and cancer. N Engl J Med *290*, 1413–1420, 1974

Basten, A., Miller, J. F. A. P., Warner, N. L., and Pye, J. Specific inactivation of thymus-derived (T) and non-thymus-derived (B) lymphocytes by ^{125}I-labelled antigen. Nature New Biol *231*, 104–106, 1971

Bataillon, G., Pross, H., and Klein, G. Comparative in vitro sensitivity of two methylcholanthrene-induced murine sarcoma lines to humoral and cellular immune cytotoxicity. Int J Cancer *16*, 255–265, 1975

Batchelor, J. R., and Silverman, M. S. Further studies on interactions between sessile and humoral antibodies in homograft reactions, pp 216–231, In Wolstenholme, G. E. W., and Cameron, M. P. (Eds): Ciba Fdn Symp—Transplantation. London: J & A Churchill, 1962

Batson, O. V. Function of vertebral veins and their roles in spread of metastases. Ann Surg *112*, 138–149, 1940

Bauer, F. W., and Robbins, S. L. Prevalence of multiple primary malignancy at the Boston City Hospital, 1955–1965, p 9, In Severi, L. (Ed): Fifth Perugia International Conference on Cancer, 1973. Perugia University, 1974

Bauer, H. Virion and tumor cell antigens of C-type RNA tumor viruses. Adv Cancer Res *20*, 275–342, 1974

Baum, H. Possible role of mitochondria in oncogenesis. Lancet *2*, 738–739, 1973

Baum, H., and Baum, M. Methylcholanthrene induced sarcomata in mice after immunisation with Corynebacterium parvum plus syngeneic subcellular membrane fractions. Lancet *2*, 1397–1398, 1974

Baum, M. The curability of breast cancer. Br Med J *1*, 439–442, 1976

Baum, M. Personal communication, 1977

Baum, M., and Breese, M. Antitumour effect of C. parvum: Possible mode of action. Br J Cancer *33*, 468–473, 1976

Baum, M., Edwards, M. H., and Magarey, C. J. Organization of clinical trial on national scale: Management of early cancer of the breast. Br Med J *4*, 476–478, 1972

Baum, M., and Fisher, B. Macrophage production by the bone marrow of tumour bearing mice. Cancer Res *32*, 2813–2817, 1972

Bayliss, W. M., and Starling, E. H. The mechanism of pancreatic secretion. J Physiol *28*, 325–353, 1902

Bean, M., Pees, H., Fogh, J. E., Grabstald, H., and Oettgen, H. F. Cytotoxicity of lymphocytes from patients with cancer of the urinary bladder: Detection by ^{3}H proline microcytotoxicity assay. Int J Cancer *14*, 186–197, 1974

Beardmore, G. L. The epidemiology of malignant melanoma in Australia, pp 39–64, In Melanoma and Skin Cancer. Sydney: NSW Government Printer, 1972

Beatson, G. T. On the treatment of inoperable cases of carcinoma of the mamma: Suggestions for a new method of treatment, with illustrative cases. Lancet *2*, 104–107, 162–165, 1896

Beck, C., and Burger, H. G. Evidence for the presence of immunoreactive growth hormone in cancers of the lung and stomach. Cancer *30*, 75–79, 1972

Becker, S., Fenyö, E. M., and Klein, E. The "natural killer" cell in the mouse does not require H-2 homology and is not directed against type or group-specific antigens of murine C-viral proteins. Eur J Immunol *6*, 882–885, 1976

Begg, R. W. Tumor-host relations. Adv Cancer Res *5*, 1–54, 1958

Beilby, J. O. W., Cameron, C. H., Catterall, R. D., and Davidson, D. Herpes-virus hominis infection of the cervix associated with gonorrhoea. Lancet *1*, 1065–1066, 1968

Bekesi, J. G., and Holland, J. F. Combined chemotherapy and immunotherapy of transplantable and spontaneous murine leukemia in DBA/2 and AKR mice. Recent Results Cancer Res *47*, 357–367, 1974

Bekesi, J. G., and Holland, J. F. Active immunotherapy of leukemia with neuraminidase-modified leukemic cells. Recent Results Cancer Res *62*, 78–89, 1977

Bekesi, J. F., and Holland, J. F. Immunotherapy of acute myelocyte leukemia, with neuraminidase-treated myeloblasts and MER, pp 375–388, In Proc Symp Immunotherapy of Malignant Diseases. New York: Schattaner-Verlag, 1978

Bekesi, G. J., Roboz, J. P., and Holland, J. F. Therapeutic effectiveness of neuraminidase treated tumor cells as immunogen in man and experimental animals with leukaemia. Ann NY Acad Sci *277*, 313–331, 1977

Bekesi, J. G., St. Arneault, G., and Holland, J. F. Increase of leukemia L1210 immunogenicity by Vibrio cholerae neuraminidase treatment. Cancer Res *31*, 2130–2132, 1971

Bekierkunst, A. Immunotherapy and vaccination against cancer with non-living BCG and cord factor (trehalose-6, 6'-dimycolate). Int J Cancer *16*, 442–447, 1975

Bekierkunst, A., Levy, I. S., Yarkoni, E., Vilkas, E., and Lederer, E. Suppression of urethan-induced lung adenomas in mice treated with trehalose-6, 6-dimycolate (cord factor) and living bacillus Calmette-Guérin. Science *174*, 1240–1242, 1971

Bekierkunst, A., Wang, L., Toubiana, R., and Lederer, E. Immunotherapy of cancer with non-living BCG and fractions derived from mycobacteria: Role of cord factor (trehalose-6,6'-dimycolate) in tumor regression. Infect Immun *10*, 1044–1050, 1974

Belisario, J. C., and Milton, G. W. The experimental local therapy of cutaneous metastases of malignant melanoblastomas with cow pox vaccine or colcemid (Demecolcine or Omaine). Australas J Dermatol *6*, 113–118, 1961

Bell, J. W., Jesseph, J. E., and Leighton, R. S. Spontaneous regression of bronchogenic carcinoma with five year survival. J Thorac Cardiovasc Surg *48*, 984–990, 1964

Bellone, C. J., and Pollard, M. A transient cytotoxic host response to the Rous sarcoma virus-induced transplantation antigen. Proc Soc Exp Biol Med *134*, 640–643, 1970

Benacerraf, B. The genetic control of specific immune responses. The Harvey Lectures, *67*, 109–141. New York: Academic Press, 1973

Benacerraf, B. A hypothesis to relate the specificity of T lymphocytes and the activity of I-region-specific Ir genes in macrophages and B lymphocytes. J Immunol *120*, 1809–1812, 1978

Bendich, A., Borenfreund, E., and Stonehill, E. Protection of adult mice against tumor challenge by immunization with irradiated adult skin or embryo cells. J Immunol *111*, 284–285, 1973

Ben-Efraim, S., Constantini-Sourojon, M., and Weiss, D. W. Potentiation and modulation of the immune response of guinea pigs to poorly immunogenic protein-hapten conjugates by pretreatement with the MER fraction of attenuated tubercle bacilli. Cell Immunol 7, 370–379, 1973

Bennett, M. Rejection of marrow allografts. Importance of H-2 homozygocity of donor cells. Transplantation 14, 289–298, 1972

Ben-Sasson, Z., Weiss, D. W., and Doljansky, F. Specific binding of factor(s) released by Rous sarcoma virus-transformed cells to splenocytes of chickens with Rous sarcoma. J Natl Cancer Inst 52, 405–412, 1974

Bentvelzen, P. Hereditary infections with mammary tumor viruses in mice, pp 309–337, In Emmelot, P., and Bentvelzen, P. (Eds): RNA Viruses and Host Genome in Oncogenesis. Amsterdam: North-Holland, 1972

Berenbaum, M. C. The last surviving cancer cell: The chances of killing it. Cancer Chemother Rep 52, 539–541, 1968

Berenbaum, M. C. Dose-response curves for agents that impair cell reproductive integrity. A fundamental difference between dose-response curves for antimetabolites and those for radiation and alkylating agents. Br J Cancer 23, 426–433, 1969a

Berenbaum, M. C. Dose-response curves for agents that impair cell reproductive integrity. The relation between dose-response curves and the design of selective regimens in cancer chemotherapy. Br J Cancer 23, 434–445, 1969b

Berenbaum, M. C. In vivo determination of the fractional kill of human tumor cells by chemotherapeutic agents. Cancer Chemother Rep 56, 563–571, 1972

Berenbaum, M. C. Synergy, additivism and antagonism in immunosuppression: A critical review. Clin Exp Immunol 28, 1–18, 1977

Berenbaum, M. C., Sheard, C. E., Reittie, J. R., and Bundick, R. V. The growth of human tumours in immunosuppressed mice and their response to chemotherapy. Br J Cancer 30, 13–32, 1974

Berenblum, I. The cocarcinogenic action of croton resin. Cancer Res 1, 44–48, 1941a

Berenblum, I. The mechanism of carcinogenesis. A study of the significance of cocarcinogenic action and related phenomena. Cancer Res 1, 807–814, 1941b

Berenblum, I. Carcinogenesis and tumor pathogenesis. Adv Cancer Res 2, 129–175, 1954

Berenblum, I. The epidemiology of cancer, p. 610, In Florey, H. (Ed): General Pathology. London: Lloyd-Luke (Medical Books), 1962

Berenblum, I. A re-evaluation of the concept of carcinogenesis. Prog Exp Tumor Res 11, 21–30, 1969

Berenblum, I., and Haran, N. The significance of the sequence of initiating and promoting actions in the process of skin carcinogenesis in the mouse. Br J Cancer 9, 268–271, 1955

Berenblum, I., and Shubik, P. A new, quantitative approach to the study of the stages of chemical carcinogenesis in the mouse's skin. Br J Cancer 1, 383–391, 1947

Berenblum, I., and Shubik, P. An experimental study of the initiating stage of carcinogenesis and a re-examination of the somatic cell mutation theory of cancer. Br J Cancer 3, 109–118, 1949

Beretta, G., Adamus, J., Aubert, C., Bonadonna, G., et al. Controlled study for prolonged chemotherapy, immunotherapy, and chemotherapy plus immunotherapy as an adjuvant to surgery in stage I-II malignant melanoma: Preliminary report, International Group for the Study of Melanoma, pp 65–72, In Terry, W. D., and Windhorst, D. (Eds): Immunotherapy of Cancer: Present Status of Trials in Man. New York: Raven Press, 1978

Berg, J. W. Inflammation and prognosis in breast cancer. A search for host resistance. Cancer 12, 714–720, 1959

Berg, J. W., Huvos, A. G., Axtell, L. M., and Robbins, G. F. A new sign of favorable prognosis in mammary cancer. Hyperplastic reactive lymph nodes in the apex of the axilla. Ann Surg 177, 8–12, 1973

Bergheden, C., and Hellström, K. E. Studies on allogeneic inhibition. II. Inhibition of mouse tumor cell growth by in vitro contact with cells containing foreign H-2 antigens. Int J Cancer 1, 361–369, 1966

Bergholtz, B. O., and Thorsby, E. Macrophage-dependent response of immune human T lymphocytes to PPD in vitro. Influence of HLA-D histocompatibility. Scand J Immunol 6, 779–786, 1977

Berkarda, F. B., d'Souza, J. P., and Bakemeier, R. F. The effect of anticoagulants on tumor growth and spread in mice. Proc Am Assoc Cancer Res 15, 99, 1974

Berke, G., and Levey, R. H. Cellular immunoabsorbents in transplantation immunity. Specific in vitro deletion and recovery of mouse lymphoid cells sensitized against allogeneic tumors. J Exp Med 135, 972–984, 1972

Berkeley, W. N. Result of three years' observation on a new form of cancer treatment. Am J Obstet Dis Wom 69, 1060–1063, 1914

Berman, L. D. On the nature of transplantation immunity in the adenovirus tumor system. J Exp Med 125, 983–1000, 1967

Berman, L. D., Allison, A. C., and Pereira, H. G. Effect of Freund's adjuvant on adenovirus oncogenesis and antibody production in hamsters. Int J Cancer 2, 539–543, 1967

Bernard, C., Geraldes, A., and Boiron, M. Action de la phytohémagglutinine "in vitro" sur les lymphocytes de leucémies lymphoïdes chroniques. Nouv Rev Fr Hematol 4, 69–76, 1964

Berney, S. N., and Gesner, B. M. The circulatory behaviour of normal and enzyme altered thymocytes in rats. Immunology 18, 681–691, 1970

Bernstein, A. Diagnostic importance of heterophile test in leukemia. J Clin Invest 13, 677–683, 1934

Bernstein, I. D., Thor, D. E., Zbar, B., and Rapp, H. J. Tumor immunity: Tumor suppression in vivo initiated by soluble products of specifically stimulated lymphocytes. Science 172, 729–731, 1971

Berry, R. J. A comparison of effects of some chemotherapeutic agents and those of x-rays on the reproductive capacity of mammalian cells. Nature 203, 1150–1153, 1964

Berson, S. A., and Yalow, R. S. Parathyroid hormone in plasma in adenomatous hyperparathyroidism, uremia and bronchogenic carcinoma. Science 154, 907–909, 1966

Bevan, M. J. The major histocompatibility complex determines susceptibility to cytotoxic T cells directed against minor histocompatibility antigens. J Exp Med 142, 1349–1364, 1975

Bevan, M. J., and Trowbridge, I. S. Aspects of tumour biology. Nature 260, 669–670, 1976

Bias, W. B., Santos, G. W., Burke, P. J., Mullins, G. M., and Humphrey, R. L. Cytotoxic antibodies in normal human serums reactive with tumor cells from acute lymphatic leukemia. Science 178, 304–306, 1972

Bichel, P., and Dombernowsky, P. On the resting stages of the JB-1 ascites tumour. Cell Tissue Kinet 6, 359–367, 1973

Bicker, U., Ziegler, B. E., and Hebold, G. 2-[2-Cyanaziridinyl-(1)]-2-[2-carbamoylaziridinyl-(1)-propane] BM 12 531. A new substance with immune stimulating action. IRCS Med Sci 5, 299, 1977

Biddle, C. Stimulation of transplanted 3-methylcholanthrene-induced sarcomas in mice by specific immune and by normal serum. Int J Cancer 17, 755–764, 1976

Bielschowsky, F. Neoplasia and internal environment. Br J Cancer 9, 80–116, 1955

Bielschowsky, F., and Hall, W. H. Carcinogenesis in thyroidectomised rats. Br J Cancer 7, 358–366, 1953

Bierman, H. R., Bryon, R. L., Kelley, K. H., and

Grady, A. Studies on the blood supply of tumors in man III. Vascular patterns of the liver by hepatic arteriography in vivo. J Natl Cancer Inst 12, 107–131, 1951

Biggs, P. M. Marek's disease pp 557–594, In Kaplan, A. S. (Ed): The Herpes-viruses. New York: Academic Press, 1973

Biggs, P. M., Jackson, C. A. W., Bell, R. A., Lancaster, F. M., and Milne, B. S. A vaccination study with an attenuated Marek's disease virus, pp 139–146, In Oncogenesis and Herpesviruses. Lyon: IARC, 1972

Biggs, P. M., and Payne, L. N. Transmission experiments with Marek's disease (fowl paralysis). Vet Rec 75, 177–180, 1963

Billingham, R. E., and Brent, L. A simple method for inducing tolerance of skin homografts in mice. Transplant Bull 4, 67–71, 1957

Billingham, R. E., Brent, L., and Medawar, P. B. Enhancement in normal homografts, with a note on the possible mechanism. Transplant Bull 3, 85–88, 1956

Billingham, R. E., and Silvers, W. K. The use of tolerance to reduce the complexity of reactions to antigen mixtures. Cancer Res 28, 1404–1409, 1968

Binder, P., Perrot, L., Beaudry, Y., Bottex, C., and Fontanges, R. Étude, chez le rat, des effets de la neuraminidase bactérienne et virale, en injection intratumorale. CR Acad Sci (D) 281, 1545–1547, 1975

Biniaminov, M., and Ramot, B. In vitro restoration by levamisole of thymus-derived lymphocyte function in Hodgkin's disease. Lancet 1, 464, 1975

Biozzi, G., Howard, J. G., Mouton, D., and Stiffel, C. Modifications of graft-versus-host reaction induced by pretreatment of the host with M. tuberculosis and C. parvum. Transplant 3, 170–177, 1965

Biozzi, G., Howard, J. G., Stiffel, C., and Mouton, D. The effect of splenectomy on the severity of graft-versus-host disease in adult mice. J Reticuloendothel Soc 1, 18–28, 1964

Biozzi, G., Stiffel, C., Halpern, B. N., and Mouton, D. Étude de la fonction phagocytaire du système réticuloendothelial au cours du développement de tumeurs malignes expérimentales chez le rat et la souris. Ann Inst Pasteur Lille 94, 681–693, 1958

Biozzi, G., Stiffel, C., Halpern, B. N., and Mouton, D. Effet de l'inoculation du bacille de Calmette Guérin sur le développement de la tumeur ascitique d'Ehrlich chez la souris. CR Soc Biol 153, 987–989, 1959

Biozzi, G., Stiffel, C., Mouton, D., Bouthillier, Y., and Decreusefond, C. A kinetic study of antibody producing cells in the spleen of mice immunized intravenously with sheep erythrocytes. Immunology *14*, 7–20, 1968

Biozzi, G., Stiffel, C., Mouton, D., Bouthillier, Y., and Decreusefond, C. Importance de l'immuité spécifique et non spécifique dans la défence antitumorale. Ann Inst Pasteur *122*, 685–694, 1972

Biran, H., Moake, J. L., Reed, R., and Freireich, E. J. Complement activation during immunotherapy with Corynebacterium parvum. Clin Res *23*, 409A, 1975

Birbeck, M. S. C., and Carter, R. L. Observations on the ultrastructure of two hamster lymphomas with particular reference to infiltrating macrophages. Int J Cancer *9*, 249–257, 1972

Biskind, M. S., and Biskind, G. R. Development of tumors in the rat ovary after transplantation into the spleen. Proc Soc Exp Biol Med *55*, 176–179, 1944

Bittner, J. J. A review of genetic studies on the transplantation of tumours. J Genet *31*, 471–487, 1935

Bittner, J. J. Some possible effects of nursing on the mammary gland tumour incidence in mice. Science *84*, 162, 1936

Bittner, J. J. Milk-influence of breast tumours in mice. Science *95*, 462–463, 1942

Bittner, J. J. The causes and control of mammary cancer in mice. Harvey Lectures *42*, 221–246, 1946

Björkland, B. A new lytic system, independent of complement (C') operating in immune lysis of human cancer cells in vitro. Acta Path Microbiol Scand (Suppl) *51*, 191–193, 1961

Björkland, B., and Björkland, V. Antigenicity of pooled human malignant and normal tissues by cyto-immunological technique: I. Presence of an insoluble, heat labile tumor antigen. Int Arch Allergy *10*, 153–184, 1957

Björkland, B., Björkland, V., and Hedlöf, I. Antigenicity of pooled human malignant and normal tissues by cytoimmunological technique: III. Distribution of tumor antigen. J Natl Cancer Inst *26*, 533–546, 1961

Björkland, B., Graham, J. B., and Graham, R. M. Effect of horse anti-human cancer serum on malignant and normal human cells. Int Arch Allergy *10*, 56–64, 1957

Björkland, B., Lundblad, G., and Björkland, V. Antigenicity of pooled human malignant and normal tissues by cyto-immunological technique: II. Nature of the tumor antigen. Int Arch Allergy *12*, 241–261, 1958

Black, M. M., Barclay, T. H., Cutler, S. J., Hankey, B. F., and Asire, A. J. Association of atypical characteristics of benign breast lesions with subsequent risk of breast cancer. Cancer *29*, 338–343, 1972

Black, M. M., Kerpe, S., and Speer, F. D. Lymph node structure in patients with cancer of the breast. Am J Pathol *29*, 505–521, 1953

Black, M.M., and Leis, H. P. Cellular responses to autologous breast cancer tissue. Correlation with the stage and lymphoreticuloendothelial activity. Cancer *28*, 263–273, 1971

Black, M. M., and Leis, H. P. Cellular responses to autologous breast cancer tissue—Sequential observations. Cancer *32*, 384–389, 1973

Black, M. M., Leis, H. P., Shore, B., and Zachra, R. E. Cellular hypersensitivity to breast cancer. Assessment by a leukocyte migration procedure. Cancer *33*, 952–958, 1974

Black, M. M., Opler, S. R., and Speer, F. D. Microscopic structure of gastric carcinomas and their regional lymph nodes in relation to survival. Surg Gynecol Obstet *98*, 725–734, 1954

Black, M. M., Opler, S. R., and Speer, F. D. Survival in breast cancer cases in relation to the structure of the primary tumor and regional lymph nodes. Surg Gynecol Obstet *100*, 543–551, 1955

Black, M. M., Opler, S. R., and Speer, F. D. Structural representations of tumor-host relationships in gastric carcinoma. Surg Gynecol Obstet *102*, 599–603, 1956

Black, M. M., and Speer, F. D. Sinus histiocytosis of lymph nodes in cancer. Surg Gynecol Obstet *106*, 163–175, 1958

Black, M. M., Zachra, R. E., Shore, B., and Leis, H. P. Biological considerations of tumor-specific and virus-associated antigens of human breast cancer. Cancer Res *36*, 769–774, 1976

Blair, P. B., Kripke, M. L., Lappé, M. A., Bonhag, R. S., and Young, L. Immunologic deficiency associated with mammary tumor virus (MTV) infection in mice: Hemagglutinin response and allograft survival. J Immunol *106*, 364–370, 1971

Blair, P. B., and Lane, M.-A. Immunologic evidence for horizontal transmission of MTV. J Immunol *113*, 1446–1449, 1974

Blamey, R. W. The effect of non-specifically sensitized lymphocytes on tumor growth. Br J Surg *53*, 152, 1966

Blamey, R. W., and Evans, D. M. D. Spleen weight in rats during tumour growth and in homograft rejection. Br J Cancer *25*, 527–532, 1971

Blanden, R. V., Lefford, J., and Mackaness, G. B. The host response to Calmette-Guérin bacillus infection in mice. J Exp Med *129*, 1079–1101, 1969

Bliznakov, E. G. Immunostimulation or immunodepression? Biomedicine *26*, 73–76, 1977

Bloom, H. J. G. The influence of delay on the natural history and prognosis of breast cancer. Br J Cancer *19*, 228–262, 1965

Bloom, H. J. G., Baker, W. H., Dukes, C. E., and Mitchley, B. C. V. Hormone-dependent tumours of the kidney. II. Effect of endocrine ablation procedures on the transplanted oestrogen-induced renal tumour of the Syrian hamster. Br J Cancer 17, 646–656, 1963a

Bloom, H. J. G., Dukes, C. E., and Mitchley, B. C. V. Hormone-dependent tumours of the kidney. I. The oestrogen-induced renal tumour of the Syrian hamster. Hormone treatment and possible relationship to carcinoma of the kidney in man. Br J Cancer 17, 611–645, 1963b

Bloom, H. J. G., Richardson, W. W., and Harries, E. J. Natural history of untreated breast cancer (1805–1933). Comparison of untreated and treated cases according to histological grade of malignancy. Br Med J 2, 213–221, 1962

Bloom, H. J. G., and Wallace, D. M. Hormones and the kidney: Possible therapeutic role of testosterone in a patient with regression of metastases from renal adenocarcinoma. Br Med J 2, 476–480, 1964

Bluming, A. Z., Vogel, L., and Ziegler, J. L. Clinical screening of systemic adjuvants of immunity. Rec Results Cancer Res 47, 415–420, 1974

Bluming, A. Z., Vogel, C. L., Ziegler, J. L., Mody, N., and Kamya, G. Immunological effects of BCG in malignant melanoma: Two modes of administration compared. Ann Intern Med 76, 405–411, 1972

Bluming, A. Z., and Ziegler, J. L. Regression of Burkitt's lymphoma in association with measles infection. Lancet 2, 105–106, 1971

Bluming, A. Z., Ziegler, J. L., Fass, L., and Herberman, R. B. Delayed cutaneous sensitivity reactions to autologous Burkitt lymphoma protein extracts. Clin Exp Immunol 9, 713–719, 1971

Boak, J. L. Local Corynebacterium parvum therapy in early breast cancer: A pilot study. Clin Oncol 4, 235–242, 1978

Boak, J. L., and Agwunobi, T. C. An in vivo study of regional lymph node phagocytic activity in benign and malignant breast cancer, pp 418–425, In James, K., McBride, B., and Stuart, A. (Eds): Proc EURES Symposium—The Macrophage and Cancer. Edinburgh Univ. Dept Surgery, 1977

Boak, J. L., Agwunobi, T. C., and Mosley, J. G. Regional lymph node phagocytic activity in experimental cancer, pp 229–307, In James, K., McBride, B., and Stuart, A. (Eds): Proc EURES Symposium—The Macrophage and Cancer. Edinburgh Univ. Dept Surgery, 1977

Boak, J. L., Dagher, R. K., Corson, J. M., and Wilson, R. E. Modification of the graft-versus-host syndrome by anti-lymphocyte serum

treatment of the host. Clin Exp Immunol 3, 801–808, 1968

Boak, J. L., and Tebbutt, S. Effect of Corynebacterium parvum on subcutaneous and skeletal methylcholanthrene sarcoma implants. Clin Oncol 3, 353–363, 1977

Boak, J. L., and Wilson, R. E. Modification of the graft-versus-host syndrome by anti-lymphocyte serum treatment of the donor. Clin Exp Immunol 3, 795–800, 1968

Bodenham, D. C. A study of 650 observed malignant melanomas in the South-West region. Ann R Coll Surg Engl 43, 218–239, 1968

Boetcher, D. A., and Leonard E. J. Abnormal monocyte chemotactic response in cancer patients. J Natl Cancer Inst 52, 1091–1099, 1974

Bolhuis, R. L. H. Cellular microcytotoxicity in a human bladder cancer system: Analysis of in vitro lymphocyte-mediated cytotoxicity against cultured target cells. Cancer Immunol Immunother 2, 245–256, 1977

Bomford, R. Active specific immunotherapy of mouse methylcholanthrene induced tumours with Corynebacterium parvum and irradiated tumour cells. Br J Cancer 32, 551–557, 1975

Bomford, R. An analysis of the factors allowing promotion (rather than inhibition) of tumour growth by Corynebacterium parvum. Br J Cancer 19, 673–679, 1977

Bomford, R. The comparative selectivity of adjuvants for humoral and cell-mediated immunity. I. Effect on the antibody response to bovine serum albumin and sheep red blood cells of Freund's incomplete and complete adjuvant, alhydrogel, Corynebacterium parvum, Bordetella pertussis, muramyl dipeptide and saponin. Clin Exp Immunol 39, 426–434, 1980a

Bomford, R. The comparative selectivity of adjuvants for humoral and cell-mediated immunity. II. Effect on delayed-type hypersensitivity in the mouse and guinea pig, and cell-mediated immunity to tumour antigens in the mouse of Freund's incomplete and complete adjuvants, alhydrogel, Corynebacterium parvum, Bordetella pertussis, muramyl dipeptide and saponin. Clin Exp Immunol 39, 435–441, 1980b

Bomford, R., and Christie, G. H. Mechanisms of macrophage activation by Corynebacterium parvum. II. In vivo experiments. Cell Immunol 17, 150–155, 1975

Bomford, R., and Moreno, R. A comparison of the antitumor activities of glucans and C. parvum. Dev Biol Stand 38, 291–295, 1978

Bomford, R., and Olivotto, M. The mechanism of inhibition by Corynebacterium parvum of the growth of lung nodules from intravenously injected tumour cells. Int J Cancer 14, 226–235, 1974

Bomford, R., Shand, F. L., and Christie, G. H. Observations on the mechanism of antitumour resistance induced by the graft-versus-host reaction. Transplantation 20, 433–435, 1975

Bonadonna, G., Brusamolino, E., Valagussa, P., Rossi, A., Brugnatelli, L., Brambilla, C., De Lena, M., Tancini, G., Bajetta, E., Musumeci, R., and Veronesi, U. Combination chemotherapy as an adjuvant treatment in operable breast cancer. N Engl J Med 294, 405–410, 1976

Bonadonna, G., Rossi, A., Valagussa, P., Banfi, A., and Veronesi, U. The CMF program for operable breast cancer with positive axillary nodes. Updated analysis on the disease-free interval, site of relapse and drug tolerance. Cancer 39, 2904–2915, 1977

Bonavida, B., and Kedar, E. Transplantation of allogeneic lymphoid cells specifically depleted of graft versus host reactive cells. Nature 249, 658–659, 1974

Bonmassar, E., Campanile, F., Houchens, D., Crino, L., and Goldin, A. Impaired growth of a radiation-induced lymphoma in intact or lethally irradiated allogeneic athymic (nude) mice. Transplantation 20, 343–346, 1975

Bonmassar, E., and Cudkowicz, G. Suppression of allogeneic lymphomas in spleen of irradiated mice—Importance of the D end of the H-2 complex. J Immunol 117, 697–700, 1976

Bonnard, G. D., Manders, E. K., Campbell, D. A., Herberman, R. B., and Collins, M. J. Immunosuppressive activity of a subline of the mouse EL-4 lymphoma. Evidence for minute virus of mice causing the inhibition. J Exp Med 143, 187–205, 1976

Boone, C. W., Brandchaft, P. R., Irving, D. N., and Gilden, R. Quantitative studies on the binding of syngeneic antibody to the surface antigens of AKR-virus-induced rat lymphoma cells. Int J Cancer 9, 685–692, 1972

Boone, C. W., Paranjpe, M., Orme, T., and Gillette, R. Virus-augmented tumor transplantation antigens: Evidence for a helper antigen mechanism. Int J Cancer 13, 543–551, 1974

Booth, S. N., Jamieson, G. C., King, J. B. G., Leonard, J., Oates, G. D., and Dykes, P. W. Carcinoembryonic antigen in management of colorectal carcinoma. Br Med J 4, 183–187, 1974

Boranic, M. Transient graft-versus-host reaction in the treatment of leukemia in mice. J Natl Cancer Inst 41, 421–437, 1968

Boranic, M., and Tonkovic, I. The effect of cyclophosphamide on the ability of graft-versus-host reaction to suppress leukaemia in mice. Rev Eur Etudes Clin Biol 17, 314–320, 1972

Borberg, H., Oettgen, H. F., Choudry, K., and

Beattie, E. J. Inhibition of established transplants of chemically induced sarcomas in syngeneic mice by lymphocytes from immunized donors. Int J Cancer 10, 539–547, 1972

Borek, C., Grob, M., and Burger, M. M. Surface alterations in transformed epithelial and fibroblastic cells in culture; A disturbance of membrane degradation versus biosynthesis? Exp Cell Res 77, 207–215, 1973

Borek, C., and Sachs, L. The difference in contact inhibition of cell replication between normal cells and cells transformed by different carcinogens. Proc Natl Acad Sci USA 56, 1705–1711, 1966

Borrie, J. Secondary lung cancer treated surgically; A nine-year study. NZ Med J 69, 71–77, 1969

Borsos, T., Colten, H. R., Spalter, J. S., Rogentine, N., and Rapp, H. J. The C'la fixation and transfer test: Examples of its applicability to the detection and enumeration of antigens and antibodies at cell surfaces. J Immunol 101, 392–398, 1968

Borsos, T., and Cooper, M. On the hemolytic activity of mouse complement. Proc Soc Exp Biol Med 107, 227–232, 1961

Borsos, T., and Rapp. H. J. Hemolysin titration based on fixation of the activated first component of complement: Evidence that one molecule of hemolysin suffices to sensitize an erythrocyte. J Immunol 95, 559–566, 1965

Borsos, T., and Rapp. H. J. Antigenic relationship between Mycobacterium bovis (BCG) and a guinea pig hepatoma. J Natl Cancer Inst 51, 1085–1086, 1973

Borst, P. Mitochondrial nucleic acids. Annu Rev Biochem 41, 333–376, 1972

Bortin, M. M. A compendium of reported human bone marrow transplants. Transplantation 9, 571–587, 1970

Bortin, M. M., Rimm, A. A., Rodey, G. E., Giller, R. H., and Saltzstein, H. C. Prolonged survival in long-passage AKR leukemia using chemotherapy, radiotherapy, and adoptive immunotherapy. Cancer Res 34, 1851–1856, 1974a

Bortin, M. M., Rimm, A. A., Rose, W. C., and Saltzstein, E. C. Graft-versus-leukemia. V. Absence of antileukemic effect using allogeneic H-2-identical immunocompetent cells. Transplantation 18, 280–283, 1974b

Bouck, N., and di Mayorca, G. Somatic mutation as the basis for malignant transformation of BHK cells by chemical carcinogens. Nature 264, 722–727, 1976

Bowen, J. G., and Baldwin, R. W. Tumour-specific antigen related to rat histocompatibility antigens. Nature 258, 75–76, 1975

Bowen, J. G., and Baldwin, R. W. Isolation and

characterization of tumour-specific antigen from the serum of rats bearing transplanted aminoazo dye-induced hepatomas. Transplantation *21*, 213–219, 1976

Boyd, W. The spontaneous regression of cancer. J Can Assoc Radiol *8*, 45–54, 1957

Boyd, W. The Spontaneous Regression of Cancer. Springfield: Charles C. Thomas, 1966

Boyer, P. J. J., and Fahey, J. L. Stimulation of lymphoid cells from normal and immune mice by syngeneic BALD/c plasma cell tumors. J Immunol *116*, 202–209, 1976

Boyle, M. D. P., and Ormerod, M. G. Destruction of allogeneic tumour cells by peritoneal macrophages. Transplantation *21*, 242–246, 1976

Boyse, E. A. The fate of mouse spleen cells transplanted into homologous and F1-hybrid hosts. Immunology *2*, 170–181, 1959

Boyse, E. A. Immune responses to experimental tumours. Active immunity against tumours induced by chemical carcinogens. Guy's Hosp Rep *112*, 433–448, 1963

Boyse, E. A. Cell membrane receptors, pp 5–30, In Smith, R. T., and Landy, M. (Eds): Immune Surveillance. New York: Academic Press, 1970

Boyse, E. A., and Old, L. J. Some aspects of normal and abnormal cell surface genetics. Annu Rev Genet *3*, 269–290, 1969

Boyse, E. A., and Old, L. J. The immunogenetics of differentiation in the mouse, pp 23–53, In The Harvey Lectures, 1975–1976, Series 71. New York: Academic Press, 1978

Boyse, E. A., Old, L. J., and Stockert, E. The TL (thymus leukemia) antigen. A review, In Grabar, P., and Miescher, P. A. (Eds): Immunopathology—IVth International Symposium. Basel: Schwabe, 1965

Boyse, E. A., Stockert, E., and Old, L. J. Modification of the antigenic structure of the cell membrane by thymus-leukemia (TL) antibody. Proc Natl Acad Sci USA *58*, 954–957, 1967

Braeman, J., and Deeley, T. J. Radiotherapy and the immune response in cancer of the lung. Br J Radiol *46*, 446–449, 1973

Brandes, L. J., Galton, D. A. G., and Wiltshaw, E. New approach to immunotherapy of melanoma. Lancet *2*, 293–295, 1971

Braun, W. Cell population dynamics and somatic change. J Cell Comp Physiol (Suppl I) *52*, 337–369, 1958

Braun, W. Influence of nucleic acid degradation products on antibody synthesis, pp 525–534, In Sterzl, J. (Ed): Molecular and Cellular Basis of Antibody Formation. New York: Academic Press, 1965

Braun, W. Some causes and repair of altered antibody formation in aged animals, In Sigel, M.

(Ed): Aging and Autoimmunity. Springfield, Ill.: C. C. Thomas, 1970

Braun, W., Firshein, W., and Whallon, A. Effects of deoxyribonucleic acid breakdown products on bacterial population changes and virulence. Science *125*, 445–447, 1957

Braun, W., Ishizuka, M., Yajima, Y., Webb, D., and Winchurch, R. Spectrum and mode of action of poly A:U in the stimulation of immune responses, pp 139–156, In Beers, R. F., and Braun, W. (Eds): Biological Effects of Polynucleotides. New York: Springer-Verlag, 1971

Braun, W., and Nakano, M. Influence of oligodeoxyribonucleotides on early events in antibody formation. Proc Soc Exp Biol Med *119*, 701–707, 1965

Braun, W., and Nakano, M. The reinforcement of immunological stimuli by oligodeoxyribonucleotides, In Smith, R., and Good, R. (Eds): Ontogeny of Immunity. Univ Florida Press, 1967a

Braun, W., and Nakano, M. Antibody formation: Stimulation by polyadenylic and polycytidylic acids. Science *157*, 819–821, 1967b

Braun, W., Nakano, M., Jaraskova, L., Yagima, Y., and Jimenez, L. Stimulation of antibody-forming cells by oligonucleotides of known composition, pp 347–363, In Plescia, O. J., and Braun, W. (Eds): Nucleic Acids in Immunology. New York: Springer-Verlag, 1968

Braun, W., and Whallon, J. The effects of DNA and enzyme-treated DNA on bacterial population changes. Proc Natl Acad Sci USA *40*, 162–165, 1954

Brawn, R. J. Possible association of embryonal antigen(s) with several primary 3-methylcholanthrene-induced murine sarcomas. Int J Cancer *6*, 245–249, 1970

Bremberg, S., Klein, E., and Stjernsward, J. Effect of heterologous antilymphoid-cell serum on tumor isografts and viral leukemogenesis. Cancer Res *27*, 2113–2118, 1967

Brennan, M. J., Prychodko, W., and Horeglad, S. Quantitative studies on the growth of spontaneous tumors, pp 739–748, In Biological Interactions in Normal and Neoplastic Growth. Henry Ford Hosp Int Symp, 1962

Brenner, H. J., and Yerushalmi, A. Combined local hyperthermia and X-irradiation in the treatment of metastatic tumours. Br J Cancer *33*, 91–95, 1975

Brenner, M. W., Holsti, L. R., and Perttala, Y. The study by graphical analysis of the growth of human tumours and metastases of the lung. Br J Cancer *21*, 1–13, 1967

Brent, L., Brown, J., and Medawar, P. B. Skin

transplantation immunity in relation to hypersensitivity. Lancet 2, 561–564, 1958

Breur, K. Growth Rate and Radiosensitivity of
Human Tumours [Thesis, in Dutch]. Haag:
Mouton, 1965

Breyere, E. J., and Williams, L. B. Antigens associated with a tumor virus: Rejection of isogenic skin grafts from leukemic mice. Science
146, 1055–1056, 1964

Brinkley, D. M., and Haybrittle, J. L. Treatment
of stage-II carcinoma of the female breast.
Lancet 2, 1086–1087, 1971

British Breast Group. Assessment of response to
treatment in advanced breast cancer. Lancet
2, 38–39, 1974

British Medical Journal. Immunotherapy of cancer.
Br Med J 2, 185–186, 1966

British Medical Journal. Cell life and death in human tumours. Br Med J 1, 177–178, 1976a

British Medical Journal. Hormone receptors and
breast cancer. Br Med J 2, 67–68, 1976b

British Medical Journal. Lung cancer and smoking:
Is there proof? Br Med J 2, 439–440, 1976c

British Medical Journal. Randomised clinical trials.
Br Med J 1, 1238–1239, 1977a

British Medical Journal. Liver tumours and the
pill. Br Med J 2, 345–346, 1977b

British Medical Journal. Skeletal scintigraphy in
carcinoma of the breast. Br Med J 2, 592–
593, 1977c

British Medical Journal. Primary treatment of prostatic cancer. Br Med J 2, 781–782, 1977d

Brittingham, T. E., and Chaplin, M. Production
of a human "antileukemic" leucocyte serum
and its therapeutic trial. Cancer 13, 412–418,
1960

Britton, D. C., Bone, G., Wright, N. A., and Camplejohn, R. S. Measurement of cell production
rates in human gastro-intestinal cancer—A
guide to treatment. Br J Surg 62, 813–815,
1975

Brncic, D., Hoecker, G., and Gasic, G. Immunity
in mice against leukaemic cells of the same
genetic constitution. Acta Unio Int Contra
Cancrum 7, 762–764, 1952

Brooks, R. F. Regulation of the fibroblast cell cycle
by serum. Nature 260, 248–250, 1976

Brooks, W. H., Netsky, M. G., Normansell, D. E.,
and Horwitz, D. A. Depressed cell-mediated
immunity in patients with primary intracranial
tumors. J Exp Med 136, 1631–1647, 1972

Broom, B. C., and Alexander, P. Mast cell and
anaphylactic antibody responses in inbred rats
to syngeneic fibrosarcomas. Int Arch Allergy
Appl Immunol 49, 627–631, 1975

Brown, G., and Greaves, M. F. Cell surface markers for human T and B lymphocytes. Eur J
Immunol 4, 302–310, 1974

Brown, J. H. The results of resection of pulmonary
metastases. Med J Aust 1, 496–497, 1963

Brown, J. M. A study of the mechanism by which
anticoagulation with warfarin inhibits blood-
borne metastases. Cancer Res 33, 1217–1224,
1973

Browning, H. C. Heterologous and homologous
growth of transplants during the course of development of spontaneous mammary tumors
in C3H mice. J Natl Cancer Inst 8, 173–189,
1948

Brozovic, B., Šljivić, V. S., and Warr, G. W. Hae-
matological changes and iron metabolism in
rats after administration of Corynebacterium
parvum. Br J Exp Pathol 56, 183–192, 1975

Bruchovsky, N., Sutherland, D. J. A., Meakin,
J. W., and Minesita, T. Androgen receptors:
Relationship to growth response and to intracellular androgen transport in nine variant
lines of the Shionogi mouse mammary carcinoma. Biochim Biophys Acta 381, 61–71,
1975

Brunner, K. W., Marthaler, T., and Muller, W.
Effects of long-term adjuvant chemotherapy
with cyclophosphamide (NSC-26271) for radi-
cally resected bronchogenic carcinoma. Cancer
Chemother Rep (Suppl) 4, 125–132, 1973

Brunschwig, A. Spontaneous regression of cancer.
Surgery 53, 423–431, 1963

Brunschwig, A., Southam, C. M., and Levin, A. G.
Host resistance to cancer. Clinical experiments
by homotransplants, autotransplants and admixture of autologous leucocytes. Ann Surg
162, 416–425, 1965

Bubenik, J. Immunity against cancerogen-induced
tumours. Neoplasma 12, 119–124, 1965

Bubenik, J., Ivanyi, J., and Koldovsky, P. Participation of 7S and 19S antibodies in enhancement and resistance to methylcholanthrene-
induced tumours. Folia Biol (Praha) 11, 426–
433, 1965

Bubenik, J., and Koldovsky, P. Detection of antitumour immunity by a cytotoxic test. Folia
Biol (Praha) 8, 363–366, 1962

Bubenik, J., and Koldovsky, P. Factors influencing
the induction of enhancement and resistance
to methylcholanthrene-induced tumours in a
syngeneic system. Folia Biol (Praha) 11, 258–
265, 1965

Bubenik, J., Perlman, P., Helmstein, K., and Mob-
erger, G. Cellular and humoral immune responses to urinary bladder carcinomas. Int J
Cancer 5, 310–319, 1970

Bubenik, J., and Turano, A. Inhibitory effect of
immune serum on carcinogenesis in mice neonatally infected with murine sarcoma virus
(Harvey). Folia Biol (Praha) 14, 433–439, 1968

Bubenik, J., Turano, A., and Fadda, G. Prevention

of carcinogenesis by murine sarcoma virus (Harvey) following injections of immune sera during the latent period. Int J Cancer 4, 648–654, 1969

Buehler, H. G., Bettaglio, A., and Kavan, L. C. Disappearance of metastases following nephrectomy for carcinoma. J Okla State Med Assoc 53, 674–677, 1960

Bull, D. M., Leibach, J. R., Williams, M. A., and Helms, R. A. Immunity to colon cancer assessed by antigen induced inhibition of mixed mononuclear cell migration. Science 181, 957–959, 1973

Bullough, W. S. Mitotic and functional homeostasis. Cancer Res 25, 1683–1727, 1965

Bullough, W. S. Mitotic control in adult mammalian tissues. Biol Rev 50, 99–127, 1975

Bullough, W. S., and Laurence, E. B. Control of mitosis in mouse and hamster melanomata by means of the melanocyte chalone. Eur J Cancer 4, 607–615, 1968

Bullough, W. S., and Laurence, E. B. The lymphocytic chalone and its antimitotic action on a mouse lymphoma in vitro. Eur J Cancer 6, 525–531, 1970

Bullough, W. S., and Rytömaa, T. Mitotic homeostasis. Nature 205, 573–578, 1965

Bumpus, H. C. The apparent disappearance of pulmonary metastases in a case of hypernephroma following nephrectomy. J Urol 20, 185–191, 1928

Burch, P. R. J. Natural and radiation carcinogenesis in man. I. Theory of initiation phase. Proc R Soc Lond B 162, 223–239, 1965a

Burch, P. R. J. Natural and radiation carcinogenesis in man. II. Natural leukaemogenesis: Initiation. Proc R Soc Lond B 162, 240–262, 1965b

Burch, P. R. J. Natural and radiation carcinogenesis in man. III. Radiation carcinogenesis. Proc R Soc Lond B 162, 263–287, 1965c

Burch, P. R. J. New approach to cancer. Nature 225, 512–516, 1970

Burchenal, J. H. Adjuvant therapy—Theory, practice and potential. Cancer 37, 46–57, 1976

Burdette, W. J. Heritable cancer of the colorectum, pp 78–97, In Burdette, W. J. (Ed): Carcinoma of the Colon and Antecedent Epithelium. Springfield, Ill.: Charles C. Thomas, 1970

Burdick, J. F., and Wells, S. A. Cross-reactivity between cell-surface antigens of different murine carcinogen-induced tumors, demonstrated by a modified isotopic antiglobulin test. J Natl Cancer Inst 51, 1149–1156, 1973

Burdick, J. F., Wells, S. A., and Herberman, R. B. Immunologic evaluation of patients with cancer by delayed hypersensitivity reactions. Surg Gynecol Obstet 141, 779–794, 1975

Burdick, K. H. Malignant melanoma treated with vaccinia injections. Arch Dermatol 82, 438–439, 1960

Burdick, K. H., and Hank, W. A. Vitiligo in a case of vaccinia virus-treated melanoma. Cancer 17, 708–712, 1964

Burger, M. M. A difference in the architecture of the surface membrane of normal and virally transformed cells. Proc Natl Acad Sci USA 62, 994–1001, 1969

Burger, M. M. Proteolytic enzymes initiating cell division and escape from contact inhibition of growth. Nature 227, 170–171, 1970

Burger, M. M., and Noonan, K. D. Restoration of normal growth by covering of agglutinin sites on tumour cell surface. Nature 228, 512–515, 1970

Burki, K., and Bresnick, E. Early morphologic alterations in mouse skin after topical application of 3-methylcholanthrene and its metabolites. J Natl Cancer Inst 55, 171–175, 1975

Burkitt, D. P. A children's cancer dependent on climatic factors. Nature 194, 232–234, 1962

Burkitt, D. P. Etiology of Burkitt's lymphoma—An alternative hypothesis to a vectored virus. J Natl Cancer Inst 42, 19–28, 1969

Burn, J. I. Should lymphadenectomy be discarded? Mechanical effects. J R Coll Surg Edinb 18, 346–350, 1973

Burn, J. I. Early breast cancer; The Hammersmith trial. Br J Surg 61, 762–765, 1974

Burnet, F. M. Cancer—A biological approach. Br Med J 1, 779–786, 841–847, 1957

Burnet, F. M. The Clonal Selection Theory of Acquired Immunity. Cambridge Univ Press, 1959

Burnet, F. M. Immunological factors in the process of carcinogenesis. Br Med Bull 20, 154–158, 1964

Burnet, F. M. Possible autoimmune processes in carcinomatous neuromyopathy. Information Exchange Group, Immunopathol Memo 70, 1965

Burnet, F. M. Immunological aspects of malignant disease. Lancet 1, 1171–1174, 1967

Burnet, F. M. Immunological Surveillance. London, New York: Pergamon Press, 1970a

Burnet, F. M. The concept of immunological surveillance. Prog Exp Tumor Res 13, 1–27, 1970b

Burnet, F. M. Immunological surveillance in neoplasia. Transplant Rev 7, 3–25, 1971

Burnet, F. M. Intrinsic Mutagenesis: A Genetic Approach to Ageing. Lancaster: Medical & Technical, 1974

Burnet, F. M. Immunology, Aging and Cancer (Medical Aspects of Mutation and Selection). San Francisco: W. H. Freeman, 1976

Burnet, F. M. Morphogenesis and cancer. Med J Aust *1*, 5–9, 1977

Burnham, T. K. Antinuclear antibodies in patients with malignancies. Lancet *2*, 436–437, 1972

Burrows, D. The Schultz-Dale test for detection of antigen in patients with carcinoma. Ann NY Acad Sci *101*, 271–273, 1962

Burstein, N. A. Immunity to murine sarcoma virus (MSV) induced tumors demonstrated by in vivo elimination of ^{51}chromium labeled tumor cells. Rev Eur Etudes Clin Biol *15*, 873–875, 1970

Burton, R. C., Chism, S. E., and Warner, N. L. In vitro induction of tumor specific immunity. III. Lack of requirement for H-2 compatibility in lysis of tumor targets by T cells activated in vitro to oncofetal and plasmacytoma antigens. J Immunol *118*, 971–980, 1977

Burton, R. C., Thompson, J., and Warner, N. L. In vitro induction of tumour-specific immunity. I. Development of optimal conditions for induction and assay of cytotoxic lymphocytes. J Immunol Meth *8*, 133–150, 1975

Burton, R. C., and Warner, N. L. Tumor immunity to murine plasma cell tumors. III. Detections of common and unique tumor-associated antigens on Balb/c, C3H and NZB plasmacytomas by in vivo and in vitro induction of tumor-immune responses. J Natl Cancer Inst *58*, 701–709, 1977a

Burton, R. C., and Warner, N. L. In vitro induction of tumor-specific immunity. IV. Specific adoptive immunotherapy with cytotoxic T cells induced in vitro to plasmacytoma antigens. Cancer Immunol Immunother *2*, 91–99, 1977b

Burton, R. C., and Warner, N. L. In vitro induction of tumor specific immunity V. Detection of common antigenic determinants of murine fibrosarcomas. Br J Cancer *37*, 159–170, 1978

Busch, H., and Smetana, K. The Nucleolus. New York: Academic Press, 1970

Busch, H., and Smetana, K. The nucleus of the cancer cell, pp 41–80, In Busch, H. (Ed): The Molecular Biology of Cancer. New York: Academic Press, 1974

Buttle, G. A. H., Eperon, J., and Menzies, D. N. Induced tumour resistance in rats. Lancet *2*, 12–14, 1964

Byers, V. S., LeCam, L., Levin, A. S., Stone, W. H., and Hackett, A. J. Identification of human populations with a high incidence of cellular immunity against breast carcinoma. Cancer Immunol Immunother *2*, 163–172, 1977

Byers, V. S., Levin, A. S., Hacket, A. J., and Fudenberg, H. H. Tumor-specific cell-mediated immunity in household contacts of cancer patients. J Clin Invest *55*, 500–513, 1975

Byfield, J. E., Weintraub, I., Klisak, I., and La-gasse, L. D. Inhibition of colony formation by cytotoxic antibodies in cervical epidermoid carcinomas. Radiology *107*, 685–686, 1973

Byrne, M., Heppner, G., Stolbach, F., Cummings, F., McDonough, E., and Calabresi, P. Tumor immunity in melanoma patients as assessed by colony inhibition and microcytotoxicity methods: A preliminary report. Natl Cancer Inst Monogr *37*, 3–8, 1973

Bystryn, J.-C. Release of tumor-associated antigens by murine melanoma cells. J Immunol *116*, 1302–1305, 1976

Bystryn, J.-C., Schenkein, I., Baur, S., and Uhr, J. W. Partial isolation and characterization of antigen(s) associated with murine melanoma. J Natl Cancer Inst *52*, 1263–1269, 1974

C

Cahan, W. G. Excision of melanoma metastases to lung: Problems in diagnosis and management. Ann Surg *178*, 703–709, 1973

Cairns, J. Mutation selection and the natural history of cancer. Nature *255*, 197–200, 1975

Calder, E. A., Irvine, W. J., and Ghaffar, A. K-cell cytotoxic activity in the spleen and lymph nodes of tumour-bearing mice. Clin Exp Immunol *19*, 393–397, 1975

Caldwell, B. V., and Wright, P. A. Neoplasm transplantation inhibition by uninvolved lymph tissue. Nature *212*, 1501, 1966

Calne, R. Y. Hepatic transplantation. Surg Clin North Am *58*, 321–333, 1978

Cameron, E. H. D., Jones, R., Jones, D., Anderson, A. B. M., and Griffiths, K. Further studies on the relationship between C_{19} and C_{20} steroid synthesis in the human adrenal gland. J Endocrinol *45*, 215–230, 1969

Campanile, F., Crino, L., Bonmassar, E., Houchens, D., and Goldin, A. Radioresistant inhibition of lymphoma growth in congenitally athymic (nude) mice. Cancer Res *37*, 394–398, 1977

Campbell, A. C., Hersey, P., Harding, B., Hollingsworth, P. M., Skinner, J., and MacLennan, I. C. M. Effects of anti-cancer agents on immunological status. Br J Cancer *28* (Suppl 1), 254–261, 1973

Canellos, G. P., and Whang-Peng, J. Philadelphia-chromosome positive preleukaemic state. Lancet *2*, 1227–1229, 1972

Cant, E. L. M., Shivas, A. A., and Forrest, A. P. M. Lymph-node biopsy during simple mastectomy. Lancet *1*, 995–997, 1975

Cantor, H., and Boyse, E. A. Functional subclasses of T lymphocytes bearing different Ly antigens. I. The generation of functionally distinct T-cell subclasses is a differentiative process independent of antigen. J Exp Med 141, 1376–1389, 1975a

Cantor, H., and Boyse, E. A. Functional subclasses of T lymphocytes bearing different Ly antigens. II. Cooperation between subclasses of Ly+ cells in the generation of killer activity. J Exp Med 141, 1390–1399, 1975b

Cantor, H., and Boyse, E. A. Regulation of cellular and humoral immune responses by T-cell subclasses. Cold Spring Harbor Symp Quant Biol 41, 23–32, 1977

Cantor, H., Kasai, M., Shen, F. W., Leclerc, J. C., and Glimcher, L. Immunogenetic analysis of "natural killer" activity in the mouse. Immunol Rev 44, 3–12, 1979

Cantor, H., and Simpson, E. Regulation of the immune response by subclasses of T lymphocytes. I. Interactions between prekiller T cells and regulatory T cells obtained from peripheral lymphoid tissues of mice. Eur J Immunol 5, 330–336, 1975

Cantor, H., and Weissman, I. Development and function of subpopulations of thymocytes and T lymphocytes. Prog Allergy 20, 1–64, 1976

Cantor, H. R., Asofsky, R., and Levy, H. B. The effect of polyinosinic-polycytidylic acid upon graft-vs-host activity in BALB/c mice. J Immunol 104, 1035–1038, 1970

Carey, R. M., Orth, D. N., and Hartmann, W. H. Malignant melanoma with ectopic production of adrenocorticotropic hormone: Palliative treatment with inhibitors of adrenal steroid biosynthesis. J Clin Endocrinol Metab 36, 482–487, 1973

Carey, R. W., Holland, J. F., Whang, H. Y., Neter, E., and Bryant, B. Clostridial oncolysis in man. Eur J Cancer 3, 37–46, 1967

Carnaud, C., Ilfeld, D., Brook, I., and Trainin, N. Increased reactivity of mouse spleen cells sensitized in vitro against syngeneic tumor cells in the presence of a thymic humoral factor. J Exp Med 138, 1521–1532, 1973

Carnes, W. H., Kaplan, H. S., Brown, M. B., and Hirsch, B. B. Indirect induction of lymphomas in irradiated mice. III. Role of the thymic graft. Cancer Res 16, 429–433, 1956

Carr, I. Macrophages in human cancer: A review, pp 364–374, In James, K., McBride, B., and Stuart, A. (Eds): Proc EURES Symposium—The Macrophage and Cancer. Edinburgh Univ Dept Surgery, 1977

Carr, I., and McGinty, F. Lymphatic metastasis and its inhibition. An experimental model. J Pathol 113, 85–95, 1974

Carr, I., and Underwood, J. C. E. The ultrastructure of the local cellular reaction to neoplasia. Int Rev Cytol 37, 329–347, 1974

Carrel, S., and Theilkaes, L. Evidence for a tumour-associated antigen in human malignant melanoma. Nature 242, 609–610, 1973

Carruthers, C., and Baumler, A. Immunological staining with fluorescein-labeled antibodies as an aid in the study of skin cancer formation. J Natl Cancer Inst 34, 191–200, 1965

Carter, S. B. Principles of cell motility: The direction of cell movement and cancer invasion. Nature 208, 1183–1187, 1965

Carter, S. K. Medical oncology. Biomedicine 26, 25–27, 1977

Cascinelli, N., Balzarine, G. P., Fontana, V., Orefice, S., and Veronesi, U. Intralymphatic administration of BCG in melanoma patients. Cancer Immunol Immunother 2, 157–161, 1977

Casey, M. J., Rabotti, G. F., Sarma, P. S., Lane, W. T., Turner, H. C., and Huebner, R. J. Complement-fixing antigens in hamster tumours induced by the Bryan strain of Rous sarcoma virus. Science 151, 1086–1088, 1966

Caspary, E. A., and Field, E. J. Specific lymphocyte sensitization in cancer: Is there a common antigen in human malignant neoplasia? Br Med J 2, 613–617, 1971

Caspersson, T., Gahrton, G., Lindsten, J., and Zech, L. Identification of the Philadelphia chromosome as a number 22 by quinacrine mustard fluorescence analysis. Exp Cell Res, 63, 238–244, 1970

Cassel, W. A., and Garrett, R. E. Tumor immunity after viral oncolysis. J Bacteriol 92, 792, 1966

Castermans-Elias, S., Simar, L., Vanwijck, R., Rustin, P., Gougnard, E., Betz, E. H., and Castermans, A. Immunosurgical treatment of stage I malignant melanoma. Cancer Immunol Immunother 2, 179–187, 1977

Castro, J. E. Human tumors grown in mice. Nature New Biol 239, 83–84, 1972

Castro, J. E. The effect of Corynebacterium parvum on the structure and function of the lymphoid system in mice. Eur J Cancer 10, 115–120, 1974a

Castro, J. E. Antitumour effects of Corynebacterium parvum in mice. Eur J Cancer 10, 121–127, 1974b

Castro, J. E. Orchidectomy and the immune response. II. Response of orchidectomized mice to antigens. Proc R Soc B 185, 437–451, 1974c

Castro, J. E. Immunological effects of hormones: A review. J R Soc Med 71, 123–125, 1978

Castro, J. E., and Hamilton, D. N. H. Adrenalectomy and orchidectomy as immunopotentiating procedures. Transplantation 13, 614–616, 1972

Castro, J. E., Hunt, R., Lance, E. M., and Medawar, P. B. Implications of the fetal antigen theory for fetal transplantation. Cancer Res *34,* 2055–2060, 1974

Castro, J. E., Lance, E. M., Medawar, P. B., Zanelli, J., and Hunt, R. Foetal antigens and cancer. Nature *243,* 225–226, 1973

Catalona, W. J., and Chretien, P. B. Abnormalities of quantitative dinitrochlorobenzene sensitization in cancer patients: Correlation with tumor stage and histology. Cancer *31,* 353–356, 1973

Catalona, W. J., Sample, W. F., and Chretien, P. B. Lymphocyte reactivity in cancer patients. Correlation with tumor and clinical stage. Cancer *31,* 65–71, 1973

Catterall, M., Bewley, D. K., and Sutherland, I. Second report on results of a randomised clinical trial of fast neutrons compared with x or gamma rays in treatment of advanced tumours of head and neck. Br Med J **1,** 1642, 1977

Cavaliere, R., Ciocatto, E. C., Giovanella, B. C., Heidelberger, C., Johnson, R. O., Margottini, M., Mondovi, B., Moricca, G., and Rossi-Fanelli, A. Selective heat sensitivity of cancer cells. Cancer *20,* 1351–1381, 1967

Cavaliere, R., Moricca, G., and Caputo, A. Regional hyperthermia by perfusion, pp 251–265, In Wizenberg, M. J., and Robinson, J. E. (Eds): Proc Intern Symp—Cancer Therapy by Hyperthermia and Radiation. Baltimore: Am Coll Radiol Press, 1976

Cavilli-Sforza, L. L., and Bodmer, W. F. The Genetics of Human Populations. San Francisco: W. H. Freeman, 1971

Ceglowski, W. S., and Friedman, H. Immunosuppression by leukemia viruses. I. Effect of Friend disease virus on cellular and humoral hemolysin responses of mice to a primary immunization with sheep erythrocytes. J Immunol *101,* 594–604, 1968

Centanni, E., and Rezzesi, F. Studio sperimentale sull' antagonismo fra tubercolosi e cancro. Riforma Med *T42,* 195–200, 1926

Cerilli, G. J., and Treat, R. C. The effect of antilymphocyte serum on the induction and growth of tumour in the adult mouse. Transplantation *8,* 774–782, 1969

Cerottini, J.-C., Nordin, A. A., and Brunner, K. T. In vitro cytotoxic activity of thymus cells sensitized to alloantigens. Nature *227,* 72–73, 1970a

Cerottini, J.-C., Nordin, A. A., and Brunner, K. T. Specific in vitro cytotoxicity of thymus-derived lymphocytes sensitized to alloantigens. Nature, *228,* 1308–1309, 1970b

Cerutti, I. Antiviral properties of Corynebacterium parvum, pp 84–90, In Halpern, B. (Ed): Corynebacterium Parvum: Applications in Experimental and Clinical Oncology. New York: Plenum Press, 1975

Chalkley, H. W. Comments on Algire, G. H., and Legallais, F. Y.: Growth and vascularization of transplanted mouse melanomas. NY Acad Sci (Special Publ) *4,* 164, 1948

Chambers, V. C., and Weiser, R. S. The ultrastructure of target cells and immune macrophages during their interaction in vitro. Cancer Res *29,* 301–317, 1969

Chambers, V. C., and Weiser, R. S. The ultrastructure of sarcoma I cells and immune macrophages during their interaction in the peritoneal cavities of immune C57B1/6 mice. Cancer Res *32,* 413–419, 1972

Champion, H. R., Wallace, I. W., and Prescott, R. J. Histology in breast cancer prognosis. Br J Cancer *26,* 129–138, 1972

Chang, K. S., Law, L. W., and Appella, E. Distinction between tumor-specific transplantation antigens and virion antigens in solubilized products from membranes of virus-induced leukemia cells. Int J Cancer *15,* 483–492, 1975

Chang, Y.-H. Investigation on human macrophage. Chin Med J (Engl) *58,* 603, 713, 1978

Chang, Y.-H., and Yao, C.-S. Investigation of the human macrophage. I. Collection and in vitro cultivation. Eur J Immunol *9,* 517–520, 1979

Char, D. H., Lepourheit, A., Leventhal, B. G., and Herberman, R. B. Cutaneous delayed hypersensitivity responses to tumour-associated and other antigens in acute leukemia. Int J Cancer *12,* 409–419, 1973

Chard, T. Immunological enhancement by mouse isoantibodies: The importance of complement fixation. Immunology *14,* 583–589, 1968

Chare, M. J. B., Webster, D. J. T., and Baum, M. Clinical experience in the use of C. parvum in the treatment of locally advanced carcinoma of the breast. Dev Biol Stand *38,* 495–499, 1978

Charney, J., and Moore, D. H. Neutralization of murine mammary tumour virus by sera of women with breast cancer. Nature *229,* 627–628, 1971

Chase, M. W. Delayed-type hypersensitivity and the immunology of Hodgkin's disease with a parallel examination of sarcoidosis. Cancer Res *26,* 1097–1120, 1966

Chassoux, D., and Salomon, J.-C. Therapeutic effect of intra-tumoral injection of BCG and other substances in rats and mice. Int J Cancer *16,* 515–525, 1975

Cheatle, G. L., and Cutler, M. Tumors of the Breast: Their Pathology, Symptoms, Diagnosis, and Treatment. Philadelphia: Lippincott, 1931

Checkik, B. E. Byull Eksp Biol Med 66, 85, 1968 [Cited by Checkik and Gelfand (1976)]

Checkik, B. E., and Gelfand, E. W. Leukaemia-associated antigen in serum of patients with acute lymphoblastic leukaemia. Lancet 1, 166–168, 1976

Chedid, L., Audibert, F., and Johnson, A. G. Biological studies of muramyl dipeptide, a synthetic glycopeptide analogous to bacterial immunoregulating agents. Prog Allergy 25, 63–105, 1978

Cheema, A. R., and Hersh, E. M. Local tumor immunotherapy with in vitro activated autochthonous lymphocytes. Cancer 29, 982–986, 1972

Cheers, C., and Cone, R. E. Effect of polyadenine:polyuridine on brucellosis in conventional and congenitally athymic mice. J Immunol 112, 1535–1539, 1974

Cheng, V. S. T., Suit, H. D., Wang, C. C., and Cummings, C. Nonspecific immunotherapy by Corynebacterium parvum. Phase I toxicity study in 12 patients with advanced cancer. Cancer 37, 1687–1695, 1976

Chernyakhovskaya, I. Y., Slavina, E. G., and Svet-Moldavsky, G. J. Antitumor effect of lymphoid cells activated by interferon. Nature 228, 71–72, 1970

Chesebro, B., and Wehrly, K. Studies on the role of the host immune response in recovery from Friend virus leukemia. I. Antiviral and antileukemia cell antibodies. J Exp Med 143, 73–84, 1976a

Chesebro, B., and Wehrly, K. Studies on the role of the host immune response in recovery from Friend virus leukemia. II. Cell-mediated immunity. J Exp Med 143, 85–99, 1976b

Chess, L., and Schlossman, S. F. Human lymphocyte subpopulations. Adv Immunol 25, 213–241, 1977

Chirigos, M. A., Fuhrman, F., and Pryor, J. Prolongation of chemotherapeutically induced remission of a syngeneic murine leukemia by 1-2,3,5,6-tetrahydro-6-phenyl-imidazole(2,1-b)thiazole hydrochloride. Cancer Res 35, 927–931, 1975

Chirigos, M. A., Pearson, J. W., and Pryor, J. Augmentation of chemotherapeutically induced remission of a murine leukemia by a chemical immuno-adjuvant. Cancer Res 33, 2615–2618, 1973

Chism, S., Burton, R., and Warner, N. L. Lymphocyte activation in vitro to murine oncofetal antigens. Nature 257, 594–596, 1975

Chism, S. E., Burton, R. C., and Warner, N. L. In vitro induction of tumor specific immunity. II. Activation of cytotoxic lymphocytes to murine oncofetal antigens. J Natl Cancer Inst 57, 377–387, 1976a

Chism, S. E., Wallis, S., Burton, R. C., and Warner, N. L. Analysis of murine oncofetal antigens as tumor associated transplantation antigens. J Immunol 117, 1870–1877, 1976b

Choi, N. W., Howe, G. R., Miller, A. B., Matthews, V., Morgan, R. W., Munan, L., Burch, J. D., Feather, J., Jain, M., and Kelly, A. An epidemiologic study of breast cancer. Am J Epidemiol 107, 510–521, 1978

Chretien, P. B., Lipson, S. D., Makuch, R., Kenady, D. E., Cohen, M. H., and Minna, J. D. Thymosin in cancer patients: In vitro effects and correlations with clinical response to thymosin immunotherapy. Cancer Treat Rep 62, 1787–1790, 1978

Christie, G. H., and Bomford, R. Mechanisms of macrophage activation by Corynebacterium parvum. I. In vitro experiments. Cell Immunol 17, 141–149, 1975

Chu, E. H. Y., Stjernsward, J., Clifford, P., and Klein, G. Reactivity of human lymphocytes against autochthonous and allogeneic normal and tumor cells in vitro. J Natl Cancer Inst 39, 595–617, 1967

Chu, T. M., Reynoso, G., and Hansen, H. J. Demonstration of carcinoembryonic antigen in normal human plasma. Nature 238, 152–153, 1972

Chuat, J.-C., Berman, L., Gunven, P., and Klein, E. Studies on murine sarcoma virus: Antigenic characterization of murine sarcoma virus-induced tumor cells. Int J Cancer 4, 465–479, 1969

Chung, E. B., Zbar, B., and Rapp, H. J. Tumor regression mediated by Mycobacterium bovis (strain BCG). Effects of isonicotinic acid hydrazide, cortisone acetate, and antithymocyte serum. J Natl Cancer Inst 51, 241–250, 1973

Churchill, W. H., and Rocklin, R. E. Studies on the detection of cellular immunity to human tumors by inhibition of macrophage migration. Natl Cancer Inst Monogr 37, 135–137, 1973

Chute, R. N., Sommers, S. C., and Warren, S. Heterotransplantation of human cancer. II. Hamster cheek pouch. Cancer Res 12, 912–914, 1952

Cinader, B., Hayley, M. A., Rider, W. D., and Warwick, O. H. Immunotherapy of a patient with choriocarcinoma. Can Med Assoc J 84, 306–309, 1961

Citrin, D. L., Bessent, R. G., Tuohy, J. B., Greig, W. R., and Blumgart, L. H. Quantitative bone scanning: A method for assessing response of bone metastases to treatment. Lancet *1*, 1132–1133, 1974

Citrin, D. L., Furnival, C. M., Bessent, R. G., Greig, W. R., Bell, G., and Blumgart, L. H. Radioactive technetium phosphate bone scanning in preoperative assessment and follow-up study of patients with primary cancer of the breast. Surg Gynecol Obstet *143*, 360–364, 1976

Clark, I. A., Cox, F. E. G., and Allison, A. C. Protection of mice against Babesia spp. and Plasmodium spp. with killed Corynebacterium parvum. Parasitology *74*, 9–18, 1977

Clarkson, B. D., Dowling, M. D., Gee, T. S., Cunningham, I. B., and Burchenal, J. H. Treatment of acute leukemia in adults. Cancer *36*, 775–795, 1975

Clarkson, B., Ota, K., Ohkita, T., and O'Connor, A. Kinetics of proliferation of cancer cells in neoplastic effusions in man. Cancer *18*, 1189–1213, 1965

Cleaver, J. E. Thymidine Metabolism and Cell Kinetics. Amsterdam: North-Holland, 1967

Cleaver, J. E. Defective repair replication of DNA in xeroderma pigmentosum. Nature *218*, 652–656, 1968

Cleaver, J. E. Xeroderma pigmentosum: A human disease in which an initial stage of DNA repair is defective. Proc Natl Acad Sci USA *63*, 428–435, 1969

Clements, D. V., Thomas, J. W., Plenderleith, I. H., Benz, C. C., Grzybowski, S., and Dorkin, E. Oral BCG sensitization, pp 135–144, In Crispen, R. G. (Ed): Neoplasm Immunity: Mechanisms. Proc Chicago Symp (1975), 1976

Clementson, K. J., Bertschmann, M., and Widner, S. Water-soluble P-815 mastocytoma membrane antigens: Separation of tumour-associated antigens from histocompatibility antigens. Immunochemistry *13*, 383–388, 1976

Cleveland, R. P., Meltzer, M. S., and Zbar, B. Tumor cytotoxicity in vitro by macrophages from mice infected with Mycobacterium bovis strain BCG. J Natl Cancer Inst *52*, 1887–1895, 1974

Clifford, P. On the epidemiology of nasopharyngeal carcinoma. Int J Cancer *5*, 287–390, 1970

Clifford, P., Singh, S., Stjernsward, J., and Klein, G. Long-term survival of patients with Burkitt's lymphoma: An assessment of treatment and other factors which may relate to survival. Cancer Res *27*, 2578–2615, 1967

Cliffton, E. E. Effect of fibrinolysin on spread of cancer. Fed Proc *25*, 89, 1966

Cliffton, E. E., and Agostino, D. Factors affecting development of metastatic cancer. Effect of alteration in clotting mechanisms. Cancer *15*, 276–283, 1962

Cliffton, E. E., and Agostino, D. The effects of fibrin formation and alterations in the clotting mechanism on the development of metastases. Vasc Dis *2*, 43–52, 1965

Cliffton, E. E., and Grossi, C. E. Effect of human plasmin on the toxic effects and growth of blood-borne metastases of the Brown-Pearce carcinoma and the V2 carcinoma of rabbit. Cancer *9*, 1147–1152, 1956

Cobb, L. M. Radiation-induced osteosarcoma in the rat as a model for osteosarcoma in man. Br J Cancer *24*, 294–296, 1970

Cobb, L. M. Metastatic spread of human tumour implanted into thymectomized, antithymocyte serum treated hamsters. Br J Cancer *26*, 183–189, 1972

Cobb, L. M. The behaviour of carcinoma of the large bowel in man following transplantation into immune deprived mice. Br J Cancer *28*, 400–411, 1973

Coca, A. F., Dorrance, G. M., and Lebredo, M. G. "Vaccination" in cancer. II. A report on the results of the vaccination therapy as applied in 79 cases of human cancer. Z Immunotatsforsch *13*, 543–585, 1912

Cochran, A. J., Diehl, V., and Stjernsward, J. Regression of primary malignant melanoma associated with a good prognosis despite metastasis to lymph nodes. Rev Eur Etudes Clin Biol *15*, 969–972, 1970

Cochran, A. J., Jehn, U. W., and Gothoskar, B. P. Cell mediated immunity in malignant melanoma. Lancet *1*, 1340–1341, 1972a

Cochran, A. J., Klein, E., and Kiessling, R. Effect of immune factors on the motility of lymphoma cells. J Natl Cancer Inst *48*, 1657–1661, 1972b

Cochran, A. J., Klein, G., Kiessling, R., and Gunven, P. Migration-inhibiting effect of sera from patients with Burkitt's lymphoma. J Natl Cancer Inst *51*, 1431–1436, 1973a

Cochran, A. J., Mackie, R. M., Jackson, A. M., Ogg, L. J., and Ross, C. E. Immunological changes in cancer patients receiving BCG. Dev Biol Stand *38*, 441–448, 1978

Cochran, A. J., Mackie, R. N., Thomas, C. E., Grant, R. M., Cameron-Mowat, D. E., and Spilg, W. G. S. Cellular immunity to breast carcinoma and malignant melanoma, In Moore, M., Nisbet, N. W., and Haigh, M. V. (Eds): Immunology of Malignancy. Br J Cancer, *28* (Suppl 1), 77–82, 1973b

Cochran, A. J., Spilg, W. G. S., Mackie, R. N., and Thomas, C. E. Post-operative depression of tumour-directed cell-mediated immunity in patients with malignant disease. Br Med J *4*, 67–70, 1972c

Coggin, J. H., Ambrose, K. R., Bellomy, B. B.,

and Anderson, N. G. Tumor immunity in hamsters immunized with fetal tissues. J Immunol 107, 526–533, 1971

Coggin, J. H., and Anderson, N. G. Phase-specific autoantigens (fetal) in model tumor systems, pp 91–102, In Anderson, N. G., and Coggin, J. H. (Eds): Embryonic and Fetal Antigens in Cancer, Vol 2. Springfield, Va.: Natl Tech Information Services, U.S. Dept Commerce, 1972

Coggin, J. H., and Anderson, N. G. Cancer, differentiation and embryonic antigens; Some central problems. Adv Cancer Res 19, 105–165, 1974

Cohen, A. Immunological method of increasing the sensitivity of primary sarcomas to local irradiation with x-rays. Lancet 1, 1163, 1964

Cohen, A. M., Ketcham, A. S., and Morton, D. L. Cellular immunity to a common human sarcoma antigen and its specific inhibition by sera from patients with growing sarcomas. Surgery 72, 560–567, 1972

Cohen, A. M., Ketcham, A. S., and Morton, D. L. Tumor-specific cellular cytotoxicity to human sarcomas: Evidence for a cell-mediated host immune response to a common sarcoma cell-surface antigen. J Natl Cancer Inst 50, 585–589, 1973

Cohen, R. B., Toll, G. D., and Castleman, B. Bronchial adenomas in Cushing's syndrome; Their relationship to thymomas and oat cell carcinomas associated with hyperadrenocorticism. Cancer 13, 812–817, 1960

Cohen, S. A., Ehrke, M. J., and Mihich, E. Mouse effector functions involved in the antibody-dependent cellular cytotoxicity to xenogeneic erythrocytes. J Immunol 115, 1007–1012, 1975

Cohen, Y., Ingrand, J., and Caro, R. A. Kinetics of the disappearance of gelatin protected radiogold colloids from the blood stream. Int J Appl Radiat Isotopes 19, 703–705, 1968

Colby, C., and Chamberlain, M. J. Specificity of interferon induction in chick embryo cells by helical RNA. Proc Natl Acad Sci USA 63, 160–167, 1969

Colby, C., Chamberlain, M. J., Duesberg, P. H., and Simon, M. I. The specificity of interferon induction, pp 79–87, In Beers, R. F., and Braun, W. (Eds): Biological Effects of Polynucleotides. New York: Springer-Verlag, 1971

Cole, L. J. Effect of reticuloendothelial cell chimerism on autochthonous and transplanted leukemias in mice, pp 335–346, In Proc IVth Int Symp Reticuloendothel Soc, 1964

Cole, L. J., Nowell, P. C., and Arnold, J. S. Late effects of x-radiation. The influence of dose fractionation on life span, leukemia, and nephrosclerosis incidence in mice. Radiat Res 12, 173–185, 1960

Cole, W. H. The mechanisms of spread of cancer. Surg Gynecol Obstet 137, 853–871, 1973

Cole, W. H., Roberts, S. S., Webb, R. S., Strehl, F. W., and Oates, G. D. Dissemination of cancer with special emphasis on vascular spread and implantation. Ann Surg 161, 753–770, 1965

Coley, W. B. A preliminary note on the treatment of inoperable sarcoma by the toxin products of erysipelas. Post-Graduate, 8, 278–286, 1893

Coley, W. B. Treatment of inoperable malignant tumors with the toxins of erysipelas and Bacillus prodigiosus. Trans Am Surg A 12, 183–212, 1894

Coley, W. B. The treatment of inoperable sarcoma with the mixed toxins of erysipelas and Bacillus prodigiosus: Immediate and final results in one hundred and forty cases. JAMA 31, 389–395, 456–465, 1898

Coley, W. B. Late results of the treatment of inoperable sarcoma with the mixed toxins of erysipelas and Bacillus prodigiosus. Trans Am Surg A 19, 27–42, 1901

Coley, W. B. Late results of the treatment of inoperable sarcoma by the mixed toxins of erysipelas and Bacillus prodigiosus. Am J Med Sci 131, 373–430, 1906

Coley, W. B. The treatment of inoperable sarcoma by bacterial toxins. Proc R Soc Med 3 (Surg Sect), 1–48, 1909/1910

Coley, W. B. Sarcoma of the long bones. Clinical lecture on end results. Exhibition of patients illustrating end results of treatment. S Clin North Am 9, 583–618, 1929

Collavo, D., Colombatti, A., Chieco-Bianchi, L., and Davies, A. J. S. T lymphocyte requirement for MSV tumour prevention or regression. Nature 249, 169–170, 1974

Collavo, D., Finco, B., and Chieco-Bianchi, L. Immune reactivity following poly I-poly C treatment in mice. Nature New Biol 237, 154–155, 1972

Collet, A. J. Experimental stimulation of alveolar macrophage production by Corynebacterium anaerobium and its quantitative evaluation. J Reticuloendothel Soc 9, 424–446, 1971

Collins, F. M., and Scott, M. T. Effect of Corynebacterium parvum treatment on the growth of Salmonella enteritidis in mice. Infect Immun 9, 863–869, 1974

Collins, V. P., Leoffler, R. K., and Tivey, H. Observation on growth rates of human tumors. Am J Roentgenol 76, 988–1000, 1956

Colnaghi, M. I., and Della Porta, G. Evidence for virus-related and unrelated antigens on murine lymphomas induced by chemical carcinogens. J Natl Cancer Inst 50, 173–180, 1973

Coman, D. R. Decreased mutual adhesiveness, a property of cells from squamous cell carcinomas. Cancer Res 4, 625–629, 1944

Coman, D. R., Eisenberg, R. B., and McCutcheon, M. Factors affecting the distribution of tumor metastases experiments with V2 carcinoma of rabbits. Cancer Res 9, 649–651, 1949

Comings, D. E. A general theory of carcinogenesis. Proc Natl Acad Sci USA 70, 3324–3328, 1973

Cone, L., and Uhr, J. W. Immunological deficiency disorders associated with chronic lymphocytic leukemia and multiple myeloma. J Clin Invest 43, 2241–2248, 1964

Cone, R. E.,and Johnson, A. G. Regulation of the immune system by synthetic polynucleotides. III. Action on antigen-reactive cells of thymic origin. J Exp Med 133, 665–676, 1971

Cone, R. E., and Johnson, A. G. Regulation of the immune system by synthetic polynucleotides. IV. Amplification of proliferation of thymus-influenced lymphocytes. Cell Immunol 3, 283–293, 1972

Cone, R. E., and Marchalonis, J. J. Adjuvant action of poly (A:U) on T-cells during the primary immune response in vitro. Aust J Exp Biol Med Sci 50, 69–77, 1972

Congdon, C. C. Pathologic findings in the delayed heterologous bone marrow reaction. Radiat Res 7, 310, 1957

Congdon, C. C., and Urso, I. S. Homologous bone marrow in treatment of radiation injury in mice. Am J Pathol 33, 749–767, 1957

Cook, J. W., Hewett, C. L., and Hieger, I. The isolation of a cancer-producing hydrocarbon from coal tar. Parts I, II, and III. J Chem Soc 395–405, 1933

Cooke, R. The Biology of Symbiotic Fungi. London: John Wiley & Sons, 1977

Cooper, E. H. The biology of cell death in tumors. Cell Tissue Kinet 6, 87–95, 1973

Cooper, E. H., Bedford, A. J., and Kenny, T. E. Cell death in normal and malignant tissues. Adv Cancer Res 21, 59–120, 1975

Cooper, E. H., Frank, G. L., and Wright, D. H. Cell proliferation in Burkitt tumours. Eur J Cancer 2, 377–384, 1966

Cooper, E. H., Peckham, M. J., Millard, R. E., Hamlin, I. M. E., and Gerard-Marchant, R. Cell proliferation in human malignant lymphomas. Analysis of labelling index and DNA content in cell populations obtained by biopsy. Eur J Cancer 4, 286–296, 1968

Cornell, C. J., Smith, K. A., Cornwell, G. G., Burke, G. P., and McIntyre, O. R. Systemic effects of intravenous polyriboinosinic-polyri-bocytidylic acid in man. J Natl Cancer Inst 57, 1211–1216, 1976

Corrin, B., Gilby, E. D., Jones, N. F., and Patrick, J. Oat cell carcinoma of the pancreas with ectopic ACTH secretion. Cancer 31, 1523–1527, 1973

Cortes, E. P., Holland, J. F., Wang, J. J., Sinks, L. F., Blom, J., Senn, H., Bank, A., and Glidewell, O. Amputation and adriamycin in primary osteosarcoma. N Engl J Med 291, 998–1000, 1974

Costanzi, J. J. Chemotherapy and BCG in the treatment of disseminated malignant melanoma, pp 87–93, In Terry, W. D., and Windhorst, D. (Eds): Immunotherapy of Cancer: Present Status of Trials in Man. New York: Raven Press, 1978

Cotchin, E. Comparative oncology: The veterinary contribution. Proc R Soc Med 69, 649–656, 1976

Court Brown, W. M., and Doll, R. Leukaemia and aplastic anaemia in patients irradiated for ankylosing spondylitis. MRC (London) Special Report Series No. 295, 1957

Cox, K. O., and Keast, D. Studies of the Corynebacterium parvum-associated anaemia in mice. Clin Exp Immunol 17, 199–207, 1974

Cox, M. L., Gourley, R. D., and Kitabchi, A. E. Acinic cell adenocarcinoma of the parotid with ectopic production of adrenocorticotropic hormone. Am J Med 49, 529–533, 1970

Cox, R., Damjanov, I., and Irving, C. C. Damage and repair of hepatic DNA by ethylating carcinogens. Proc Am Assoc Cancer Res 14, 28, 1973

Crain, R. C. Spontaneous tumors in the Rochester strain of the Wistar rat. Am J Pathol 34, 311–335, 1958

Creech, O. Metastatic melanoma of the lung treated by pulmonary resection: Report of a case. Med Rec Ann 45, 426, 1951

Crile, G. Heat as an adjunct to the treatment of cancer. Clinical studies. Cleve Clin Q 28, 75–89, 1961a

Crile, G. Simplified treatment of cancer of the breast. Early results of a clinical study. Ann Surg 153, 745–761, 1961b

Crile, G. Selective destruction of cancers after exposure to heat. Ann Surg 156, 404–407, 1962

Crile, G. Results of simplified treatment of breast cancer. Surg Gynecol Obstet 118, 517–523, 1964

Crile, G. Rationale of simple mastectomy without radiation for clinical stage 1 cancer of the breast. Surg Gynecol Obstet 120, 975–982, 1965

Crile, G. Endocrine dependence of papillary carcinomas of the thyroid. JAMA *195,* 721–724, 1966a

Crile, G. Metastases from involved lymph nodes after removal of various primary tumors: Evaluation of radical and of simple mastectomy for cancers of the breast. Ann Surg *163,* 267–271, 1966b

Crile, G. Results of simple mastectomy without irradiation in the treatment of operative stage 1 cancer of the breast. Ann Surg *168,* 330–336, 1968

Crile, G. The case for local excision of breast cancer in selected cases. Lancet *1,* 549–551, 1972

Crile, G. Results of conservative treatment of breast cancer at ten and fifteen years. Ann Surg *181,* 26–30, 1975

Crile, G., and Turnbull, R. B. The role of electrocoagulation in the treatment of carcinoma of the rectum. Surg Gynecol Obstet *135,* 391–396, 1972

Crile, G. W. Excision of cancer of the head and neck. With special reference to the plan of dissection based on one hundred and thirty-two operations. JAMA *47,* 1780–1786, 1906

Crisler, C., Rapp, H. J., Weintraub, R. M., and Borsos, T. Forssman antigen content of guinea pig hepatomas induced by diethylnitrosamine: A quantitative approach to the search for tumour-specific antibodies. J Natl Cancer Inst *36,* 529–538, 1966

Criss, W. E. A review of isozymes in cancer. Cancer Res *31,* 1523–1542, 1971

Croce, C. M., Aden, D., and Koprowski, H. Somatic cell hybrids between mouse peritoneal macrophages and simian-virus-40-transformed human cells: II. Presence of human chromosome 7 carrying simian virus 40 genome in cells of tumors induced by hybrid cells. Proc Natl Acad Sci USA *72,* 1397–1400, 1975

Croce, C. M., and Koprowski, H. Positive control of the transformed phenotype in hybrids between SV40 transformed and normal cells. Science *184,* 1288–1289, 1974

Crum, E. D., and McGregor, D. D. Induction of tumor resistance with BCG-associated tumor antigen. Int J Cancer *20,* 805–812, 1977

Csaba, G., Korosa, K., Horvath, K., and Mold, T. Effect of heparin-bound alkylating agents and enzyme inhibitors on neoplastic growth. Neoplasma *11,* 137–143, 1964

Cudkowicz, G., and Bennett, M. Peculiar immunobiology of bone marrow allografts. I. Graft rejection by irradiated responder mice. J Exp Med *134,* 83–102, 1971a

Cudkowicz, G., and Bennett, M. Peculiar immunobiology of bone marrow allografts. II. Rejection of parental grafts by resistant F1 hybrid mice. J Exp Med *134,* 1513–1528, 1971b

Cudkowicz, G., and Hochman, P. Do natural killer cells engage in regulatory reactions against self to ensure homeostasis? Immunol Rev *44,* 13–41, 1979

Cudkowicz, G., and Rossi, G. B. Hybrid resistance to parental DBA/2 grafts: Independence from H-2 locus. I. Studies with normal haematopoietic cells. J Natl Cancer Inst *48,* 131–139, 1972

Cudkowicz, G., and Stimpfling, J. H. Hybrid resistance to parental marrow grafts: Association with the K region of H-2. Science, *144,* 1339–1340, 1964a

Cudkowicz, G., and Stimpfling, J. H. Induction of immunity and of unresponsiveness to parental marrow grafts in adult F1 hybrid mice. Nature *204,* 450–453, 1964b

Cullen, P. R., and Mason, D. Y. Leukaemia-associated antigens in man. Detection by antibodies in maternal sera. Clin Exp Immunol *17,* 571–586, 1974

Cunningham, T. J., Olson, K. B., Laffin, R., Horton, J., and Sullivan, J. Treatment of advanced cancer with active immunization. Cancer *24,* 932–937, 1969

Cunningham, T. J., Schoenfeld, D., Nathanson, L., Wolter, J., Patterson, W. B., and Cohen, M. H. A controlled study of adjuvant therapy in patients with stage I and II malignant melanoma, pp 19–26, In Terry, W. D., and Windhorst, D. (Eds): Immunotherapy of Cancer: Present Status of Trials in Man. New York: Raven Press, 1978

Cunningham-Rundles, W. F., Hirshaut, Y., Pinsky, C. M., and Oettgen, H. F. Phase I trial of intralesional Corynebacterium parvum. Clin Res *23,* 337A, 1975

Currie, G. A. Masking of antigens on the Landschutz ascites tumour. Lancet *2,* 1336–1338, 1967

Currie, G. A. Eighty years of immunotherapy: A review of immunological methods used for the treatment of human cancer. Br J Cancer *26,* 141–153, 1972

Currie, G. A. Serum lysozyme as a marker of host resistance. II. Patients with malignant melanoma, hypernephroma or breast carcinoma. Br J Cancer *33,* 593–599, 1976

Currie, G. A. Activated macrophages kill tumour cells by releasing arginase. Nature *273,* 758–759, 1978

Currie, G. A., and Alexander, P. Spontaneous shedding of TSTA by viable sarcoma cells: Its possible role in facilitating metastatic spread. Br J Cancer *29,* 72–75, 1974

Currie, G. A., and Bagshawe, K. D. The masking of antigens on trophoblast and cancer cells. Lancet *1*, 708–710, 1967

Currie, G. A., and Bagshawe, K. D. The effect of neuraminidase on the immunogenicity of the Landschutz ascites tumour: Site and mode of action. Br J Cancer *22*, 588–594, 1968a

Currie, G. A., and Bagshawe, K. D. The role of sialic acid in antigenic expression: Further studies of the Landschutz ascites tumour. Br J Cancer *22*, 843–853, 1968b

Currie, G. A., and Bagshawe, K. D. Tumour specific immunogenicity of methylcholanthrene-induced sarcoma cells after incubation in neuraminidase. Br J Cancer *23*, 141–149, 1969

Currie, G. A., and Bagshawe, K. D. Active immunotherapy with Corynebacterium parvum and chemotherapy in murine fibrosarcomas. Br Med J *1*, 541–544, 1970

Currie, G. A., and Basham, C. Serum mediated inhibition of the immunological reactions of the patient to his own tumour: A possible role for circulating antigen. Br J Cancer *26*, 427–438, 1972

Currie, G. A., and Basham, C. Differential arginine dependence and the selective cytotoxic effects of activated macrophages for malignant cells in vitro. Br J Cancer *38*, 653–659, 1978

Currie, G. A., and Eccles, S. A. Serum lysozyme as a marker of host resistance. I. Production by macrophages resident in rat sarcomata. Br J Cancer *33*, 51–99, 1976

Currie, G. A., and Gage, J. O. Influence of tumour growth on the evolution of cytotoxic lymphoid cells in rats bearing a spontaneously metastasizing syngeneic fibrosarcoma. Br J Cancer *28*, 136–146, 1973

Currie, G. A., Gyure, L., and Cifuentes, L. Microenvironmental arginine depletion by macrophages in vivo. Br J Cancer *39*, 613–620, 1979

Currie, G. A., Lejeune, F., and Fairley, G. H. Immunization with irradiated tumour cells and specific lymphocyte cytotoxicity in malignant melanoma. Br Med J *2*, 305–310, 1971

Currie, G. A., and Sime, G. C. Syngeneic immune serum specifically inhibits the motility of tumour cells. Nature New Biol *241*, 284–285, 1973

Cushing, H., and Wolback. S. B. The transformation of a malignant paravertebral sympathicoblastoma into a benign ganglioneuroma. Am J Pathol *5*, 203–216, 1927

Custer, R. P., Outzen, H. C., Eaton, G. J., and Prehn, R. T. Does the absence of immunologic surveillance affect the tumor incidence in "nude" mice? First recorded spontaneous lymphoma in a nude mouse. J Natl Cancer Inst *51*, 707–711, 1973

Cuttner, J., Glidewell, O., Holland, J. F., and Beski, J. G. Chemoimmunotherapy of acute myelocytic leukemia with MER, pp 405–412, In Terry, W. D., and Windhorst, D. (Eds): Immunotherapy of Cancer: Present Status of Trials in Man. New York: Raven Press, 1978

Czajkowski, N. P., Rosenblatt, M., Cushing, F. R., Vazquez, J., and Wolf, P. L. Production of active immunity to malignant neoplastic tissue. Cancer *19*, 739–749, 1966

Czajkowski, N. P., Rosenblatt, M., Wolf, P. L., and Vazquez, J. A new method of active immunisation to autologous human tumour tissue. Lancet *2*, 905–909, 1967

D

Daams, J. H., Timmermans, A., van der Gugten, A., and Bentvelzen, P. Genetical resistance of inbred strain C57BL mice against mammary tumour inciting virus. II. Resistance by means of a repressed provirus. Genetica *38*, 400–402, 1968

Da Fano, C. A. A cytological analysis of the reaction in animals resistant to implanted carcinoma. 5th Scientific Report, Imp Cancer Res Fund, pp 57–78, 1912

Dailey, J. E., and Marcuse, P. A. Gonadotropin secreting giant cell carcinoma of the lung. Cancer *24*, 388–396, 1969

Dalton, A. RNA tumour viruses and ultrastructural aspects of virion morphology and replication. J Natl Cancer Inst *49*, 323–325, 1972

Dao, T. L., and Sunderland, J. Mammary carcinogenesis by 3-methylcholanthrene. I. Hormonal aspects in tumor incidence and growth. J Natl Cancer Inst *23*, 567–585, 1959

Dargeon, H. W., Eversole, J. W., and Del Duca, V. Malignant melanoma in an infant. Cancer *3*, 299–306, 1950

Dausset, J., Degos, L., Estampe, B., and Bernard, J. Rapport entre le nombre des grossesses et le risque de leucémie aiguë. Nouv Rev Fr Hematol *10*, 55–62, 1970

David, C. S. Role of Ia antigens in immune response. Transplant Proc *11*, 677–682, 1979

David, J., and Burkitt, D. Burkitt's lymphoma: Remissions following seemingly non-specific therapy. Br Med J *4*, 288–291, 1968

Davies, C. J., Griffiths, P. A., Preston, B. J., Morris, A. H., Elston, C. W., and Blamey, R. W. Staging breast cancer: Role of bone scanning. Br Med J *2*, 603–605, 1977

Davies, D. A. L. The combined effect of drugs

and tumor-specific antibodies in protection against a mouse lymphoma. Cancer Res *34*, 3040–3043, 1974

Davies, D. A. L. What are tumour-specific antigens? Nature *254*, 653–654, 1975

Davies, D. A. L., Baugh, V. S. G., Buckham, S., and Manstone, A. J. Separation of the specific antigen of a mouse lymphoma from histocompatibility antigens. Eur J Cancer *10*, 781–786, 1974a

Davies, D. A. L., Buckham, S., and Manstone, A. J. Protection of mice against syngeneic lymphomata: II. Collaboration between drugs and antibodies. Br J Cancer *30*, 305–311, 1974b

Davies, D. A. L., Manstone, A. J., and Buckham, S. Protection of mice against syngeneic lymphomata: I. Use of antibodies. Br J Cancer *30*, 297–304, 1974c

Davies, D. A. L., and O'Neill, G. J. In vivo and in vitro effects of tumour specific antibodies with chlorambucil. Br J Cancer *28*, 285–298, 1973

Davies, D. A. L., and O'Neill, G. J. Methods of cancer immunotherapy (drab and drac) using antisera against tumour specific cell membrane antigens, pp 218–221, In Proc XI Int Cancer Congr, Florence, 1974

Davignon, L., Lemonde, P., Robillard, P., and Frappier, A. B.C.G. vaccination and leukaemia mortality. Lancet *2*, 638–640, 1970

Davignon, L., Lemonde P., St.-Pierre, J., and Frappier, A. B.C.G. vaccination and leukaemia mortality. Lancet *1*, 80–81, 1971a

Davignon, L., Lemonde, P., St.-Pierre, J., and Frappier, A. B.C.G. vaccination and leukaemia mortality. Lancet *1*, 799, 1971b

Davis, H. H., Simons, M., and Davis, J. B. Cystic disease of the breast; Relationship to carcinoma. Cancer *17*, 957–978, 1964

Davis, N. C. Personal communication, based on data from the Queensland Melanoma Project, Princess Alexandra Hospital, Brisbane, 1975

Dawe, D. L., Segre, D., and Myers, W. L. Passive transfer of the action of Freund's adjuvant by serum of rabbits injected with the adjuvant. Science *148*, 1345–1347, 1965

Dawes, J., and McBride, W. H. Analysis of anaerobic coryneform cell wall antigens by radioimmunoassay. Immunochemistry *12*, 855–860, 1975

Dean, J. H., Wallen, W. C., and Lucas, D. O. Polyinosinic-polycytidylic acid activation of mouse spleen cells in vitro. Nature New Biol *237*, 218–219, 1972

De Bracco, M. M. DeE., Isturiz, M. A., and Manni, J. A. Cell-mediated cytotoxicity. Characterization of the effector cells. Immunology *30*, 325–333, 1976

de Carvalho, S. Preliminary experimentation with specific immunotherapy of neoplastic disease in man. I. Immediate effects of hyperimmune equine gamma globulins. Cancer *16*, 306–330, 1963

Deckers, P. J., and Pilch, Y. H. RNA-mediated transfer of tumor immunity—A new model for the immunotherapy of cancer. Cancer *28*, 1219–1228, 1971a

Deckers, P. J., and Pilch, Y. H. Transfer of immunity to tumor isografts by the systemic administration of xenogeneic "immune" RNA. Nature New Biol *231*, 181–183, 1971b

Deckers, P. J., and Pilch, Y. H. Mediation of immunity to tumour-specific transplantation antigens by RNA inhibition of isograft growth in rats. Cancer Res *32*, 839–846, 1972

DeClercq, E., and Merigan, T. C. Requirement of a stable secondary structure for antiviral activity of polynucleotides. Nature *222*, 1148–1152, 1969

DeClercq, E., and Merigan, T. C. Moloney sarcoma virus-induced tumours in mice: Inhibition or stimulation by (PolyrI) (PolyrC). Proc Soc Exp Biol Med *137*, 590–594, 1971

DeCosse, J., and Gelfant, S. Effect of hydrocortisone on cell division of tumor cells. Surg Forum *18*, 80–81, 1967

DeCosse, J., and Gelfant, S. Noncycling tumor cells: Mitogenic response to antilymphocytic serum. Science *162*, 698–699, 1968

Defendi, V. Effect of SV40 virus immunization on growth of transplantable SV40 and polyoma virus tumors in hamsters. Proc Soc Exp Biol Med *113*, 12–16, 1963

Defendi, V., Ephrussi, B., Koprowski, H., and Yoshida, M. C. Properties of hybrids between polyoma-transformed and normal mouse cells. Proc Natl Acad Sci USA *57*, 299–305, 1967

DeGast, G. C., The, T. H., Koops, H. S., Huiges, H. A., Oldhoff, J., and Nieweg, H. O. Humoral and cell-mediated immune response in patients with malignant melanoma. Cancer *36*, 1289–1297, 1975

Degre, M., and Ejgjo, K. Methylcholanthrene-induced mouse skin carcinogenesis modified by treatment with polyinosinic:polycytidylic acid (poly I:C). Acta Pathol Microbiol Scand A *79*, 687–688, 1971

DeJager, R., Pinsky, C., Kaufman, R., Ochoa, M., Oettgen, H. F., and Krakoff, I. H. Chemotherapy of advanced breast cancer with a combination of cyclophosphamide, Adriamycin, methotrexate and 5-fluorouracil (CAMF) with and without C. parvum. Proc Am Soc Clin Oncol *17*, 296, 1976

DeLaPava, S., Nigogosyan, G., and Pickren, J. W. Fatal glomerulonephritis after receiving horse anti-human-cancer serum. Arch Intern Med *109*, 391–399, 1962

de Long, R. P., and Coman, D. R. Relative susceptibility of various organs to tumor transplantation. Cancer Res *10*, 513–515, 1950

Delorme, E. J., and Alexander, P. Treatment of primary fibrosarcoma in the rat with immune lymphocytes. Lancet *2*, 117–120, 1964

Denham, S., Grant, C. K., Hall, J. G., and Alexander, P. The occurrence of two types of cytotoxic lymphoid cells in mice immunized with allogeneic tumor cells. Transplantation *9*, 366–382, 1970

Denham, S., Wrathmell, A. B., and Alexander, P. Evidence of cytotoxic T and B immunoblasts in the thoracic duct of rats bearing tumor grafts. Transplantation *19*, 102–114, 1975

Denlinger, R. H., Swenberg, J. A., Koestner, A., and Wechsler, W. Differential effect of immunosuppression on the induction of nervous system and bladder tumors by N-methyl N-nitrosourea. J Natl Cancer Inst *50*, 87–93, 1973

Dennert, G., and Lennox, E. S. Phagocytic cells as effectors in a cell-mediated immunity system. J Immunol *111*, 1844–1854, 1973

Dennert, G., and Tucker, D. F. Selective priming of T cells by chemically altered cell antigens. J Exp Med *136*, 656–661, 1972

Den Otter, W., Dullens, H. F. J., vanLoveren, H., and Pels, E. Anti-tumor effects of macrophages injected into animals: A review, pp 119–140, In James, K., McBride, B., and Stuart, A. (Eds): Proc EURES Sympos—The Macrophage and Cancer. Edinburgh Univ Dept Surgery, 1977

Den Otter, W., Evans, R., and Alexander, P. Cytotoxicity of murine peritoneal macrophages in tumour allograft immunity. Transplantation *14*, 220–226, 1972

Den Otter, W., Evans, R., and Alexander, P. Differentiation of immunologically specific cytotoxic macrophages into two types on the basis of radiosensitivity. Transplantation *18*, 421–428, 1974

Dent, R. I., Cruickshank, J. G., Gordon, J. A., and Swanepole, R. An investigation of the effects of inoculated and intralymphatic vaccinia virus on primary and secondary deposits of malignant melanoma. Cent Afr J Med *18*, 173–176, 1972

Deodhar, S. D., Crile, G., and Esselstyn, C. B. Study of the tumor cell-lymphocyte interaction in patients with breast cancer. Cancer *29*, 1321–1325, 1972

Deodhar, S. D., Kuklinea, A. G., Vidt, D. G., Robertson, A.L., and Hazard, J. B. Development of reticulum cell sarcoma at the site

of antilymphocyte globulin injection in a patient with renal transplant. N Engl J Med *280*, 1104–1106, 1969

DePace, N. Sulla scomparsa di en enorme cancro vegetante del colle dell'utero senza cura chirurgica. Ginecologia (Firenze) *9*, 82–88, 1912

DeSouza, I., Morgan, L., Lewis, U. J., Raggatt, P. R., Salih, H., and Hobbs, J. R. Growth-hormone dependence among human breast cancers. Lancet *2*, 182–184, 1974

Dethlefsen, L. A. An evaluation of radioiodine labeled 5-iodo-2'-deoxyuridine as a tracer for measuring cell loss from solid tumours. Cell Tissue Kinet *4*, 123–138, 1971

Dethlefsen, L. A., Prewitt, J. M. S., and Mendelsohn, M. L. Analysis of tumor growth curves. J Natl Cancer Inst *40*, 389–405, 1968

Detre, S. I., and Gazet, J. C. Transplantation of human tumour to immune deprived mice. Br J Cancer *28*, 412–416, 1973

DeVita, V., Canellos, G., Carbone, P., Baron, S., Levy, H., and Gralnick, H. Clinical trials with the interferon inducer, polyinosinic-polycytidilic acid. Proc Am Assoc Cancer Res *11*, 21, 1970

De Vita, V. T., Young, R. C., and Canellos, G. P. Combination versus single agent chemotherapy: A review of the basis for selection of drug treatment of cancer. Cancer *35*, 98–110, 1975

DeVries, M. J., and Vos, O. Treatment of mouse lymphosarcoma by total body irradiation and by injection of bone marrow and lymph node cells. J Natl Cancer Inst *21*, 1117–1129, 1958

Dhar, P., Moore, T., Zamchek, N., and Kupchik, H. Z. Carcinoembryonic antigen (CEA) in colon cancer. JAMA *221*, 31–35, 1972

Dickson, J. A. Effects of hyperthermia in animal tumour systems. Rec Results Cancer Res *59*, 43–111, 1977

Dickson, J. A., and Calderwood, S. K. In vivo hyperthermia of Yoshida tumour induces entry of non-proliferating cells into cycle. Nature *263*, 772–774, 1976

Dickson, J. A., and Ellis, H. A. Stimulation of tumour cell dissemination by raised temperature (42°C) in rats with transplanted Yoshida tumours. Nature *248*, 354–358, 1974

Dickson, J. A., and Ellis, H. A. The influence of tumor volume and the degree of heating on the response of the solid Yoshida sarcoma to hyperthermia (40–42°C). Cancer Res *36*, 1188–1195, 1976

Dickson, J. A., and Muckle, D. S. Total body hyperthermia versus primary tumour hyperthermia in the treatment of the rabbit VX2 carcinoma. Cancer Res *32*, 1916–1923, 1972

Dickson, J. A., and Shah, S. A. Technology for the hyperthermic treatment of large solid tumours at 50°C. Clin Oncol *3,* 301–318, 1977

Dickson, J. A., and Suzanger, M. A predictive in vitro assay for the sensitivity of human solid tumours to hyperthermia (42°C) and its value in patient management. Clin Oncol *2,* 141–155, 1976

Diehl, V., Jereb, B., Stjernsward, J., O'Toole, C., and Ahstrom, L. Cellular immunity to nephroblastoma. Int J Cancer *7,* 277–284, 1971

Di Luzio, N. R., and Morrow, H. S. Comparative behavior of soluble and particulate antigens and inert colloids in reticuloendothelial-stimulated or depressed mice. J Reticuloendothel Soc *9,* 273–287, 1971

Di Luzio, N. R., and Riggi, S. J. The development of a lipid emulsion for the measurement of reticuloendothelial function. J Reticuloendothel Soc *1,* 136–149, 1964

Dimitrov, N. V., André, S., Eliopoulos, G., and Halpern, B. Effect of Corynebacterium parvum on bone marrow cell cultures. Proc Soc Exp Biol Med *148,* 440–442, 1975a

Dimitrov, N. V., Conroy, J., Suhrland, L. G., Singh, T., and Teitlebaum, H. Combination therapy with Corynebacterium parvum and doxorubin hydrochloride in patients with lung cancer, pp 181–189, In Terry, W. D., and Windhorst, D. (Eds): Immunotherapy of Cancer: Present Status of Trials in Man. New York: Raven Press, 1978

Dimitrov, N. V., Israel, L., and Peltier, A. Immunological monitoring of cancer patients during treatment with Corynebacterium parvum. Proc Am Soc Clin Oncol *16,* 258, 1975b

Disaia, P. J., Sinkovics, J. G., Rutledge, R. N., and Smith, J. P. Cell mediated immunity to human malignant cells. Am J Obstet Gynecol *114,* 979–989, 1972

Dixon, W. J., Longmire, W. P., and Holden, W. D. Use of triethylenethiophosphoramide as an adjuvant to the surgical treatment of gastric and colorectal carcinoma: Ten year follow-up. Ann Surg *173,* 26–39, 1971

Dizon, Q. S., and Southam, C. M. Abnormal cellular response to skin abrasion in cancer patients. Cancer *16,* 1288–1292, 1963

Djerassi, I., and Kim, J. S. Methotrexate and citrovorum factor rescue in the management of childhood lymphosarcoma and reticulum cell sarcoma (non-Hodgkin's lymphomas). Prolonged unmaintained remission. Cancer *38,* 1043–1051, 1976

Djerassi, I., Kim, J. S., and Suvansri, U. "Pulse" methotrexate and citrovorum factor "rescue" in common solid tumors (including lung and pancreas cancer of the adult). Proc Am Assoc Cancer Res *15,* 78, 1974

Djeu, J. Y. Unpublished observation [*Cited by Herberman and Holden (1978)*], 1978

Dmochowski, L. The milk agent in the origin of mammary tumors in mice. Adv Cancer Res *1,* 103–172, 1953

Doak, P. B., Montgomerie, J. Z., North, J. D. K., and Smith, F. Reticulum cell sarcoma after renal homotransplantation and azathioprine and prednisone therapy. Br Med J *4,* 746–748, 1968

Doherty, P. C., Blanden, R. V., and Zinkernagel, R. M. Specificity of virus-immune effector T cells for H-2K or H-2D compatible interactions: Implications for H-antigen diversity. Transplant Rev *29,* 89–124, 1976

Doll, R. Etiology of lung cancer. Adv Cancer Res *3,* 1–50, 1955

Doll, R. Strategy for detection of cancer hazards to man. Nature *265,* 589–596, 1977

Doll, R., and Hill, A. B. Smoking and carcinoma of the lung; Preliminary report. Br Med J *2,* 739–748, 1950

Doll, R., and Hill, A. B. Mortality in relation to smoking; Ten years' observations of British doctors. Br Med J *1,* 1399–1410, 1964a

Doll, R., and Hill, A. B. Mortality in relation to smoking; Ten years' observations of British doctors. Br Med J *1,* 1460–1467, 1964b

Doll, R., and Peto, R. Mortality among doctors in different occupations. Br Med J *1,* 1433–1436, 1977

Dolton, E. G. Combined surgery and chemotherapy for carcinoma of bronchus. Lancet *1,* 40–41, 1970

Donahower, G. F., Schumacher, O. R., and Hazard, J. B. Two cases of medullary thyroid carcinoma causing Cushing's syndrome. Clin Res *14,* 430, 1966

Doniach, I. The effect of radioactive iodine alone and in combination with methylthiouracil upon tumour production in the rat's thyroid gland. Br J Cancer *7,* 181–202, 1953

Doniach, I., Crookston, J. H., and Cope, T. I. Attempted treatment of a patient with choriocarcinoma by immunization with her husband's cells. J Obstet Gynaecol Br Commonw *65,* 553–556, 1958

Dore, J. F., Guibout, C., Bertoglio, J., and Liabeuf, A. Cytotoxic antibodies to human leukaemia cells in normal human sera. Biomedicine *25,* 382–384, 1976

Dore, J. F., Hadjiyamiakis, M. J., Guibout, C., and Coudert, A. Use of enzyme-treated cells in immunotherapy of a murine leukemia. Lancet *1,* 600–601, 1973

Dore, J. F., Motta, R., Marholev, L., Hrsak, I., De La Noue, H. C., Seman, G., De Vassal, F., and Mathé, G. New antigens in human leukaemic cells, and antibody in the serum of leukaemic patients. Lancet 2, 1396–1398, 1967

Double, J. A. Human tumour xenografts. Biomedicine 22, 461–465, 1975

Douglas, H. C., and Gunter, S. E. The taxonomic position of Corynebacterium acnes. J Bacteriol 52, 15–23, 1946

Douglass, H. O., Wang, J., Takita, H., Wallace, H. J., Friedman, M., and Mindell, E. Improvement in the results of treatment of osteogenic sarcoma. Surg Gynecol Obstet 140, 693–700, 1975

Drake, J. W. The Molecular Basis of Mutation. San Francisco: Holden Day, 1970

Drake, W. P., LeGendre, S., and Mardiney, M. R. Depression of complement activity in three strains of mice after tumor transfer. Int J Cancer 11, 719–724, 1973

Drake, W. P., and Mardiney, M. R. Parameters of serum complement in relation to tumor therapy. Biomedicine 21, 206–209, 1974

Drake, W. P., Roberts, G. C., Pendergrast, W. J., and Mardiney, M. R. The kinetics of the interaction of heterologous anti-tumor serum and heterologous complement in non-tumor bearing mice. Biomedicine 22, 502–508, 1975

Drake, W. P., Ungaro, P. C., and Mardiney, M. R. Passive administration of antiserum and complement in producing anti-EL4 cytotoxic activity in the serum of C57Bl/6 mice. J Natl Cancer Inst 50, 909–914, 1973

Dresser, D. W. Preparation of highly radioactive bovine anti-mouse lymphocyte antibody. Nature 229, 630–632, 1971

Dubois, J. B., and Serrou, B. Treatment of the mouse Lewis tumor by the association of radiotherapy and immunotherapy with bacillus Calmette-Guérin. Cancer Res 36, 1731–1734, 1976

Duclos, H., Schwarzenberg, L., Duclos, S. H., Hugues, H., and Kuss, R. Cutaneous response to dinitrochlorobenzene in patients with genito-urinary cancer. Biomedicine 27, 43–47, 1977

Duffy, B. J., and Fitzgerald, P. J. Cancer of the thyroid in children; A report of 28 cases. J Clin Endocrinol 10, 1296–1308, 1950

Dukes, C. E. Familial intestinal polyposis. Ann Eugen Lond 17, 1–29, 1952

Dulbecco, R. Topoinhibition and serum requirement of transformed and untransformed cells. Nature 227, 802–806, 1970

Dulbecco, R. Cell transformation by viruses and

the role of viruses in cancer. J Gen Microbiol 79, 7–17, 1973

Dullens, H. F. J., and Den Otter, W. Eradication of lymphoma cells with allogeneic immune peritoneal cells. Experientia 29, 479–481, 1973

Dullens, H. F. J., and Den Otter, W. Therapy with allogeneic immune peritoneal cells. Cancer Res 34, 1726–1730, 1974

Dullens, H. F. J., deWeger, R. A., Woutersen, R. A., and DenOtter, W. Therapy with antibody-coated immune and hyperimmune peritoneal cells in a murine lymphoma system. J Natl Cancer Inst 54, 77–82, 1975

Dullens, H. F. J., Kingma, F. J., and Den Otter, W. Immunotherapy with allogeneic hyperimmune peritoneal cells in a murine lymphoma system. Eur J Cancer 10, 41–47, 1974a

Dullens, H. F. J., Woutersen, R. A., deWeger, R. A., and DenOtter, W. Eradication of tumour cells by successive injections of allogeneic immune and hyperimmune peritoneal cells in a murine lymphoma system. Eur J Cancer 10, 701–706, 1974b

Dumonde, D. C., Wolstencroft, R. A., Panayi, G. S., Matthew, M., Morley, J., and Howson, W. T. "Lymphokines:" Non-antibody mediators of cellular immunity generated by lymphocyte activation. Nature 224, 38–42, 1969

Dunning, W. F., and Curtis, M. R. The respective roles of longevity and genetic specificity in the occurrence of spontaneous tumors in the hybrids between two inbred lines of rats. Cancer Res 6, 61–81, 1946

Dunphy, J. E. Some observations on the natural behavior of cancer in man. N Engl J Med 242, 167–172, 1950

Duplan, J. F. Dimunuition de la leucogenèse spontanée chez les souris AKR irradiées en totalité et greffées avec des cellules hémopoïétiques homologues. C R Acad Sci 247, 662–664, 1958

Dupont, B., Ballow, M., Hansen, J. A., Quick, C., Yunis, E. J., and Good, R. A. Effect of transfer factor therapy on mixed lymphocyte culture reactivity. Proc Natl Acad Sci USA 71, 867–871, 1974

Dupuy, J. M., Kourilsky, F. M., Fradelizzi, D., Feingold, N., Jacquillat, C. L., Bernard, J., and Dausset, J. Depression of immunologic reactivity of patients with acute leukemia. Cancer 27, 323–331, 1971

Dustin, P. Cell differentiation and carcinogenesis: A critical review. Cell Tissue Kinet 5, 519–533, 1972

Dutton, R. W. Suppressor T cells. Transplant Rev 26, 39–55, 1975

Dux, A., and Muhlbock. O. Susceptibility of mammary tissues of different mice to tumor development. J Natl Cancer Inst *40*, 1259–1265, 1968

Dwight, R. W., Humphrey, E. W., Higgins, G. A., and Keehn, R. J. FUDR as an adjuvant to surgery in cancer of the large bowel. J Surg Oncol *5*, 243–249, 1973

Dykes, P. W., and Trejdosiewicz, L. K. Intra-tumor C. parvum therapy in gastric carcinoma: A pilot study. Dev Biol Stand *38*, 547–552, 1978

E

Eagle, H., and Levine, E. M. Growth regulatory effects of cellular interaction. Nature *213*, 1102–1106, 1967

East, J., and Harvey, J. J. The differential action of neonatal thymectomy in mice infected with murine sarcoma virus-Harvey (MSV-H). Int J Cancer *3*, 614–627, 1968

Easty, G. C., Easty, D. M., and Ambrose, E. J. Studies of cellular adhesiveness. Exp Cell Res *19*, 539–547, 1960

Eccles, S. A. Studies on the effect of rat sarcomata on the migration of mononuclear phagocytes in vitro and in vivo, pp 308–319, In James, K., McBride, B., and Stuart, A. (Eds): Proc EURES Symp—The Macrophage and Cancer. Edinburgh Univ Dept Surgery, 1977

Eccles, S. A., and Alexander, P. Macrophage content of tumours in relation to metastatic spread and host immune reaction. Nature *250*, 667–669, 1974a

Eccles, S. A., and Alexander, P. Sequestration of macrophages in growing tumours and its effect on the immunological capacity of the host. Br J Cancer *30*, 42–49, 1974b

Eccles, S. A., and Alexander, P. Immunologically-mediated restraint of latent tumour metastases. Nature *257*, 52–53, 1975

Eccles, S. A., Bandlow, B., and Alexander, P. Monocytosis associated with the growth of transplanted syngeneic rat sarcomata differing in immunogenicity. Br J Cancer *34*, 20–27, 1976

Eckner, R. J., and Stevens, R. A. A classification of the murine leukemia viruses. J Exp Med *136*, 832–850, 1972

Economides, F., Bruley-Rosset, M., and Mathé, G. Effect of pre- and post-surgical active BCG immunotherapies on murine EaKR lymphosarcoma. Biomedicine *25*, 372–376, 1976

Edington, G. M., Maclean, C. M. U., and Okubadejo, O. A. One-hundred and one necropsies on tumours of the reticulo-endothelial system in Ibadan, Nigeria, with special reference to childhood lymphosarcoma, pp 236–252, In Symposium—Lymph Tumors in Africa (Paris, 1963). Basel: S. Karger, 1964

Edlich, R. F., Shea, M. A., Foker, J. E., Grondin, C., Castaneda, A. R., and Varco, R. L. A review of 26 years experience with pulmonary resection for metastatic cancer. Dis Chest *49*, 587–594, 1966

Edwards, A. J. The response of the reticulo-endothelial system to a transplanted cancer. Br J Surg *51*, 470, 1964

Edwards, M. H., Baum, M., and Magarey, C. J. Regression of axillary lymph-nodes in cancer of the breast. Br J Surg *59*, 776–779, 1972

Edynak, E. M., Old, L. J., Vrana, M., and Lardis, M. P. A fetal antigen associated with human neoplasia. N Engl J Med *286*, 1178–1183, 1972

Ehrlich, P. Experimentelle Carcinomstudien an Mäusen. Inst Exp Ther Frankf *1*, 75–102, 1906

Ehrlich, P. Experimentelle Studien an Mäusetumoren. Z Krebsforsch *5*, 59–81, 1907

Ehrlich, P. Über den jetzigen Stand der Karzinomforschung. Ned Tijdschr Geneesk *1*, 273–290, 1909 [*Reprinted in* Himmelweit, F. (Ed): The Collected Papers of Paul Ehrlich, Vol 3, pp 560–562. London, New York: Pergamon Press, 1960

Eichmann, K. Idiotype suppression. I. Influence of the dose and of effector functions of anti-idiotypic antibody on the production of an idiotype. Eur J Immunol *4*, 296–302, 1974

Eichmann, K. Expression and functions of idiotypes on lymphocytes. Adv Immunol *26*, 195–254, 1978

Eichmann, K., and Rajewsky, K. Induction of T and B cell immunity by anti-idiotypic antibody. Eur J Immunol *5*, 661–666, 1975

Eilber, F. R., and Morton, D. L. Impaired immunologic reactivity and recurrence following cancer surgery. Cancer *25*, 362–367, 1970a

Eilber, F. R., and Morton, D. L. Immunologic studies of human sarcomas: Additional evidence suggesting an associated sarcoma virus. Cancer *26*, 588–596, 1970b

Eilber, F. R., and Morton, D. L. Sarcoma-specific antigens: Detection by complement fixation with serum from sarcoma patients. J Natl Cancer Inst *44*, 651–656, 1970c

Eilber, F. R., and Morton, D. L. Immunologic response to human sarcomas: Relation of antitumor antibody to the clinical course, pp 951–957, In Progress in Immunology (First International Congress of Immunology). New York, London: Academic Press, 1971

Eilber, F. R., Morton, D. L., Holmes, E. C., Sparks, F. C., and Ramming, K. P. Adjuvant immunotherapy with BCG in treatment of regional lymph node metastases from malignant melanoma. N Engl J Med *294*, 237–240, 1976

Eilber, F. R., Townsend, C. M., and Morton, D. L. Adjuvant immunotherapy of osteosarcoma with BCG and allogeneic tumor cells, pp 299–303, In Terry, W. D., and Windhorst, D. (Eds): Immunotherapy of Cancer: Present Status of Trials in Man. New York: Raven Press, 1978

Eisen, H. N., Sakato, N., and Hall, S. J. Myeloma proteins as tumor-specific antigens. Transplant Proc *7*, 209–214, 1975

Ekert, H., Jose, D. G., Waters, K. D., Smith, P. J., and Matthews, R. N. Intermittent chemotherapy and BCG in continuation therapy of children with acute lymphocytic leukemia, pp 483–492, In Terry, W. D., and Windhorst, D. (Eds): Immunotherapy of Cancer: Present Status of Trials in Man. New York: Raven Press, 1978

El-Domeiri, A. A., and Shroff, S. Role of preoperative bone scan in carcinoma of the breast. Surg Gynecol Obstet *142*, 722–724, 1976

El Hassan, A. M., and Stuart, A. E. Changes in the lymphoreticular tissues of mice bearing the Landschutz tumour. Br J Cancer *19*, 343–352, 1965

Elias, E. G., and Elias, L. L. Some immunologic characteristics of carcinoma of the colon and rectum. Surg Gynec Obstet *141*, 715–718, 1975

Elkind, M. M., and Sutton, H. Radiation response of mammalian cells grown in culture. I. Repair of x-ray damage in surviving Chinese hamster cells. Radiat Res *13*, 556–593, 1960

Ellerman, V., and Bang, O. Experimentalle Leukämie bei Hühnern. Centralb F Bacter Parasit Infektionskr *46*, 595–609, 1908

Ellis, H. Should lymphadenectomy be discarded? Historical developments. J R Coll Surg Edinb *18*, 342–345, 1973

Ellison, M. L. Cell differentiation and the biological significance of inappropriate tumour products. Proc R Soc Med *70*, 845–850, 1977

Ellman, L., Katz, D. H., Green, I., Paul, W. E., and Benacerraf, B. Mechanism involved in the antileukemic effect of immunocompetent allogeneic lymphoid cell transfer. Cancer Res *32*, 141–148, 1972

Elston, C. W., and Bagshawe, K. D. Cellular reaction in trophoblastic tumours. Br J Cancer *28*, 245–256, 1973

Elves, M. W. (Ed): The Biological Effects of Phytohaemagglutinin. Oswestry: Charles Salt Research Centre Symposium, 1970

Embleton, M. J. Effect of BCG on cell-mediated cytotoxicity and serum blocking factor during

growth of rat hepatoma. Br J Cancer *33*, 584–592, 1976

Engelbart, K., and Gericke, D. Transplanted tumors of the hamster. Cancer Res *24*, 239–243, 1964

Engell, H. C. Cancer cells in circulating blood: Clinical study on occurrence of cancer cells in peripheral blood and in venous blood draining tumor area at operation. Acta Chir Scand (Suppl) *201*, 1–70, 1955

Engell, H. C. Cancer cells in blood; 5 to 9 year follow up study. Ann Surg *149*, 457–461, 1959

Engelsman, E., Korsten, C. B., Persijn, J. P., and Cleton, F. J. Oestrogen and androgen receptors in human breast cancer. Br J Cancer *30*, 177, 1974

Engeset, A. The route of peripheral lymph to the blood stream. An x-ray study of the barrier theory. J Anat *93*, 96–100, 1959a

Engeset, A. Intralymphatic injections in the rat. Cancer Res *19*, 277–278, 1959b

Engstrom, P. F., Paul, A. R., Catalano, R. B., Mastrangelo, M. J., and Creech, R. H. Fluorouracil versus fluorouracil + BCG in colorectal adenocarcinoma, pp 587–595, In Terry, W. D., and Windhorst, D. (Eds): Immunotherapy of Cancer: Present Status of Trials in Man. New York: Raven Press, 1978

Enker, W. E., and Jacobitz, J. L. The definitive value of active-specific immunotherapy for experimental carcinoma of the colon. Surgery *80*, 164–170, 1976

Ennis, R. S., Granda, J. L., and Posner, A. S. Effect of gold salts and other drugs on the release and activity of lysosomal hydrolases. Arthritis Rheum *11*, 756–764, 1968

Epstein, M. A. Aspects of the EB virus. Adv Cancer Res *13*, 383–411, 1970

Epstein, M. A., Achong, B. G., and Barr, Y. M. Virus particles in cultured lymphomablasts from Burkitt's lymphoma. Lancet *2*, 702–703, 1964

Epstein, M. A., Achong, B. G., and Pope, J. H. Virus in cultured lymphoblasts from a New Guinea Burkitt lymphoma. Br Med J *2*, 290–291, 1967

Erb, P., and Feldman, M. Role of macrophages in in vitro induction of T-helper cells. Nature *254*, 352–354, 1975

Essex, M. Horizontally and vertically transmitted oncornaviruses of cats. Adv Cancer Res *21*, 175–248, 1975

Essex, M., Sliski, A., Cotter, S. M., Jakowski, R. M., and Hardy, W. D. Immunosurveillance of naturally occurring feline leukemia. Science *190*, 790–792, 1975

Evans, C. A., Gorman, L. R., Ito, Y., and Weiser,

R. S. Antitumor immunity in the Shope papilloma-carcinoma complex of rabbits. I. Papilloma regression induced by homologous and autologous tissue vaccines. J Natl Cancer Inst 29, 277–285, 1962a

Evans, C. A., and Ito, Y. Antitumor immunity in the Shope papilloma-carcinoma complex of rabbits. III. Response to reinfection with viral nucleic acid. J Natl Cancer Inst 36, 1161–1166, 1966

Evans, C. A., Weiser, R. S., and Ito, Y. Antiviral and antitumor immunologic mechanisms operative in the Shope papilloma-carcinoma system. Cold Spring Harbor Symp Quant Biol 27, 453–462, 1962b

Evans, C. R., and Pierrepoint C. G. Tissue-steroid interactions in canine hormone-dependent tumours. Vet Rec 97, 464–467, 1976

Evans, R. Macrophages in syngeneic animal tumours. Transplantation 14, 468–473, 1972

Evans, R. Macrophages and the tumour bearing host. Br J Cancer 28 (Suppl I), 19–25, 1973

Evans, R. Macrophage-mediated cytotoxicity: Its possible role in rheumatoid arthritis. Ann NY Acad Sci 256, 275–287, 1975

Evans, R. Macrophages in Solid Tumours: A review, pp 321–329, In James, K., McBride, B., and Stuart, A. (Eds): Proc EURES Symp—The Macrophage and Cancer. Edinburgh Univ Dept Surgery, 1977

Evans, R., and Alexander, P. Cooperation of immune lymphoid cells with macrophages in tumour immunity. Nature 228, 620–622, 1970

Evans, R., and Alexander, P. Rendering macrophages specifically cytotoxic by a factor from immune lymphoid cells. Transplantation 12, 227–229, 1971

Evans, R., and Alexander, P. Role of macrophages in tumour immunity. I. Cooperation between macrophages and lymphoid cells in syngeneic tumour immunity. Immunology 23, 615–626, 1972a

Evans, R., and Alexander, P. Role of macrophages in tumour immunity. II. Involvement of a macrophage cytophilic factor during syngeneic tumour growth inhibition. Immunology 23, 627–636, 1972b

Evans, R., and Alexander, P. Mechanism of immunologically specific killing of tumour cells by macrophages. Nature 236, 168–170 [Erratum 237, 60], 1972c

Evans, R., and Alexander, P. Mechanisms of extracellular killing of nucleated mammalian cells by macrophages, pp 535–576, In Nelson, D. S. (Ed): Immunobiology of the Macrophage. New York: Academic Press, 1976

Evans, R., Grant, C. K., Cox, H., Steele, K., and Alexander, P. Thymus-derived lymphocytes produce an immunologically specific macrophage-arming factor. J Exp Med 136, 1318–1322, 1972

Everall, J. D., O'Doherty, C. J., Wand, J., and Dowd, P. M. Treatment of primary melanoma by intralesional vaccinia before excision. Lancet 2, 583–586, 1975

Everson, T. C., and Cole, W. H. Spontaneous regression of cancer: Preliminary report. Ann Surg 144, 366–380, 1956

Everson, T. C., and Cole, W. H. Spontaneous Regression of Cancer. Philadelphia: W. B. Saunders, 1966

Ewing, J. Neoplastic Diseases (4th Ed). Philadelphia, London: W. B. Saunders, 1940

Ezdinli, E. Z., Sokal, J. E., Crosswhite, B. S., and Sandberg, A. A. Philadelphia-chromosome-positive and -negative chronic myelocytic leukemia. Ann Intern Med 72, 175–182, 1970

F

Faiman, C., Colwell, J. A., Ryan, R. J., Hershman, J. M., and Shields, T. W. Gonadotropin secretion from a bronchogenic carcinoma; Demonstration by radioimmunotherapy. N Engl J Med 277, 1395–1399, 1967

Fairley, G. H., and Freeman, J. E. Blood and neoplastic diseases. Treatment of the lymphomas. Br Med J 4, 761–765, 1974

Fairley, G. H., and Matthias, J. Q. Cortisone and skin sensitivity to tuberculin in reticuloses. Br Med J 2, 433–436, 1960

Fakhri, O., and Hobbs, J. R. Target cell death without added complement after co-operation of 7S antibodies with nonimmune lymphocytes. Nature New Biol 235, 177–178, 1972

Falk, H. L. Anticarcinogenesis—An alternative. Prog Exp Tumor Res 14, 105–137, 1971

Falk, R. E., MacGregor, A. B., Landi, S., Ambus, U., and Langer, B. Immunostimulation with intraperitoneally administered bacille Calmette Guérin for advanced malignant tumors of the gastrointestinal tract. Surg Gynecol Obstet 142, 363–368, 1976

Faraci, R. P., Barone, J. J., Marrone, J. C., and Chour, L. In vitro evidence of specific BCG-induced immunity to malignant melanoma in BALB/c mice. J Natl Cancer Inst 52, 1913–1915, 1974

Faraci, R. P., Marrone, J. A. C., and Ketcham, A. S. Antitumor immune response following injection of neuraminidase-treated sarcoma cells. Ann Surg *181*, 359–362, 1975

Farber, E. Biochemistry of carcinogenesis. Cancer Res *28*, 1859–1869, 1968

Farber, S. Chemotherapy in the treatment of leukemia and Wilms' tumor. JAMA *198*, 826–836, 1966

Farrow, J. H., and Adair, F. E. Effect of orchidectomy on skeletal metastases from cancer of male breast. Science *95*, 654, 1942

Fass, L., and Fefer, A. Studies of adoptive chemoimmunotherapy of a Friend virus-induced lymphoma. Cancer Res *32*, 997–1001, 1972

Fass, L., Herberman, R. B., and Ziegler, J. Delayed cutaneous hypersensitivity reactions to autologous extracts of Burkitt-lymphoma cells. N Engl J Med *282*, 776–780, 1970a

Fass, L., Herberman, R. B., Ziegler, J. L., and Kiryabwire, J. W. M. Cutaneous hypersensitivity to autologous extracts of malignant melanoma cells. Lancet *1*, 116–118, 1970b

Fass, L., Herberman, R. B., Ziegler, J., and Morrow, R. H. Evaluation of the effect of remission plasma on untreated patients with Burkitt's lymphoma. J Natl Cancer Inst *44*, 145–149, 1970c

Fauve, R. M. Influence of synthetic polynucleotides on the bacterial power of mouse macrophages against Listeria monocytogenes, pp 215–224, In Beers, R. F., and Braun, W. (Eds): Biological Effects of Polynucleotides. New York: Springer-Verlag, 1971

Fauve, R. M. Stimulating effect of Corynebacterium parvum and C. parvum extract on the macrophage activities against Salmonella typhimurium and Listeria monocytogenes, pp 77–83; In Halpern, B. (Ed): Corynebacterium Parvum: Applications in Experimental and Clinical Oncology. New York: Plenum Press, 1975

Fauve, R. M., and Hevin, M. B. Pouvoir bactéricide des macrophages spléniques et hépatiques de souris envers Listeria monocytogenes. Ann Inst Pasteur *120*, 399–411, 1971

Fauve, R. M., and Hevin, B. Immunostimulation with bacterial phospholipid extracts. Proc Natl Acad Sci USA *71*, 573–577, 1974

Fefer, A. Immunotherapy and chemotherapy of Moloney sarcoma virus-induced tumors in mice. Cancer Res *29*, 2177–2183, 1969

Fefer, A. Immunotherapy of primary Moloney sarcoma-virus-induced tumors. Int J Cancer *5*, 327–337, 1970

Fefer, A. Adoptive chemoimmunotherapy of a Moloney lymphoma. Int J Cancer *8*, 364–373, 1971

Fefer, A. Adoptive tumor immunotherapy in mice as an adjunct to whole-body x-irradiated and chemotherapy. Isr J Med Sci *9*, 350–365, 1973

Fefer, A. Tumor immunotherapy, pp 528–554, In Sartorelli, A. C., and Johns, D. G. (Eds): Antineoplastic and Immunosuppressive Agents. New York: Springer-Verlag, 1974

Fefer, A., Buckner, C. D., Clift, R. A., Fass, L., Lerner, K. G., Mickelson, E. M., Neiman, P., Rudolph, R. Storb, R., and Thomas, E. D. Marrow grafting in identical twins with hematologic malignancies. Transplant Proc *5*, 927–931, 1973

Fefer, A., Einstein, A. B., and Cheever, M. A. Adoptive chemoimmunotherapy of cancer in animals: A review of results, principles, and problems. Ann NY Acad Sci *277*, 492–502, 1976

Fefer, A., Einstein, A. B., Thomas, E. D., Buckner, C. D., Clift, R. A., Glucksberg, H., Neiman, P. E., and Storb, R. Bone-marrow transplantation for hematologic neoplasia in 16 patients with identical twins. N Engl J Med *290*, 1389–1393, 1974

Fefer, A., McCoy, J. L., and Glynn, J. P. Antigenicity of a virus-induced murine sarcoma (Moloney). Cancer Res *27*, 962–967, 1967

Fefer, A., McCoy, J. L., Kalman, P., and Glynn, J. P. Immunologic, virologic and pathologic studies of autochthonous Moloney sarcoma virus-induced tumors in mice. Cancer Res *28*, 1577–1585, 1968

Feigin, I., Allen, L. B., and Lipkin, O. The endothelial hyperplasia of the cerebral blood vessels with brain tumors and its sarcomatous transformation. Cancer *11*, 264–277, 1958

Feinleib, M. Breast cancer and artificial menopause: A cohort study. J Natl Cancer Inst *41*, 315–329, 1968

Fel, V. J., and Tsikarishvili, T. N. Reduction of normal muscle antigens in rat tumors of muscle origin induced by intramuscular injections of 20-methylcholanthrene. Cancer Res *24*, 1675–1677, 1964

Feldberg, W. Body temperature and fever: Changes in our views during the last decade (Ferrier Lecture, 1974). Proc R Soc Lond B *191*, 199–229, 1975

Feldman, M., Globerson, A., and Nachtigal, D. The reactivation of the immune response in immunologically suppressed animals, pp 427–449, In Conceptual Advances in Immunology and Oncology. New York: Hoeber Med Div, Harper & Row, 1963

Feneley, R. C. L., Eckert, H., Riddell, A. G., Symes, M. O., and Tribe, C. R. The treatment of advanced bladder cancer with sensitised pig lymphocytes. Br J Surg *61*, 825–827, 1974

Fennely, J. J., McBride, A., and O'Connell, L. G. Maintenance immunotherapy of acute nonlymphocytic leukaemia using unirradiated blast cells and BCG. Biomedicine 25, 198–200, 1976

Feraci, R. P., and Schour, L. Parabiotic inhibition of murine sarcoma growth. Surgery 75, 430–435, 1974

Ferluga, J. Increased cytolytic activity of a subcellular fraction from mouse liver after BCG infection. Lancet 2, 1476–1477, 1973

Fialkow, P. J. Use of genetic markers to study cellular origin and development of tumors in human females. Adv Cancer Res 15, 191–226, 1972

Fialkow, P. J. The origin and development of human tumors studied with cell markers. N Engl J Med 291, 26–35, 1974

Fialkow, P. J., Klein, G., Gartler, S. M., and Clifford, P. Clonal origin for individual Burkitt tumours. Lancet 1, 384–386, 1970

Fialkow, P. J., Klein, E., Klein, G., Clifford, P., and Singh, S. Immunoglobulin and glucose-6-phosphate dehydrogenase as markers of cellular origin in Burkitt lymphoma. J Exp Med 138, 89–102, 1973

Fialkow, P. J., Sagebiel, R. W., Gartler, S. M., and Rimoin, D. L. Multiple cell origin of hereditary neurofibromas. N Engl J Med 284, 298–300, 1971a

Fialkow, P. J., Thomas, E. D., Bryant, J. I., and Neiman, P. E. Leukaemic transformation of engrafted human marrow cells in vivo. Lancet 1, 251–255, 1971b

Fidler, I. J. In vitro studies of cellular-mediated immunostimulation of tumor growth. J Natl Cancer Inst 50, 1307–1312, 1973

Fidler, I. J. Inhibition of pulmonary metastasis by intravenous injection of specifically activated macrophages. Cancer Res 34, 1074–1078, 1974

Field, A. K., Tytell, A. A., Lampson, G. P., and Hilleman, M. R. Inducers of interferon and host resistance. II. Multistranded synthetic polynucleotide complexes. Proc Natl Acad Sci USA 58, 1001–1010, 1967

Field, E. J., and Caspary, E. A. Lymphocyte sensitisation: An in vitro test for cancer? Lancet 2, 1337–1341, 1970

Field, E. J., and Caspary, E. A. Lymphocyte sensitization in advanced malignant disease: A study of serum lymphocyte depressive factor. Br J Cancer 26, 164–173, 1972

Field, E. J., Caspary, E. A., and Smith, K. S. Macrophage electrophoretic mobility (MEM) test in cancer: A critical evaluation. Br J Cancer 28 (Suppl 1), 208–218, 1973

Fingerhut, B., and Veenema, R. J. Observations on possible autoimmune therapeutic effects in experimentally produced rat bladder tumors. Urol Int 30, 255–265, 1975

Finkel, M. P., Bergstrand, P. J., and Biskis, B. O. The latent period, incidence, and growth of Sr90-induced osteosarcomas in CF1 and CBA mice. Radiology 77, 269–281, 1961

Finkel, M. P., and Biskis, B. O. Experimental induction of osteosarcomas. Prog Exp Tumor Res 10, 72–111, 1968

Finkel, M. P., Biskis, B. O., and Farrell, C. Osteosarcomas appearing in Syrian hamsters after treatment with extracts of human osteosarcomas. Proc Natl Acad Sci USA 60, 1223–1230, 1968

Finney, J. W., Byers, E. H., and Wilson, R. H. Studies in tumor auto-immunity. Cancer Res 20, 351–356, 1960

Firshein, W., and Benson, R. C. Influence of oligonucleotides of known composition on rates of DNA synthesis in pneumococci, pp 364–378, In Prescia, O. J., and Braun, W. (Eds): Nucleic Acids in Immunology. New York: Springer-Verlag, 1968

Firshein, W., Benson, C., and Sease, M. Deoxycytidylate and deoxyguanylate kinase activity in pneumococci after exposure to known polyribonucleotides. Science 157, 821–822, 1967

Fisher, B. Status of adjuvant therapy: Results of the National Surgical Adjuvant Breast Cancer Project studies on oophorectomy, post operative radiation therapy, and chemotherapy. Cancer 28, 1654–1658, 1971

Fisher, B. In discussion, p 632, In Terry, W. D., and Windhorst, D. (Eds): Immunotherapy of Cancer: Present Status of Trials in Man. New York: Raven Press, 1978

Fisher, B., Carbone, P., Economou, S. G., Frelick, R., Glass, A., Lerner, H., Redmond, C., Zelen, M., Band, P., Katrych, D. L., Wolmark, N., and Fisher, E. R. L-phenylalanine mustard (L-PAM) in the management of primary breast cancer. A report of early findings. N Engl J Med 292, 117–122, 1975a

Fisher, B., and Fisher, E. R. Experimental studies of factors influencing hepatic metastases. III. Effect of surgical trauma with special reference to liver injury. Ann Surg 150, 731–744, 1959a

Fisher, B., and Fisher, E. R. Experimental evidence in support of the dormant tumor cell. Science 130, 918–919, 1959b

Fisher, B., and Fisher, E. R. The effect of alteration of liver blood flow upon experimental hepatic metastases. Surg Gynecol Obstet 112, 11–18, 1961a

Fisher, B., and Fisher, E. R. Experimental studies of factors influencing hepatic metastases. VIII.

Effect of anticoagulants. Surgery *50*, 240–247, 1961b

Fisher, B., and Fisher, E. R. Local factors affecting tumor growth. I. Effect of tissue homogenates. Cancer Res *23*, 1651–1657, 1963

Fisher, B., and Fisher, E. R. Transmigration of lymph nodes by tumor cells. Science *152*, 1397–1398, 1966a

Fisher, B., and Fisher, E. R. The interrelationship of hematogenous and lymphatic tumor cell dissemination. Surg Gynecol Obstet *122*, 791–798, 1966b

Fisher, B., and Fisher, E. R. Anticoagulants and tumor cell lodgement. Cancer Res *27*, 421–425, 1967

Fisher, B., and Fisher, E. R. Studies concerning the regional lymph node in cancer. II. Maintenance of immunity. Cancer *29*, 1496–1501, 1972

Fisher, B., Glass, A., Redmond, C., Fisher, E. R., Barton, B., Such, E., Carbone, P., Economou, S., Foster, R., Frelick, R., Lerner, H., Levitt, M., Margolese, R., MacFarlane, J., Plotkin, D. et al. L-phenylalanine mustard (L-PAM) in the management of primary breast cancer. Cancer *39*, 2883–2903, 1977

Fisher, B., Hanlon, J. T., Linta, J., and Fisher, E. R. Natural history of breast cancer: A brief overview, pp 621–634, In Terry, W. D., and Windhorst, D. (Eds): Immunotherapy of Cancer: Present Status of Trials in Man. New York: Raven Press, 1978

Fisher, B., Ravdin, R. G., Austman, R. K., Slack, N. H., Moore, G. E., and Noer, R. J. Surgical adjuvant chemotherapy in cancer of the breast: Results of a decade of cooperative investigations. Ann Surg *168*, 337–356, 1968

Fisher, B., Rubin, H., Saffer, E., and Wolmark, N. Further observations on the inhibition of tumour growth by Corynebacterium parvum with cyclophosphamide. II. Effect of cortisone acetate. J Natl Cancer Inst *56*, 571–574, 1976a

Fisher, B., Rubin, H., Sartiano, G., Ennis, L., and Wolmark, N. Observations following C. parvum administration to patients with advanced malignancy. A phase I study. Cancer *38*, 119–138, 1976b

Fisher, B., Saffer, E., and Fisher, E. R. Studies concerning the regional lymph node in cancer. IV. Tumor inhibition by regional lymph node cells. Cancer *33*, 631–636, 1974a

Fisher, B., Taylor, S., Levine, M., Saffer, E., and Fisher, E. R. Effect of Mycobacterium bovis (strain of bacillus Calmette-Guérin) on macrophage production by the bone marrow of tumor-bearing mice. Cancer Res *34*, 1668–1670, 1974b

Fisher, B., Wolmark, N., and Coyle, J. Effect of Corynebacterium parvum on cytotoxicity of regional and nonregional lymph node cells from animals with tumors present or removed. J Natl Cancer Inst *53*, 1793–1801, 1974c

Fisher, B., Wolmark, N., Rubin, H., and Saffer, E. Further observations on the inhibition of tumor growth by Corynebacterium parvum with cyclophosphamide. I. Variation in administration of both agents. J Natl Cancer Inst *55*, 1147–1153, 1975b

Fisher, B., Wolmark, N., Saffer, E., and Fisher, E. R. Inhibitory effect of prolonged Corynebacterium parvum and cyclophosphamide administration on the growth of established tumors. Cancer *35*, 134–143, 1975c

Fisher, E. R., and Fisher. B. Experimental studies of factors influencing hepatic metastases. IV. Effect of cirrhosis. Cancer *13*, 860–864, 1960

Fisher, E. R., and Fisher. B. Experimental studies of factors influencing hepatic metastases. VII. Effect of reticuloendothelial interference. Cancer Res *21*, 275–280, 1961

Fisher, E. R., and Fisher, B. Experimental studies of factors influencing hepatic metastases. X. Effect of reticuloendothelial stimulation. Cancer Res *22*, 478–483, 1962

Fisher, E. R., and Fisher, B. Local lymphoid response as an index of tumor immunity. Arch Pathol Lab Med *94*, 137–146, 1972

Fisher, E. R., Gregorio, R. M., and Fisher, B. The pathology of invasive breast cancer. J Natl Cancer Inst *36*, 1–85, 1975a

Fisher, E. R., Gregorio, R., Redmond, C., Vellios, F., Sommers, S. C., and Fisher, B. Pathologic findings from the National Surgical Adjuvant Breast Project (Protocol No. 4). I. Observations concerning the multicentricity of mammary cancer. Cancer *35*, 247–254, 1975b

Fisher, E. R., and Turnbull, R. B. The cytologic demonstration and significance of tumor cells in the mesenteric venous blood in patients with colorectal carcinoma. Surg Gynecol Obstet *100*, 102–108, 1955

Fisher, J. C., Cooperband, S. R., and Mannick, J. A. The effect of polyinosinic-polycytidylic acid on the immune response of mice to antigenically distinct tumors. Cancer Res *32*, 889–892, 1972

Fisher, J. C., Davis, R. C., and Mannick, J. A. The effects of immunosuppression on the induction and immunogenicity of chemically induced sarcomas. Surgery *68*, 150–157, 1970

Fisher, J. C., Grace, W. R., and Mannick, J. A. The effect of nonspecific immune stimulation with Corynebacterium parvum on patterns of tumor growth. Cancer *26*, 1379–1382, 1970

Fisher, J. C., and Holloman, J. H. Hypothesis for origin of cancer foci. Cancer *4*, 916–918, 1951

Fisher, R. A. In vitro and in vivo effects of Corynebacterium parvum on lymphocyte transformation. Dev Biol Stand *38*, 461–466, 1978

Fishman, M. Antibody formation in vitro. J Exp Med *114*, 837–856, 1961

Flanagan, S. P. 'Nude,' a new hairless gene with pleiotropic effects in the mouse. Genet Res *8*, 295–309, 1966

Flax, H., Salih, H., Newton, K., and Hobbs, J. R. Are some women's breast cancers androgen dependent? Lancet *1*, 1204–1207, 1973

Floersheim, G. L. Treatment of Moloney lymphoma with lethal doses of dimethyl myleran combined with injection of hemopoietic cells. Lancet *1*, 228–233, 1969

Floersheim, G. L. Treatment of hyperacute graftversus-host disease in mice with cytosine arabinoside. Transplantation *14*, 325–330, 1972

Florentin, I., Huchet, R., Bruley-Rosset, M., Halle-Pannenko, O., and Mathé, G. Studies on the mechanisms of action of BCG. Cancer Immunol Immunother *1*, 31–39, 1976

Fogh, J., and Giovanella, B. The Nude Mouse in Experimental and Clinical Research. New York: Academic Press, 1978

Foley, E. J. Attempts to induce immunity against mammary adenocarcinoma in inbred mice. Cancer Res *13*, 578–580, 1953a

Foley, E. J. Antigenic properties of methylcholanthrene-induced tumours in mice of strain of origin. Cancer Res *13*, 835–837, 1953b

Folkman, J. Anti-angiogenesis: New concept for therapy of solid tumors. Ann Surg *175*, 409–416, 1972

Folkman, J. Tumor angiogenesis. Adv Cancer Res *19*, 331–358, 1974

Folkman, J., and Hochberg, M. Self-regulation of growth in three dimensions. J Exp Med *138*, 745–753, 1973

Folkman, J., Merler, E., Abernathy, C., and Williams, G. Isolation of a tumor factor responsible for angiogenesis. J Exp Med *133*, 275–288, 1971

Foote, F. W., and Stewart, F. W. Comparative studies of cancerous versus non-cancerous breasts. Ann Surg *121*, 197–222, 1945

Forbes, I. J. Mitosis in mouse peritoneal macrophages. J Immunol *96*, 734–743, 1966

Forbes, I. J. Measurement of immunological function in clinical medicine. Aust NZ J Med *2*, 160–170, 1971

Forbes, J. F. The application of clinical trials to solid tumour management. An introduction. Aust NZ J Surg *47*, 617–627, 1977a

Forbes, J. F. Guidelines for planning clinical trials. Aust NZ J Surg *47*, 628–636, 1977b

Forbes, J. T., Nakao, Y., and Smith, R. T. Tumor-specific immunity to chemically induced tumors. Evidence for immunologic specificity and shared antigenicity in lymphocyte responses to soluble tumor antigens. J Exp Med *141*, 1181–1200, 1975

Forni, G., and Comoglio, P. M. Growth of syngeneic tumours in unimmunized newborn and adult hosts. Br J Cancer *27*, 120–127, 1973

Forni, G., and Comoglio, P. M. Effect of solubilized membrane antigens and tumour bearer serum on tumour growth in syngeneic hosts. Br J Cancer *30*, 365–369, 1974

Forrest, A. P. M., Roberts, M. M., Cant, E., and Shivas, A. A. Simple mastectomy and pectoral node biology. Br J Surg *63*, 569–575, 1976

Forrest, A. P. M., Roberts, M. M., Preece, P., Henk, J. M., Campbell, H., Hughes, L. E., Desai, S., and Hulbert, M. The Cardiff–St Mary's trial. Br J Surg *61*, 766–769, 1974

Forscher, B. K., and Houch, J. C. Chalones: Concepts and current researches. Natl Cancer Inst Monogr *38*, 1–233, 1973

Foster, R. S., MacPherson, B. R., and Browdie, D. A. Effect of C. parvum on colony-stimulation factor of granulocyte-macrophage colony formation. Cancer Res *37*, 1349–1357, 1977

Foulds, L. Mammary tumours in hybrid mice: Growth qnd progression of spontaneous tumours. Br J Cancer *3*, 345–375, 1949

Foulds, L. Experimental study of the course and regulation of tumour growth. Ann R Coll Surg Engl *9*, 93–101, 1951

Foulds, L. The histologic analysis of mammary tumors of mice. I. Scope of investigations and general principles of analysis. J Natl Cancer Inst *17*, 701–712, 1956a

Foulds, L. The histologic analysis of mammary tumors of mice. II. The histology of responsiveness and progression. J Natl Cancer Inst *17*, 713–754, 1956b

Foulds, L. The histologic analysis of mammary tumors of mice. III. Organoid tumors. J Natl Cancer Inst *17*, 755–782, 1956c

Foulds, L. The histologic analysis of mammary tumors of mice. IV. Secretion. J Natl Cancer Inst *17*, 783–802, 1956d

Foulds, L. Neoplastic development. London: Academic Press, 1969

Franks, C. R., Perkins, F. T., and Holmes, J. T. Growth of human tumours in immune-suppressed mice. Proc R Soc Med *68*, 287–290, 1975

Franks, L. M. The spread of prostatic carcinoma to the bones. J Pathol *66*, 91–93, 1953

Franks, L. M. Latency and progression in tumours. The natural history of prostatic cancer. Lancet *2*, 1037–1039, 1956a

Franks, L. M. The spread of prostatic cancer. J Pathol *72*, 601–611, 1956b

Fraser, H. Astrocytomas in an inbred mouse strain. J Pathol *103*, 266–270, 1971

Fraser, J., and Gill, W. Cryosurgery. J R Coll Surg Edinb *12*, 207–216, 1967

Fraumeni, J. F., and Miller, R. W. Breast cancer from breastfeeding. Lancet *2*, 1196–1197, 1971

Fredette, V. Le meilleur chimiste du cancer. Le Saguenay Med *20*, 129–138, 1973

Fredette, V., McSween, G., Vinet, G., and Chagnon, A. Production and purification of the oncolytic principle from Clostridium oncolyticum culture filtrates, pp 719–720. Proc VIIth Int Congr Chemother Prague, 1971

Fredette, V., and Plante, C. Oncolytic activity of clostridium M55 spores. Can J Microbiol *16*, 249–252, 1970

Fredette, V., and Plante, C. Effect of clostridium M55 spore extracts on Ehrlich solid tumor in the mouse. Can J Microbiol *18*, 367–369, 1972

Freedman, H. H., and Braun, W. Influence of oligodeoxyribonucleotides on phagocytic activity of the reticuloendothelial system. Proc Soc Exp Biol Med *120*, 222–225, 1965

Freeman, C. B., Harris, R., Geary, C. G., Leyland, M. J., MacIver, J. E., and Delamore, I. W. Active immunotherapy used alone for maintenance of patients with acute myeloid leukaemia. Br Med J *4*, 571–572, 1973

Frei, J. V. Toxicity, tissue changes and tumor induction in inbred Swiss mice by methylnitrosamine and -amide compounds. Cancer Res *30*, 11–17, 1970

Frei, J. V., Iwasutiak, R., and Viragos, G. Lack of significant visible C-type virus activation in the bone marrow and thymus of mice given a leukaemogenic dose of methylnitrosourea. Chem Biol Interactions *6*, 333–337, 1973

Frenster, J. H., and Rogoway, W. M. In-vitro activation and reinfusion of autologous human lymphocytes. Lancet *2*, 979–980, 1968

Freund, H., Biran, S., Laufer, N., and Eyal, Z. Breast cancer arising in thoracotomy scars. Lancet *1*, 97, 1976

Fridman, W. H., and Kourilsky, F. M. Stimulation of lymphocytes by autologous leukaemia cells in acute leukaemia. Nature *224*, 277–279, 1969

Friedell, G. H. Anaemia in cancer. Lancet *1*, 356–359, 1965

Friedewald, W. F., and Rous, P. The initiating and promoting elements in tumor production. An analysis of the effects of tar, benzpyrene, and methylcholanthrene on rabbit skin. J Exp Med *80*, 101–144, 1944

Friedman, J. M., and Fialkow, P. J. Cell marker studies of human tumorigenesis. Transplant Rev *28*, 17–33, 1976

Frindel, E., Malaise, E., and Tubiana, M. Cell proliferation kinetics in five human solid tumors. Cancer *22*, 611–620, 1968

Friou, G. J., and Teague, P. A. Spontaneous autoimmunity in mice. Antibodies to nucleoprotein in strain A/J. Science *143*, 1333–1334, 1964

Fritsche, R., and Mach, J. P. Identification of a new oncofoetal antigen associated with several types of human carcinomas. Nature *258*, 734–737, 1975

Fritze, D., Kern, D. H., Chow, N., and Pilch, Y. H. Production of cytotoxic antibody to a benz(a)pyrene-induced sarcoma in mice receiving xenogeneic antitumor immune RNA. Cancer Immunol Immunother *1*, 245–250, 1976a

Fritze, D., Kern, D. H., Humme, J. A., Drogemuller, C. R., and Pilch, Y. H. Detection of private and common tumor-associated antigens in murine sarcomas induced by different chemical carcinogens. Int J Cancer *17*, 138–147, 1976b

Froese, G., Berczi, I., and Sehon, A. H. Neuraminidase-induced enhancement of tumor growth in mice. J Natl Cancer Inst *52*, 1905–1908, 1974

Frøland, S. S., and Natvig, J. B. Identification of three different human lymphocyte populations by surface markers. Transplant Rev *16*, 114–162, 1973

Frost, M.J., Rogers, G. T., and Bagshawe, K. D. Extraction and preliminary characterisation of a human bronchogenic carcinoma antigen. Br J Cancer *31*, 379–386, 1975

Frost, P. Further evidence for the role of macrophages in the initiation of lymphocyte trapping. Immunology *27*, 609–616, 1974

Frost, P., and Lance, E. M. The relation of lymphocyte trapping to the mode of action of adjuvants, pp 29–45, In Wolstenholme, G. E. W., and Knight, J. (Eds): Ciba Fdn Symp—Immunopotentiation, New Series 18. Amsterdam: ASP, 1973

Frost, P., and Lance, E. M. The cellular origin of the lymphocyte trap. Immunology *26*, 175–186, 1974

Fuchs, W. A., Davidson, J. A., and Fisher, H. E. (Eds): Lymphography in Cancer. Recent Results Cancer Res, *23*. New York: Springer-Verlag, 1969

Fujimoto, S., Greene, M. I., and Sehon, A. H. Regulation of the immune response to tumor antigens. I. Immunosuppressor cells in tumor-bearing hosts. J Immunol *116*, 791–799, 1976a

Fujimoto, S., Greene, M. I., and Sehon, A. H. Regulation of the immune response to tumor antigens. II. The nature of immunosuppressor cells in tumor-bearing hosts. J Immunol *116*, 800–806, 1976b

Fukuhara, S., Shirakawa, S., and Uchino, H. Specific marker chromosome 14 in malignant lymphomas. Nature *259*, 210–211, 1976

Fuller, P. C., and Winn, H. J. Immunochemical and biological characterization of alloantibody activity in immunological enhancement. Transplant Proc *5*, 585–587, 1973

Fullerton, J. M., and Hill, R. D. Spontaneous regression of cancer. Br Med J *2*, 1589–1590, 1963

Furth, J. Influence of host factors on the growth of neoplastic cells. Cancer Res *23*, 21–34, 1963

Furth, J., and Kahn, M. C. The transmission of leukemia of mice with a single cell. Am J Cancer *31*, 276–282, 1937

Fusco, F. D., and Rosen, S. N. Gonadotrophin-producing anaplastic large cell carcinomas of the lung. N Engl J Med *275*, 507–515, 1966

G

Gabrilove, J. L., Nicolis, G. L., and Kirschner, P. A. Cushing's syndrome in association with carcinoid tumor. Ann Surg *169*, 240–248, 1969

Galasko, C. S. B. The detection of skeletal metastases from mammary cancer by gamma camera scintigraphy. Br J Surg *56*, 757–764, 1969

Galasko, C. S. B. The detection of skeletal metastases from carcinoma of the breast. Surg Gynecol Obstet *132*, 1019–1024, 1971

Galasko, C. S. B. Skeletal metastases and mammary cancer. Ann R Coll Surg Engl *50*, 3–28, 1972

Galasko, C. S. B. The significance of occult skeletal metastases, detected by skeletal scintigraphy in patients with otherwise apparently 'early' mammary carcinoma. Br J Surg *62*, 694–696, 1975

Galasko, C. S. B., and Doyle, F. H. The response to therapy of skeletal metastases from mammary cancer. Assessment by scintigraphy. Br J Surg *59*, 85–88, 1972

Galasko, C. S. B., Westerman, B., Li, J., Sellwood, R. A., and Burn, J. I. Use of the gamma camera for early detection of osseous metastases from mammary cancer. Br J Surg *55*, 613–615, 1968

Gale, R. P., and Zighelboim, J. Polymorphonuclear leukocytes in antibody-dependent cellular cytotoxicity. J Immunol, *114*, 1047–1051, 1975

Gallily, R. Allogeneic recognition and killing capacity of immune macrophages in mixed macrophage cultures (MMC). Cell Immunol *15*, 419–431, 1975

Gallily, R., and Ben-Ishay, Z. Immune cytolysis of mouse macrophages in vitro. J Reticuloendothel Soc *18*, 44–52, 1975

Gallin, J. I., and Kirkpatrick. C. H. Chemotactic activity in dialyzable transfer factor. Proc Natl Acad Sci USA *71*, 498–502, 1974

Garb, S., Stein, A. A., and Sims, G. The production of anti-human leukaemia serum in rabbits. J Immunol *88*, 142–152, 1962

Gardner, P. S., Trench, C. A. H., Green, C. A., and Bird, T. Inhibition of tumour growth in irradiated mice by sensitized homologous spleen cells. Nature *203*, 1295, 1964

Gardner, R. J., and Preston, F. W. Prolonged skin homograft survival in advanced cancer and cirrhosis of the liver. Surg Gynecol Obstet *115*, 399–402, 1962

Garland, H., Coulson, W., and Wollin, E. The rate of growth and apparent duration of untreated primary bronchial carcinoma. Cancer *16*, 694–707, 1963

Garner, F. B., Meyer, C. A., White, D. S., and Lipton, A. Aerosol BCG treatment of carcinoma metastatic to the lung: A phase I study. Cancer *35*, 1088–1094, 1975

Gasic, G., Gasic, T., and Stewart, C. C. Antimetastatic effects associated with platelet reduction. Proc Natl Acad Sci USA *61*, 46–52, 1968

Gatti, R. A., Ostborn, A., and Fagraeus, A. Selective impairment of cell antigenicity by fixation. J Immunol *113*, 1361–1368, 1974

Gauci, C. L., and Alexander, P. The macrophage content of some human tumours. Cancer Lett *1*, 29–32, 1975

Gaudin, D., Gregg, R. S., and Yielding, K. L. Inhibition of DNA repair by cocarcinogens. Biochem Biophys Res Commun *48*, 945–949, 1972

Gautherie, M., Armand, M.-O., and Gros, Ch. Thermogénèse des épithéliomes mammaires. IV. Étude lors d'évolutions spontanées, de l'influence de la vitesse de croissance et des corrélations avec la probabilité de dissémination lymphatique. Biomedicine *22*, 328–336, 1975

Gee, T. S., Dowling, M. D., Cunningham, I., Oettgen, H. S., Armstrong, D., and Clarkson, B. D. Evaluation of Pseudomonas aeruginosa vaccine for prolongation of remissions in adults with acute nonlymphoblastic leukemia treated with the L-12 protocol: A preliminary report, pp 415–421, In Terry, W. D., and Windhorst, D. (Eds): Immunotherapy of Cancer: Present

Status of Trials in Man. New York: Raven Press, 1978

Geffard, M., and Orbach-Arbouys, S. Enhancement of T suppressor activity in mice by high doses of BCG. Cancer Immunol Immunother 1, 41–43, 1976

Gehan, E. A. A generalized Wilcoxon test for comparing arbitrarily singly-censored samples. Biometrika 52, 203–223, 1965

Gehan, E. A. Statistical methods for survival time studies, pp 7–35, In Staquet, M. J. (Ed): Cancer Therapy: Prognostic Factors and Criteria of Response. New York: Raven Press, 1975

Gehan, E. A., Sutow, W. W., Uribe-Botero, G., Romsdahl, M., and Smith, T. L. Osteosarcoma: The M. D. Anderson experience, 1950–1974, pp 271–282, In Terry, W. D., and Windhorst, D. (Eds): Immunotherapy of Cancer: Present Status of Trials in Man. New York: Raven Press, 1978

Gelboin, H. V. Carcinogens, enzyme induction and gene action. Adv Cancer Res 10, 1–82, 1967

Gelboin, H. V., and Levy, H. B. Polyinosinic-polycytidylic acid inhibits chemically induced tumorigenesis in mouse skin. Science 167, 205–207, 1970

Gelboin, H. V., and Wiebel, F. J. Studies on the mechanism of aryl hydrocarbon hydroxylase induction and its role in cytotoxicity and tumorigenicity. Ann NY Acad Sci 179, 529–547, 1971

Gensler, W. T., and Alam, I. Trehalose covalently conjugated to bovine serum albumin. J Org Chem 42, 130–135, 1977

Gentile, J. M., and Flickinger, J. T. Isolation of a tumor-specific antigen from adenocarcinoma of the breast. Surg Gynecol Obstet 135, 69–73, 1972

Gerber, P., and Birch, S. M. Complement-fixing antibodies in sera of human and non-human primates to viral antigens derived from Burkitt's lymphoma. Proc Natl Acad Sci USA 58, 478–484, 1967

Gericke, D. Bösartige Geschwülste und Mikroorganismen. Fortschr Med 89, 32–35, 1971

Gericke, D., and Engelbart, K. Oncolysis by clostridia. II. Experiments on a tumor spectrum with a variety of clostridia in combination with heavy metal. Cancer Res 24, 217–221, 1964

Gershon, R. K. A disquisition on suppressor T cells. Transplant Rev 26, 170–185, 1975

Gershon, R. K., and Kondo, K. Cell interactions in the production of tolerance: The role of thymic lymphocytes. Immunology 18, 723–737, 1970

Gershon, R. K., and Kondo, K. Infectious immunological tolerance. Immunology 21, 903–914, 1971

Gewirtz, G., and Yalow, R. S. Ectopic ACTH production in carcinoma of the lung. J Clin Invest 53, 1022–1032, 1974

Ghaffar, A., Calder, E. A., and Irvine, W. J. K cell cytotoxicity against antibody-coated chicken erythrocytes in tumor-bearing mice: Its development with progressively growing tumor and the effect of immunization against the tumor. J Immunol 116, 315–318, 1976

Ghaffar, A., Cullen, R. T., Dunbar, N., and Woodruff, M. F. A. Anti-tumour effect in vitro of lymphocytes and macrophages from mice treated with Corynebacterium parvum. Br J Cancer 29, 199–205, 1974

Ghaffar, A., Cullen, R. T., and Woodruff, M. F. A. Further analysis of the anti-tumour effect in vitro of peritoneal exudate cells from mice treated with Corynebacterium parvum. Br J Cancer 31, 15–24, 1975

Ghose, T., Cerini, M., Carter, M., and Nairn, R. C. Immunoradioactive agent against cancer. Br Med J 1, 90–93, 1967

Ghose, T., Guclu, A., Tai, J., MacDonald, A. S., Norvell, S. T., and Aquino, J. Antibody as carrier of ^{131}I in cancer diagnosis and treatment. Cancer 36, 1646–1657, 1975a

Ghose, T., Guclu, A., Tai, J., Mammen, N., and Norwell, S. T. Immunoprophylaxis and immunotherapy of EL4 lymphoma. Eur J Cancer 13, 925–935, 1977

Ghose, T., and Nigam, S. P. Antibody as a carrier of chlorambucil. Cancer 29, 1398–1400, 1972

Ghose, T., Norvell, S. T., Guclu, A., Cameron, D., Bodurtha, A., and MacDonald, A. S. Immunochemotherapy of cancer with chlorambucil-carrying antibody. Br Med J 3, 495–499, 1972

Ghose, T., Norvell, S. T., Guclu, A., and MacDonald, A. S. Immunochemotherapy of human malignant melanoma with chlorambucil-carrying antibody. Eur J Cancer 11, 321–326, 1975b

Giannelli, F. DNA repair and tumours of the skin: Xeroderma pigmentosum as a model. Proc R Soc Med 70, 388–395, 1977

Gidlund, M., Ojo, E., Örn, A., Wigzell, H., and Murgita, R. A. Severe suppression of the B-cell system has no impact on the maturation of natural killer cells in mice. Scand. J. Immunol, 162–173, 1979

Gidlund, M., Örn, A., Wigzell, H., Senik, A., and Gresser, I. Enhanced NK cell activity in mice injected with interferon and interferon inducers. Nature 273, 759–761, 1978

Gilden, R. V. Interrelationships among RNA tumor viruses and host cells. Adv Cancer Res 22, 157–202, 1975

Gill, P. G., Waller, C. A., Clarke, J., Darley, J.,

and Morris, P. J. The effect of Corynebacterium parvum on human effector cells in peripheral blood. Dev Biol Stand *38*, 455–460, 1978

Gillespie, A. V. Detection of a tumour-specific antigen (Gross) with the mixed antiglobulin reaction using erythrocytes from NZB/Bl mice. Immunology *15*, 855–862, 1968

Gillette, R. W., and Boone, C. W. Changes in phytohemagglutinin response due to presence of tumors. J Natl Cancer Inst *50*, 1391–1393, 1973

Gillette, R. W., and Boone, C. W. Kinetic studies of macrophages. VI. The effect of the presence of a solid tumor. J Reticuloendothelial Soc *15*, 126–131, 1974

Gimbrone, M. A., Cotran, R. S., Leapman, S. B., and Folkman, J. Tumor growth and neovascularization. An experimental model using the rabbit cornea. J Natl Cancer Inst *52*, 413–427, 1974

Giovanella, B. C., Stehlin, J. S., and Williams, I. J. Heterotransplantation of human malignant tumors in "nude" thymus-less mice. II. Malignant tumors induced by injections of cell cultures derived from human solid tumors. J Natl Cancer Inst *52*, 921–927, 1974

Girardi, A. J., Repucci, P., Dierlam, P., Rutala, W., and Coggin, J. H. Prevention of simian virus 40 tumors by hamster fetal tissue: Influence of parity status of donor females on immunogenicity of fetal tissue and on immune cell cytotoxicity. Proc Natl Acad Sci USA *70*, 183–186, 1973

Girmann, G., Pees, H., Schwarze, G., and Scheurlen, P. G. Immunosuppression by micromolecular fibrinogen degradation products in cancer. Nature *259*, 399–401, 1976

Glaser, M., Bonnard, G. D., and Herberman, R. B. In vitro generation of secondary cell-mediated cytotoxic response against a syngeneic Gross virus-induced lymphoma in rats. J Immunol *116*, 430–436, 1976

Glaser, R., Ablashi, D. V., Nonoyama, M., Henle, W., and Easton, J. Enhanced oncogenic behavior of human and mouse cells after cellular hybridization with Burkitt tumor cells. Proc Natl Acad Sci USA *74*, 2574–2578, 1977

Glaser, R., deThe, G., Lenoir, G., and Ho, J. H. C. Superinfection of epithelial nasopharyngeal carcinoma cells with Epstein-Barr virus. Proc Natl Acad Sci USA *73*, 960–963, 1976

Glasgow, A. H., Nimberg, R. B., Menzoian, J. O., Saporoschetz, I., Cooperband, S. R., Schmid, K., and Mannick, J. A. Association of anergy with an immunosuppressive peptide fraction in the serum of patients with cancer. N Engl J Med *291*, 1263–1267, 1974

Gleichmann, E., Gleichmann, H., and Schwartz, R. S. Immunologic induction of malignant lymphoma: Genetic factors in the graft-versus-host model. J Natl Cancer Inst *49*, 793–804, 1972

Gleichmann, E., Gleichmann, H., Schwartz, R. S., Weinblatt, A., and Armstrong, M. Y. K. Immunologic induction of malignant lymphoma: Identification of donor and host tumors in the graft-versus-host model. J Natl Cancer Inst *54*, 107–116, 1975a

Gleichmann, E., Peters, K., Lattmann, E., and Gleichmann, H. Immunologic induction of reticulum cell sarcoma: Donor-type lymphomas in the graft-versus-host model. Eur J Immunol *5*, 406–412, 1975b

Glick, J. L. Induction of an allogeneic-like inhibition by means of DNA obtained from untreated cells, pp 414–428, In Plescia, O. J., and Braun, W. (Eds): Nucleic Acids in Immunology. New York: Springer-Verlag, 1968

Glick, J. L., and Goldberg, A. R. Inhibition of L1210 tumor growth by thymus DNA. Science *149*, 997–998, 1965

Glick, J. L., and Goldberg, A. R. The action of thymus DNA on L1210 leukemia cells. Trans NY Acad Sci *28*, 741–753, 1966

Gliedman, M. L., Horowitz, S., and Lewis, F. J. Lung resection for metastatic cancer. Surgery *42*, 521–532, 1957

Glimcher, L., and Cantor, H. [*Cited by Cantor and Boyse (1978) as in preparation.*] 1978

Glimcher, L., Shen, F. W., and Cantor, H. Identification of a cell-surface antigen selectively expressed on the natural killer cell. J Exp Med *145*, 1–9, 1977

Globerson, A., and Feldman, M. Antigenic specificity of benzo(a)pyrene-induced sarcomas. J Natl Cancer Inst *32*, 1229–1243, 1964

Glynn, J. P., Bianco, A. R., and Goldin, A. Studies on induced resistance against isotransplants of virus-induced leukemia. Cancer Res *24*, 502–508, 1964

Godrick, E. A., Michaelson, J. S., Vanwijck, R., and Wilson, R. E. Immunotherapy combined with primary resection of murine fibrosarcoma: Correlation of immunological status of the host with prevention of metastases. Ann Surg *176*, 544–553, 1972

Gold, P., and Freedman, S. O. Demonstration of tumor-specific antigens in human colonic carcinomata by immunological tolerance and absorption techniques. J Exp Med *121*, 439–462, 1965

Golde, D. W., Byers, L. A., and Finley, T. N. Proliferative capacity of human alveolar macrophage. Nature *247*, 373–375, 1974a

Golde, D. W., Schambelan, M., Weintraub, B. D.,

and Rosen, S. W. Gonadotropin secreting renal carcinoma. Cancer *33*, 1048–1053, 1974b

Goldenberg, D. M. Unusual metastasis of a human colonic tumour xenograft in the hamster brain. Nature *226*, 550–552, 1970

Goldenberg, D. M. Human tumours in the hamster cheek pouch, p 18, In Mihich, E., Laurance, D. J. R., Laurance, D. M., and Echardt, S. (Eds): IUCC Workshop of New Animal Models for Chemotherapy of Human Solid Tumours. UICC Technical Report Service, Vol 15, 1974

Goldenberg, D. M., Bhan, R. D., and Pavia, R. A. In vivo human-hamster somatic cell fusion indicated by glucose 6-phosphate dehydrogenase and lactate dehydrogenase profiles. Cancer Res *31*, 1148–1152, 1971

Goldenberg, D. M., Pant, K. D., and Dahlman, H. A new oncofetal antigen associated with gastrointestinal cancer. Proc Am Assoc Cancer Res *17*, 155, 1976

Goldenberg, G. H., and Brandes, L. J. Immunotherapy of nasopharyngeal carcinoma with transfer factor from donors with previous infectious mononucleosis. Clin Res *20*, 947, 1972

Goldman, L., Siler, V. E., and Blaney, D. Laser therapy of melanomas. Surg Gynecol Obstet *124*, 49–56, 1967

Goldman, R., and Hogg, N. Enhanced susceptibility of virus-infected cells to starch-induced peritoneal exudate cells, pp 97–107, In James, K., McBride, B., and Stuart, A. (Eds): Proc EURES Symp—The Macrophage and Cancer. Edinburgh Univ Dept Surgery, 1977

Goldsmith, H. S., Levin, A. G., and Southam, C. M. A study of the cellular responses in cancer patients by qualitative and quantitative Rebuck test. Surg Forum *16*, 102–104, 1965

Goldstein, M. Thymosin: Basic properties and clinical potential in the treatment of patients with immunodeficiency and cancer. Antibiot Chemother *24*, 47–59, 1978

Goligher, J. C., Dukes, C. E., and Bussey, H. J. R. Preservation of the anal sphincters in the radical treatment of rectal cancer. Ann R Coll Surg Engl *22*, 311–329, 1958

Golstein, P., and Smith, E. T. The lethal hit stage of mouse T and non-T cell-mediated cytolysis: Differences in cation requirements and characterization of an analytical "cation pulse" method. Eur J Immunol *6*, 31–37, 1976

Golstein, P., Svedmyr, E. A. J., and Wigzell, H. Cells mediating specific in vitro cytotoxicity. I. Detection of receptor-bearing lymphocytes. J Exp Med *134*, 1385–1402, 1971

Golstein, P., Wigzell, H., Blomgren, H., and Svedmyr, E. A. J. Cells mediating specific in vitro

cytotoxicity. II. Probable autonomy of thymus processed lymphocytes (T cells) for the killing of allogeneic target cells. J Exp Med *135*, 890–906, 1972

Golub, S. H., and Morton, D. L. Sensitisation of lymphocytes in vitro against human melanoma associated antigens. Nature 251, 161–163, 1974

Golub, S. H., O'Connell, T. X., and Morton, D. L. Correlation of in vivo and in vitro assays of immunocompetence in cancer patients. Cancer Res 34, 1833–1837, 1974

Gomard, E., LeClerc, J. C., and Levy, J. P. Murine leukemia and sarcoma viruses: Further studies on the antigens of the viral envelope. J Natl Cancer Inst *50*, 955–961, 1973

Gompertz, B. On the nature of the function expressive of the law of human mortality, and on a new mode of determining the value of life contingencies. Philos Trans R Soc *115*, 513–585, 1825

Good, R. A. Chairman's introduction, Session V: Clinical implications of the data base concerning the tumor-host relationship. New York: Academic Press pp 279–286, In Smith, R. T., and Landy, M. (Eds): Immunobiology of the Tumor-Host Relationship, 1975

Good, R. A. [*Cited in* Editorial: Immunological deficiency and cancer. Br Med J *2*, 654, 1977]

Goodwin, B. C. Analytical Physiology of Cells and Developing Organisms. London, New York: Academic Press, 1976

Gordon, D. S. Clinical immunotherapy experiences in the Southeastern Cancer Study Group. Dev Biol Stand *38*, 567–572, 1978

Gordon, J. Isoantigenicity of liver tumours induced by an azo dye. Br J Cancer *19*, 387–391, 1965

Gordon, R. D., Simpson, E., and Samelson, L. E. In vitro cell-mediated immune response to the male (H-Y) antigen in mice. J Exp Med *142*, 1108–1120, 1975

Gordon, S., Todd, J., and Cohn, Z. A. In vitro synthesis and secretion of lysozyme by mononuclear phagocytes. J Exp Med *139*, 1228–1248, 1974

Gordon-Taylor, G. The incomputable factor in cancer prognosis. Br Med J *1*, 455–462, 1959

Gorer, P. A. The significance of studies with transplanted tumours. Br J Cancer *2*, 103–107, 1948

Gorer, P. A. Some recent work on tumor immunity. Adv Cancer Res *4*, 149–186, 1956

Gorer, P. A. The antigenic structure of tumours. Adv Immunol *1*, 345–393, 1961

Gorer, P. A., and Amos, D. B. Passive immunity in mice against C57Bl leukosis EL4 by means of isoimmune serum. Cancer Res *16*, 338–343, 1956

Gorer, P. A., Tuffrey, M. A., and Batchelor, J. R. Serological studies on the X antigens. Ann NY Acad Sci *101*, 5–11, 1962

Gorodilova, V. V., Silino, I. G., and Soraeva, Z. M. The first experience in vaccination against metastases in patients with breast cancer. Vop Onkol *2*, 22–26, 1965

Gotohda, E., Sendo, F., Hosokawa, M., Kodama, T., and Kobayashi, H. Combination of active and passive immunisation and chemotherapy to transplantation of methylcholanthrene-induced tumor in WKA rats. Cancer Res *34*, 1947–1951, 1974

Gottlieb, J. A., Frei, E., and Luce, J. K. An evaluation of the management of patients with cerebral metastases from malignant melanoma. Cancer *29*, 701–705, 1972

Goudie, R. B., and McCallum, H. M. Loss of tissue-specific autoantigen in thyroid tumours. A demonstration by immunofluorescence. Lancet *2*, 1035–1038, 1963

Gough, I. R., and Furnival, C. M. Corynebacterium parvum and hyperthermia. Lancet *2*, 999–1000, 1978

Goulmy, E., Termijtelen, A., Bradley, B. A., and Van Rood, J. J. Y-antigen killing by T cells of women is restricted by HLA. Nature *266*, 544–545, 1976

Grace, J. T., and Kondo, T. Investigations of host resistance in cancer patients. Ann Surg *148*, 633–641, 1958

Grace J. T., and Lehoczky, A. Tumor-host relationship factors in man. Surgery *46*, 238–246, 1959

Graff, R. J., Lappé, M. A., and Snell, G. D. The influence of the gonads and adrenal glands on the immune response to skin grafts. Transplantation *7*, 105–111, 1969

Grage, T., Cornell, G., Strawitz, J., Jonas, K., Frelick, R., and Metter, G. Adjuvant therapy with 5-FU after surgical resection of colorectal cancer. Proc Amer Soc Clin Oncol *16*, 258, 1975

Graham, F. L. Biological activity of tumor virus DNA. Adv Cancer Res *25*, 1–51, 1977

Graham, J. B., and Graham, R. M. Antibodies elicited by cancer in patients. Cancer *8*, 409–416, 1955

Graham, J. B., and Graham, R. M. Vaccine in cancer patients. Surg Gynecol Obstet *109*, 131–138, 1959

Graham, J. B., and Graham, R. M. Autogenous vaccine in cancer patients. Surg Gynecol Obstet *114*, 1–4, 1962

Graham, S., Levin, M. L., Lilienfeld, A. M., Schuman, L. M., Gibson, R., Dowd, J. E., and Hemplemann, L. Preconception, intrauterine and postnatal irradiation as related to leuke-mia. Natl Cancer Inst Monogr *19*, 347–371, 1966

Graham-Pole, J., Ogg, L. J., Ross, C. E., and Cochran, A. J. Sensitisation of neuroblastoma patients and related and unrelated contacts to neuroblastoma extracts. Lancet *1*, 1376–1379, 1976

Granger, R. A., and Weiser, R. S. Homograft target cells: Specific destruction in vitro by contact interaction with immune macrophages. Science *145*, 1427–1429, 1964

Granger, R. A., and Weiser, R. S. Homograft target cells: Contact destruction in vitro by immune macrophages. Science *151*, 97–99, 1966

Grant, G. A., and Miller, J. F. A. P. Effect of neonatal thymectomy on the induction of sarcomata in C57BL mice. Nature *205*, 1124–1125, 1965

Grant, G. A., Roe, F. J. C., and Pike, M. C. Effect of neonatal thymectomy on the induction of papillomata and carcinomata by 3,4 benzopyrene in mice. Nature *210*, 603–604, 1966

Grant, J. P., Bigner, D. D., Fischinger, P. J., and Bolognesi, D. P. Expression of murine leukemia virus structural antigens on the surface of chemically induced murine sarcomas. Proc Natl Acad Sci USA *71*, 5037–5041, 1974a

Grant, J. P., Ladisch, S., and Wells, S. A. Immunologic similarities between fetal cell antigens and tumor cell antigens in guinea pigs. Cancer *33*, 376–383, 1974b

Grant, R. M., Mackie, R., Cochran, A. J., Murray, E. L., Hoyle, D., and Ross, C. Results of administering BCG to patients with melanoma. Lancet *2*, 1096–1100, 1974

Graw, R. G., Buckner, C. D., Whang-Peng, J., Leventhal, B. D., Krueger, G., Berard, C., and Henderson, E. S. Complication of bone-marrow transplantation. Graft-versus-host disease resulting from chronic-myelogenous-leukaemia leucocyte transfusions. Lancet *2*, 338–346, 1970

Graw, R. G., Lohrmann, H.-P., Bull, M.I., Decter, J., Herzig, G. P., Bull, J. M., Leventhal, B. G. Yankee, R. A., Herzig, R. H., Krueger, G. R. F., Bleyer, W. A., Buja, M. L., McGinniss, M. H., Alter, H. J., Whang-Peng, J., Gralnick, H. R., Kirkpatrick, C. H., and Henderson, E. S. Bone-marrow transplantation following combination chemotherapy immunosuppression (B.A.C.T.) in patients with acute leukemia. Transplant Proc *6*, 349–354, 1974

Graw, R. G., and Santos, G. W. Bone marrow transplantation in patients with leukemia. Transplantation *11*, 197–199, 1971

Graw, R. G., Yankee, R. A., Rogentine, G. N., Levanthal, B. G., Herzig, G. P., Halterman, R. H., Merritt, C. B., McGinniss, M. H., Krueger, G. R. D., Whang-Peng, J., Carolla, R. L. Gullion, D. S., Lippman, M. E., Gralnick, H. R., Berard, C. W., Terasaki, P. I., and Henderson, E. S. Bone marrow transplantation from HL-A matched donor to patients with acute leukemia. Transplantation 14, 79–90, 1972

Gray, G. R., Ribi, E., Granger, D., Parker, R., Azuma, I., and Yamamoto, K. Tumor suppression and regression by cell walls of Mycobacterium phlei attached to oil droplets. J Natl Cancer Inst 55, 727–730, 1975

Green, H. N. An immunological concept of cancer: A preliminary report. Br Med J 2, 1374–1380, 1954

Green, H. N. Immunological aspects of cancer, p 1, In Raven, R. W. (Ed): Cancer (3rd Ed). London: Butterworths, 1958

Green, H. N., Wakefield, J., and Littlewood, G. The nature of cancer anaemia and its bearing on the immunological theory of cancer. Br Med J 2, 779–784, 1957

Greenberg, A. H., Hudson, L., Shen, L., and Roitt, I. M. Antibody-dependent cell-mediated cytotoxicity due to a "null" lymphoid cell. Nature New Biol 242, 111–113, 1973

Greenberg, A. H., Shen, L., and Medley, G. Characteristics of the effector cells mediating cytotoxicity against antibody-coated target cells. I. Phagocytic and non-phagocytic effector cell activity against erythrocyte and tumour target cells in a 51-Cr release cytotoxicity assay and (125-I) IUdr growth inhibition assay. Immunology 29, 719–730, 1975

Greene, H. S. N. Heterologous transplantation of human and other mammalian tumors. Science 88, 357–358, 1938

Greene, H. S. N. Heterologous transplantation of mammalian tumors. II. The transfer of human tumors to alien species. J Exp Med 73, 475–485, 1941

Greene, H. S. N. The microscope or the guinea pig? Yale J Biol Med 18, 239–242, 1946

Greene, H. S. N. The heterologous transplantation of human melanomas. Yale J Biol Med 22, 611–620, 1950

Greene, H. S. N. The significance of the heterologous transplantability of human cancer. Cancer 5, 24–44, 1952

Greene, H. S. N., and Harvey, E. K. The relationship between the dissemination of tumor cells and the distribution of metastases. Cancer Res 24, 799–811, 1964

Greene, H. S. N., and Lund, P. K. The heterologous transplantation of human cancers. Cancer Res 4, 352–363, 1944

Greene, M.I., Dorf, M. E., Pierres, M., and Benacerraf, B. Reduction of syngeneic tumor growth by an anti-I-J alloantiserum. Proc Natl Acad Sci USA 74, 5118–5121, 1977

Gresser, I. Interferon and cancer: Therapeutic prospects. Rev Eur Etudes Clin Biol 15, 23–27, 1972

Gresser, I. (Ed). Interferon 1979 Vol I. London/New York: Academic Press 1979.

Gresser, I., and Bourali, C. Antitumor effects of interferon preparations in mice. J Natl Cancer Inst 45, 365–376, 1970

Gresser, I., and Bourali-Maury, C. The antitumor effect of interferon in lymphocyte- and macrophage-depressed mice. Proc Soc Exp Biol Med 144, 896–901, 1973

Gresser, I., Bourali, C., Chouroulinkov, I., Fontaine-Brouty-Boyé, D., and Thomas, M. T. Treatment of neoplasia in mice with interferon preparations. Ann NY Acad Sci 173, 694–707, 1970a

Gresser, I., Bourali, C., Levi, J. P., Fontaine-Brouty-Boyé, D., and Thomas, M. T. Increased survival in mice inoculated with tumor cells and treated with interferon preparations. Proc Natl Acad Sci USA 63, 51–57, 1969

Gresser, I., Brouty-Boyé, D., Thomas, M. T., and Macieira-Coelho, A. Interferon and cell division. II. Influence of various experimental conditions on the inhibition of L1210 cell multiplication in vitro by interferon preparations. J Natl Cancer Inst 5, 1145–1153, 1970b

Gresser, I. J., Coppey, D., Fontaine-Brouty-Boyé, D., Falcoff, E., Falcoff, R., Zajdela, F., Bourali, C., and Thomas, M. T. The effect of interferon preparations on Friend leukaemia in mice, pp 240–248, In Wolstenholme, G. E. W., and O'Connor, M. (Eds): Ciba Fdn Symp—Interferon. London: Churchill, 1968

Gresser, I., Maury, C., and Brouty-Boyé, D. Mechanisms of the antitumor effect of interferon in mice. Nature 239, 167–168, 1972

Griesbach, W. E., Kennedy, T. H., and Purves, H. D. Studies on experimental goitre; Thyroid adenomata in rats on Brassica seed diet. Br J Exp Pathol 26, 18–24, 1945

Griffin, A. C., Rinfert, A. P., and Corsigilia, V. F. Inhibition of liver carcinogenesis with 3-methyl-4-dimethylaminoazobenzene in hypophysectomised rats. Cancer Res 13, 77–79, 1953

Griffith, A. H., and Regamey, R. H. (Eds): Int Symp—Biological Preparations in the Treatment of Cancer. Developments in Biological Standardization, Vol 38. Basel: S. Karger, 1978

Griffiths, J. D., McKinna, J. A., Rowbotham, H. D., Tsolakidis, P., and Salsbury, A. J. Carcinoma of the colon and rectum: Circulating malignant cells and five-year survival. Cancer *31,* 226–236, 1973

Griffiths, J. D., and Salsbury, A. J. Circulating Cancer Cells. Springfield, Ill., Charles C. Thomas, 1965

Griscelli, C., Revillard, J. P., Betuel, H., Herzog, C., and Touraine, J. L. Transfer factor in immuno-deficiencies. Biomedicine *18,* 220–227, 1973

Grob, P. J., and Herold, G. E. Immunological abnormalities and hydantoins. Br Med J *2,* 561–563, 1972

Gross, L. Intradermal immunization of C3H mice against sarcoma that originated in animal of same line. Cancer Res *3,* 326–333, 1943

Gross, L. Specificity of acquired tumor immunity. J Immunol *50,* 91–99, 1945

Gross, L. Immunological relationship of mammary carcinomas developing spontaneously in female mice of high-tumor line. J Imminol *55,* 297–307, 1947

Gross, L. Effect of thymectomy on development of leukemia in C3H mice inoculated with leukemic "passage" virus. Proc Soc Exp Biol Med *100,* 325–328, 1959

Gross, L. Oncogenic Viruses. New York: Pergamon Press, 1961

Gross, L., and Dreyfuss, Y. How is the mouse leukemia virus transmitted from host to host under natural life condition? p 9, In Carcinogenesis: A Broad Critique. 20th Annual Symposium, 1967

Gross, L., Roswit, B., Mada, E. R., Dreyfuss, Y., and Moore, L. A. Studies on radiation-induced leukemia in mice. Cancer Res *19,* 316–320, 1959

Grosser, N., and Thomson, D. M. P. Cell-mediated antitumor immunity in breast cancer patients evaluated by antigen-induced leukocyte adherence inhibition in test tubes. Cancer Res *35,* 2571–2579, 1975

Guérin, C. The history of BCG. In Rosenthal, S. (Ed), BCG Vaccination Against Tuberculosis, pp. 48–53. Boston: Little, Brown and Co., 1957.

Guillou, P. J., Brennan, T. G., and Giles, G. R. Phytohaemagglutinin-stimulated transformation of peripheral and lymph-node lymphocytes in patients with gastro-intestinal cancer. Br J Surg *60,* 745–749, 1973

Gunven, P., Klein, G., Henle, G., Henle, W., and Clifford, P. Antibodies to EBV associated membrane and viral capsid antigens in Burkitt lymphoma patients. Nature *228,* 1053–1056, 1970

Gurdon, J. B. Egg cytoplasm and gene control in development. Proc R Soc Lond B *198,* 211–247, 1977

Gurland, J., and Johnson, R. O. How reliable are tumor measurements? JAMA *194,* 973–978, 1965

Gurrioch, D. B., Good, R. A., and Gatti, R. A. Lymphocyte response to P.H.A. in patients with non-lymphoid tumours. Lancet *1,* 618, 1970

Guthrie, D., and Way, S. Immunotherapy of non-clinical vaginal cancer. Lancet *2,* 1242–1243, 1975

Gutterman, J. U. Cancer systemic active immunotherapy today—Prospects for tomorrow. Cancer Immunol Immunother *2,* 1–9, 1977

Gutterman, J. U., Cardenas, J. O., Blumenschein, G. R., Hortobagyi, G., Burgess, M. A., Livingston, R. B., Mavligit, G. M., Freireich, E. J., Gottlieb, J. A., and Hersh, E. M. Chemoimmunotherapy of advanced breast cancer: Prolongation of remission and survival with BCG. Br Med J *4,* 1222–1225, 1976a

Gutterman, J. U., Hersh, E. M., Mavligit, G. M., Burgess, M. A., Chemoimmunotherapy of disseminated malignant melanoma with BCG: Follow-up report, pp 103–111, In Terry, W. D., and Windhorst, D. (Eds): Immunotherapy of Cancer: Present Status of Trials in Man. New York: Raven Press, 1978a

Gutterman, J. U., Hersh, E. M., Rodriguez, V., McCredie, K. B., Mavligit, G., Reed, R., Burgess, M. A., Smith, T., Gehan, E., Bodey, G. P., and Freireich, E. J. Chemotherapy of adult acute leukaemia. Lancet *2,* 1405–1409, 1974a

Gutterman, J. U., Mavligit, G. M., Burgess, M. A., Cardenas, J. O., Blumenschein, G. R., Gottlieb, J. A., McBride, C. M., McCredie, K. B., Bodey, G. P., Rodriguez, V., Freireich, E. J., and Hersh, E. M. Immunotherapy of breast cancer, malignant melanoma and acute leukemia with BCG: Prolongation of disease free interval and survival. Cancer Immunol Immunother *1,* 99–107, 1976b

Gutterman, J. U., Mavligit, G., Gottlieb, J. A., Burgess, M. A., McBride, C. E., Einhorn, L., Freireich, E. J., and Hersh, E. M. Chemoimmunotherapy of disseminated malignant melanoma with dimethyl triazeno imidazole carboxamide and bacillus Calmette-Guérin. N Engl J Med *291,* 592–597, 1974b

Gutterman , J. U., Mavligit, G. M., McBride, C. M., Richman, S. P., Burgess, M. A., and Hersh, E. M. Postoperative immunotherapy for recurrent malignant melanoma: An updated report, pp 35–36, In Terry, W. D., and

Windhorst, D. (Eds): Immunotherapy of Cancer: Present Status of Trials in Man. New York: Raven Press, 1978b

Gutterman, J. U., Mavligit, G., McCredie, K. B., Bodey, G. P., Freireich, E. J., and Hersh, E. M. Antigen solubilized from human leukemia. Lymphocyte stimulation. Science *177*, 1114–1115, 1972

Gutterman, J. U., Mavligit, G., McCredie, K. B., Freireich, E. J., and Hersh, E. M. Auto-immunization with acute leukaemia cells: Demonstration of increased lymphocyte responsiveness. Int J Cancer *11*, 521–526, 1973

Gutterman, J. U., Rodriguez, V., McCredie, K. B., Hester, J. P., Bodey, G. P., Freireich, E. J., and Hersh, E. M. Chemoimmunotherapy of acute myeloblastic leukemia: Four-year follow-up with BCG, pp 375–381, In Terry, W. D., and Windhorst, D. (Eds): Immunotherapy of Cancer: Present Status of Trials in Man. New York: Raven Press, 1978c

Guyer, R. J., and Crowther, D. Active immunotherapy in treatment of acute leukaemia. Br Med J *4*, 406–407, 1969

Gynning, I., Langeland, P., Lindberg, S., and Waldeskog, B. Localization with Sr-85 of spinal metastases in mammary cancer and changes in uptake after hormone and roentgen therapy. Acta Radiol *55*, 119–128, 1961

H

Haagensen, C. D. The choice of treatment for operable carcinoma of the breast. Surgery *76*, 685–714, 1974

Habel, K. Resistance of polyoma virus immune animals to transplanted polyoma tumors. Proc Soc Exp Biol Med *106*, 722–725, 1961

Habel, K. Immunological determinants of polyoma virus oncogenesis. J Exp Med *115*, 181–193, 1962

Habel, K., and Eddy, B. E. Specificity of resistance to tumor challenge of polyoma and SV40 virus-immune hamsters. Proc Soc Exp Biol Med *113*, 1–4, 1963

Hackett, E., and Beech, M. Immunological treatment of a case of choriocarcinoma. Br Med J *2*, 1123–1126, 1961

Haddow, A. Oncology: Its scope and prospects. Proc R Soc Med *64*, 323–328, 1971

Haddow, A. Molecular repair, wound healing, and carcinogenesis: Tumor production a possible overhealing? Adv Cancer Res *16*, 181–234, 1972

Haddow, A. Addendum to "Molecular repair, wound healing, and carcinogenesis: Tumor production a possible overhealing?" Adv Cancer Res *20*, 343–366, 1974

Haddow, A., and Alexander, P. An immunological method of increasing the sensitivity of primary sarcomas to local irradiation with x-rays. Lancet *1*, 452–457, 1964

Haddow, A., Watkinson, J. M., and Paterson, E. Influence of synthetic oestrogens upon advanced malignant disease. Br Med J *2*, 393–398, 1944

Hadfield, G. The dormant cancer cell. Br Med J *2*, 607–610, 1954

Hageman, P. C., Links, J., and Bentvelzen, P. Biological properties of B particles from C3H and C3HF mouse milk. J Natl Cancer Inst *40*, 1319–1324, 1968

Hagmar, B. Effect of heparin, ε-aminocaproic acid and coumarin on tumour growth and spontaneous metastasis formation. Pathol Eur *3*, 622–630, 1968

Hagmar, B. Experimental tumour metastases and blood coagulation. Acta Path Microbiol Scand (Suppl) *211*, 1–38, 1970

Hagmar, B., and Boeryd, B. Effect of heparin, ε-amino-caproic acid and coumarin on tumour growth and spontaneous metastasis formation. Pathol Eur *3*, 509–520, 1968

Hakkinen, I. An immunochemical method for detecting carcinomatous secretion from human gastric juice. Scand J Gastroenterol *1*, 28–32, 1966

Hakkinen, I. P. Immunological relationship of the carcinoembryonic antigen and the fetal sulphoglycoprotein antigen. Immunochemistry *9*, 1115–1119, 1972

Hall, R. R., Schade, R. O. K., and Swinney, J. Effects of hyperthermia on bladder cancer. Br Med J *2*, 593–594, 1974

Hallahan, J. D. Spontaneous remission of metastatic renal cell carcinoma. J Urol *81*, 522–555, 1959

Halle-Pannenko, O., Bourut, C., and Kamel, M. Comparison of various BCG preparations in the EORTC-ICIG experimental screening for systemic immunity adjuvants applicable to cancer immunotherapy. Cancer Immunol Immunother *1*, 17–23, 1976

Haller, O., Hansson, M., Kiessling, R., and Wigzell, H. Non conventional natural killer cells may play a decisive role in providing resistance against syngeneic tumor cells in vivo. Nature *270*, 609–611, 1977a

Haller, O., Kiessling, R., Örn, A., Kärre, K., Nilsson, K., and Wigzell, H. Natural cytotoxicity to human leukemia mediated by mouse non-T cells. Int J Cancer *20*, 93–103, 1977b

Haller, O., Kiessling, R., Örn, A., and Wigzell, H. Generation of natural killer cells: An autonomous function of the bone marrow. J Exp Med *145*, 1411–1416, 1977c

Halpern, B. N., Biozzi, C., Stiffel, C., and Mouton, D. Corrélation entre l'activité phagocytaire du système réticuloendothélial et la production d'anticorps antibactérien. CR Soc Biol *152*, 758–761, 1958

Halpern, B. N., Biozzi, G., Stiffel, C., and Mouton, D. Effet de la stimulation du système retio uloendothélial par l'inoculation du bacille de Calmette-Guérin sur le développement de l'épithélioma atypique T-8 de Guérin chez le rat. CR Soc Biol *153*, 919–923, 1959

Halpern, B. N., Biozzi, G., Stiffel, C., and Mouton, D. Inhibition of tumour growth by administration of killed Corynebacterium parvum. Nature 212, 853–854, 1966

Halpern, B., Crepin, Y., and Rabourdin, A. An analysis of the increase in host resistance to isogenic tumor invasion in mice by treatment with Corynebacterium parvum, pp 191–201, In Halpern, B. (Ed): Corynebacterium Parvum: Applications in Experimental and Clinical Oncology. New York: Plenum Press, 1975

Halpern, B., and Fray, A. Déclenchement de l'anémie hémolytique autoimmune chez de jeunes souriceaux NZB par l'administration de C. parvum. Ann Inst Pasteur *117*, 778, 1969

Halpern, B., Fray, A., Crepin, Y., Platica, O., Lorinet, A. M., Rabourdin, A., Sparros, L., and Isac, R. Corynebacterium parvum, a potent immunostimulant in experimental infections and in malignancies, pp 217–236, In Wolstenholme, G. E. W., and Knight, J. (Eds): Ciba Fdn Symp—Immunopotentiation, New Series 18. Amsterdam: ASP, 1973a

Halpern, M. B., Fray, A., Crepin, Y., Platica, O., Sparros, L., Lorinet, A. M., and Rabourdin, A. Immunologie: Action inhibitrice du Corynebacterium parvum sur le développement des tumeurs malignes syngéniques et son mécanisme. CR Acad Sci (Paris) *276*, 1911–1915, 1973b

Halpern, B., and Israel, L. Etude de l'action d'une immunostimuline associée aux Corynebactéries anaérobies dans les néoplasies expérimentales et humaines. CR Acad Sci *273*, 2186–2190, 1971

Halpern, B. N., Prévot, A. R., Biozzi, G., Stiffel, C., Mouton, D., Morard, J.-C., Bouthillier, Y., and Decreusefond, C. Stimulation de l'activité phagocytaire du système réticuloendothélial provoquée par Corynebacterium parvum. J Reticuloendothel Soc *1*, 77–96, 1963

Halsted, W. S. The treatment of wounds with especial reference to the value of blood clot in the management of dead spaces. Johns Hopkins Hosp Rep 2, 255–314, 1891

Halsted, W. S. A clinical and histological study of certain adenocarcinomata of the breast: And a brief consideration of the supraclavicular operation and of the results of operation for cancer of the breast from 1889 to 1898 at the Johns Hopkins Hospital. Ann Surg 28, 557–576, 1898

Halterman, R. H., Leventhal, B. G., and Mann, D. L. An acute-leukemia antigen. Correlation with clinical status. N Engl J Med 287, 1272–1274, 1972

Hamaoka, T., and Katz, D. H. Mechanism of adjuvant activity of poly A:U on antibody responses to hapten-carrier conjugates. Cell Immunol 7, 246–260, 1973

Hamburg, V. P., Loizner, A. L., and Svet-Moldavsky, G. Artificial induction of transplantation viral antigens in the course of chemical carcinogenesis. Nature *212*, 1495, 1966

Hamilton, J. M. A review of recent advances in the study of the aetiology of canine mammary tumors. Vet Annu *15*, 276–283, 1975

Hamilton, M. S. Cell-mediated immunity to embryonic antigens of syngeneically and allogeneically mated mice. Transplantation *21*, 261–263, 1976

Hamilton, T., Langlands, A.O., and Prescott, R. J. The treatment of operable cancer of the breast: A clinical trial in the South-East region of Scotland. Br J Surg *61*, 758–761, 1974

Hamlin, I. M. E. Possible host resistance in carcinoma of the breast: A histological study. Br J Cancer *22*, 383–401, 1968

Hammond, C. B., Hertz, R., Ross, G. T., Lipsett, M. B., and Odell, W. D. Primary chemotherapy for nonmetastatic gestational trophoblastic neoplasms. Am J Obstet Gynecol *98*, 71–78, 1967

Hammond, W. G., Fisher, J. C., and Rolley, R. J. Tumor-specific transplantation immunity to spontaneous mouse tumors. Surgery *62*, 124–133, 1967

Han, T., and Takita, H. Immunologic impairment in bronchogenic carcinoma: A study of lymphocyte response to phytohemagglutinin. Cancer *30*, 616–620, 1972

Han, T., and Wang, J. 'Antigenic' disparity between leukemic lymphoblasts and normal lymphocytes in identical twins. Clin Exp Immunol *12*, 171–175, 1972

Hanau, A. Erfolgreiche experimentelle Übertragung von Karzinom. Fortschr Med *7*, 321–329, 1889

Handler, A. H., Davis, S., and Sommers, S. C. Heterotransplantation experiments with human cancers. Cancer Res *16*, 32–36, 1956

Handler, H. I., Daniel, B. G., and Platt, R. D.

The induction of ATP energized mitochondrial volume changes by carcinogenic N-hydroxy-N-acetylaminofluorine when combined with Showdomycin. A unitary hypothesis for carcinogenesis. J Antibot (Tokyo) *24*, 405–417, 1971

Handley, R. S. Further observations on the internal mammary lymph chain in carcinoma of the breast. Proc R Soc Med *45*, 565–566, 1952

Handley, R. S. The early spread of breast carcinoma and its bearing on operative treatment. Br J Surg *51*, 206–208, 1964

Handley, W. S. The pathology of melanotic growths in relation to their operative treatment. Lancet *1*, 927–933, 1907

Handley, W. S. Lecture on the natural cure of cancer. Br Med J *1*, 582–589, 1909

Handley, W. S. Cancer of the Breast. London: John Murray, 1922

Hanna, M. G., Peters, L. C., Gutterman, J. U., and Hersh, E. M. Evaluation of BCG administered by scarification for immunotherapy of metastatic hepatocarcinoma in the guinea pig. J Natl Cancer Inst *56*, 1013–1017, 1976

Hanna, M. G., Snodgrass, M. J., Zbar, B., and Rapp, H. J. Histopathology of tumour regression after intralesional injection of Mycobacterium bovis. IV. Development of immunity to tumor cells and BCG. J Natl Cancer Inst *51*, 1897–1909, 1973

Hanna, M. G., Tennant, R. W., Coggin, J. H., and Treber, J. A. Immunization with mouse fetal antigens: suppressive effect on growth of leukemia-virus-infected cells and on plasma cell tumors, pp 267–269, In Anderson, N. G., and Coggin, J. H. (Eds): Embryonic and Fetal Antigens in Cancer, Vol 1. Springfield, Va.: U.S. Dept Commerce, 1971

Hanna, M. G., Tennant, R. W., Yuhas, J. M., Clapp, N. K., Batzing, B. L., and Snodgrass, M. J. Autogenous immunity to endogenous RNA tumor virus antigens in mice with a low natural incidence of lymphoma. Cancer Res *32*, 2226–2234, 1972

Haran, N., and Berenblum, I. The induction of the initiating phase of skin carcinogenesis in the mouse by oral administration of urethane (ethyl carbamate). Br J Cancer *10*, 57–60, 1956

Hard, G. C., and Grasso, P. Nephroblastoma in the rat: Histology of a spontaneous tumor, identity with respect to renal mesenchymal neoplasms, and a review of previously recorded cases. J Natl Cancer Inst *57*, 323–329, 1976

Harder, F. H., and McKhann, C. F. Demonstration of cellular antigens on sarcoma cells by an indirect ^{125}I-labelled antibody technique. J Natl Cancer Inst *40*, 231–241, 1968

Harding, B., Pudifin, D. J., Gotch, F., and Mac-

Lennan, I. C. M. Cytotoxic lymphocytes from rats depleted of thymus-processed cells. Nature New Biol *232*, 80–81, 1971

Hardisty, R. N., Kay, H. E. M., et al. Report to Medical Research Council by the Working Party on Leukaemia in Childhood Treatment of acute lymphoblastic leukaemia: Effect of variation in length of treatment on duration of remission. Br Med J *2*, 495–497, 1977

Harnden, D. G. Chromosome abnormalities and predisposition towards cancer. Proc R Soc Med *69*, 41–43, 1976

Harnden, D. G., MacLean, N., and Langlands, A. O. Carcinoma of the breast and Klinefelter's syndrome. J Med Genet *8*, 460–461, 1971

Harris, H. Cell fusion and the analysis of malignancy. Proc R Soc Lond B *179*, 1–20, 1971

Harris, H., Miller, O. J., Klein, G., Worst, P., and Tachibana, T. Suppression of malignancy by cell fusion. Nature *223*, 363–368, 1969

Harris, N. S., Jagarlamoody, S. M., McKhann, C. F., and Najarian, J. S. The effect of antiplasma cell sera on the primary immune response. J Immunol *108*, 958–964, 1972

Hartley, J. W., and Rowe, W. P. Production of altered cell in tissue culture by defective Moloney sarcoma virus particles. Proc Natl Acad Sci USA *55*, 780–786, 1966

Hartman, J. T., and Crile, G. Heat treatment of osteogenic sarcoma. Clin Orthop *61*, 269–276, 1968

Hartmann, D., Lewis, M. G., Proctor, J. W., and Lyons, H. In-vitro interactions between antitumour antibodies and anti-antibodies in malignancy. Lancet *2*, 1481–1483, 1974

Hartveit, F. The complement content of the serum of normal as opposed to tumor bearing mice. Br J Cancer *18*, 714–720, 1964

Harvey, H. A., Schochat, S., Lipton, A., Miller, C., White, D., and Hepner, G. Immuno-chemotherapy with cyclophosphamide and Corynebacterium parvum—A clinical trial, pp 97–107, In Crispen, R. G. (Ed): Neoplasm Immunity: Mechanisms. Proc Chicago Symp, 1975

Haskell, E. M., Ossorio, C., Sarna, G. P., and Fahey, J. L. Chemoimmunotherapy of metastatic breast cancer with Corynebacterium parvum (CP): A double-blind randomized trial. Proc Am Soc Clin Oncol *17*, 265, 1976

Haskill, J. S., and Fett, J. W. Possible evidence for antibody-dependent macrophage-mediated cytotoxicity directed against murine adenocarcinoma cells in vivo. J Immunol *117*, 1992–1998, 1976

Haskill, J. S., Yamamura, Y., and Radov, L. A. Host responses within solid tumors: Non-thymus-derived specific cytotoxic cells within a murine mammary adenocarcinoma. Int J Cancer 16, 798–809, 1975

Hattan, D., and Cerilli, G. J. Spontaneous reticulum cell sarcomas developing in C3H/HeJ mice on prolonged immunosuppressive therapy. Transplantation 11, 580–581, 1971

Hattori, T., and Mori, A. Antitumor activity of anaerobic corynebacterium isolated from the bone marrow. Gann 64, 15–27, 1973

Hattori, T., Mori, A., and Hirata, K. Five-year survival rate of gastric cancer patients treated by gastrectomy, large dose of mitomycin-C, and/or allogeneic bone marrow transplantation. Gann 63, 517–522, 1972

Haughton, G. Moloney virus-induced leukemias of mice: Measurement in vitro of specific antigen. Science 147, 506–507, 1965

Hausman, M. S., Brosman, S., Snyderman, R., Mickey, M. R., and Faney, J. Defective monocyte function in patients with genitourinary carcinoma. J Natl Cancer Inst 55, 1047–1054, 1975

Haybittle, J. L. The cured group in series of patients treated for cancer. Anglo-German Med Rev 2, 422–436, 1964

Hays, E. F., and White, E. M. The development of leukemia in lethally irradiated mice protected with cells from mice of a high incidence leukemia strain. Blood 23, 557–563, 1964

Hayward, J. Conservative treatment in the treatment of early breast cancer. Br J Surgery 61, 770–771, 1974

Haywood, G. R., and McKhann, C. F. Relationship between tumor-specific and H-2 antigens on mouse sarcomas. Fed Proc 29, 371, 1970

Haywood, G. R., and McKhann, C. F. Antigenic specificities on murine sarcoma cells. Reciprocal relationship between normal transplantation antigens (H-2) and tumor specific immunogenicity. J Exp Med 133, 1171–1187, 1971

Healey, J. E. Vascular patterns in human metastatic liver tumors. Surg Gynecol Obstet 120, 1187–1193, 1955

Heidelberger, C. Chemical oncogenesis in culture. Adv Cancer Res 18, 317–366, 1973

Heinonen, O. P., Shapiro, S., Tuominen, L., and Turunen, M. I. Reserpine use in relation to breast cancer. Lancet 2, 675–677, 1974

Hellström, I. A colony inhibition (CI) technique for demonstration of tumor cell destruction by lymphoid cells in vitro. Int J Cancer 2, 65–68, 1967

Hellström, I., Evans, C. A., and Hellström, K. E. Cellular immunity and its serum-mediated inhibition in Shope-virus-induced rabbit papillomas. Int J Cancer 4, 601–607, 1969a

Hellström, I., and Hellström, K. E. Recent studies on the mechanisms of the allogeneic inhibition phenomenon. Ann NY Acad Sci 129, 724–734, 1966

Hellström, I., and Hellström, K. E. Studies on cellular immunity and its serum-mediated inhibition in Moloney-virus-induced mouse sarcomas. Int J Cancer 4, 587–600, 1969

Hellström, I., and Hellström, K. E. Colony inhibition studies on blocking and nonblocking serum effects on cellular immunity to Moloney sarcomas. Int J Cancer 5, 195–201, 1970

Hellström, I., and Hellström, K. E. Some aspects of the immune defence against cancer. Cancer 28, 1269–1271, 1971

Hellström, I., and Hellström, K. E. Cytotoxic effect of lymphocytes from pregnant mice on cultivated tumor cells. I. Specificity, nature of effector cells and blocking by serum. Int J Cancer 15, 1–16, 1975

Hellström, I., Hellström, K. E., Bill, A. H., Pierce, G. E., and Yang, J. P. S. Studies on cellular immunity to human neuroblastoma cells. Int J Cancer 6, 172–188, 1970

Hellström, I., Hellström, K. E., Evans, C. A., Heppner, G. H., Pierce, G. E., and Yang, J. P. S. Serum mediated protection of neoplastic cells from inhibition by lymphocytes immune to their tumor-specific antigens. Proc Natl Acad Sci USA 62, 362–368, 1969b

Hellström, I., Hellström, K. E., Kall, M. A., Nelson, K., and Pollack, S. Suppression of cell-mediated cytotoxicity by lymphocytes from tumor-bearing animals. Transplant Proc 8, 255–264, 1976

Hellström, I., Hellström, K. E., and Pierce, G. E. In vitro studies of immune reactions against autochthonous and syngeneic mouse tumors induced by methylcholanthrene and plastic discs. Int J Cancer 3, 467–482, 1968a

Hellström, I., Hellström, K. E., Pierce, G. E., and Bill, A. H. Demonstration of cell-bound and humoral immunity against neuroblastoma cells. Proc Nat Acad Sci USA 60, 1231–1238, 1968b

Hellström, I., Hellström, K. E., Pierce, G. E., and Fefer, A. Studies on immunity to autochthonous mouse tumors. Transplant Proc 1, 90–94, 1969c

Hellström, I., Hellström, K. E., Sjögren, H. O., and Warner, G. A. Demonstration of cell-mediated immunity to human neoplasms of various histological types. Int J Cancer 7, 1–16, 1971a

Hellström, I., Hellström, K. E., Sjögren, H. O., and Warner, G. A. Destruction of cultivated melanoma cells by lymphocytes from healthy black (North American Negro) donors. Int J Cancer 11, 116–122, 1973

Hellström, I., and Sjögren, H. O. Demonstration of common specific antigens in mouse and hamster polyoma tumors. Int J Cancer *1*, 481–489, 1966

Hellström, I., and Sjögren, H. O. In vitro demonstration of humoral and cell-bound immunity against common specific transplantation antigen(s) of adenovirus 12-induced mouse and hamster tumors. J Exp Med *125*, 1105–1118, 1967

Hellström, I., Sjögren, H. O., Warner, G. A., and Hellström, K. E. Blocking of cell mediated tumor immunity by sera from patients with growing neoplasms. Int J Cancer *7*, 226–237, 1971b

Hellström, K. E. Differential behaviour of transplanted mouse lymphoma lines in genetically compatible homozygous and F1 hybrid mice. Nature *199*, 614–615, 1963

Hellström, K. E. Growth inhibition of sarcoma and carcinoma cells of homozygous origin. Science *143*, 477–478, 1964

Hellström, K. E., and Hellström, I. Syngeneic preference and allogeneic inhibition, pp 79–91, In Palm, J. (Ed): Isoantigens and Cell Interactions. Philadelphia, Wistar Institute Press Monograph, 1965

Hellström, K. E., and Hellström, I. Some aspects of the immune defense against cancer. I. In vitro studies on animal tumors. Cancer *28*, 1266–1268, 1971

Hellström, K. E., and Hellström, I. Lymphocyte-mediated cytotoxicity and blocking serum activity to tumor antigens. Adv Immunol *18*, 209–277, 1974

Hellström, K. E., Hellström, I., and Bergheden, C. Studies on allogeneic inhibition. II. Inhibition of mouse tumor cell colony formation in vitro by contact with lymphoid cells containing foreign H-2 antigens. Int J Cancer *2*, 286–296, 1967

Hellström, K. E., Hellström, I., and Haughton, G. Demonstration of syngeneic preference in vitro. Nature *204*, 661–664, 1964

Helm, F., and Klein, E. Effects of allergic contact dermatitis on basal cell epithelium. Arch Dermatol *91*, 142–144, 1965

Helpap, B., and Maurer, W. Autoradiografische Untersuchung zur Frage der Vergleichbarkeit des einbaus von markierten Thymidin unter In vivo-bedin gungen und bei Inkubation von Gewebeproben. Virchows Arch (Cell Pathol) *4*, 102–118, 1969

Hems, G., and Stuart, A. BCG and leukaemia. Lancet *1*, 183, 1971

Henderson, B. E., Powell, D., Rosario, I., Keys, C., Hanisch, R., Young, M., Casagrande, J., Gerkins, V., and Pike, M. C. An epidemiologic study of breast cancer. J Natl Cancer Inst *53*, 609–614, 1974

Henderson, M. A., and Pettigrew, R. T. Induction of controlled hyperthermia in treatment of cancer. Lancet *1*, 1275–1277, 1971

Henle, G., and Henle, W. Immunofluorescence in cells derived from Burkitt's lymphoma. J Bacteriol *91*, 1248–1256, 1966

Henle, G., Henle, W., Diehl, W. Relation of Burkitt's tumor associated herpes-type virus to infectious mononucleosis. Proc Natl Acad Sci USA *59*, 94–101, 1968

Henney, C. S., and Bubbers, J. E. Studies on the mechanism of lymphocyte-mediated cytolysis. I. The role of divalent cations in cytolysis by T lymphocytes. J Immunol *110*, 63–72, 1973

Henon, P., Gerota, I., and Palacios, S. Functional abnormalities of neutrophils in cancer patients: Inefficient phagocytosis and reverse endocytosis. Biomedicine *27*, 261–266, 1977

Heppner, F. Grundlagenforschung und praktische Erfahrungen mit dem Clostridienstaam "M55," pp 623–626, In Spitzy, K. H., and Haschek, H. (Eds): Fifth Int Cong Chemotherapy. Vienna: Verlag der Wiener Medizinischen Akademie, 1967

Herberman, R. B., and Aoki, T. Immune and natural antibodies to syngeneic murine plasma cell tumors. J Exp Med *136*, 94–111, 1972

Herberman, R. B., Djeu, J. Y., Kay, H. D., Ortaldo, J. R., Riccardi, C., Bonnard, G. D., Holden, H. T., Fagnani, R., Santoni, A., and Puccetti, P. Natural killer cells: Characteristics and regulation of activity. Immunol Rev *44*, 43–70, 1979

Herberman, R. B., and Fahey, J. L. Cytotoxic antibody in Burkitt's tumor and normal human serum reactive with cultures of lymphoid cells. Proc Soc Exp Biol Med *127*, 938–940, 1968

Herberman, R. B., and Gaylord, C. E. (Eds): Conference and Workshop on Cellular Immune Reactions to Human Tumor-associated Antigens. Natl Cancer Inst Monogr No. 37, 1973

Herberman, R. B., and Holden, H. T. Natural cell-mediated immunity. Adv Cancer Res *27*, 305–377, 1978

Herberman, R. B., Hollinshead, A. C., Alford, T. C., McCoy, J. L., Halterman, R. H., and Leventhal, B. G. Delayed cutaneous hypersensitivity reactions to extracts of human tumors. Natl Cancer Inst Monogr *37*, 189–195, 1973a

Herberman, R. B., Nunn, M. E., and Holden, H. J. Low density of Thy 1 antigen on mouse effector cells mediating natural cytotoxicity against tumor cells. J Immunol *121*, 304–309, 1978

Herberman, R. B., Nunn, M. E., Holden, H. T.,

Staal, S. and Djeu, J. Y. Augmentation of natural cytotoxic reactivity of mouse lymphoid cells against syngeneic and allogeneic target cells. Int J Cancer 19, 555–564, 1977

Herberman, R. B., Nunn, M. E., and Lavrin, D. H. Natural cytotoxic reactivity of mouse lymphoid cells against syngeneic and allogeneic tumors. I. Distribution of reactivity and specificity. Int J Cancer 16, 216–229, 1975

Herberman, R. B., Nunn, M. E., Lavrin, D. H., and Asofsky, R. Effect of antibody to theta antigen on cell mediated immunity induced in syngeneic mice by murine sarcoma virus. J Natl Cancer Inst 51, 1509–1512, 1973b

Herberman, R. B., Rosenberg, E. D., and Halterman, R. H. Cellular immune reactions to human leukemia. Natl Cancer Inst Monogr 35, 259–266, 1972

Herberman, R. B., Ting, C. C., Kirchner, H., Holden, H., Glaser, M., Bonnard, G. D., and Lavrin, D. Effector mechanism in tumour immunity. Prog Immunol 2, 285–295, 1974

Herberman, R. B., Ting, C. C., and Lavrin, D. Immune reactions to virus-induced leukemia in animals immunized with fetal tissues, pp 259–266, In Anderson, N. G., and Coggin, J. H. (Eds): Embryonic and Fetal Antigens in Cancer, Vol 1. Springfield, Va: U.S. Dept Commerce, 1971

Herbst, A. L., Ulfelder, H., and Poskanzer, D. C. Adenocarcinoma of the vagina. Association of maternal stilbestrol therapy with tumor appearance in young women. N Engl J Med 284, 878–881, 1971

Héricourt, J., and Richet, C. De la sérothérapie dans le traitement du cancer. CR Acad Sci D (Paris) 121, 567–569, 1895

Herrera, M., Chu, T. M., and Holyoke, E. D. Carcinoembryonic antigen (CEA) as a prognostic and monitoring test in clinically complete resection of colorectal carcinoma. Ann Surg 183, 5–9, 1976

Herrera, M. A., Chu, T. M., Holyoke, E. D., and Mittleman, A. CEA monitoring of palliative treatment for colorectal carcinoma. Ann Surg 185, 23–30, 1977

Hersey, P. New look at antiserum therapy of leukaemia. Nature New Biol 244, 22–24, 1973

Hersey, P., Edwards, A., and Edwards, J. Characterization of mononuclear effector cells in human blood. Clin Exp Immunol 23, 104–113, 1976a

Hersey, P., Edwards, A., Edwards, J., Adams, E., Milton, G. W., and Nelson, D. S. Specificity of cell-mediated cytotoxicity against human melanoma lines: Evidence for "non-specific" killing by activated T-cells. Int J Cancer 16, 173–183, 1975

Hersey, P., Isbister, J., Edwards, A., Murray, E., Adams, E., Biggs, J., and Milton, G. W. Antibody-dependent, cell-mediated cytotoxicity against melanoma cells induced by plasmapheresis. Lancet 1, 825–828, 1976b

Hersh, E. M., Whitecar, J. P., McCredie, K. B., Bodey, G. P., and Freireich, E. J. Chemotherapy, immunocompetence, immunosuppression and prognosis in acute leukemia. N Engl J Med 285, 1211–1216, 1971

Hershorn, K., Schreibman, R. R., Bach, F. H., and Silzbach, L. E. In-vitro studies of lymphocytes from patients with sarcoidosis and lymphoproliferative diseases. Lancet 2, 842–843, 1964

Heslop, B. F., and Little, V. A. Hyperplasia of donor cells in rejecting weakly antigenic skin grafts. Proc R Soc B 193, 209–215, 1976

Heston, W. E. The genetic aspects of human cancer. Adv Cancer Res 23, 1–21, 1976

Hewitt, H. B., and Blake, E. Quantitative studies of translymphnodal passage of tumour cells naturally disseminated from a non-immunogenic murine squamous carcinoma. Br J Cancer 31, 25–35, 1975

Hewitt, H. B., and Blake, E. R. Failure of preoperative C. parvum vaccine to modify secondary disease following excision of two non-immunogenic murine sarcomas. Br J Cancer 38, 219–223, 1978

Hewitt, H. B., Blake, E. R., and Walder, A. S. A critique of the evidence for active host defence against cancer, based on personal studies of 27 murine tumours of spontaneous origin. Br J Cancer 33, 241–259, 1976

Hewlett, J. S., Balcerzak, S., Gutterman, J. U., Freireich, E. J., Gehan, E. A., and Kennedy, A. Remission maintenance in adult acute leukemia with and without BCG. A Southwest Oncology Study Group, pp 383–390, In Terry, W. D., and Windhorst, D. (Eds): Immunotherapy of Cancer: Present Status of Trials in Man. New York: Raven Press, 1978

Heyes, J., Catherall, E. J., and Harnden, M. R. Antitumor evaluation of a ribonuclease resistant double-stranded RNA-poly-quaternary ammonium complex (BRL 10793). Eur J Cancer 10, 431–435, 1974

Heyn, R. M., Joo, P., Karon, M., Nesbit, M., Shore, N., Breslow, N., Weiner, J., Reed, A., and Hammond, D. BCG in the treatment of acute lymphocytic leukemia. Blood 46, 431–442, 1975

Heyn, R. M., Joo, P., Karon, M., Nesbit, M., Shore, N., Breslow, N., Weiner, J., Reed, A., Sather, H., and Hammond, D. BCG in the treatment of acute lymphocytic leukemia, pp 503–510, In Terry, W. D., and Windhorst, D. (Eds):

Immunotherapy of Cancer: Present Status of Trials in Man. New York: Raven Press, 1978

Hibbs, J. B. Macrophage nonimmunologic recognition: Target cell factors related to contact inhibition. Science 180, 868–870, 1973

Hibbs, J. B. Heterocytolysis by macrophages activated by bacillus Calmette-Guérin: Lysosome exocytosis into tumor cells. Science 184, 468–471, 1974a

Hibbs, J. B. Discrimination between neoplastic and non-neoplastic cells in vitro by activated macrophages. J Natl Cancer Inst 53, 1487–1492, 1974b

Hibbs, J. B. Activated macrophages as cytotoxic effector cells. I. Inhibition of specific and non-specific tumor resistance by trypan blue. Transplantation 19, 77–81, 1975

Hibbs, J. B., Lambert, L. H., and Remington, J. S. Possible role of macrophage mediated nonspecific cytotoxicity in tumour resistance. Nature New Biol 235, 48–50, 1972a

Hibbs, J. B., Lambert, L. H., and Remington, J. S. In vitro non immunologic destruction of cells with abnormal growth characteristics by adjuvant activated macrophages. Proc Soc Exp Biol Med 139, 1049–1052, 1972b

Hibbs, J. B., Lambert, L. H., and Remington, J. S. Control of carcinogenesis: A possible role for the activated macrophage. Science 177, 998–1000, 1972c

Higgins, G. A. Use of chemotherapy as an adjuvant to surgery for bronchogenic carcinoma. Cancer 30, 1383–1387, 1972

Higgins, G. A., Dwight, R. W., Smith, J. V., and Keehn, R. J. Fluorouracil as an adjuvant to surgery in carcinoma of the colon. Arch Surg 102, 339–343, 1971

Higgins, G. A., Humphrey, E., Juler, G. L., Le-Veen, H. H., McCaughan, J., and Keehn, R. J. Adjuvant chemotherapy in the surgical treatment of large bowel cancer. Cancer 38, 1461–1467, 1976

Hiles, R. W. Should lymphadenectomy be discarded? Malignant melanoma. J R Coll Surg Edinb 18, 368–372, 1973

Hilf, R., Burnett, F. F., and Borman, A. The effect of sarcoma 180 and other stressing agents upon adrenal and plasma corticosterone in mice. Cancer Res 20, 1389–1393, 1960

Hilgard, P., and Thornes, R. D. Anticoagulants in the treatment of cancer. Eur J Cancer 12, 755–762, 1976

Hill, A. B. Medical ethics and controlled trials. Br Med J, 1, 1043–1049, 1963

Hill, G. J. Treatment of murine leukaemia with heterologous antiserum or cyclophosphamide. Nature 232, 196–197, 1971

Hill, G. J., Johnson, R. O., Metter, G., Wilson, W. L., Davis, H. L., Grage, T., Fletcher, W. S., Golomb, F. M., and Gruz, A. B. Multimodal surgical adjuvant therapy for a broad spectrum of tumors in humans. Surg Gynecol Obstet 142, 882–892, 1976

Hill, G. J., and Littlejohn, K. Comparison of heterologous antiserum and cyclophosphamide in therapy of mouse leukemia. Proc Am Assoc Cancer Res 11, 37, 1970

Hill, G. J., and Littlejohn, K. B16 melanoma in C57Bl/6J mice: Kinetics and effects of heterologous serum. J Surg Oncol 3, 1–7, 1971

Hill, L. E., Nunn, A. J., and Fox, W. Matching quality of agents employed in 'double-blind' controlled clinical trials. Lancet 1, 352–356, 1976

Hill, M., and Hillova, J. Genetic transformation of animal cells with viral DNA or RNA tumor viruses. Adv Cancer Res 23, 237–297, 1976

Hill, M. J., Crowther, J. S., Drasar, B. S., Hawksworth, G., Aries, V., and Williams, R. E. O. Bacteria and aetiology of cancer of the large bowel. Lancet 1, 95–100, 1971

Hilleman, M. R. Double-stranded RNA's (poly I:C) in the prevention of viral infections. Arch Intern Med 126, 109–124, 1970

Hilleman, M. R., Lampson, G. P., Tytell, A. A., Field, A. K., Nemes, M. M., Krakoff, I. H., and Young, C. W. Double-stranded RNA's in relation to interferon induction and adjuvant activity, pp 27–44, In Beers, R. F., and Braun, W. (Eds): Biological Effects of Polynucleotides. New York: Springer-Verlag, 1971

Hines, J. R., and Williams, J. S. Nitrogen mustard as adjunctive chemotherapy for breast carcinoma. Br J Surg 62, 497–500, 1975

Hirano, M., Sinkovics, J. G., Shullenberger, C. C., and Howe, C. D. Murine lymphoma: Augmented growth in mice with pertrussis vaccine-induced lymphocytosis. Science 158, 1061–1064, 1967

Hirayama, T., and Wynder, E. L. A study of the epidemiology of cancer of the breast. II. The influence of hysterectomy. Cancer 15, 28–38, 1962

Hirsch, H. M. Some aspects of the problem of immunity against transplanted and spontaneous tumors. Bact Rev 26, 336–353, 1962

Hirsch, H. M., Bittner, J. J., Cole, H., and Iversen, I. Can the inbred mouse be immunized against its own tumor? Cancer Res 18, 344–346, 1958

Hirsch, M. S., Ellis, D. A., Black, P. H., Monaco, A. P., and Wood, M. L. Leukemia virus activation during homograft rejection. Science 180, 500–502, 1973

Hirshaut, Y., Pinsky, C., Cunningham-Rundles,

W., Rao, B., Fried, J., and Oettgen, H. Phase I clinical trial of C. parvum. Proc Am Assoc Cancer Res *16*, 181, 1975

Hirshaut, Y., Pinsky, C., Marquardt, H., and Oettgen, H. F. Effects of levamisole on delayed hypersensitivity reactions in cancer patients. Proc Am Assoc Cancer Res *14*, 109, 1973

Hiu, I. J. Water-soluble and lipid free fraction from BCG with adjuvant and antitumor activity. Nature New Biol *238*, 241–242, 1972

Hoag, W. G. Spontaneous cancer in mice. Ann NY Acad Sci *108*, 805–831, 1963

Hochman, P., and Cudkowicz, G. Different sensitivities to hydrocortisone of natural killer cell activity and hybrid resistance to parental marrow grafts. J Immunol *119*, 2013–2015, 1977

Hodgkinson, A. Hyperparathyroidism and cancer. Br Med J *2*, 444, 1964

Hodson, M. E., and Turner-Warwick, M. Autoantibodies in patients with bronchial carcinoma. Thorax *30*, 367–370, 1975

Hoebeke, J., and Franchi, G. Influence of tetramisole and its optical isomers on the mononuclear phagocytic system: Effect on carbon clearance in mice. J Reticuloendothel Soc *14*, 317–323, 1973

Hoerni, B., Chauvergne, J., Hoerni-Simon, G., Durand, M., Brunet, R., and Lagarde, C. BCG in the immunotherapy of Hodgkin's disease and non-Hodgkin's lymphomas. Cancer Immunol Immunother *1*, 109–112, 1976

Hofer, K. G., Prensky, W., and Highes, W. L. Death and metastatic distribution of tumor cells in mice monitored with ^{125}I-ododeoxyuridine. J Natl Cancer Inst *43*, 763–773, 1969

Hoffken, K., Meredith, I. D., Robins, R. A., Baldwin, R. W., Davies, C. J., and Blamey, R. W. Circulating immune complexes in patients with breast cancer. Br Med J *2*, 218–220, 1977

Hoffken, K., Price, M. R., McLaughlin, P. J., Moore, V. E., and Baldwin, R. W. Circulating immune complexes in rats bearing chemically induced tumors. I. Sequential determination during the growth of tumors at various body sites. Int J Cancer *21*, 496–504, 1978

Hoffmann, G. W. A theory of regulation and self-nonself discrimination in an immune network. Eur J Immunol *5*, 638–647, 1975

Holden, H. T., Haskill, J. S., Kirchner, H., and Herberman, R. B. Two functionally distinct anti-tumor effector cells isolated from primary murine sarcoma virus-induced tumors. J Immunol *117*, 440–446, 1976

Holland, E. Case of transplacental metastasis of malignant melanoma from mother to fetus. J Obstet Gynaecol Br Empire *56*, 529–536, 1949

Holland, J. F., and Bekesi, J. G. Comparisons of chemotherapy with chemotherapy plus VCN-treated cells in acute myeloid leukemia, pp 347–352, In Terry, W. D., and Windhorst, D. (Eds.): Immunotherapy of Cancer: Present Status of Trials in Man. New York: Raven Press, 1978

Holland, J. F., St. Arneault, G., and Bekesi, G. Combined chemo- and immunotherapy of transplantable and spontaneous murine leukemia. Proc Am Assoc Cancer Res *13*, 83, 1972

Hollinshead, A., Glew, P., Bunnag, R., Gold, P., and Herberman, R. Skin-reactive soluble antigen from intestinal cancer-cell-membranes and relationship to carcinoembryonic antigens. Lancet *1*, 1191–1195, 1970

Hollinshead, A. C., Jaffurs, W. T., Alpert, L. K., Harris, J. E., and Herberman, R. B. Isolation and identification of soluble skin-reactive membrane antigens of malignant and normal human breast cells. Cancer Res *34*, 2961–2968, 1974

Hollmann, K. H. Human mammary tumor virus. Biomedicine *18*, 103–108, 1973

Holm, G., Perlmann, P., and Johansson, B. Impaired phytohemagglutinin-induced cytotoxicity in vitro of lymphocytes from patients with Hodgkin's disease or chronic lymphatic leukemia. Immunol Exchange Group No. 5, Sci Memo 273, 1966

Holmes, E. C., and Morton, D. L. Detection of antibodies against the mammary tumor virus with the antiglobulin consumption test. J Natl Cancer Inst *42*, 733–738, 1969

Holmes, E. C., Morton, D. L., Schidlovsky, B. S., and Trahan, E. Cross-reacting tumor-specific transplantation antigens in methylcholanthrene-induced guinea pig sarcomas. J Natl Cancer Inst *46*, 693–697, 1971

Holtermann, O. A., Klein, E., and Casale, G. P. Selective cytotoxicity of peritoneal leucocytes for neoplastic cells. Cell Immunol *9*, 339–352, 1973

Holtermann, O. A., Lisafield, B. A., and Klein, E. Selective cytotoxicity of peritoneal leucocytes. A preliminary report. J Med (Basel) *3*, 359–362, 1972

Holtermann, O. A., Lisafeld, B. A., Klein, E., and Klostergaard, J. Cytocidal and cytostatic effects of activated peritoneal leukocytes. Nature *257*, 228–229, 1975

Hoover, H. C., Ketcham, A. S., Millar, R. C., and Gralnick, H. R. Osteosarcoma; Improved survival with anticoagulation and amputation. Cancer *41*, 2475–2480, 1978

Hoover, R., and Fraumeni, J. F. Risk of cancer in renal-transplant recipients. Lancet *2*, 55–57, 1973

Hopper, D. G., and Pimm, M. V. Antitumour effects of macrophages in BCG contact therapy of rat tumours, pp 182–187, In James, K., McBride, B., and Stuart, A. (Eds): Proc EURES Symp—The Macrophage and Cancer. Edinburgh Univ Dept Surgery, 1977

Hopper, D. G., Pimm, M. V., and Baldwin, R. W. Methanol extraction residue of BCG in the treatment of transplanted rat tumours. Br J Cancer 31, 176–181, 1975a

Hopper, D. G., Pimm, M. V., and Baldwin, R. W. Levamisole treatment of local and metastatic growth of transplanted rat tumours. Br J Cancer 32, 345–351, 1975b

Hopper, D. G., Pimm, M. V., and Baldwin, R. W. Silica abrogation of mycobacterial adjuvant contact suppression of tumor growth in rats and mice. Cancer Immunol Immunother 1, 143–144, 1976

Hopper, D. G., Robins, R. A., and Baldwin, R. W. [Cited by Baldwin and Pimm (1978)] 1978

Horn, L., and Horn, H. L. An immunological approach to the therapy of cancer? Lancet 2, 466–469, 1971

Horsfall, F. L. Heritance of acquired characters. Science 136, 472–476, 1962

Hortobagyi, G. N., Gutterman, J. U., Blumenschein, G. R., and Buzdar, A. Chemoimmunotherapy of advanced breast cancer with BCG, pp 655–663, In Terry, W. D., and Windhorst, D. (Eds): Immunotherapy of Cancer: Present Status of Trials in Man. New York: Raven Press, 1978

Horwitz, K. B., and McGuire, W. L. Specific receptors in human breast cancer. Steroids 25, 497–505, 1975

Houchens, D. P., and Gaston, M. R. Therapy of experimental tumors with Corynebacterium parvum (CP) alone and in combination with Adriamycin (ADR). Proc Am Assoc Cancer Res 17, 53, 1976

Houck, J. C., Attallah, A. M., and Lilly, J. R. Immunosuppressive properties of the lymphocyte chalone. Nature 245, 148–149, 1973

Hough, D. W., Eady, R. P., Hamblin, T. J., Stevenson, F. K., and Stevenson, G. T. Antiidiotype sera raised against surface immunoglobulin of human neoplastic lymphocytes. J Exp Med 144, 960–969, 1976

Howard, J. G. Mechanisms concerned with endotoxin sensitivity during graft-versus-host reaction, pp 331–340, In: Chedid, L. (Ed): Structure et Effet Biologiques de Produits Bactériens Provenant de Bacilles Gram Négatifs. Paris: CNRS, 1969

Howard, J. G., Biozzi, G., Halpern, B. N., Stiffel,

C., and Mouton, D. The effect of mycobacterium tuberculosis (B.C.G.) infection on the resistance of mice to bacterial endotoxin and salmonella enteritidis infection. Br J Exp Pathol 40, 281–290, 1959

Howard, J. G., Biozzi, G., Stiffel, C., Mouton, D., and Liacopoulos, P. An analysis of the inhibitory effect of Corynebacterium parvum on graft-versus-host disease. Transplant 5, 1510–1524, 1967

Howard, J. G., Christie, G. H., and Scott, M. T. Biological effects of the adjuvant Corynebacterium parvum. IV. Adjuvant and inhibitory activities. Cell Immunol 7, 290–301, 1973a

Howard, J. G., Scott, M. T., and Christie, G. H. Cellular mechanisms underlying the adjuvant activity of Corynebacterium parvum: Interactions of activated macrophages with T and B lymphocytes, pp 101–120, In Wolstenholme, G. E. W., and Knight, J. (Eds): Ciba Fdn Symp—Immunopotentiation, New Series 18. Amsterdam: ASP, 1973b

Howard, J. M. Studies of autotransplantation of incurable cancer. Surg Gynecol Obstet 117, 567–572, 1963

Howe, G. M. The geography of lung-bronchus cancer and stomach cancer in the United Kingdom. Scott Geogr Mag 87, 202–220, 1971

Howell, K. M. The failure of antibody formation in leukemia. Arch Intern Med 26, 706–714, 1920

Huber, B., Devinsky, O., Gershon, R. K., and Cantor, H. Cell-mediated immunity; Delayed-type hypersensitivity and cytotoxic responses are mediated by different T-cell subclasses. J Exp Med 143, 1534–1539, 1976

Hudson, C. N., Levin, L., McHardy, J. E., Poulton, T. A., Curling, O. M., Crowther, M., English, P. E., and Leighton, M. Active specific immunotherapy for ovarian cancer. Lancet 2, 877–879, 1976

Huebner, R. J., and Todaro, G. J. Oncogenes of RNA tumor viruses as determinants of cancer. Proc Natl Acad Sci USA 64, 1087–1094, 1969

Hueper, W. C. Carcinogens in the human environment. Arch Pathol 71, 237–267, 355–380, 1961

Hueper, W. C., and Russell, M. Some immunologic aspects of leukemia. Arch Intern Med 49, 113–122, 1932

Huggins, C. Endocrine-induced regression of cancers. Science 156, 1050–1054, 1967

Huggins, C., and Bergenstal, D. M. Inhibition of human mammary and prostatic cancers by adrenalectomy. Cancer Res 12, 134–141, 1952

Huggins, C., Briziarelli, G., and Sutton, H. Rapid

induction of mammary carcinoma in the rat and the influence of hormones on the tumors. J Exp Med *109,* 25–42, 1958

Huggins, C., and Clark, P. J. Quantitative studies of prostatic secretion: Effect of castration and of estrogen injection on the normal and on the hyperplastic prostate glands of dogs. J Exp Med *72,* 747–762, 1940

Huggins, C., and Fukunishi, R. Cancer in the rat after single exposure to irradiation or hydrocarbons. Age and strain factors. Hormone dependence of the mammary cancers. Radiat Res *20,* 493–503, 1963

Huggins, C., Grand, L. C., and Brillantes, F. P. Mammary cancer induced by a single feeding of polynuclear hydrocarbons, and its suppression. Nature *189,* 204–207, 1961

Huggins, C., and Hodges, C. V. Studies on prostatic cancer: Effect of castration, of estrogen, and of androgen on serum phosphatases in metastatic carcinoma of prostate. Cancer Res *1,* 293–297, 1941

Huggins, C., Moon, R. C., and Morii, S. Extinction of experimental mammary cancer I. Estradiol-17β and progesterone. Proc Natl Acad Sci USA *48,* 379–386, 1962

Huggins, C., Stevens, R. E., and Hodges, C. V. Studies on prostatic cancer: Effects of castration on advanced carcinoma of prostate gland. Arch Surg *43,* 209–223, 1941

Hughes, L. E. Treatment of malignant disease with protamine sulphate. Lancet *1,* 408–409, 1964

Hughes, L. E. Tuberculin sensitivity in malignant disease. Aust NZ J Surg *35,* 159, 1965

Hughes, L. E., Kearney, R., and Tully, M. A study in clinical cancer immunotherapy. Cancer *26,* 269–278, 1970

Hughes, L. E., and Lytton, B. Antigenic properties of human tumours: Delayed cutaneous hypersensitivity reactions. Br Med J *1,* 209–212, 1964

Hughes, L. E., and Mackay, W. D. Suppression of the tuberculin response in malignant disease. Br Med J *2,* 1346–1348, 1965

Hughes, P. E. Chemical carcinogen and oncogenic virus: A possible interaction mechanism. Nature *205,* 871–872, 1965

Humble, J. G., Jayne, W. H. W., and Pulvertaft, R. J. V. Biological interaction between lymphocytes and other cells. Br J Haematol *2,* 283–294, 1956

Humphrey, G., Nitschke, R., Oleinick, S., Wells, J., Cox, C., and Lankford, J. Clinical toxicity immuno-hematological effect of Corynebacterium parvum immunostimulation in children. Proc Am Assoc Cancer Res *17,* 198, 1976

Humphrey, L. J. The role of cell receptors in tumor biology. Surg Gynecol Obstet *143,* 289–296, 1976

Humphrey, L. J., Boehm, B., Jewell, W. R., and Boehm, O. R. Immunologic response of cancer patients modified by immunization with tumor vaccine. Ann Surg *176,* 554–558, 1972

Humphrey, L. J., Jewell, W. R., Murray, D. R., and Griffin, W. O. Immunotherapy for the patient with cancer. Ann Surg *173,* 47–54, 1971a

Humphrey, L. J., Lincoln, P. M., and Griffin, W. O. Immunologic response in patients with disseminated cancer. Ann Surg *168,* 374–381, 1968

Humphrey, L. J., Murray, D. R., and Boehm, O. R. Effect of tumor vaccines in immunizing patients with cancer. Surg Gynecol Obstet *132,* 437–442, 1971b

Hung, W., Blizzard, R. M., Migeon, C. J., Camacho, A. M., and Nyhan, W. L. Precocious puberty in a boy with hepatoma and circulating gonadotropin. J Pediatr *63,* 895–903, 1963

Hunter-Craig, I., Newton, K. A., Westbury, G., and Lacey, B. W. Use of vaccine virus in the treatment of metastatic malignant melanoma. Br Med J *2,* 512–515, 1970

Hustu, H. O., Pinkel, D., and Pratt, C. B. Treatment of clinically localized Ewing's sarcoma with radiotherapy and combination chemotherapy. Cancer *30,* 1522–1527, 1972

Hutchin, P., Amos, D. B., and Prioleau, W. H. Interactions of humoral antibodies and immune lymphocytes. Transplantation *5,* 68–75, 1967

Huvos, A. G., Hutter, R. V. P., and Berg, J. W. Significance of axillary macrometastases and micrometastases in mammary cancer. Ann Surg *173,* 44–46, 1971

Hyman, R., Ralph, P., and Sarkar, S. Cell-specific antigens and immunoglobulin synthesis of murine myeloma cells and their variants. J Natl Cancer Inst *48,* 173–184, 1972

I

IARC. Monographs on the Evaluation of Carcinogenic Risk of Chemicals to Man, Vols 1–9, (1972–)1975

Iio, M., Wagner, H. N., Scheffel, U., and Jabbour, B. Studies of the reticulo-endothelial system (RES). I. Measurement of the phagocytic capacity of the RES in man and dog. J Clin Invest 42, 417–426, 1963

Ikonopisov, R. L., Lewis, M. G., Hunter-Craig, I. D., Bodenham, D. C., Phillips, T. M., Colling, C. I., Proctor, J., Hamilton Fairley, G., and Alexander, P. Autoimmunization with irradiated tumour cells in human malignant melanoma. Br Med J 2, 752–754, 1970

Ilfeld, D., Carnaud, C., Cohen, I. R., and Trainin, N. In vitro cytotoxicity and in vivo tumor enhancement induced by mouse spleen cells autosensitised in vitro. Int J Cancer 12, 213–222, 1973

Im, H. M., and Simmons, R. L. Modification of graft-versus-host disease by neuraminidase treatment of donor cells. Decreased tolerogenicity of neuraminidase-treated cells. Transplantation 12, 472–478, 1971

Invernizzi, G., and Parmiani, G. Tumor associated transplantation antigens of chemically induced sarcomata cross reacting with allogeneic histocompatibility antigens. Nature 254, 713–714, 1975

Ioachim, H. L. The stromal reaction of tumors: An expression of immune surveillance. J Natl Cancer Inst 57, 465–475, 1976

Ioachim, H. L., Dorsett, B. H., and Paluch, E. The immune response at the tumor site in lung carcinoma. Cancer 38, 2296–2309, 1976

Iorio, A., Campanile, F., Neri, M., Spreafico, F., Goldin, A., and Bonmassar, E. Inhibition of lymphoma growth in the spleen and liver of lethally irradiated mice. J Immunol 120, 1679–1685, 1978

Irino, S., Ota, Z., Sezaki, T., Suzaki, M., and Hiraki, K. Cell-free transmission of 20-methylcholanthrene-induced RF mouse leukemia and electron microscopic demonstration of virus particles in its leukemia tissue. Gann 54, 225–237, 1963

Irvin, G. L., and Eustace, J. C. The enhancement and rejection of tumor allografts by immune lymph node cells. Transplantation 10, 555–557, 1970

Irvin, G. L., and Eustace, J. C. A study of tumor allograft-sensitized lymph nodes in mice. I. Biologic activities of transferred cell and antibody titers of donor and recipient mice. J Immunol 106, 956–961, 1971

Irvin, G. L., Eustace, J. C., and Fahey, J. L. Enhancement activity of mouse immunoglobulin classes. J Immunol 99, 1085–1091, 1967

Isa, A. M., and Sanders, B. R. Enhancement of tumor growth in allogeneic mice following impairment of macrophage function. Transplantation 20, 296–302, 1975

Isaacs, A., and Lindenmann, J. Virus interference.

I. The interferon. Proc R Soc Lond B 147, 258–267, 1957

Isaacs, A., Lindenmann, J., and Valentine, R. C. Virus interference. II. Some properties of interferon. Proc R Soc Lond B 147, 268–273, 1957

Ishizuka, M., Braun, W., and Matsumoto, T. Cyclic AMP and immune responses. I. Influence of polyA:U and cAMP on antibody formation in vitro. J Immunol, 107, 1027–1035, 1971

Ishmael, D. R., Bottomley, R. H., Hoge, A. F., and Zieren, J. D. Preliminary results in the treatment of surgically resected melanoma with adjuvant immunotherapy using BCG or Corynebacterium parvum. Proc Am Assoc Cancer Res 17, 105, 1976

Israel, L. Report on 414 cases of human tumors treated with Corynebacterium parvum, pp 389–401, In Halpern, B. (Ed): Corynebacterium Parvum: Applications in Experimental and Clinical Oncology. New York: Plenum Press, 1975

Israel, L., Bouvrain, A., Cros-Decam, J., and Mugica, J. Contribution a l'étude des phénomènes d'immunité cellulaire chez les cancéraux pulmonaires avant traitement palliatif ou chirurgical. Poumon Coeur 24, 339–350, 1968

Israel, L., and Edelstein, R. Nonspecific immunostimulation with Corynebacterium parvum in human cancer, p 485, In Symp Houston, Texas, March 1973—Immunological Aspects of Neoplasia. Baltimore: Williams & Wilkins, 1975

Israel, L., Edelstein, R., Depierre, A., and Dimitrov, N. Daily intravenous infusions of Corynebacterium parvum in twenty patients with disseminated cancer: A preliminary report of clinical and biologic findings. J Natl Cancer Inst 55, 29–33, 1975

Israel, L., Edelstein, R., Mannoni, P., and Radot, E. Plasmapheresis and immunological control of cancer. Lancet 2, 642–643, 1976

Israel, L., and Halpern, B. N. Le Corynébactérium parvum dans les cancers avancés. Nouv Pr Med 1, 19–23, 1972

Israel, L., Mannoni, P., Gineste, J., Kriegel, A., Delobel, J., and Sors, C. L'immunothérapie des cancers avancés. Modalités pratiques et résultats à court terme. Sem Hop Paris 42, 1822–1824, 1966

Israel, L., Mannoni, P., Mawas, C., Gineste, J., Gross, B., and Sors, C. 70 perfusions de lymphocytes homolgues dans 25 cas de cancers avancés. Pathol Biol (Paris) 15, 603–606, 1967a

Israel, L., Mawas, C., Bouvrain, A., Mannoni, P., and Sors, C. Etude de l'hypersensibilité retardée à la tuberculine chez 130 cancéraux adultes: Effets du BCG. Pathol Biol (Paris) 15, 597–601, 1967b

Israels, L. G., and Linford, J. H. Some observations on the reactions of chlorambucil, azo-mustard (CB1414), and cyclophosphamide. Canad. Cancer Conf. 5, 399–415, 1963

Itoh, T., and Southam, C. M. Isoantibodies to human cancer cells in healthy recipients of cancer homotransplants. J Immunol 91, 469–483, 1963

Iversen, O. H. Kinetics of cellular proliferation and cell loss in human carcinomas. A discussion of methods available for in vivo studies. Eur J Cancer 3, 389–394, 1967

Iversen, O. H., Iversen, U., Ziegler, J. L., and Bluming. A. Z. Cell kinetics in Burkitt lymphoma. Eur J Cancer 10, 155–163, 1974

Ivins, J. C., and Pritchard, D. J. Management of ostogenic sarcoma at the Mayo Clinic. Recent Results Cancer Res 54, 221–230, 1976

Ivins, J. C., Ritts, R. E., Pritchard, D. J., Gilchrist, G. S., Miller, G. C., and Taylor, W. F. Transfer factor versus combination chemotherapy: A preliminary report of a randomized postsurgical adjuvant treatment study in osteogenic sarcoma. Ann NY Acad Sci 277, 558–574, 1976

Iwasaki, T. Histological and experimental observations on the destruction of tumor cells in blood vessels. J Pathol Bacteriol 20, 85–105, 1915

Izawa, T., Sakurai, M., Atsuta, Y., and Yoshizuma, T. Antigenicity of leukemia and antiserum therapy. Ann Paediatr Jpn 12, 346–360, 1966

J

Jacob, F., and Monod, J. Genetic regulatory mechanisms in the synthesis of proteins. J Mol Biol 3, 318–356, 1961

Jacobs, D. M., and Kripke, M. L. Accelerated development of transplanted mammary tumors in mice pretreated with the methanol extraction residue of BCG and prevention of acceleration by concomitant specific immunization. J Natl Cancer Inst 52, 219–224, 1974

Jacobs, J. B., Edelstein, L. M., Snyder, L. M., and Fortier, N. Ultrastructural evidence for destruction in the halo nevus. Cancer Res 35, 352–357, 1975

Jaffe, N., Frei, E., Traggis, D., and Bishop, Y. Adjuvant methotrexate and citrovorum-factor treatment of osteogenic sarcoma. N Engl J Med 291, 994–997, 1974

Jagarlamoody, S. M., Aust, J. C., Tew, R. H., and McKhann, C. F. In vitro detection of cytotoxic cellular immunity against tumor-specific antigens by a radioisotope technique. Proc Natl Acad Sci USA 68, 1346–1350, 1971

Jakoubková, J., Koldovsky, P., Bek, V., Májský, A., Schneid, V., and Vopatova, M. To the problem of immunotherapy of choriocarcinoma. Neoplasma 12, 531–542, 1965

James, K. The influence of tumour cell products on macrophage function in vitro and in vivo, pp 225–246, In James, K., McBride, B., and Stuart, A. (Eds): Proc EURES Symp—The Macrophage and Cancer. Edinburgh Univ Dept Surgery, 1977

James, K., Clunie, G. J. A., Woodruff, M. F. A., McBride, W. H., Stimson, W. H., Drew, R., and Catty, D. The effect of Corynebacterium parvum therapy on immunoglobulin class and IgG subclass levels in cancer patients. Br J Cancer 32, 310–322, 1975

James, K., Ghaffar, A., and Milne, I. The effect of transplanted methylcholanthrene induced fibrosarcomata and Corynebacterium parvum on the immune response of CBA and A/HeJ mice to thymus dependent and indepndent antigens. Br J Cancer 29, 11–20, 1974

James, K., Merriman, J., Woodruff, M. F. A., McCormick, J. N., McBride, W. H., Innes, J., and Horne, N. W. Further studies on the serological effects of C. parvum immunotherapy in cancer patients. Dev Biol Stand 38, 501–506, 1978

James, K., Willmott, N., Milne, I., and McBride, W. H. Antitumor antibodies and immunoglobulin class and subclass levels in C. parvum-treated mice. J Natl Cancer Inst 56, 1035–1040, 1976

James, K., Woodruff, M. F. A., McBride, W. H., and Willmott, N. Serological changes associated with C. parvum treatment in nude mice. Br J Cancer 35, 684–686, 1977

Jamieson, C. W. Enhancement of antigenicity of syngeneic murine melanoma by neuraminidase, p 233, Workshop 1 Abstracts, Int Cancer Congr, Florence, 1974

Jandiski, J., Cantor, H., Tadakuma, T., Peavy, D. L., and Pierce, C. W. Separation of helper T cells from suppressor T cells expressing different Ly components. I. Polyclonal activation: Suppressor and helper activities are inherent properties of distinct T-cell subclasses. J Exp Med 143, 1382–1390, 1976

Jaroslow, B. N. Nucleic acids and induction of

antibody synthesis in inhibited systems, pp 404–413, In Plescia, O. J., and Braun, W. (Eds.): Nucleic Acids in Immunology. New York: Springer, Verlag, 1968

Jarrett, O., Laird, H. M., and Hay, D. Growth of feline leukaemia virus in human cells. Nature 224, 1208–1209, 1969

Jarrett, W., Jarrett, O., Mackey, L., Laird, H., Hardy, W., and Essex, M. Horizontal transmission of leukemia in the cat. J Natl Cancer Inst 51, 833–841, 1973

Jeejeebhoy, H. F. Stimulation of tumor growth by the immune response. Int J Cancer 13, 665–678, 1974

Jehn, U. W., Nathanson, L., Schwartz, R. S., and Skinner, M. In vitro lymphocyte stimulation by a soluble antigen from malignant melanoma. N Engl J Med 283, 329–333, 1970

Jenkins, G. D. Regression of pulmonary metastases from carcinoma of the kidney after nephrectomy. J Urol 82, 37–40, 1959

Jennette, J. C., and Feldman, J. D. Sequential quantitation of circulating immune complexes in syngeneic and allogeneic rats bearing Moloney sarcomas. J Immunol 118, 2269–2274, 1977

Jensen, C. O. Experimentelle Untersuchungen uber Krebs bei Mäusen. Centralbl Bakt 34, 28–34, 122–143, 1903

Jensen, E. V., Block, G. E., Smith, S., Kyser, K., and DeSombre, E. R. Estrogen receptors and hormone dependency. Estrogen receptors and breast cancer response to adrenalectomy. Natl Cancer Inst Monogr 34, 55–70, 1971

Jensen, E. V., DeSombre, E. R., and Jungblut, P. W. Estrogen receptors in hormone responsive tissues and tumors, pp 15–30, In Wissler, R. W., Dao, T. L., and Wood, S. (Eds): Endogenous Factors Affecting Host-Tumour Balance. Chicago Univ Press, 1967

Jensen, E. V., Numata, M., Smith, S., Suzuki, T., Brecher, P. A., and DeSombre, E. R. Estrogen-receptor interaction in target tissues. Dev Biol Suppl 3, 151–171, 1969

Jerne, N. K. What precedes clonal selection? pp 1–10, In Porter, R., and Knight, J. (Eds): Ontogeny of Acquired Immunity. CIBA Fdn Symp New Series. Amsterdam: Associated Scientific Publishers, 1972

Jerne, N. K. Towards a network theory of the immune system. Ann Immunol (Inst Pasteur) 125C, 373–389, 1974

Jick, H. Reserpine and breast cancer. Lancet 2, 669–671, 1974

Johnson, A. G., Schmidtke, J., Merritt, K., and Han, I. Enhancement of antibody formation by nucleic acids and their derivatives, pp 379–385, In Plescia, O. J., and Braun, W. (Eds): Nucleic Acids in Immunology. New York: Springer-Verlag, 1968

Johnson, H. G., and Johnson, A. G. Enhancement of antibody synthesis in mice by macrophages stimulated in vitro with antigen and polyadenylic, polyuridylic acids. Bacteriol Proc, p. 75, 1968

Johnson, H. G., and Johnson, A. G. Regulation of the immune system by synthetic polynucleotides. II. Action on peritoneal exudate cells. J Exp Med 133, 649–664, 1971

Johnson, J. L., and Cummins, C. S. Cell wall composition and deoxyribonucleic acid similarities among the anaerobic coryneforms, classical propionibacteria and strains of Arachnia propionica. J Bacteriol 109, 1047–1066, 1972

Johnson, P. R., and Hersey, P. Anti-leukaemia activity as a bystander effect of graft-versus-host reactions. Br J Cancer 33, 370–378, 1976

Johnson, R. M., and Lindskog, G. E. 100 cases of tumor metastatic to lung and mediastinum. Treatment and results. JAMA 202, 94–98, 1967

Johnson, S. The effect of thymectomy and of the dose of 3-methylcholanthrene on the induction and antigenic properties of sarcomas in C57B1 mice. Br J Cancer 22, 93–104, 1968a

Johnson, S. Effect of thymectomy on the induction of skin tumours by dibenzanthracene, and of breast tumors by dimethylbenzanthracene, in mice of the IF strain. Br J Cancer 22, 755–761, 1968b

Jolles, P., Migliore Samour, D., Korontzis, M., Folch, F., Maral, R., and Werner, G. H. Study on soluble substances extracted from Corynebacterium parvum, pp 40–47, In Halpern, B. (Ed): Corynebacterium Parvum and Its Application in Experimental and Clinical Oncology. New York: Plenum Press, 1975

Jondal, M., and Gunven, P. Antibody-dependent cellular cytotoxicity (ADCC) against Epstein-Barr virus-determined antigens. III. Reactivity in sera from patients with Burkitt's lymphoma in relation to tumour development. Clin Exp Immunol 29, 11–15, 1977

Jondal, M., Holm, G., and Wigzell, H. Surface markers on human T and B lymphocytes. I. A large population of lymphocytes forming nonimmune rosettes with sheep red blood cells. J Exp Med 136, 207–215, 1972

Jondal, M., Svedmyr, E., Klein, E., and Singh, S. Killer T cells in a Burkitt's lymphoma biopsy. Nature 255, 405–407, 1975

Jondal, M., Wigzell, H., and Aiuti, F. Human lymphocyte populations: Classification according to surface markers and/or functional characteristics. Transplant Rev 16, 163–195, 1973

Jones, B. M., and Turnbull, A. R. In vitro cellular immunity in mammary carcinoma. Br J Cancer 29, 337–339, 1974

Jones, J. E., Shane, S. R., Gilbert, E., and Flunk, E. B. Cushing's syndrome induced by the ectopic production of ACTH by a bronchial carcinoid. J Clin Endocrinol Metab 29, 1–5, 1969

Jones, P. D. E., and Castro, J. E. Immunological mechanism in metastatic spread and the antimetastatic effects of C. parvum. Br J Cancer 35, 519–527, 1977

Jones, S. E., Salmon, S. E., Moon, T. E., and Butler, J. Chemoimmunotherapy of non-Hodgkin's lymphoma with BCG: A preliminary report, pp 519–527, In Terry, W. D., and Windhorst, D. (Eds): Immunotherapy of Cancer: Present Status of Trials in Man. New York: Raven Press, 1978

Jonsson, N., and Sjögren, H. O. Further studies on specific transplantation antigens in Rous sarcoma of mice. J Exp Med 122, 403–421, 1965

Jonsson, N., and Sjögren, H. O. Specific transplantation immunity in relation to Rous sarcoma virus tumorigenesis in mice. J Exp Med 123, 487–503, 1966

Joshi, V. V., and Frei, J. V. Effects of dose and schedule of methylnitrosourea on incidence of malignant lymphoma in adult female mice. J Natl Cancer Inst 46, 751–762, 1970

Jurin, M. Persistance of a resistance to the tumour following injection of lymphoid cells from specifically sensitized allogeneic donors. Period Biol 74, 53–56, 1972

K

Kahn, M. F., Ryckewaert, A., Cannat, A., Solnica, J., and de Seze, S. Systemic lupus erythematosus and ovarian dysgerminoma: Remission of the systemic lupus erythematosus after extirpation of the tumour. Clin Exp Immunol 1, 355–359, 1966

Kaliss, N. The transplanted tumor as a research tool in cancer immunology. Cancer Res 21, 1203–1208, 1961

Kaliss, N., and Suter, R. B. Altered survival times of murine skin allografts from cancer-bearing donors. Transplantation 6, 844–848, 1968

Kall, M. A., and Hellstrom, I. Specific stimulatory and cytotoxic effects of lymphocytes sensitised in vitro to either alloantigens or tumor antigens. J Immunol 114, 1083–1088, 1975

Kallman, R. F., Silini, G., and van Putten, L. M. Factors influencing the quantitative estimation of the in vivo survival of cells from solid tumors. J Natl Cancer Inst 39, 539–549, 1967

Kamo, I., and Friedman, H. Immunosuppression and the role of suppressive factors in cancer. Adv Cancer Res 25, 271–321, 1977

Kampschmidt, R. F., and Clabaugh, W. A. Effect of Jensen sarcoma upon the reticuloendothelial system of rats of different ages. Proc Soc Exp Biol Med 115, 681–684, 1964

Kaplan, A. M., and Morahan, P. S. Macrophage mediated tumor cell cytotoxicity. Ann NY Acad Sci 276, 134–145, 1975

Kaplan, A. M., Morahan, P. S., and Baird, L. G. Macrophage regulation of tumor-cell growth and nitogen induced blastogenesis. Fogarty International Center Proceedings. Washington, D.C.: U.S. Govt Printing Office, 1976

Kaplan, E. L., and Meier, P. Nonparametric estimation from incomplete observations. J Am Stat Assoc 53, 457–481, 1958

Kaplan, H. S. Observations on radiation-induced lymphoid tumors of mice. Cancer Res 7, 141–147, 1947

Kaplan, H. S. Influence of thymectomy, splenectomy and gonadectomy on incidence of radiation-induced lymphoid tumors in strain C57 black mice. J Natl Cancer Inst 11, 83–90, 1950

Kaplan, H. S. On the natural history of the murine leukemias: Presidential address. Cancer Res 27, 1325–1340, 1967

Kaplan, H. S., and Brown, M. B. Further observations on inhibition of lymphoid tumor development by shielding and partial body irradiation of mice. J Natl Cancer Inst 12, 427–436, 1951

Kaplan, H. S., and Brown, M. B. Effect of peripheral shielding on lymphoid tissue response to irradiation in C57 black mice. Science 116, 195–196, 1952a

Kaplan, H. S., and Brown, M. B. Protection against radiation-induced lymphoma development by shielding and partial-body irradiation of mice. Cancer Res 12, 441–444, 1952b

Kaplan, H. S., and Brown, M. B. Development of lymphoid tumors in nonirradiated thymic grafts in thymectomized irradiated rats. Science 119, 439–446, 1954

Kaplan, H. S., Brown, M. B., and Paull, J. Influence of bone marrow injections on involution and neoplasia of mouse thymus after systemic irradiation. J Natl Cancer Inst 14, 303–316, 1953

Kaplan, H. S., Carnes, W. H., Brown, M. B., and Hirsh, B. B. Indirect induction of lymphomas in irradiated mice. I. Tumor incidence and morphology in mice bearing nonirradiated thymic grafts. Cancer Res *16*, 422–425, 1956

Kaplan, H. S., and Smithers, D. W. Autoimmunity in man and homologous disease in mice in relation to the malignant lymphomas. Lancet *2*, 1–4, 1959

Kappas, A., Jones, H. E. H., and Roitt, I. M. Effect of steroid sex hormones on immunological phenomena. Nature *198*, 902, 1963

Karlson, A. G., and Mann, F. C. The transmissible venereal tumor of dogs: Observations on forty generations of experimental transfers. Ann NY Acad Sci *54*, 1197–1213, 1952

Kaschka-Dierich, C., Adams, A., Lindahl, T., Bornkamm, G. W., Bjursell, G., Glein, G., Giovanelli, B. C., and Singh, S. Intracellular forms of Epstein-Barr virus DNA in human tumour cells in vivo. Nature *260*, 302–306, 1976

Katsuki, H., Shimada, K., Koyama, A., Okita, M., Yamaguchi, Y., and Okamoto, T. Long-term intermittent adjuvant chemotherapy for primary, resected lung cancer. J Thorac Cardiovasc Surg *70*, 590–605, 1975

Katz, D. H., and Benacerraf, B. The regulatory influence of activated T cells on B cell responses to antigen. Adv Immunol *15*, 1–94, 1972

Katz, D. H., and Benacerraf, B. The function and interrelationship of T cell receptors, Ir genes and other histocompatibility gene products. Transplant Rev *22*, 175–195, 1975

Katz, D. H., Ellman, L., Paul, W. E., Green, I., and Benacerraf, B. Resistance of guinea pigs to leukemia following transfer of immunocompetent allogeneic lymphoid cells. Cancer Res *32*, 133–140, 1972

Katz, D. H., Order, S. E., Graves, M., and Benacerraf, B. Purification of Hodgkin's disease tumor-associated antigens. Proc Natl Acad Sci USA *70*, 396–400, 1973

Katz, D. H., and Skidmore, B. J. Self recognition as the predominate mechanism for communication in the immune system. Prog Immunol *3*, 322–329, 1977

Katz, D. H., and Unanue, E. R. Critical role of determinant presentation in the induction of specific responses in immunocompetent lymphocytes. J Exp Med *137*, 967–990, 1973

Katz, J., Currie, G. A., and Oliver, R. T. D. Inhibition of leukaemia blast cell motility as a test for specific antibody in acute adult myelogenous leukaemia. Br J Haematol *36*, 59–66, 1977

Kay, H. E. M. Acute lymphoblastic leukemia: 5-year follow-up of the Concord Trial, pp 493–

496, In Terry, W. D., and Windhorst, D. (Eds): Immunotherapy of Cancer: Present Status of Trials in Man. New York: Raven Press, 1978

Kearney, R., Basten, A., and Nelson, D. S. Cellular basis for the immune response to methylcholanthrene-induced tumors in mice. Heterogeneity of effector cells. Int J Cancer *15*, 438–450, 1975

Kedar, E., Raanan, Z., and Schwartzbach, M. In vitro induction of cell-mediated immunity to murine leukemia cells. VI. Adoptive immunotherapy in combination with chemotherapy of leukemia in mice, using lymphocytes sensitized in vitro to leukemia cells. Cancer Immunol Immunother *4*, 161–169, 1978a

Kedar, E., Schwartzbach, M., Hefetz, S., and Raanan, Z. In vitro induction of cell-mediated immunity to murine leukemia cells. V. Adoptive immunotherapy of leukemia in mice with lymphocytes sensitized in vitro to leukemia cells. Cancer Immunol Immunother *4*, 151–159, 1978b

Kedar, E., Unger, E., and Schwartzbach, M. In vitro induction of cell-mediated immunity to murine leukemia cells. I. Optimization of tissue culture conditions for the generation of cytotoxic lymphocytes. J Immunol Methods *13*, 1–19, 1976

Keeler, C. E. Albinism, xeroderma pigmentosum, and skin cancer. Natl Cancer Inst Monogr *10*, 349–356, 1963

Keller, A. R., Kaplan, H. S., Lukes, R. J., and Rappaport, H. Correlation of histopathology with other prognostic indicators in Hodgkin's disease. Cancer *22*, 487–499, 1968

Keller, R. Cytostatic elimination of syngeneic rat tumor cells in vitro by nonspecifically activated macrophages. J Exp Med *138*, 625–644, 1973

Keller, R. Mechanisms by which activated normal macrophages destroy syngeneic rat tumour cells in vitro. Cytokinetics, non-involvement of T lymphocytes, and effect of metabolic inhibitors. Immunology *27*, 285–298, 1974

Keller, R. Promotion of tumor growth in vivo by antimacrophage agents. J Natl Cancer Inst *57*, 1355–1361, 1976

Keller, R. Mononuclear phagocytes and antitumour resistance: A discussion, pp 31–48, In James, K., McBride,B., and Stuartl A. (Eds): Proc EURES Sympos—The Macrophage and Cancer. Edinburgh Univ Dept Surgery, 1977

Kellock. T. H., Chambers, H., and Russ, S. An attempt to produce immunity to malignant disease in man. Lancet *1*, 217–219, 1922

Kelly, J. F., Snell, M. E., and Berenbaum, M. C.

Photodynamic destruction of human bladder carcinoma. Br J Cancer 31, 237–244, 1975

Kelly, M. T. Activation of guinea pig macrophages by cell walls of Mycobacterium bovis, strain BCG. Cell Immunol 26, 254–263, 1976

Kelly, P. A., Bradley, C., Shiu, R. P. C., Meites, J., and Friesen, H. G. Prolactin binding to rat mammary tumor tissue. Proc Soc Exp Biol Med 146, 816–819, 1974

Kelly, W. D., Good, R. A., and Varco, R. L. Anergy and skin homograft survival in Hodgkin's disease. Surg Gynecol Obstet 107, 565–570, 1958

Kenis, Y. Chemotherapy of residual disease in solid tumours. Rev Eur Etudes Clin Biol 16, 103–107, 1971

Kennaway, E. L., and Hieger, I. Carcinogenic substances and their fluorescence spectra. Br Med J 1, 1044–1046, 1930

Kennaway, E., and Lindsey, A. J. Some possible exogenous factors in the causation of lung cancer. Br Med Bull 14, 124–131, 1958

Kennedy, C. T. C., Cater, D. B., and Hartveit, F. Protection of C3H mice against BP8 tumour by RNA extracted from lymphnodes and spleens of specifically sensitised mice. Preliminary communication. Acta Pathol Microbiol Scand 77, 196–200, 1969

Kerbel, R. S. Mechanisms of tumor-induced immunological deficiencies and their possible significance in relation to the use of immunopotentiators in tumor-bearing hosts. Biomedicine 20, 253–261, 1974

Kerbel, R. S., and Davies, A. J. S. The possible biological significance of F_C receptors on mammalian lymphocytes and tumor cells. Cell 3, 105–112, 1974

Kerbel, R. S., Pross, H. F., and Elliott, E. V. Origin and partial characterization of F_C receptor-bearing cells found within experimental carcinomas and sarcomas. Int J Cancer 15, 918–932, 1975

Kerman, R. H., and Stefani, S. S. Effect of BCG immunotherapy on the active-T and total T-RFC in patients with lung cancer. Cancer Immunol Immunother 4, 41–47, 1978

Kern, D. H., Drogemuller, C. R., Chow, N., Holleman, D. D., and Pilch, Y. H. Specificity of antitumor immune reactions mediated by xenogeneic immune RNA. J Natl Cancer Inst 58, 117–121, 1977

Kern, D., Drogemuller, C. R., and Pilch, Y. H. Immune cytolysis of rat tumor cells mediated by syngeneic "immune" RNA. J Natl Cancer Inst 52, 299–302, 1974

Kern, D. M., Fritze, D., Drogemuller, C. R., and Pilch, Y. H. Mediation of cytotoxic immune responses against human tumor-associated antigens by xenogeneic immune RNA. J Natl Cancer Inst 57, 97–103, 1976a

Kern, D. H., Fritze, D., Schick, P. M., Chow, N., and Pilch, Y. H. Mediation of cytotoxic immune responses against human tumor-associated antigens by allogeneic immune RNA. J Natl Cancer Inst 57, 105–109, 1976b

Kern, D. H., and Pilch, Y. H. Immune cytolysis of murine tumor cells mediated by xenogeneic "immune" RNA. Int J Cancer 13, 679–688, 1974

Kerr, J. F. R., and Searle, J. A suggested explanation for the paradoxically slow growth rate of basal-cell carcinomas that contain numerous mitotic figures. J Pathol 107, 41–44, 1972

Kerr, J. F. R., Wyllie, A. H., and Currie, A. R. Apoptosis: A basic biological phenomenon with wide-ranging implications in tissue kinetics. Br J Cancer 26, 239–257, 1972

Kersey, J. H., Spector, B. D., and Good, R. A. Primary immunodeficiency disease and cancer: The immunodeficiency cancer registry. Int J Cancer 12, 333–347, 1973a

Kersey, J. H., Spector, B. D., and Good, R. A. Immunodeficiency and cancer. Adv Cancer Res 18, 211–230, 1973b

Kessel, J. Spontaneous disappearance of bilateral pulmonary metastases from carcinoma of the kidney. JAMA 169, 1737–1739, 1959

Ketcham, A. S., and Chretien, P. B. Therapeutic implications of cellular immune defects in operable cancer patients revealed by dinitrochlorobenzene skin contact sensitivity. Pan Med 17, 174–178, 1975

Kiang, D. T., Bauer, G. E., and Kennedy, B. J. Immunoassayable insulin in carcinoma of the cervix associated with hypoglycemia. Cancer 31, 801–805, 1973

Kidd, J. G., and Toolan, H. W. Effect of "sensitized" lymphocytes on transplanted cancer cells. Fed Proc 9, 385, 1950

Kieler, J., Radzikowski, C., Moore, J., and Ulrich, K. Tumorigenicity and isoimmunizing properties of C3H mouse cells undergoing spontaneous malignant conversion in vitro. J Natl Cancer Inst 48, 393–405, 1972

Kiessling, R., Bataillon, G., Lamon, E. W., and Klein, E. The lymphocyte response to primary Moloney sarcoma virus tumors: Definition of a nonspecific component of the in vitro cellular hyporeactivity of tumor-bearing hosts. Int J Cancer 14, 642–648, 1974

Kiessling, R., Haller, O., Fenyo, E. M., Steinitz, M., and Klein, G. Mouse natural killer (NK)

cell activity against human cell lines is not influenced by superinfection of the target cells with xenotropic murine C-type virus. Int J Cancer *21*, 460–465, 1978

Kiessling, R., Hochman, P. S., Haller, O., Shearer, G. M., Wigzell, H., and Cudkowicz, G. Evidence for a similar or common mechanism for natural killer cell activity and resistance to haemopoietic grafts. Eur J Immunol *7*, 655–663, 1977

Kiessling, R., Klein, E., Pross, H., and Wigzell, H. "Natural" killer cells in the mouse. II. Cytotoxic cells with specificity for mouse Moloney leukemia cells. Characteristics of the killer cell. Eur J Immunol *5*, 117–121, 1975a

Kiessling, R., Klein, E., and Wigzell, H. "Natural" killer cells in the mouse. I. Cytotoxic cells with specificity for mouse Moloney leukemia cells. Specificity and distribution according to genotype. Eur J Immunol *5*, 112–117, 1975b

Kiessling, R., Petranyi, G., Klein, G., and Wigzell, H. Genetic variation of in vitro cytolytic activity and in vivo rejection potential of non-immunized semi-syngeneic mice against a mouse lymphoma line. Int J Cancer *15*, 933–940, 1975c

Kiessling, R., and Wigzell, H. An analysis of the murine NK cell as to structure, function and biological relevance. Immunol Rev *44*, 165–208, 1979

Kiger, N., et al. [*Cited by Mathé, Olsson et al.* (1980)] 1978

Kikuchi, K., Kikuchi, Y., Phillips, M. E., and Southam, C. M. Tumor-specific cell mediated immune resistance to autochthonous tumors. Cancer Res *32*, 516–521, 1972

Kilburn, D. G., Smith, J. B., and Gorczynski, R. M. Nonspecific suppression of T lymphocyte responses in mice carrying progressively growing tumours. Eur J Immunol *4*, 784–788, 1974

Killion, J. J. Immunotherapy with tumor cell subpopulations. I. Active, specific immunotherapy of L1210 leukemia. Cancer Immunol Immunother *4*, 115–119, 1978

Killion, J. J., and Kollmorgen, G. M. Isolation of immunogenic tumor cells by cell-affinity chromatography. Nature *259*, 674–676, 1976

Kim, C.-A. H., and Reif, A. E. Immunization schedules for potent rabbit antisera to leukemia L1210. Cancer Res *31*, 7–11, 1971

King, T. J., and DiBerardino, M. A. Transplantation of nuclei from the frog renal adenocarcinoma. I. Development of tumor nuclear-transplant embryos. Ann NY Acad Sci *126*, 115–126, 1965

Kingston, A., Harnden, D. G., Woodruff, M. F.A.,

Nolan, B., and Robson, J. S. Studies on the lymphocytes of patients with renal homografts. Transplantation *12*, 305–309, 1971

Kinlen, L. J. The epidemiology of leukaemias and lymphomas: A review. Proc R Soc Med *70*, 553–556, 1977

Kinlen, L. J., Sheil, A. G. R., Peto, J., and Doll, R. Collaborative United Kingdom-Australian study of cancer in patients treated with immunosuppressive drugs. Br Med J *2*, 1461–1466, 1979

Kirchner, H., Glaser, M., and Herberman, R. B. Suppression of cell-mediated tumour immunity by Corynebacterium parvum. Nature *257*, 396–398, 1975

Kirchner, H., Glaser, M., Holden, H. T., and Herberman, R. B. Mixed lymphocyte/tumor-cell interaction in a murine sarcoma virus (Moloney)-induced tumor system. Comparison between lymphoproliferation and lymphocyte cytotoxicity. Int J Cancer *17*, 362–369, 1976

Kirchner, H., Holden, H. T., and Herberman, R. B. Splenic suppressor macrophages induced in mice by injection of Corynebacterium parvum. J Immunol *115*, 1212–1216, 1975

Kirsch, R., and Schmidt, D. Erste Experimentelle und Klinische Erfahrungen mit der Ganz-korper-Extrem-Hyperthermi. Aktuelle Probleme aus dem Gebeit der Cancerologie, p 53. Heidelberg: Springer-Verlag, 1966

Kleenman, M. S., and Turner, M. D. Radioimmunoassay of carcinoembryonic antigen in serum of normal subjects and patients with colonic carcinoma. Gut *13*, 390–394, 1972

Klein, E. Tumors of the skin. X. Immunotherapy of cutaneous and mucosal neoplasms. NY State Med *68*, 900–911, 1968a

Klein, E. Local cytostatic chemotherapy and immunotherapy. Geriatrics *23*, 154–175, 1968b

Klein, E. Hypersensitivity reactions at tumor site. Cancer Res *29*, 2351–2362, 1969

Klein, E. The cell surface in immune response. Eur J Cancer *6*, 15–22, 1970

Klein, E., Eskeland, T., Inoue, M., Strom, R., and Johansson, B. Surface immunoglobulin-moieties on lymphoid cells. Exp Cell Res *62*, 133–148, 1970

Klein, E., and Klein, G. Antigenic properties of lymphomas induced by the Moloney agent. J Natl Cancer Inst *32*, 547–568, 1964

Klein, E., Klein, G., Nadkarni, J. S., Nadkarni, J. J., Wigzell, H., and Clifford, P. Surface IgM specificity on cells derived from a Burkitt's lymphoma. Lancet *2*, 1068–1070, 1967

Klein, E., Klein, G., Nadkarni, J. S., Nadkarni, J. J., Wigzell, H., and Clifford, P. Surface IgM-Kappa specificity on a Burkitt lymphoma cell in vivo and in derived culture lines. Cancer Res 28, 1300–1310, 1968

Klein, E., and Möller, E. Relationship between host range and isoantigenic properties in different sublines of the same sarcoma. J Natl Cancer Inst 31, 347–364, 1963

Klein, E., and Sjögren, H. O. Humoral and cellular factors in homograft and isograft immunity against sarcoma cells. Cancer Res 20, 452–461, 1960

Klein, G. The usefulness and limitations of tumor transplantation in cancer research: A review. Cancer Res 19, 343–358, 1959

Klein, G. Tumor antigens. Annu Rev Microbiol 20, 223–252, 1966a

Klein, G. Recent trends in tumor immunology. Isr J Med Sci 2, 135–142, 1966b

Klein, G. Tumor-specific transplantation antigens: G. H. A. Clowes Memorial Lecture. Cancer Res 28, 625–635, 1968

Klein, G. Immunological aspects of Burkitt's lymphoma. Adv Immunol 14, 187–250, 1971

Klein, G. pp 56–57, In Smith, R. T., and Landy, M. (Eds): Immunobiology of the Tumor-Host Relationship. New York: Academic Press, 1975a

Klein, G. Immunological surveillance against neoplasia. Harvey Lect 69, 71–102, 1975b

Klein, G., Clifford, P., Klein, E., Smith, R. T., Minowada, J., Kourilsky, F. M., and Burchenal, J. H. Membrane immunofluorescence reactions of Burkitt lymphoma cells from biopsy specimens and tissue cultures. J Natl Cancer Inst 39, 1027–1044, 1967

Klein, G., Clifford, P., Klein, E., and Stjernsward, J. Search for tumor specific immune reactions in Burkitt lymphoma patients by the membrane immunofluorescence reaction. Proc Natl Acad Sci USA 55, 1628–1635, 1966a

Klein, G., Friberg, S., Wiener, F., and Harris, H. Hybrid cells derived from fusion of TA3-Ha ascites carcinoma with normal fibroblasts. I. Malignancy, karyotype and formation of isoantigenic variants. J Natl Cancer Inst 50, 1259–1268, 1973

Klein, G. Giovanella, B. C., Lindahl, T., Fialkow, P. J., Singh, S., and Stehlin, J. S. Direct evidence for the presence of Epstein-Barr virus DNA and nuclear antigen in malignant epithelial cells from patients with poorly differentiated carcinoma of the nasopharynx. Proc Natl Acad Sci USA 71, 4737–4741, 1974

Klein, G., and Klein, E. Antigenic properties of other experimental tumors. Cold Spring Harbor Symp Quant Biol 27, 463–470, 1962

Klein, G., and Klein, E. Are methylcholanthrene-induced sarcoma-associated, rejection-inducing (TSTA) antigens, modified forms of H-2 or linked determinants? Int J Cancer 15, 879–887, 1975

Klein, G., and Klein, E. Immune surveillance against virus-induced tumors and nonrejectability of spontaneous tumors: Contrasting consequences of host versus tumor evolution. Proc Natl Acad Sci USA 74, 2121–2125, 1977

Klein, G., Klein, E., and Haughton, G. Variation of antigenic characteristics between different mouse lymphomas induced by the Moloney virus. J Natl Cancer Inst 36, 607–621, 1966b

Klein, G., and Oettgen, H. F. Immunologic factors involved in the growth of primary tumors in human or animal hosts. Cancer Res 29, 1741–1746, 1969

Klein, G., Pearson, G., Henle, G., Diehl, V., and Niederman, J. C. Relation between Epstein-Barr viral and cell membrane immunofluorescence in Burkitt tumor cells. II. Comparison of cells and sera from patients with Burkitt's lymphoma and infectious mononucleosis. J Exp Med 128, 1021–1030, 1968a

Klein, G., Pearson, G., Nadkarni, J. S., Nadkarni, J. J., Klein, E. Henle, G., Henle, W., and Clifford, P. Relation between Epstein-Barr viral and cell membrane immunofluorescence of Burkitt tumor cells. I. Dependence of cell membrane immunofluorescence on presence of EB virus. J Exp Med 128, 1011–1020, 1968b

Klein, G., and Revesz, L. Quantitative studies on the multiplication of neoplastic cells in vivo. I. Growth curves of the Ehrlich and MCIM ascites tumors. J Natl Cancer Inst 14, 229–277, 1953

Klein, G., Sjögren, H. O., and Klein, E. Demonstration of host resistance against isotransplantation of lymphomas induced by the Gross agent. Cancer Res 22, 955–961, 1962

Klein, G., Sjögren, H. O., and Klein, E. Demonstration of host resistance against sarcomas induced by implantation of cellophane films in isologous (syngeneic) recipients. Cancer Res 23, 84–92, 1963

Klein, G., Sjögren, H. O., Klein, E., and Hellström, K. E. Demonstration of resistance against methylcholanthrene-induced sarcomas in the primary autochthonous host. Cancer Res 20, 1561–1572, 1960

Klein, H. O. Synchronisation of tumor cell proliferation and the timing of cytostatic drugs. Rev Eur Etudes Clin Biol 17, 835–838, 1972

Klein, J. Genetic control of virus susceptibility, pp 389–410, In Biology of the Mouse Histocompatibility-2 Complex. New York: Springer-Verlag, 1976

Klemperer, M. R., Ganick, D., Shigeoka, A., Lee,

H., and Segel, G. Attempted treatment of a child with metastatic neuroblastoma employing syngeneic marrow transplantation. Transplantation *21*, 161–164, 1976

Knill-Jones, R. P., Buckle, R. M., and Parson, V. Hypercalacemia and increased parathyroid hormone activity in a primary hepatoma. N Engl J Med *282*, 704–708, 1970

Knudson, A. G. Mutation and human cancer. Adv Cancer Res *17*, 317–352, 1973

Knudson, A. G. Genetic and environmental interactions in the origin of human cancer, pp 391–399, In Mulvihill, J. J., Miller, R. W., and Fraumeni, J. F. (Eds): Genetics of Human Cancer. New York: Raven Press, 1976

Knudson, A. G., Strong, L. C., and Anderson, D. E. Heredity and cancer in man. Prog Med Genet *9*, 113–158, 1973

Kobayashi, H., Kodama, T., and Gotohda, E. Xenogenization of Tumor Cells. Hokkaido Univ School Medicine, 1977

Kobayashi, H., Sendo, F., Kaji, H., Shirai, T., Saito, H., Takeichi, N., Hosokawa, M., and Kodama, T. Inhibition of transplanted rat tumors by immunization with identical tumor cells infected with Friend virus. J Natl Cancer Inst *44*, 11–19, 1970

Koch, M. A., and Sabin, A. B. Specificity of virus-induced resistance to transplantation of polyoma and SV40 tumors in adult hamsters. Proc Soc Exp Biol Med *113*, 4–12, 1963

Kohler, G. and Milstein, C. Derivation of specific anti-body-producing tissue culture and tumour cell lines by cell fusion. Eur J Immunol, *6*, 511–519, 1976

Kohn, J., Orr, A. H., McElwain, T. J., Bentall, M., and Peckham, M. J. Serum-alpha₁-fetoprotein in patients with testicular tumours. Lancet *2*, 433–436, 1976

Koldovsky, P. Combined surgical removal and specific immunotherapy of experimental tumours. Folia Biol (Praha) *8*, 90–94, 1962

Koldovsky, P. Immunity against tumour tissue. Neoplasma *12*, 113–118, 1965

Koldovsky, P. An attempt at in vitro sensitization of immunologically competent cells against tumour specific antigen. Folia Biol (Praha) *12*, 238–240, 1966a

Koldovsky, P. Dangers and limitations of the immunological treatment of cancer. Lancet *1*, 654–655, 1966b

Koldovsky, P., and Bubenik, J. Occurrence of tumours in mice after inoculation of Rous sarcoma and antigenic changes in these tumours. Folia Biol (Praha) *10*, 81–89, 1964

Koldovsky, P., and Bubenik, J. Resistance to RSV-induced tumours in mice. Folia Biol (Praha) *11*, 198–202, 1965

Koldovsky, P., and Lengerova, A. A combination of specific anti-tumor therapy and x-ray irradiation. Folia Biol (Praha) *6*, 441–444, 1960

Koldovsky, P., and Svoboda, J. On the question of the role of heterologous tolerance in possibility to immunize against tumour antigen. Folia Biol (Praha) *8*, 101–104, 1962

Koldovsky, P., and Svoboda, J. Cross-reaction between benzpyrene-induced tumours in rats and mice. Folia Biol (Praha) *9*, 233–236, 1963

Koldovsky, P., and Svoboda, J. Induction of tumours by Rous sarcoma virus in adult mice. Folia Biol (Praha) *11*, 203–207, 1965

Koldovsky, P., Svoboda, J., and Bubenik, J. Further studies on the immunobiology of tumour RVA2 induced by RSV in C57BL strain mice. Folia Biol (Praha) *12*, 1–10, 1966

Koller, P. C., and Doak, S. M. Serial transfer of donor marrow in radiation mouse chimaeras. Int J Rad Biol *2*, 1–7, 1960

Kölsch, E., Stumpf, R., and Weber, G. Low zone tolerance and suppressor T cells. Transplant Rev *26*, 56–86, 1975

Komuro, K., Itakura, K., Boyse, E. A., and John. M. Ly-5: A new T-lymphocyte antigen system. Immunogenetics *1*, 452–456, 1975

Koprowski, H., Love, R., and Koprowska, I. Enhancement of susceptibility to viruses in neoplastic tissues. Tex Rep Biol Med *15*, 559, 1957

Korenman, S. G., and Dukes, B. A. Specific estrogen binding by the cytoplasm of human breast carcinoma. J Clin Endocrinol Metab *30*, 639–645, 1970

Kouznetzova, B., Bizzini, B., Chermann, J. C., DeGrand, F., Prévot, A. R., and Raynaud, M. Immunostimulating activity of whole cells, cell-walls and fractions of anaerobic corynebacteria. Recent Results Cancer Res *47*, 275–293, 1974

Krahenbuhl, J. L., and Lambert, L. H. Cytokinetic studies of the effect of activated macrophages on tumor target cells. J Natl Cancer Inst *54*, 1433–1439, 1975

Krahenbuhl, J. L., Lambert, L. H., and Remington, J. S. Effects of Corynebacterium parvum treatment and Toxoplasma gondii infection on macrophage-mediated cytostasis of tumour target cells. Immunology *31*, 837–846, 1976

Krahenbuhl, J. L., and Remington, J. S. The role of activated macrophages in specific and nonspecific cytostasis of tumor cells. J Immunol *113*, 507–516, 1974

Krant, M. J., Manskoff, G., Brandrup, C. S., and

Madoff, M. A. Immunologic alterations in bronchogenic cancer. Cancer 21, 623–631, 1968

Krebs, C., Rask-Nielsen, H. C., and Wagner, A. The origin of lymphosarcomatosis and its relation to other forms of leucosis in white mice. Acta Radiol (Suppl) (Stockh) 10, 1–53, 1930

Krebs, J. A., Roenigh, H. H., Deodhar, S. D., and Barna, B. Halo nevus: Competent surveillance of potential melanoma. Cleve Clin Q 43, 11–15, 1976

Kreider, J. W., and Benjamin, S. A. Tumor immunity and the mechanism of polyinosinic-polycytidylic acid inhibition of tumor growth. J Natl Cancer Inst 49, 1303–1310, 1972

Krementz, E. T., Mansell, P. W. A., Hornung, M. O., Samuels, M. S., Sutherland, C. A., and Benes, E. N. Immunotherapy of malignant disease: The use of viable sensitized lymphocytes or transfer factor prepared from sensitized lymphocytes. Cancer 33, 394–401, 1974

Krementz, E. T., and Ryan, R. F. Chemotherapy of melanoma of the extremities by perfusion: Fourteen years clinical experience. Ann Surg 175, 900–917, 1972

Krementz, E. T., Samuels, M. S., Wallace, J. H., and Benes, E. N. Clinical experiences in immunotherapy of cancer. Surg Gynecol Obstet 133, 209–217, 1971

Kripke, M. L., Budmen, M. B., and Fidler, I. J. Production of specific macrophage activating factor by lymphocytes from tumor-bearing mice. Cell Immunol 30, 341–352, 1977

Kruger, G. Morphologic studies of lymphoid tissues during the growth of an isotransplanted mouse tumor. J Natl Cancer Inst 39, 1–15, 1967

Kufe, D., MacGrath, I. T., Ziegler, J. L., and Spiegelman, S. Burkitt's tumors contain particles encapsulating RNA-instructed DNA polymerase and high molecular weight virus-related RNA. Proc Natl Acad Sci USA 70, 737–740, 1973

Kumar, S., and Taylor, G. Non-organ-specific and tumour-specific antibodies in children with Wilms' tumour. Int J Cancer 16, 448–455, 1975

Kung, J. T., Brooks, S. D., Jakway, J. P., Leonard, L. L., and Talmage, D. W. Suppression of in vitro cytotoxic response by macrophages due to induced arginase. J Exp Med 146, 665–672, 1977

Kuper, S. W. A., and Bignall, J. R. Tritiated-thymidine uptake by tumour cells in blood. Lancet 1, 1412–1414, 1964

Kuper, S. W. A., Bignall, J. R., and Luckcock, E. D. A quantitative method for studying tumour cells in blood. Lancet 1, 852–853, 1961

Kuperman, O., Feigis, M., and Weiss, D. W. Reversal by the MER tubercle bacillus fraction of the suppressive effects of heterologous antilymphocytic serum (ALS) on the allograft reactivity of mice. Cell Immunol 8, 484–489, 1973

Kuperman, O., Fortner, G. W., and Lucas, Z. J. Immune response to a syngeneic mammary adenocarcinoma. II. In vitro generation of cytotoxic lymphocytes. J Immunol 115, 1277–1281, 1975b

Kurnick, N. B. Experiences with infusion of autologous and isologous bone marrow in man, In Abstracts of Conference on Bone Marrow Transplantation and Chemical Protection in Large Animals and Man (Veterans Admin Hospital, Long Beach, Calif., June 1962). 1962

Kurnick, N. B. Intensive radiotherapy of lymphoma with the aid of frozen autologous bone marrow. In Protection and Recovery Discussion Meeting, Abstracts. Blood 24, 658–659, 1964

Kurnick, N. B., Montano, A., Gerdes, J. C., and Feder, B. H. Preliminary observations on the treatment of postirradiation hematopoietic depression in man by the infusion of stored autogenous bone marrow. Ann Intern Med 49, 973–986, 1958

Kurth, R., and Bauer, H. Avian oncornavirus-induced tumor antigens of embryonic and unknown origin. Virology 56, 496–504, 1973

Kurth, R., Teich, N. M., Weiss, R. A., and Oliver, R. T. D. Natural human antibodies reactive with primate type-C viral antigens. Proc Natl Acad Sci USA 74, 1237–1241, 1977

L

Lachmann, P. J., and Sikora, K. Coupling PPD to tumor cells enhances their antigenicity in BCG-primed mice. Nature 271, 463–464, 1978

Lacour, F., Spira, A., Lacour, J., and Prade, M. Polyadenylic-polyuridylic acid an adjunct to surgery in the treatment of spontaneous mammary tumors in C3H/He mice and transplantable melanoma in the hamster. Cancer Res 32, 648–649, 1972

Lagrange, P. H. Comparative studies of different strains of BCG vaccine in mice: T-cell dependent immuno responses. Dev Biol Stand 38, 223–229, 1978

Lagrange, P. H., Mackaness, G. B., and Miller, T. E. Influence of dose and route of antigen injection on the immunological induction of T cells. J Exp Med *139*, 528–542, 1974

Lagrange, P. H., Miller, T. E., and Mackaness, G. B. Parameters conditioning the potentiating effect of BCG on the immune response, pp 23–26, In Lamoureux, G., Turcotte, R., and Portelance, V. (Eds): BCG in Cancer Immunotherapy. New York: Grune & Stratton, 1976

Laing, C. A., Heppner, G. H., and Bekesi, J. G. Tumor antigens: Biological activity of components of soluble antigens of MTV-induced mammary tumors. Cancer Immunol Immunother *4*, 5–13, 1978

Laird, A. K. Cell fractionation of normal and malignant tissues. Exp Cell Res *6*, 30–44, 1954

Laird, A. K. Dynamics of tumour growth. Br J Cancer *18*, 490–502, 1964

Laird, A. K. Dynamics of tumour growth: Comparison of growth rates and extrapolation of growth curve to one cell. Br J Cancer *19*, 278–291, 1965a

Laird, A. K. Dynamics of relative growth. Growth *29*, 249–263, 1965b

Laird, A. K., and Barton, A. D. Cell population in precancerous liver: Relation to presence and dose of carcinogen. J Natl Cancer Inst *27*, 827–839, 1961

Laird, A. K., Tyler, S. A., and Barton, A. D. Dynamics of normal growth. Growth *29*, 233–248, 1965

Laki, K., Tyler, H. M., and Yancey, S. T. Clot forming and clot stabilizing enzymes from the mouse tumor YPC-1. Biochem Biophys Res Commun *24*, 776–781, 1966

Lala, P. K. Studies on tumor cell population kinetics, pp 3–95, In Busch, H. (Ed): Methods in Cancer Research. New York: Academic Press, 1971

Lala, P. K. Evaluation of the mode of cell death in Ehrlich ascites tumor. Cancer *29*, 261–266, 1972

Lala, P. K. Cell kinetics and cancer, pp 29–35, In Proc XI Intern Cancer Congress, Vol 1. Cell Biology and Tumor Immunology. Amsterdam: Excerpta Medica, 1974a

Lala, P. K. Changes in antigenicity of the Ehrlich ascites tumor by propagation in different host strains. Proc Am Assoc Cancer Res *15*, 117, 1974b

Lala, P. K. Dynamics of leukocyte migration into the mouse ascites tumor. Cell Tissue Kinet *7*, 293–304, 1974c

Lala, P. K. Effects of tumor bearing on the dynamics of host homopoietic cells. Cancer Treat Rep (Suppl) *60*, 1781–1789, 1976a

Lala, P. K. Homopoietic stem cells in tumor bearing hosts, pp 343–355, In Cairnie, A. B., Lala, P. K., and Osmond, D. G. (Eds): Stem Cells in Renewing Cell Populations. New York: Academic Press, 1976b

Lala, P. K. Growth kinetics of malignant cells in ascites and solid forms. Proc 29th Annu Symp on Cancer Research, 1977

Lala, P. K., and Kaiser, L. Kinetics of host mononuclear cells in TA-3(St) solid tumours. Anat Rec *184*, 455, 1976

Lamb, D., Pilney, F., Kelly, W. D., and Good, R. A. A comparative study of the incidence of anergy in patients with carcinoma, leukemia, Hodgkin's disease and other lymphomas. J Immunol *89*, 555–558, 1962

Lamensans, A., Stiffel, C., Millier, M. F., Laurent, M., Mouton, D., and Biozzi, G. Effet protecteur de corynebacterium parvum contre la leucémie greffée AKR. Relations avec l'activité catalasique hépatique et la fonction phagocytaire du système réticulo-endothélial. Rev Fr Etudes Clin Biol *13*, 773–779, 1968

Lamerton, L. F. Tumor cell kinetics. Br Med Bull *29*, 23–28, 1973

Lamerton, L. F., and Fry, R. J. (Eds): Cell Proliferation. Oxford: Blackwell, 1963

Lamon, E. W., Andersson, B., Wigzell, H., Fenyö, E. M., and Klein, E. The immune response to primary Moloney sarcoma virus tumors in Balb/c mice: Cellular and humoral activity of long-term regressors. Int J Cancer *13*, 91–104, 1974

Lamon, E. W., Klein, E., Andersson, B., Fenyö, E. M., and Skurzak, H. M. The humoral antibody response to a primary viral neoplasm (MSV) through its entire course in Balb/c mice. Int J Cancer *12*, 637–645, 1973a

Lamon, E. W., Skurzak, H. M., Klein, E., and Wigzell, H. In vitro cytotoxicity by a nonthymus-processed lymphocyte population with specificity for a virally determined tumor cell surface antigen. J Exp Med *136*, 1072–1079, 1972

Lamon, E. W., Whitten, H. D., Skurzak, H. M., Andersson, B., and Lindin, B. IgM antibody-dependent cell-mediated cytotoxicity in the Moloney sarcoma virus system. The involvement of T and B lymphocytes as effector cells. J Immunol *115*, 1288–1294, 1975

Lamon, E. W., Wigzell, H., Andersson, B., and Klein, E. Antitumor activity in vitro dependent on immune B lymphocytes. Nature New Biol *244*, 209–211, 1973b

Lamon, E. W., Wigzell, H., Klein, E., Andersson, B., and Skurzak, H. M. The lymphocyte response to primary Moloney sarcoma virus tumors in Balb/c mice. Definition of the active subpopulations at different times after infection. J Exp Med *137*, 1472–1493, 1973c

Lampson, G. P., Tytell, A. A., Field, A. K., Nemes, M. M., and Hilleman, M. R. Inducers of interferon and host resistance. I. Double-stranded RNA from extracts of Penicillium funiculosum. Proc Natl Acad Sci USA *58*, 782–789, 1967

Lancet. Spontaneous regression of cancer. Lancet *2*, 896, 1966

Lancet. Cancer in cats and dogs. Lancet *2*, 618 619, 1968

Lancet. Testing anti-cancer drugs. Lancet *1*, 827, 1972a

Lancet. Prolactin and breast cancer. Lancet *2*, 1129–1130, 1972b

Lancet. How double blind? Lancet *1*, 348–349, 1976

Landi, S., Barbara, C., Przykuta, K., and Held, H. R. Comparison of freeze-dried vaccines prepared from four different strains of BCG. Dev Biol Stand *38*, 19–28, 1978

Laroye, G. J. How efficient is immunological surveillance against cancer and why does it fail? Lancet *1*, 1097–1100, 1974

Larsen, V., Morgensen, B., Amzis, C. J., and Storm, O. Fibrinolytic enzyme in the treatment of patients with cancer. Dan Med Bull *11*, 137–140, 1961

Larson, D. L., and Tomlinson, L. J. Quantitative antibody studies in man. III. Antibody response in leukemia and other malignant lymphomata. J Clin Invest *32*, 317–321, 1953

Laszlo, J., Buckley, C. E., and Amos, D. B. Infusion of isologous immune plasma in chronic lymphocytic leukemia. Blood *31*, 104–110, 1968

Lauder, I., and Aherne, W. The significance of lymphocytic infiltration in neuroblastoma. Br J Cancer *26*, 321–330, 1972

Lavrin, D. H., Blair, P. B., and Weiss, D. W. Immunology of spontaneous mammary carcinomas in mice. III. Immunogenicity of C3H preneoplastic hyperplastic alveolar nodules in C3Hf hosts. Cancer Res *26*, 293–304, 1966

Lavrin, D. H., Rosenberg, S. A., Connor, R. J., and Terry, W. D. Immunoprophylaxis of methylcholanthrene-induced tumors in mice with bacillus Calmette-Guérin and methanol-extracted residue. Cancer Res *33*, 472–477, 1973

Law, L. W. Neoplasms in thymectomized mice following room infection with polyoma virus. Nature *205*, 672–673, 1965

Law, L. W. Studies of the significance of tumour antigens in induction and repression of neoplastic diseases: Presidential address. Cancer Res *29*, 1–21, 1969

Law, L. W., and Chang, S. S. Effects of antilymphocyte serum (ALS) on the induction of lymphocytic leukemia in mice. Proc Soc Exp Biol Med *136*, 420–425, 1971

Law, L. W., and Miller, J. H. Observations on the effect of thymectomy on spontaneous leukemias of the high-leukemia strains RIL and C58. J Natl Cancer Inst *11*, 253–262, 1950a

Law, L. W., and Miller, J. H. The influence of thymectomy on the incidence of carcinogen-induced leukemia in strain DBA mice. J Natl Cancer Inst *11*, 425–438, 1950b

Law, L. W., Ting, R. C., and Allison, A. C. Effects of antilymphocyte serum on induction of tumours and leukaemia by murine sarcoma virus. Nature *220*, 611–612, 1968

Law, L. W., Ting, R. C., and Stanton, M. F. Some biologic, immunogenic and morphologic effects in mice after infection with a murine sarcoma virus. I. Biologic and immunogenic studies. J Natl Cancer Inst *40*, 1101–1112, 1968

Lawrence, H. S. The transfer in humans of delayed skin sensitivity to streptococcal M substance and to tuberculin with disrupted leukocytes. J Clin Invest *34*, 219–230, 1955

Lawrence, H. S. Transfer factor. Adv Immunol *11*, 195–266, 1969

Lawrence, H. S. Transfer factor in cellular immunity. Harvey Lect Series *68*, 239–350, 1974

Lawrence, W., Terz, J. J., Horsley, S., Donaldson, M., Lovett, W. L., Brown, P. W., Ruffner, B. W., and Regelson, W. Chemotherapy as an adjuvant to surgery for colorectal cancer. Ann Surg *181*, 616–622, 1975

Leclerc, C., Lamensans, A., Chedid, L., Drapier, J.-C., Petit, J.-F., Wietzerbin, J., and Lederer, E. Nonspecific immunoprevention of L1210 leukemia by cord factor (6-6′dimycolate of trehalose) administered in a metabolizable oil. Cancer Immunol Immunother *1*, 227–232, 1976

LeClerc, J. C., Gomard, E., and Levy, J. P. Cell-mediated reaction against tumors induced by oncornaviruses. I. Kinetics and specificity of the immune response in murine sarcoma virus (MSV)-induced tumors and transplanted lymphomas. Int J Cancer *10*, 589–601, 1972

LeClerc, J. C., Gomard, E., Plata, F., and Levy, J. P. Cell-mediated immune reaction against tumors induced by oncorna viruses. II. Nature of the effector cells in tumor-cell cytolysis. Int J Cancer *11*, 426–432, 1973

Leditschke, J. F. Surgery and metastatic hypernephroma. Aust NZ J Surg *34*, 136–139, 1964

Lee, A. K. Y., Rowley, M., and Mackay, I. R. Antibody-producing capacity in human cancer. Br J Cancer *24*, 454–463, 1970

Lee, J. A. H., and Merrill, J. M. Sunlight and the aetiology of malignant melanoma: A synthesis. Med J Aust 2, 846–851, 1970

Lee, J. C., and Ihle, J. N. Characterization of the blastogenic and cytotoxic responses of normal mice to ecotropic C-type viral gp71. J Immunol 118, 928–934, 1977

Le Fever, A. V., Killion, J. J., and Kollmorgen, G. M. Active immunotherapy of L1210 leukemia with neuraminidase-treated, drug-resistant L1210 sublines. Cancer Immunol Immunother 1, 211–217, 1976

LeGarrec, Y., Sablovic, D., Toujas, L., Dazord, L., Guelfi, J., and Pilet, C. Activity of inactivated Brucella on murine tumors: Prophylactic effect and combination with specific immunostimulation. Biomedicine 21, 40–43, 1974

Lehmann, A. R., Kirk-Bell, S., Arlett, C. F., Paterson, M. C., Lohman, P. H. M., DeWeerd-Kastelein, E. A., and Bootsma, D. Xeroderma pigmentosum cells with normal levels of excision repair have a defect in DNA synthesis after UV-irradiation. Proc Natl Acad Sci USA 72, 219–223, 1975

Leiberman, M., and Kaplan, H. S. Leukemogenic activity of filtrates from radiation induced lymphoid tumors of mice. Science 130, 387–388, 1959

LeMevel, B. P., and Wells, S. A. Foetal antigens cross-reactive with tumour specific transplantation antigens. Nature New Biol 244, 183–184, 1973

Lemonde, P., and Clode-Hyde, M. Influence of bacille Calmette-Guérin infection on polyoma in hamsters and mice. Cancer Res 26, 585–589, 1966

Leonard, B. J., Eccleston, E., and Jones, D. Toxicity of interferon inducers of the double stranded RNA type. Nature 224, 1023–1024, 1969

Lespinats, G. Induction d'une immunité vis-à-vis de la greffe de plasmacytosarcomes chez la souris Balb/c. Eur J Cancer 5, 421–426, 1969

LeVeen, H. H., Wapnick, S., Piccone, V., Falk, G., and Ahmed, N. Tumor eradication by radiofrequency therapy. JAMA 235, 2198–2200, 1976

Leventhal, B. G., Halterman, R. H., Rosenberg, E. B., and Herberman, R. B. Immune reactivity of leukemia patients to autologous blast cells. Cancer Res 32, 1820–1825, 1972

Leventhal, B. G., Poplack, D. G., Johnson, E. G., Simon, R., Bowles, C., and Steinberg, S. The effect of chemotherapy and immunotherapy on the response to mitogens in acute lymphatic

leukemia, pp 613–623, In Oppenheim, J., and Rosentreich, D. (Eds): Mitogens in Immunobiology. New York: Academic Press, 1976

Levi, E., and Schechtman, A. M. The preparation in immunologically tolerant rabbits of antisera against the Ehrlich ascites tumor. Cancer Res 23, 1566–1570, 1963

Levi, E., Schechtman, A., Sherins, R. S., and Tobias, S. Tumor specificity and immunological suppression. Nature 185, 563–565, 1959

Levi, E. L., Cooper, E. H., Anderson, C. K., Path, M. C., and Williams, R. E. Analysis of DNA content, nuclear size and cell proliferation of transitional cell carcinoma in man. Cancer 23, 1074–1085, 1969

Levij, I. S., and Polliack, A. Inhibition of chemical carcinogenesis in the hamster cheek pouch by topical chlorpromazine. Nature 228, 1096–1097, 1970

Levin, A. G., Cunningham, M. P., Steers, A. K., Miller, D. G., and Southam, C. M. Production of 19S and 7S antibodies by cancer patients. Clin Exp Immunol 7, 839–849, 1970

Levin, A. G., Custadio, D. B., Mandel, E. E., and Southam, C. M. Rejection of cancer homotransplants by patients with debilitating nonneoplastic diseases. Ann NY Acad Sci 120, 410–423, 1964

Levin, A. S., Byers, V. S., Fudenberg, H. H., Wegban, J., Hackett, A. J., Johnston, J. O., and Spitler, L. E. Immunologic parameters before and during immunotherapy with tumor specific transfer factor. J Clin Invest 55, 487–499, 1975

Levine, P. H. Introduction. Conference and Workshop on Cellular Immune Reactions to Human Tumor-associated Antigens. Natl Cancer Inst Monogr 37, ix–xii, 1973

Levine, R. J., and Metz, S. A. A classification of ectopic hormone-producing tumors. Ann NY Acad Sci 230, 533–546, 1974

Levinthal, J. D., Buffett, R. F., and Furth, J. Prevention of viral leukemia of mice by thymectomy. Proc Soc Exp Biol Med 100, 610–614, 1959

Levis, A. G. X-irradiation sensitivity of nitrogen mustard-resistant mammalian cells in vitro. Nature 198, 498–499, 1963

Levy, H. B., Adamson, R., Carbone, P., DeVita, V., Gazdar, A., Rhim, J., Weinstein, A., and Riley, F. Studies on the anti-tumor action of poly I: poly C, pp 55–65, In Beers, R. F., and Braun, W. (Eds): Biological Effects of Polynucleotides. New York: Springer-Verlag, 1971

Levy, H. B., Baer, G., Baron, S., Buckler, C. E.,

Gibbs, C. J., Indarola, M. J., London, W. T., and Rice, J. A modified polyriboinosinic: polyribocytidylic acid complex that induces interferon in primates. J Infect Dis *132*, 434–439, 1975

Levy, H. B., Law, L. W., and Rabson, A. S. Inhibition of tumor growth by polyinosinic-polycytidylic acid. Proc Natl Acad Sci USA *62*, 357–361, 1969

Levy, J. P., and LeClerc, J. C. Immune rejection of tumor cells: "In vivo" significance of anti-tumor "in vitro" immune reactions. Biomedicine *22*, 249–254, 1975

Levy, J. P., and LeClerc, J. C. The murine sarcoma virus-induced tumor: Exception or general model in tumor immunology? Adv Cancer Res *24*, 2–66, 1977

Levy, M. H., and Wheelock, E. F. The role of macrophages in defense against neoplastic disease. Adv Cancer Res *20*, 131–165, 1974

Levy, N. L., Mahaley, M. S., and Day, E. D. In vitro demonstration of cell-mediated immunity to human brain tumors. Cancer Res *32*, 477–482, 1972

Lewis, M. G., Hartman, D., and Jerry, L. M. Antibodies and anti-antibodies in human malignancy: An expression of deranged immune regulation. Ann NY Acad Sci *276*, 316–327, 1976a

Lewis, M. G., Ikonopisov, R. L., Nairn, R. C., Phillips, T. M., Fairley, G. H., Bodenham, D. C., and Alexander, P. Tumour-specific antibodies in human malignant melanoma and their relationship to the extent of the disease. Br Med J *3*, 547–552, 1969

Lewis, M. G., Jerry, L. M., Rowden, G., Phillips, T. M., Shibata, H., and Capek, A. Some effects of oral administration of BCG on immune responses in cancer patients, pp 339–358, In Lamoureux, G., et al. (Eds): BCG in Cancer Immunotherapy. New York: Grune & Stratton, 1976b

Lewis, M. G., McCloy, E., and Blake, J. The significance of humoral antibodies in the localization of human malignant melanoma. Br J Surg *60*, 443–446, 1973

Lewis, M. G., and Phillips, T. M. The specificity of surface membrane immunofluorescence in human malignant melanoma. Int J Cancer *10*, 105–111, 1972

Lewis, M. G., Phillips, T. M., Cook, K. B., and Blake, J. Possible explanation for loss of detectable antibody in patients with disseminated malignant melanoma. Nature *232*, 52–54, 1971

Libansky, J. Study of immunologic reactivity in hemoblastosis. Circulating antibody formation as a response to antigenic stimulus in leukemia, malignant lymphoma, myeloma and myelofibrosis. Blood *25*, 169–178, 1965

Liddle, G. W., Island, D., and Meador, C. K. Normal and abnormal regulation of corticotropin secretion in man. Recent Prog Horm Res *18*, 125–166, 1962

Liddle, G. W., Nicholson, W. E., and Island, D. P. Clinical and laboratory studies of ectopic humoral syndromes. Recent Prog Horm Res *25*, 283–314, 1969

Lieberman, M. W., and Forbes, P. D. Demonstration of DNA repair in normal and neoplastic tissues after treatment with proximate chemical carcinogens and ultraviolet radiation. Nature New Biol *241*, 199–201, 1973

Lieberman, R., Wybran, J., and Epstein, W. The immunologic and histopathologic changes of BCG-mediated tumor regression in patients with malignant melanoma. Cancer *35*, 756–777, 1975

Likhite, V. V. Rejection of tumors and metastases in Fischer 344 rats following intratumor administration of killed Corynebacterium parvum. Int J Cancer *14*, 684–690, 1974

Likhite, V. V. Suppression of the incidence of death with spontaneous tumours in DBA/2 mice after Corynebacterium parvum-mediated rejection of syngeneic tumours. Nature *259*, 397–399, 1976

Likhite, V. V. Rejection of tumor metastases in Fischer 344 rats following the administration of killed Corynebacterium parvum. Cancer Immunol Immunother *2*, 173–178, 1977

Likhite, V. V., and Halpern, B. N. The delayed rejection of tumors formed from the administration of tumor cells mixed with killed Corynebacterium parvum. Int J. Cancer *12*, 699–704, 1973

Likhite, V. V., and Halpern, B. N. Lasting rejection of mammary adenocarcinoma cell tumors in DBA/2 mice with intratumor injection of killed Corynebacterium parvum. Cancer Res *34*, 341–344, 1974

Lilly, F., and Pincus, T. Genetic control of murine viral leukemogenesis. Adv Cancer Res *17*, 231–277, 1974

Lindenmann, J. Resistance of mice to mouse-adapted influenza A virus. Virology *16*, 203–204, 1962

Lindenmann, J. Viral oncolysis with host survival. Proc Soc Exp Biol Med *113*, 85–91, 1963

Lindenmann, J. Immunity to transplantable tumors following viral oncolysis. I. Mechanism of immunity to Ehrlich ascites tumor. J Immunol *92*, 912–919, 1964

Lindenmann, J. The use of viruses as immunological potentiators, pp 197–214, In Wolstenholme, G. E. W., and Knight, J. (Eds): Ciba Fdn Symp, New Series 18—Immunopotentiation. Amsterdam: ASP, 1973

Lindenmann, J. Viruses as immunological adjuvants in cancer. Biochim Biophys Acta 355, 49–75, 1974

Lindenmann, J., and Klein, P. A. Immunological aspects of viral oncolysis. Recent Results Cancer Res 9, 1–75, 1967a

Lindenmann, J., and Klein, P. A. Viral oncolysis: Increased immunogenicity of host cell antigens associated with influenza virus. J Exp Med 126, 93–108, 1967b

Linder, D., and Gartler, S. M. Glucose-6-phosphate dehydrogenase mosaicism: Utilization as a cell marker in the study of leiomyomas. Science 150, 67–69, 1965

Linder, O. E. A. Survival of skin homografts in methylcholanthrene treated mice and in mice with spontaneous mammary cancers. Cancer Res 22, 380–383, 1962

Lindstrom, G. A. An experimental study of myelotoxic sera. Therapeutic attempts in myeloid leukemia. Acta Med Scand (Suppl) 22, 1–169, 1927

Linn, J. E., Bowdoin, B., Farmer, T. B., and Meador, C. K. Observations and comments on failure of dexamethasone suppression. N Engl J Med 277, 403–405, 1967

Linscott, W. D. An antigen density effect on the hemolytic efficiency of complement. J Immunol 104, 1307–1309, 1970a

Linscott, W. D. Effect of cell surface antigen density on immunological enhancement. Nature 228, 824–827, 1970b

Lipscomb, H. S., Wilson, C., Retiene, K., Matsen, F., and Ward, D. N. The syndrome of inappropriate secretion of antidiuretic hormone in oat cell carcinoma of lung. Cancer Res 28, 378–383, 1968

Livnat, S., and Cohen, I. R. Recruitment of effector lymphocytes by initiator lymphocytes: Role of a trypsin-sensitive membrane component. Eur J Immunol 5, 357–360, 1975a

Livnat, S., and Cohen, I. R. Recruitment of effector lymphocytes by initiator lymphocytes. In vivo migration of in vitro sensitized initiator T lymphocytes. Eur J Immunol 5, 389–394, 1975b

LoBuglio, A., and Neidhart, J. A. Transfer factor: A potential agent for cancer therapy. Med Clin North Am 60, 585–590, 1976

LoBuglio, A. E., Neidhart, J. A., Helberg, R. W., Metz, E. N., and Balcerzak, S. P. The effect of transfer factor therapy on tumor immunity in alveolar soft part sarcoma. Cell Immunol 7, 159–165, 1973

Loeb, L. Über Entstehung eines Sarkoms nach Transplantation eines Adenocarcinoms einer japanischen Maus. Z Krebsforsch 7, 80–110, 1909

Logan, J. The delayed type of allergic reaction in cancer: Altered response to tuberculin and mumps virus. NZ Med J 55, 408–410, 1956

LoGerfo, P., Hansen, H. J., and Krupey, J. Demonstration of common tumor neoplastic antigen. N Engl J Med 285, 138–143, 1971

LoGerfo, P., Herter, F. P., Braun, J., and Hansen, H. J. Tumor associated antigen with pulmonary neoplasms. Ann Surg 175, 495–500, 1972

Lohmann-Matthes, M. L., and Fischer, H. T-cell cytotoxicity and amplification of the cytotoxic reaction by macrophages. Transplant Rev 17, 150–171, 1973

Lohmann-Matthes, M. L., Schipper, H., and Fischer, H. Macrophage-mediated cytotoxicity against allogeneic target cells in vitro. Eur J Immunol 2, 45–49, 1972

Lonai, P., Clark, W. R., and Feldman, M. Participation of θ-bearing cell in an in vitro assay of transplantation immunity. Nature 229, 566–567, 1971

Londner, M. V., Morini, J. C., Font, M. T., and Rabasa, S. L. RNA-induced immunity against rat sarcoma. Experientia 24, 598–599, 1968

London Hospital Clinical Trials Unit. Aide-memoire for preparing clinical trial protocols. Br Med J 1, 1323–1324, 1977

Loor, F., Hagg, L.-B., Mayor, K. S., and Roelants, G. E. θ positive cells in nude mice born from homozygous nu/nu mother. Nature 255, 657–658, 1975

Loor, F., and Roelants, G. E. High frequency of T lineage lymphocytes in nude mouse spleen. Nature 251, 229–230, 1974

Lorenz, E. K., and Congdon, C. C. Some aspects of the role of haematopoietic tissues in the pathogenesis and treatment of experimental leukemia. Rev Hematol 10, 476–484, 1955

Lotzová, E., and Cudkowicz, G. Hybrid resistance to parental NZW bone marrow grafts. Association with the D end of H-2. Transplantation 12, 130–138, 1971

Lotzová, E., and Cudkowicz, G. Hybrid resistance to parental WB/Re bone marrow grafts. Association with genetic markers of linkage group IX. Transplantation 13, 256–264, 1972

Lotzová, E., and Cudkowicz, G. Resistance of irradiated Fl hybrid and allogeneic mice to bone marrow grafts of NZB donors. J Immunol 110, 791–800, 1973

Lotzová, E., and Cudkowicz, G. Abrogation of resistance to bone marrow grafts by silica particles. Prevention of the silica effect by the macrophage stabilizer poly-2-vinylpyridine N-oxide. J Immunol *113,* 798–803, 1974

Lotzová, E., Gallagher, M. T., and Trentin, J. J. Involvement of macrophages in genetic resistance to bone marrow grafts. Studies with two specific antimacrophage agents, carrageenan and silica. Biomedicine *22,* 387–392, 1975

Lotzová, E., and Savary, C. Possible involvement of natural killer cells in bone marrow graft rejection. Biomedicine *27,* 341–344, 1977

Loutit, J. F., and Ash, P. J. N. D. Radiation leukaemogenesis: Is virus really necessary? Br J Cancer *38,* 24–33, 1978

Loutit, J. F., and Carr, T. E. F. Lymphoid tumours and leukaemia induced in mice by bone seeking radionucleides. Int J Radiat Biol *33,* 245–263, 1978

Lozzio, B. B., Machado, E. A., Lozzio, C. B., and Lair, S. Hereditary asplenic-athymic mice: Transplantation of human myelogenous leukemic cells. J Exp Med *143,* 225–231, 1976

Lüben, G., Sedlacek, H. H., and Seiler, F. R. Quantitative experiments on the cell membrane binding of neuraminidase. Behring Inst Mitt *59,* 30–37, 1976

Ludwig Lung Cancer Study Group. Search for the possible role of 'immunotherapy' in operable bronchial non-small cell carcinoma (stage I and II): A phase I study with Corynebacterium parvum intrapleurally. Cancer Immunol Immunother *4,* 69–75, 1978

Luft, R., Olivecrona, H., and Sjögren, B. Hypophysectomy in man. Nord Med *47,* 351–354, 1952

Lundak, R. L., and Raidt, D. J. Cellular immune response against tumor cells. I. In vitro immunisation of allogeneic and syngeneic mouse spleen cell suspensions against DBA mastocytoma cells. Cell Immunol *9,* 60–66, 1973

Lundgren, G., and Möller, G. Non-specific induction of cytotoxicity in normal human lymphocytes in vitro: Studies of mechanism and specificity of the reaction. Clin Exp Immunol *4,* 435–452, 1969

Lynch, H. T., Guirgis, H. A., Brodkey, F., Lynch, J., Maloney, K., Rankin, L., and Mulcahy, G. M. Genetic heterogeneity and familial carcinoma of the breast. Surg Gynecol Obstet **142,** 693–699, 1976

Lynch, N. R., and Salomon, J.-C. Tumor growth inhibition and potentiation of immunotherapy by indomethacin in mice. J Natl Cancer Inst *62,* 117–121, 1979

Lyons, M. J., and Moore, D. H. Isolation of the mouse mammary tumor virus: Chemical and morphological studies. J Natl Cancer Inst *35,* 549–565, 1965

Mc

McBean, M. A., Pees, H., Rosen, G., and Oettgen, H. F. Prelabelling target cells with ^{3}H-proline as a method for studying lymphocyte cytotoxicity. Natl Cancer Inst Monogr *37,* 41–48, 1973

McBride, W. H., Dawes, J., Dunbar, N., Ghaffar, A., and Woodruff, M. F. A. A comparative study of anaerobic coryneforms. Attempts to correlate their anti-tumour activity with their serological properties and ability to stimulate the lymphoreticular system. Immunology *28,* 49–58, 1975a

McBride, W. H., Dawes, J., and Tuach, S. Antitumor activity of Corynebacterium parvum extracts. J Natl Cancer Inst *56,* 437–439, 1976

McBride, W. H., Jones, J. T., and Weir, D. M. Increased phagocytic cell activity and anaemia in corynebacterium parvum treated mice. Br J Exp Pathol *55,* 38–46, 1974

McBride, W. H., Tuach, S., and Marmion, B. P. The effect of gold salts on tumour immunity and its stimulation by Corynebacterium parvum. Br J Cancer *32,* 558–567, 1975b

McBride, W. H., Weir, D. M., Kay, A. B., Pearce, D., and Caldwell, J. R. Activation of the classical and alternate pathways of complement by Corynebacterium parvum. Clin Exp Immunol *19,* 143–147, 1975c

McCarthy, R. E. Modification of the immune response of mice to skin homografts and heterografts by Ehrlich ascites carcinoma. Cancer Res *24,* 915–919, 1964

McCarthy, R. E., Coffin, J. M., and Gates, S. L. Selective inhibition of the secondary immune response to mouse skin allografts by cell-free Ehrlich ascites carcinoma fluid. Transplant *6,* 737–743, 1968

McCarthy, R. E., and Russfield, A. B. Tumor-induced accelerated skin graft rejection. Transplantation *6,* 358–362, 1968

McCollester, D. L. Isolation of Meth A cell surface membranes possessing tumor-specific transplantation antigen activity. Cancer Res *30,* 2832–2840, 1970

McCorquodale, D. W., Thayer, S. A., and Doisey,

E. A. Isolation of principal estrogenic substance of liquor folliculi. J Biol Chem *115*, 435–448, 1936

McCoy, J. L., Dean, J. H., Law, L. W., Williams, J., McCoy, N. T., and Holiman, B. J. Immunogenicity, antigenicity and mechanisms of tumor rejection of mineral-oil-induced plasmacytomas in syngeneic Balb/c mice. Int J Cancer *14*, 264–276, 1974

McCoy, J. L., Fefer, A., McCoy, N. T., and Kirsten, W. H. Immunobiologic studies of tumors induced by murine sarcoma virus (Kirsten). Cancer Res *32*, 343–349, 1972a

McCoy, J. L., Herberman, R. B., Rosenberg, E. B., Donnelly, F. C., Levine, P. H., and Alford, C. [51]Chromium-release assay for cell-mediated cytotoxicity of human leukemia and lymphoid tissue-culture cells. Natl Cancer Inst Monogr *37*, 59–67, 1973

McCoy, J. L., Ting, R. C., Morton, D. L., and Law, L. W. Immunologic and virologic studies of nonproducer tumor induced by murine sarcoma virus (Harvey). J Natl Cancer Inst *48*, 383–391, 1972b

McCracken, A., McBride, W. H., and Weir, D. M. Adjuvant-induced anti-red blood cell activity in CBA mice. Clin Exp Immunol *8*, 949–955, 1971

McCredie, J. A., Brown, E. R., and Cole, W. H. Immunologic treatment of tumors. Proc Soc Exp Biol Med *100*, 31–33, 1959

McCredie, J. A., Inch, W. R., Kruuv, J., and Watson, T. A. The rate of tumor growth in animals. Growth *29*, 331–347, 1965

McDermott, M. V., and Hensle, T. W. Metastatic carcinoid to the liver treated by hepatic dearterialization. Ann Surg *180*, 305–308, 1974

MacDonald, H. R. Early detection of potentially lethal events in T cell-mediated cytolysis. Eur J Immunol *5*, 251–254, 1975

MacDonald, H. R. Effect of hyperthermia on the functional activity of cytotoxic T-lymphocytes. J Natl Cancer Inst *59*, 1263–1268, 1977

MacDowell, E. C., Potter, J. S., Richeter, M. N., Victor, J., Bovarnick, M., Taylor, M. J., Ward, E. N., Laanes, T., and Wintersteiner, M. P. [Cited by Gorer (1956).]Carnegie Inst Wash Yearbook *37*, 47, 1938

McEndy, D. P., Boon, M. C., and Furth, J. On the role of thymus, spleen and gonads in the development of leukemia in a high leukemia stock of mice. Cancer Res *4*, 377–383, 1944

McEwen, L. M. The Schultz-Dale anaphyactic test for carcinoma antigen. Br Med J *2*, 615–617, 1959

McFarland, W., Granville, N. B., and Dameshek, W. Autologous bone marrow infusion as an adjunct in therapy of malignant disease. Blood *14*, 503–521, 1959

MacGregor, A. B., and Falk, R. E. Immunotherapy of malignant disease (Parts 1 and 2). J R Coll Surg Edinb *21*, 43–49, 1976

MacGregor, A. B., Falk, R. E., Landi, S., Ambus, U., and Langer, B. Oral bacille Calmette Guérin immunostimulation in malignant melanoma. Surg Gynecol Obstet *141*, 747–754, 1975

McGuigan, J. E., and Trudeau, W. L. Immunochemical measurements of elevated levels of gastrin in the serum of patients with pancreatic tumors of the Zollinger-Ellison variety. N Engl J Med *278*, 1308–1313, 1968

McGuire, W. L. Current status of estrogen receptors in human breast cancer. Cancer *36*, 638–644, 1975

McGuire, W. L., Carbone, P. P., Sears, M. E., and Escher, G. C. Estrogen receptors in human breast cancer—An overview, pp 1–7, In McGuire, W. L., Carbone, P. P., and Vollmer, E. P. (Eds): Estrogen Receptors in Human Breast Cancer. New York: Raven Press, 1975

McIllmurray, M. B., Embleton, M. J., Reeves, W. G., Langman, M. J. S., and Deane, M. Controlled trial of active immunotherapy in management of stage IIB malignant melanoma. Br Med J *1*, 540–542, 1977

McIntyre, R. O., Rai, K., Glidewell, O., and Holland, J. F. Polyriboinosinic:polyribocytidylic acid as an adjunct to remission maintenance therapy in acute myelogenous leukemia, pp 423–431, In Terry, W. D., and Windhorst, D. (Eds): Immunotherapy of Cancer: Present Status of Trials in Man. New York: Raven Press, 1978

McIvor, K. L., and Weiser, R. S. Mechanisms of target cell destruction by alloimmune peritoneal macrophages. II. Release of a specific cytotoxin from interacting cells. Immunology *20*, 315–322, 1971

Mackaness, G. B., Auclair, D. J., and Lagrange, P. H. Immunopotentiation with BCG. I. Immune response to different strains and preparations. J Natl Cancer Inst *51*, 1655–1669, 1974a

Mackaness, G. B., Lagrange, P. H., and Ishibashi, T. The modifying effect of BCG on the immunological induction of T cells. J Exp Med *139*, 1540–1552, 1974b

MacKay, E. N., and Sellars, A. H. Breast cancer at the Ontario Cancer Clincs, 1938–1956. A statistical review. Ontario: Medical Statistics Branch, Ontario Dept Health, 1965

Mackay, W. D. Role of splenomegaly in tumour-bearing mice. Nature *205*, 918–919, 1965

McKearn, T. J., Hamada, Y., Stuart, F. P., and

Fitch, F. W. Anti-receptor antibody and resistance to graft-versus-host disease. Nature *251*, 648–650, 1974

McKhann, C. F., Cleveland, P. H., and Burk, M. W. Some problems involving in vitro cellular cytotoxicity assays. Natl Cancer Inst Monogr *37*, 37–39, 1973

McKhann, C. F., and Harder, F. H. Tumor-specific antigens of methylcholanthrene-induced sarcomas. Transplantation *6*, 655–656, 1968

McKhann, C. F., and Jagarlamoody, S. M. Evidence for immune reactivity against neoplasms. Transplant Rev *7*, 55–57, 1971a

McKhann, C. F., and Jagarlamoody, S. M. In vitro immunization for immunotherapy, pp 539–544, In Lindhal-Kiessling et al. (Eds): Functional Morphological Aspects of Immunity. New York: Plenum Press, 1971b

McKhann, C. F., and Jagarlamoody, S. M. Manipulation of the immune response towards immunotherapy in cancer, pp 577–599, In Day, S. B., and Good, R. A. (Eds): Membranes and Viruses in Immunopathology. New York, London: Academic Press, 1972

Macklin, M. T. Comparison of the number of breast-cancer deaths observed in relatives of breast-cancer patients, and the number expected on the basis of mortality rates. J Natl Cancer Inst *22*, 927–951, 1959

McKneally, M. F., Maver, C., and Kausel, H. W. Regional immunotherapy of lung cancer with intrapleural BCG. Lancet *1*, 377–379, 1976

McKneally, M. F., Maver, C. M., and Kausel, H. W. Regional immunotherapy of lung cancer using postoperative intrapleural BCG, pp 161–171, In Terry, W. D., and Windhorst, D. (Eds): Immunotherapy of Cancer: Present Status of Trials in Man. New York: Raven Press, 1978

McLaren, A. Mammalian Chimaeras. Cambridge Univ Press, 1976

McLaughlin, J. F., Ruddle, N. H., and Waksman, B. H. Relationship between activation of peritoneal cells and their cytopathogenicity. J Reticuloendothel Soc *12*, 293–304, 1972

MacLennan, I. C. M. Competition for receptors for immunoglobulin on cytotoxic lymphocytes. Clin Exp Immunol *10*, 275–283, 1972

MacLennan, I. C. M., and Harding, B. The role of immunoglobulins in lymphocyte-mediated cell damage in vitro: II. The mechanism of target cell damage by lymphoid cells from immunized rats. Immunology *18*, 405–412, 1970

MacLennan, I. C. M., Loewi, G., and Harding, B. The role of immunoglobulins in lymphocyte-mediated cell damage in vitro: I. Comparison of the effects of target cell specific antibody and normal serum factors on cellular damage by immune and non-immune lymphocytes. Immunology *18*, 397–404, 1970

MacLennan, I. C., Loewi, G., and Howard, A. A human serum immunoglobulin with specificity for certain homologous target cells, which induces target cell damage by normal human lymphocytes. Immunology *17*, 897–910, 1969

McLeod, G. R., Beardmore, G. L., Little, J. H., Quinn, R. L., and Davis, N. C. Results of treatment of 361 patients with malignant melanoma in Queensland. Med J Aust *1*, 1211–1216, 1971

MacMahon, B., Cole, P., and Brown, J. Etiology of human breast cancer: A review. J Natl Cancer Inst *50*, 21–42, 1973

MacMahon, B., Cole, P., and Lin, T. N. Age at first birth and breast cancer risk. Bull WHO *43*, 209–221, 1970

McPeak, C. J. Intralymphatic therapy with immune lymphocytes. Cancer *28*, 1126–1128, 1971

McQuarrie, I. The Experiments of Nature and Other Essays. Lawrence: Univ Kansas, 1944

McWhirter, R. Simple mastectomy and radiotherapy in the treatment of breast cancer. Br J Radiol *28*, 128–139, 1955

McWhirter, R. Some factors influencing prognosis in breast cancer. J Fac Radiol *8*, 220–234, 1957

McWhirter, R. On the management of osteosarcoma. Health Bulletin (Scot Home Health Dept) *24*, 91–93, 1966

M

Maciera-Coehlo, A. Dissociation between inhibition of movement and inhibition of division in RSV transformed human fibroblasts. Exp Cell Res *47*, 193–200, 1967

Madden, J. L., Kandaloft, S., and Bourque, R. A. Modified radical mastectomy. Ann Surg *175*, 624–634, 1972

Madoc-Jones, H., and Bruce, W. R. Sensitivity of L cells in exponential and stationary phase to 5-fluorouracil. Nature *215*, 302–303, 1967

Maeda, Y. Y., and Chihara, G. Lentinan, a new immunoaccelerator of cell-mediated responses. Nature *229*, 634, 1971

Maeda, Y. Y., and Chihara, G. The effect of neonatal thymectomy on the antitumour activity of lentinan carboxymethylpachymaran and zymosan, and their effects on various immune responses. Int J Cancer *11*, 153–161, 1973

Maeda, Y. Y., Hamuro, J., and Chihara, G. The mechanisms of antitumor polysaccharides. I. The effect of antilymphocyte serum on the antitumor activity of lentinan. Int J Cancer 8, 41–46, 1971

Maeda, Y. Y., Hamuro, J., Yamada, Y. O., Ishimura, K., and Chihara, G. The nature of immunopotentiation by the antitumor polysaccharide lentinan and the significance of biogenic amines in its action, pp 259–281, In Wolstenholme, G. E. W., and Knight, J. (Eds): Ciba Fdn Symp—Immunopotentiation, New Series 18. Amsterdam: ASP, 1973

Maeda, Y. Y., Ishimura, K., Takasuka, N., Sasaki, T., and Chihara, G. Antitumor polysaccharides and host defence against cancer, pp 181–195, In Mizuno, D., et al. (Eds): Host Defence Against Cancer and Its Potentiation. Baltimore: Univ Park Press, 1975

Magarey, C. J., and Baum, M. Reticulo-endothelial activity in humans with cancer. Br J Surg 57, 748–752, 1970

Magarey, C. J., and Baum, M. Oestrogen as a reticuloendothelial stimulant in patients with cancer. Br Med J 2, 367–370, 1971

Magee, P. N. Carcinogens in the environment. Proc R Soc Med 67, 741–743, 1974

Magee, P. N., and Barnes, J. N. Carcinogenic nitrogen compounds. Adv Cancer Res 10, 164–247, 1967

Magrath, I. T., Lwanga, S., Carswell, W., and Harrison, N. Surgical reduction of tumour bulk in management of abdominal Burkitt's lymphoma. Br Med J 2, 308–312, 1974

Magrath, I. T., and Ziegler, J. L. Failure of BCG immunostimulation to affect the clinical course of Burkitt's lymphoma. Br Med J 1, 615–618, 1976

Maguire, H., Outzen, H. C., Custer, P. R., and Prehn, R. T. Invasion and metastasis of a xenogeneic tumor in nude mice. J Natl Cancer Inst 57, 439–442, 1976

Mahaley, M. S. Chemotherapy and immunology of brain tumors. Penn Med J 68, 45–46, 1965

Mahé, E., Bourdin, J. S., Gest, J., Saracino, R., Brunet, M., Halpern, G., Debaud, B., and Roth, F. Therapeutic trial with reticulo-stimulin in patients with ear, nose, or throat cancers, pp 376–382, In Halpern, B. (Ed): Corynebacterium Parvum: Applications in Experimental and Clinical Oncology. New York: Plenum Press, 1975

Maher, V. M., and McCormick, J. J. Effect of DNA repair on the cytotoxicity and mutagenicity of UV radiation and of chemical carcinogens in normal and xeroderma

pigmentosum cells, pp 129–145, In Yuhas, J. M., Tennant, R. W., and Regan, J. D. (Eds): Biology of Radiation Carcinogenesis. New York: Raven Press, 1976

Maini, M. M., and Stich, H. F. Chromosomes of tumor cells. II. Effect of various liver carcinogens on mitosis of hepatic cells. J Natl Cancer Inst 26, 1413–1424, 1961

Maini, M. M., Stich, H. F., and McCulloch, E. A. Changes in cell populations of precancerous lesions of rats. Proc Am Assoc Cancer Res 3, 341, 1962

Makari, J. G. Use of Schultz-Dale test for detection of specific antigens in sera of patients with carcinoma. Br Med J 2, 1291–1295, 1955

Makari, J. G. Detection of antigens in sera of patients with neoplastic disease by Schultz-Dale test. Br Med J 1, 359–361, 1958

Makari, J. G. Determination of tumor antigens and antibodies by the Schultz-Dale reaction and of cutaneous autohypersensitivity in subjects with tumors. Ann NY Acad Sci 101, 274–318, 1962

Mallucci, L. Cell response to surface stimulation. Nature New Biol 240, 60–61, 1972

Malmgren, R. A., and Flanigan, C. C. Localization of the vegetative form of Clostridium tetani in mouse tumors following intravenous spore administration. Cancer Res 15, 473–478, 1955

Malmgren, R. A., Rabson, A. S., and Carney, P. G. Immunity and viral carcinogenesis. Effect of thymectomy on polyoma virus carcinogenesis in mice. J Natl Cancer Inst 33, 101–104, 1964

Malpas, J. S., Freeman, J. E., Paxton, A., Walker Smith, J., Stansfield, A. G., and Wood, C. B. S. Radiotherapy and adjuvant combination chemotherapy for childhood rhabdomyosarcoma. Br Med J 1, 247–249, 1976

Maluish, A., and Halliday, W. L. Cell-mediated immunity and specific serum factors in human cancer: The leukocyte adherence inhibition test. J Natl Cancer Inst 52, 1415–1420, 1974

Manes, C. Phasing of gene products during development. Cancer Res 34, 2044–2052, 1974

Mankiewicz, E., Kurti, V., Munro, D. D., Wilson, J. A. S., and Papenburg, R. Immunologic responses in patients with pulmonary carcinoma receiving immunotherapy. Cancer Immunol Immunother 2, 27–39, 1977

Mann, D. L., Halterman, R., and Leventhal, B. G. Cross-reactive antigens on human cells injected with Rauscher leukemia virus and on human acute leukemia cells. Proc Natl Acad Sci USA 70, 495–497, 1973

Mann, D. L., Rogentine, G. N., Halterman, R., and Leventhal, B. Detection of an antigen associated with acute leukemia. Science *174*, 1136–1137, 1971

Mann, L. T. Spontaneous disappearance of pulmonary metastases after nephrectomy for hypernephroma. J Urol *59*, 564–566, 1948

Mannick, J. A., and Egdahl, R. H. Ribonucleic acid in "transformation" of lymphoid cells. Science *137*, 976–977, 1962a

Mannick, J. A., and Egdahl, R. H. Transformation on nonimmune lymph node cells to state of transplantation immunity by RNA. A preliminary report. Ann Surg *156*, 356–366, 1962b

Mannick, J. A., and Egdahl, R. H. Transfer of heightened immunity to skin homografts by lymphoid RNA. J Clin Invest *43*, 2166–2177, 1964

Manning, D. D., and Jutila, J. W. Immunosuppression in mice injected with heterologous anti-immunoglobulin antisera. J Immunol *108*, 282–285, 1972a

Manning, D. D., and Jutila, J. W. Effect of anti-immunoglobulin antisera on homograft rejection in mice. Nature New Biol *237*, 58–59, 1972b

Manning, D. D., and Jutila, J. W. Immunosuppression of mice injected with heterologous anti-immunoglobulin heavy chain antisera. J Exp Med *135*, 1316–1333, 1972c

Mansell, P. W., and DiLuzio, N. R. The in vivo destruction of human tumor by glucan activated macrophages, pp 227–243, In Fink, M. A. (Ed): The Macrophage in Neoplasia. New York: Academic Press, 1976

Mansell, P. W. A., Krementz, E. T., and DiLuzio, N. R. Clinical experiences with immunotherapy of malignant melanoma. Behring Inst Mitt *56*, 256–262, 1975

Manson, L. A., and Palmer, J. C. Induction of the immune response to cell surface antigens in vitro. In Vitro *11*, 186–204, 1975

Marchant, J. Prolonged survival of allogeneic skin from tumour-bearing mice. Int J Cancer *1*, 557–564, 1966

Marcove, R. C., Miké, V., Huvos, A. G., Southam, C. M., and Levin, A. G. Vaccine trials for osteogenic sarcoma. A preliminary report. Cancer *23*, 74–80, 1973

Mark, J., Levan, G., and Mitelman, F. Identification by fluorescence of the G-chromosome lost in human meningiomas. Hereditas *71*, 163–168, 1972

Marks, L. J., Berde, B., Klein, L. A., Roth, J., Goonan, S. R. Blumen, D., and Nasbeth, D. C. Inappropriate vasopressin secretion and car-cinoma of the pancreas. Am J Med *45*, 967–974, 1968

Marquardt, H. Polyriboinosinic-polyribocytidylic acid prevents chemically-induced malignant transformation in vitro. Nature New Biol *246*, 228–229, 1973

Marsh, B., Flynn, L., and Enneking, W. Immunologic aspects of osteosarcoma and their application to therapy. A preliminary report. J Bone Joint Surg *54*, 1367–1397, 1972

Marshall, A. H. E., and Dayan, A. D. An immune reaction in man against seminomas, dysgerminomas, pinealomas, and the mediastinal tumours of similar hostological appearance? Lancet *2*, 1102–1104, 1964

Marshall, G. D., Low, T. L., Thurman, G. B., Hu, S. K. Rossio, J. L., Trivers, G., and Goldstein, A. L. Overview of thymosin activity. Cancer Treat Rep *62*, 1731–1737, 1978

Marshall, V. C. Skin tumours in immunosuppressed patients. Aust NZ J Surg *43*, 214–222, 1973

Marshall, V. C. Premalignant and malignant skin tumours in immunosuppressed patients. Transplantation *17*, 272–275, 1974

Martensson, L. On a 'key point of modern biochemical genetics.' Lancet *1*, 946–947, 1963

Martin, D. S., Stolfi, R. L., and Fugmann, R. A. Animal models for tumor immunotherapy—A commentary. Cancer Immunol Immunother *2*, 77–79, 1977

Martin, M., Bourut, C., Halle-Pannenko, O., and Mathé, G. Routes other than I. V. injection to mice for BCG administration in active immunotherapy of L1210 leukemia. Biomedicine *23*, 339–340, 1975

Martin, M. S., Martin, F., Michiels, R., Bastien, H., Justrabo, E., Bordes, M., and Viry, B. An experimental model for cancer of the colon and rectum. Intestinal carcinoma induced in the rat by 1,2-dimethylhydrazine. Digestion *8*, 22–34, 1973

Martin, S. E., and Martin, W. J. Anti-tumour antibodies in normal mouse sera. Int J Cancer *15*, 658–664, 1975

Martin, W. J., Esber, E., Cotton, G. W., and Price, J. M. Depression of alloantigens in malignancy. Evidence for tumour susceptibility alloantigens and for possible self-reactivity of lymphoid cells active in the microcytotoxicity assay. Br J Cancer *28* (Suppl 1), 48–61, 1973

Martin, W. J., and Martin, S. E. Naturally occurring cytotoxic anti-tumour antibodies in sera of congenitally athymic (nude) mice. Nature *249*, 564–565, 1974

Martinez, C. Effect of early thymectomy on development of mammary tumours in mice. Nature *203*, 1188, 1964

Martinez, J., Winternitz, F., and Vindel, J. Nouvelles synthèses et propriétés de la tuftsine. Eur J Med Chem *12*, 511–516, 1978

Martland, H. S., and Humphries, R. E. Osteogenic sarcoma in dial painters using luminous paint. Arch Pathol *7*, 406–417, 1929

Martz, E. Early steps in specific tumor cell lysis by sensitized mouse T lymphocytes. I. Resolution and characterization. J Immunol *115*, 261–267, 1975

Martz, E. Multiple target cell killing by the cytolytic T-lymphocyte and the mechanism of cytotoxicity. Transplantation *21*, 5–11, 1976

Martz, E., and Benacerraf, B. An effector-cell independent step in target cell lysis by sensitized mouse lymphocytes. J Immunol *111*, 1538–1545, 1973

Masina, M. H. Biological assay of human kidney tumors by means of heterologous ocular transplantations; A study of clear-cell carcinoma, granular-cell carcinoma and papilliferous epithelioma of the kidney. J Urol *58*, 1–9, 1947

Mastrangelo, M. J., Bellet, R. E., Berd, D., and Lustbader, E. A randomized prospective trial comparing methyl-CCNU + vincristine to methyl-CCNU + vincristine + BCG + allogeneic tumor cells in patients with metastatic malignant melanoma, pp 95–102, In Terry, W. D., and Windhorst, D. (Eds): Immunotherapy of Cancer: Present Status of Trials in Man. New York: Raven Press, 1978

Mathé, G. Application of hematopoietic cell grafts to the treatment of leukemias and allied diseases. A critical review. Blood *16*, 1073–1088, 1960

Mathé, G. Immunothérapie adoptive locale de la tumeur BP8 sous forme ascitique chez la souris. Rev Fr Etudes Clin Biol *11*, 1027–1029, 1966

Mathé, G. Immunothérapie active de la leucémie L1210 appliquée après la greffe tumorale. Rev Fr Etudes Clin Biol *13*, 881–883, 1968

Mathé, G. Lymphocyte inhibitors fulfilling the definition of chalones and immunosuppression. Rev Eur Etudes Clin Biol *17*, 548–551, 1972

Mathé, G. General discussion, p 331, In Wolstenholme, G. E. W., and Knight, J. (Eds): Ciba Fdn Symp, New Series 18—Immunopotentiation. Amsterdam: ASP, 1973

Mathé, G. Cancer Active Immunotherapy. Recent Results in Cancer Research, Vol 55. New York: Springer-Verlag, 1976a

Mathé, G. Surviving in company of BCG. Cancer Immunol Immunother *1*, 3–5, 1976b

Mathé, G., Amiel, J. L., and Bernard, J. Traitement de souris AKR a l'age de six mois par irradiation totale suivie de transfusion de cellules hématopoietiques allogéniques: Incidences respectives de la leucémie et du syndrome secondaire. Bull Cancer (Paris) *47*, 331–340, 1960a

Mathé, G., Amiel, J. L., Schwarzenberg, L., Cattan, A., and Schneider, M. Haematopoietic chimera in man after allogenic (homologous) bone-marrow transplantation (Control of the secondary syndrome. Specific tolerance due to the chimerism). Br Med J *2*, 1633–1635, 1963

Mathé, G., Amiel, J. L., Schwarzenberg, L., Cattan, A., Schneider, M., deVries, M. J., Tubiana, M., Lalanne, C., Binet, J. L., Papiernik, M., Seman, G., Matsukura, M., Mery, A. M., Schwarzmann, V., and Flaisler, A. Successful allogenic bone marrow transplantation in man: Chimerism, induced specific tolerance and possible anti-leukemic effects. Blood *25*, 179–196, 1965

Mathé, G., Amiel, J. L., Schwarzenberg, L., Choay, J., Trolard, P., Schneider, M., Hayat, M., Schlumberger, J. R., and Jasmin, C. Bone marrow graft in man after conditioning by antilymphocytic serum. Br Med J *2*, 131–136, 1970a

Mathé, G., Amiel, J. L., Schwarzenberg, L., Schneider, M., Cattan, A., Schlumberger, J. R., Hayat, M., and DeVassal, F. Démonstration de l'efficacité de l'immunothérapie active dans la leucémie aigué lymphoblastique humaine. Rev Franc Etudes Clin Biol *13*, 454–459, 1968

Mathé, G., Amiel, J. L., Schwarzenberg, L., Schneider, M., Cattan, A., Schlumberger, J. R., Hayat, M., and DeVassal, F. Active immunotherapy for acute lymphoblastic leukaemia. Lancet *1*, 697–699, 1969a

Mathé, G., Amiel, J. L., Schwarzenberg, L., Schneider, M., Cattan, A., Schlumberger, J. R., Hayat, M., and DeVassal, F. Follow-up of the first (1962) pilot study on active immunotherapy of acute lymphoid leukaemia: A critical discussion. Biomedicine *26*, 29–35, 1977a

Mathé, G., Amiel, J. L., Schwarzenberg, L., Schneider, M., Hayat, M., DeVassal, F., Jasmin, C., Rosenfeld, C., and Pouillart, P. Preliminary result of a new protocol for the active immunotherapy of acute lymphoblastic leukaemia: Inhibition of the immunotherapeutic effect by vincristine or adamantadine. Eur J Clin Biol Res *16*, 216–224, 1971

Mathé, G., Amiel, J. L., Schwarzenberg, L., Schneider, M., Hayat, M., DeVassal, F., Jasmin, C., Rosenfeld, C., Sakouhi, M., and Choay, J. Remission induction with polyIC in patients with acute lymphoblastic leukaemia (preliminary results). Eur J Clin Biol Res *15*, 671–673, 1970b

Mathé, G., Belpomme, D., Pouillart, P., Schwarzenberg, L., Misset, J. L., Jasmin, C., Musset, M., Cattan, A., Amiel, J. L., and Schneider, M. Preliminary results of an immunotherapy trial on terminal leukaemic lymphosarcoma. Biomedicine *23*, 465–467, 1975a

Mathé, G., and Bernard, J. Essai de traitement par l'irradiation X suivie de greffe de cellules myeloïdes homologues de souris AK atteintes de leucémie spontanée très avancée. Bull Cancer *45*, 289–300, 1958

Mathé, G., and Bernard, J. Essais de traitement de la leucémie greffe 1210 par l'irradiation x suivie de transfusion de cellules hématopoiétiques normales (isologues ou homologues, myeloïdes ou lymphoïdes, adultes ou embryonnaires). Rev Eur Etudes Clin Biol *4*, 442–446, 1959a

Mathé, G., and Bernard, J. Essai de traitement de leucémie experimentales par la greffe de cellules hématopoiétiques normales. Sang *30*, 789–801, 1959b

Mathé, G., Bernard, J., DeVries, M. J., Schwarzenberg, L., Larrieu, M. J., Lalanne, C. M., Dutreix, A., Amiel, J. L., and Surmont, J. Nouveaux essais de greffe de moelle osseuse homologue après irradiation totale chez des enfants atteints de leucémie aigué en rémission. Le problème du syndrome secondaire chez l'homme. Rev Hematol *15*, 115–161, 1960b

Mathé, G., Bernard, J., Schwarzenberg, L., Larrieu, M. J., Lalanne, C., Dutreix, A., Denoix, P., Surmont, J., Schwarzmann, V., and Ceoara, B. Essai de traitement de sujets atteints de leucémie aigué en rémission par l'irradiation totale suivie de transfusion de moelle osseuse homologue. Rev Franc Etudes Clin Biol *4*, 675–704, 1959

Mathé, G., DeVassal, F., Delgado, M., Pouillart, P., Belpomme, D., Joseph, R., Schwarzenberg, L., Amiel, J. L., Schneider, M., Cattan, A., Musset, M., Misset, J. L., and Jasmin, C. 1975 current results of the first 100 cytologically typed acute lymphoid leukemia submitted to BCG active immunotherapy. Cancer Immunol Immunother *1*, 77–86, 1976

Mathé, G., DeVassal, F., Schwarzenberg, L., Delgado, M., Weiner, R., Gil, M. A., Pena-Angulo, J., Belpomme, D., Pouillart, P., Machover, D., Misset, J. L., Pico, J. L., Jasmin, C., Hayat, M., Schneider, M., Cattan, A., Amiel, J. L., Musset, M., and Rosenfeld, C. Results in children of acute lymphoid leukaemia. Protocol ICIG-ALL 9 consisting of

chemotherapy for only nine months followed by active immunotherapy. Comparison with the results of more prolonged chemotherapy protocols. Recognition of two groups of acute lymphoid leukaemias from prognostic parameters. Cancer Immunol Immunother *2*, 225–232, 1977b

Mathé, G., Halle-Pannenko, O., and Bourut, C. Immune manipulation by BCG administered before or after cyclophosphamide for chemoimmunotherapy of L1210 leukaemia. Eur J Cancer *10*, 661–666, 1974a

Mathé, H., Hayat, M., Sakouhi, M., and Choay, J. L'action immuno-adjuvante du poly IC chez la souris et son application au traitement de la leucémie L1210. CR Acad Sci *272*, 170–173, 1970c

Mathé, G., Kamel, M., Dezfulian, M., Halle-Pannenko, O., and Bourut, C. An experimental screening for "systemic adjuvants of immunity" applicable to cancer immunotherapy. Cancer Res *33*, 1987–1997, 1973

Mathé, G., Loc, T. B., and Bernard, J. Effet sur la Leucémie L1210 de la souris d'une combinaison par diazotization d'A-methoptérine et de γ-globulines de hamsters porteurs de cette leucémie par hétérogreffe. CR Acad Sci *246*, 1626–1628, 1958

Mathé, G., Musset, M., Schwarzenberg, L., Hayat, M., DeVassal, F., Amiel, J. L., Pouillart, P., and Misset, J. L. Phase II trial of active immunotherapy of acute myeloid leukemia. Biomedicine *23*, 291–293, 1975b

Mathé, G., Olsson, L. Florentin, I., Kiger, N., Bruley-Rosset, M., Orbach-Arbuoys, S., and Schulz, J. I. From BCG to more quantifiable immunity systemic adjuvants in active immunotherapy of cancer minimal residual disease. Proc Chicago Symp (sponsored by Univ Illinois) (Sept 1978) (in press), 1980

Mathé, G., Pouillart, P., and Lapeyraque, F. Active immunotherapy of L1210 leukemia applied after the graft of tumor cells. Br J. Cancer *23*, 814–824, 1969b

Mathé, G., Schwarzenberg, L., Amiel, J. L., Schneider, M., Cattan, M., and Schlumberger, J. R. The role of immunology in the treatment of leukemias and haematosarcomas. Cancer Res *27*, 2542–2553, 1967

Mathé, G., Schwarzenberg, L., DeVassal, F., and Delgado, M. Chemotherapy followed by active immunotherapy in the treatment of acute lymphoid leukemias for patients of all ages: Results of ICIG protocols 1, 9 and 10, prognostic factors and therapeutic indications, pp 451–468. In Terry, W. D., and Windhorst, D. (Eds): Immunotherapy of Cancer: Present Status of Trials in Man. New York: Raven Press, 1978

Mathé, G., Schwarzenberg, L., Kiger, N., Florentin, I., Halle-Pannenko, O., and Garcia-Giralt, E. Bone marrow transplantation for aplasias and leukemias. Clin Immunobiol 2, 33–62, 1974b

Matsumoto, T. Antigenicity of a crude lipopolysaccharide fraction of the methylcholanthrene-induced tumor, with special reference to isologous immunity in inbred rats. Gann 56, 1–11, 1965

Matsumoto, T., Otsu, K., and Komeda, T. Induction of host resistance against isotransplantation of C-1498 leukemia by spleen cells from tumor-bearing donors. Gann 57, 143–153, 1966

Maurer, A. M., Saunders, E. F., and Lampkin, C. B. Possible significance of nonproliferating leukemic cells. Natl Cancer Inst Monogr 30, 63–79, 1969

Mavligit, G. M., Gutterman, J. U., Burgess, M. A., Khankhanian, N., Seibert, G. B., Speer, J. F., Reed, R. C., Jubert, A. V., Martin, R. C., McBride, C. M., Copeland, F. M., Gehan, E. A., and Hersh, E. M. Adjuvant immunotherapy and chemoimmunotherapy in colorectal cancer of the Dukes' C classification. Cancer 36, 2421–2427, 1975

Mavligit, G. M., Gutterman, J. U., Burgess, M. A., Khankhanian, N., Seibert, G. B., Speer, J. F., Jubert, A. V., Martin, R. C., McBride, C. M., Copeland, E. M., Gehan, E. A., and Hersh, E. M. Prolongation of postoperative disease-free interval and survival in human colorectal cancer by BCG or BCG plus 5-fluorouracil. Lancet 1, 871–875, 1976

Mavligit, G. M., Gutterman, J. U., McBride, C. M., and Hersh, E. M. Cell-mediated immunity to human solid tumors: In vitro detection by lymphocyte blastogenic responses to cell-associated and solubilized tumor antigens. Natl Cancer Inst Monogr 37, 167–176, 1973

Mavligit, G. M., Gutterman, J. U., Malahy, M. A., Burgess, M. A., McBride, C. M., Jubert, A., and Hersh, E. M. Systemic adjuvant immunotherapy and chemoimmunotherapy in patients with colorectal cancer (Dukes' C Class): Prolongation of disease free interval and survival, pp 597–604, In Terry, W. D., and Windhorst, D. (Eds): Immunotherapy of Cancer: Present Status of Trials in Man. New York: Raven Press, 1978

Mayneord, W. V. On a law of growth of Jensen's rat sarcoma. Am J Cancer 16, 841–846, 1932

Mayr, A. C., Senn, H. J., Gallmeier, W. M., Drings, P., and Queisser, W. Randomized trial in advanced breast cancer using combination chemotherapy with or without C. parvum; Preliminary results. Dev Biol Stand 38, 553–557, 1978a

Mayr, A. C., Westerhausen, M., and Senn, H. J. Toxic and immunologic side effects of daily C. parvum-infusion in treatment-resistant cancer patients. Dev Biol Stand 38, 523–527, 1978b

Mazurek, C., Chalvet, H., Stiffel, C., and Biozzi, G. Study of the mechanism of Corynebacterium parvum anti-tumour activity. I. Protective effect on the growth of two syngeneic tumours. Int J Cancer 17, 511–517, 1976

Medawar, P. B., and Hunt, R. Vulnerability of methylcholanthrene-induced tumors to immunity aroused by syngeneic foetal cells. Nature 271, 164–165, 1978

Medical Research Council. Streptomycin in Tuberculosis Trials Committee Report. Br Med J 2, 769–782, 1948

Medical Research Council's Working Party on Leukaemia in Childhood. Treatment of acute lymphoblastic leukaemia. Comparison of immunotherapy (BCG), intermittent methotrexate, and no therapy after a five-month intensive cytotoxic regimen (Concord trial). Br Med J 4, 189–194, 1971

Meerpohl, H.-G., Lohmann-Matthes, M. L., and Fischer, H. Studies on the activation of mouse bone marrow-derived marcophages by the macrophage cytotoxicity factor (MCF). Eur J Immunol 6, 213–217, 1976

Meier, H. Etiologic considerations of spontaneous tumors in animals with special reference to the endocrine system. Ann NY Acad Sci 108, 881–889, 1963

Meier, H., Myers, D. D., and Huebner, R. J. Ineffectiveness of poly rI:rC on transplanted tumors induced by methylcholanthrene. Naturwissenschaften 57, 248–249, 1970

Mellors, R. C. Autoimmune disease in NZB/BL mice. II. Autoimmunity and malignant lymphoma. Blood 27, 435–448, 1966

Mellstedt, H. In vitro activation of human T and B lymphocytes by pokeweed mitogen. Clin Exp Immunol 19, 75–82, 1975

Mellstedt, H., Ahre, A., Bjorkholm, M., Holm, G., Johansson, B. and Strander, H. Interferon therapy in myelomatosis. Lancet 1, 245–247, 1979

Meltzer, M. S. Tumoricidal responses in vitro of peritoneal macrophages from conventionally housed and germ-free nude mice. Cell Immunol 22, 176–181, 1976

Meltzer, M. S., Jones, E. E., and Boetcher, D. A. Increased chemotactic response of macrophages from BCG infected mice. Cell Immunol *17*, 268–276, 1975a

Meltzer, M. S., Tucker, R. W., and Breuer, A. C. Interaction of BCG-activated macrophages with neoplastic and nonneoplastic cell lines in vitro: Cinemicrographic analysis. Cell Immunol *17*, 30–42, 1975b

Mempel, W., and Thierfelder, S. Die Wirkung von Antilymphozytenserum allein oder in Verbindung mit einem Zytostatikum auf eine Mäuselukämie. Blut *20*, 37–43, 1970

Menard, S., and Colnaghi, M. I. Embryonic antigens shared between chemically induced lymphosarcomas and fibrosarcomas of the mouse. J Natl Cancer Inst *54*, 479–481, 1975

Menard, S., Colnaghi, M. I., and Della Porta, G. In vitro demonstration of tumour-specific common antigens and embryonal antigens in murine fibrosarcomas induced by 7,12-dimethylbenz(a)anthrene. Cancer Res *33*, 478–481, 1973

Menard, S., Colnaghi, M. I., and Della Porta, G. Embryonic antigens and growth of murine fibrosarcomata. Br J Cancer *30*, 524–531, 1974

Mendelsohn, M. L. Autoradiographic analysis of cell proliferation in spontaneous breast cancer of C3H mouse. III. The growth fraction. J Natl Cancer Inst *28*, 1015–1029, 1962

Mendelsohn, M. L. Cell proliferation and tumour growth, pp 190–210, In Lamerton, L. F., and Fry, R. J. M. (Eds): Cell Proliferation. Oxford: Blackwell, 1963

Mendelsohn, M. L., and Takahashi, M. A critical evaluation of the fraction of labeled mitoses method as applied to the analysis of tumor and other cell cycles, pp 58–95, In Baserga, R. (Ed): The Cell Cycle and Cancer. New York: Marcel Dekker, 1971

Meriadec de Byans, B., Ducimetière, P., Richard, J. L., Salard, J. L., and Henry, R. Variations in carcinoembryonic antigen levels correlated with tobacco consumption in normal subjects. Biomedicine *25*, 197–198, 1976

Merigan, T. C., DeClercq, E., Eckstein, F., and Wells, R. D. Molecular requirements for synthetic RNA to act in interferon stimulation, pp 67–78, In Beers, R. F., and Braun, W. (Eds): Biological Effects of Polynucleotides. New York: Springer-Verlag, 1971

Merigan, T. C., Sikora, K., Breeden, J. H. Levy, R. and Rosenberg, S. A. Preliminary observations on the effect of human leukocyte interferon in non-Hodgkins lymphoma patients. New Engl J Med, *299*, 1449–1453, 1978

Merrill, J. P., Murray, J. E., Harrison, J. H., Friedman, E. A., Dealy, J. B., and Dammin, G. J. Successful homotransplantation of the kidney between nonidentical twins. N Engl J Med *262*, 1251–1260, 1960

Merritt, C. B., Darrow, C. C., Vaal, L., Herzig, G. P., and Rogentine, G. N. Rescue of rhesus monkeys from acute lethal graft-versus-host disease using cyclophosphamide and frozen autologous bone marrow. Transplantation *15*, 154–159, 1973

Merritt, K., and Johnson, A. G. Studies on the adjuvant action of bacterial endotoxins on antibody formation. VI. Enhancement of antibody formation by nucleic acids. J Immunol *94*, 416–422, 1965

Metcalf, D. Thymus grafts and leukemogenesis. Cancer Res *24*, 1952–1957, 1964

Metcalf, D. Human leukaemia: Recent tissue culture studies on the nature of myeloid leukaemia. Br J Cancer *27*, 191–202, 1973

Metcalf, W., Analysis of cancer survival as an exponential phenomenon. Surg Gynecol Obstet *138*, 731–740, 1974

Metchnikoff, O. The Life of Eli Metchnikoff, 1845–1916. London: Constable, 1921

Metzgar, R. S., Mohanakumar, T., and Bolognesi, D. P. Relationship between membrane antigens of human leukemic cells and oncogenic RNA virus structural components. J Exp Med *143*, 47–63, 1976

Meyer, T. J., Ribi, E. E., Azuma, I., and Zbar, B. Biologically active components from mycobacterial cell walls. II. Suppression and regression of strain-2 guinea pig hepatoma. J Natl Cancer Inst *52*, 103–112, 1974

Michaels, L. Cancer incidence and mortality in patients having anti-coagulant therapy. Lancet *2*, 832–835, 1964

Mider, G. B. Neoplastic diseases: Some metabolic aspects. Annu Rev Med *4*, 187–198, 1953

Mihich, E. Combined effects of chemotherapy and immunity against leukemia L1200 in DBA/2 mice. Cancer Res *29*, 848–854, 1969

Miké, V., and Marcove, R. C. Osteogenic sarcoma under the age of 21: Experience at the Memorial Sloan-Kettering Cancer Center, pp 283–292, In Terry, W. D., and Windhorst, D. (Eds): Immunotherapy of Cancer: Present Status of Trials in Man. New York: Raven Press, 1978

Mikulska, Z. B., Smith, C., and Alexander P. Evidence for an immunological reaction of the host directed against its own actively growing primary tumor. J Natl Cancer Inst *36*, 29–35, 1966

Milas, L., Basic, I., Kogelnik, H. D., and Withers, H. R. Effects of Corynebacterium granulosum on weight and histology of lymphoid organs, response to mitogens, skin allografts, and a syngeneic fibrosarcoma in mice. Cancer Res *35*, 2365–2374, 1975a

Milas, L., Gutterman, J. U., Basic, I., Hunter, N., Mavligit, G. M., Hersh, E. M., and Withers, H. R. Immunoprophylaxis and immunotherapy for a murine fibrosarcoma with C. granulosum and C. parvum. Int J Cancer *14*, 493–503, 1974a

Milas, L., Hunter, N., Basic, I., Mason, K., Grdina, D. J., and Withers, H. R. Nonspecific immunotherapy of murine solid tumors with Corynebacterium granulosum. J Natl Cancer Inst *54*, 895–902, 1975b

Milas, L., Hunter, N., Basic, I., and Withers, H. R. Protection by Corynebacterium granulosum against radiation-induced enhancement of artificial pulmonary metastases of a murine fibrosarcoma. J Natl Cancer Inst *52*, 1875–1880, 1974b

Milas, L., Hunter, N., Basic, I., and Withers, H. R. Complete regressions of an established murine fibrosarcoma induced by systemic application of Corynebacterium granulosum. Cancer Res *34*, 2470–2475, 1974c

Milas, L., Hunter, N., Stone, H. B., and Withers, R. H. Corynebacterium parvum: Effect on radiocurability of murine tumors. Cancer Immunol Immunother *5*, 109–117, 1978

Milas, L., Hunter, N., and Withers, H. R. Corynebacterium granulosum-induced protection against artificial pulmonary metastases of a syngeneic fibrosarcoma in mice. Cancer Res *34*, 613–620, 1974d

Milas, L., Hunter, N., and Withers, H. R. Combination of local irradiation with systemic application of anaerobic corynebacteria in therapy of a murine fibrosarcoma. Cancer Res *35*, 1274–1277, 1975c

Milas, L., Kogelnik, H. D., Basic, I., Mason, K., Hunter, N., and Withers, H. R. Combination of C. parvum and specific immunization against artificial pulmonary metastases in mice. Int J Cancer *16*, 738–746, 1975d

Milas, L., Mason, K., and Withers, H. R. Therapy of spontaneous pulmonary metastases of a murine mammary carcinoma with anaerobic corynebacteria. Cancer Immunol Immunother *1*, 233–237, 1976

Milas, L., and Mujagic, H. Protection by corynebacterium parvum against tumour cells injected intravenously. Rev Eur Etudes Clin Biol *17*, 498–500, 1972

Milas, L., and Scott, M. T. Antitumor activity of Corynebacterium parvum. Adv Cancer Res *26*, 257–306, 1977

Miles, C. P. Non-random chromosome changes in human cancer. Br J Cancer *30*, 73–85, 1974

Miles, W. E. A method of performing abdominoperineal excision for carcinoma of the rectum and of the terminal portion of the pelvic colon. Lancet *2*, 1812–1813, 1908

Milhaud, G., Calmettes, C., Taboulet, J., Julienne, A., and Moukhtar, M. S. Hypersecretion of calcitonin in neoplastic conditions. Lancet *1*, 462–463, 1974

Miller, B. J., and Rosenbaum, A. S. The vascular supply to metastatic tumors of the lung. Surg Gynecol Obstet *125*, 1009–1012, 1967

Miller, D. G., Molovanu, G., Kaplan, A., and Tocci, S. Antilymphocytic leukemic serum and chemotherapy in the treatment of murine leukemia. Cancer *22*, 1192–1198, 1968

Miller, E. C., and Miller, J. A. In vivo combinations between carcinogens and tissue constituents and their possible role in carcinogenesis. Cancer Res *12*, 547–556, 1952

Miller, E. C., and Miller, J. A. Mechanisms of chemical carcinogenesis: Nature of proximate carcinogens and interactions with macromolecules. Pharmacol Rev *18*, 805–838, 1966

Miller, E. C., and Miller, J. A. The mutagenicity of chemical carcinogens: Correlations, problems and interpretations, pp 83–119, In Hollaender, A. (Ed): Chemical Mutagens, Vol 1. New York, London: Plenum Press, 1971

Miller, H. C., Woodruff, M. W., and Gambacorta, J. P. Spontaneous regression of pulmonary metastases from hypernephroma. Ann Surg *156*, 852–856, 1962

Miller, J. A. Carcinogenesis by chemicals: An overview—GHA Clowes Memorial Lecture. Cancer Res *30*, 559–576, 1970

Miller, J. F. A. P. Role of the thymus in murine leukaemia. Nature *183*, 1069, 1959

Miller, J. F. A. P. Etiology and pathogenesis of mouse leukemia. Adv Cancer Res *6*, 292–368, 1961

Miller, J. F. A. P. Selective activation of T lymphocytes. Its possible application in the immunomanipulation of tumors. Biomedicine *18*, 81–85, 1973

Miller, J. F. A. P., Brunner, K. T., Sprent, J., Russell, P. J., and Mitchell, G. F. Thymus-derived cells as killer cells in cell-mediated immunity. Transplant Proc *3*, 915–917, 1971

Miller, J. F. A. P., Grant, G. A., and Roe, F. J. C. Effect of thymectomy on the induction of skin tumours by 3,4-benzopyrene. Nature *199*, 920–922, 1963

Miller, J. F. A. P., and Osoba, D. Current concepts of the immunological function of the thymus. Physiol Rev *47*, 437–520, 1967

Miller, J. F. A. P., Ting, R. C., and Law, L. W. Influence of thymectomy on tumor induction by polyoma virus in C57BL mice. Proc Soc Exp Biol Med *116*, 323–327, 1964

Miller, J. F. A. P., and Vadas, M. A. The major histocompatibility complex: Influence on immune reactivity and T-lymphocyte activation. Scand J Immunol *6*, 771–778, 1977

Miller, J. J., Gaffney, P. R., Rees, J. A., and Symes, M. O. Lymphocyte reactivity in patients with carcinoma of the breast and large bowel. Br. J. Cancer *32*, 16–20, 1975

Miller, R. G., and Dunkley, M. Quantitative analysis of the ^{51}Cr release cytotoxicity assay for cytotoxic lymphocytes. Cell Immunol *14*, 284–302, 1974

Miller, T. E., Mackaness, G. B., and Lagrange, P. H. Immunopotentiation with BCG. II. Modulation of the response to sheep red blood cells. J Natl Cancer Inst *51*, 1669–1677, 1973

Miller, T. R., and Nicholson, J. T. End results in reticulum cell sarcoma of bone treated by bacterial toxin therapy alone or combined with surgery and/or radiotherapy (47 cases) or with concurrent infection (5 cases). Cancer *27*, 524–548, 1974

Miller, W. R., and Forrest, A. P. M. Oestradiol synthesis by a human breast carcinoma. Lancet *2*, 866–868, 1974

Miller, W. R., and Forrest, A. P. M. Oestradiol synthesis from C19 seroids by human breast cancers. Br J Cancer *33*, 116–118, 1976

Millman, I., Scott, A. W., and Halbherr, T. Antitumor activity of Propionibacterium acnes (Corynebacterium parvum) and isolated cytoplasmic fractions. Cancer Res *37*, 4150–4155, 1977

Milton, G. W. Some methods used in the management of metastatic malignant melanoma. Australas J Dermatol *7*, 15–22, 1963

Milton, G. W. Malignant melanoma and a study of some aspects of cancer. J R Coll Surg Edinb *14*, 193–202, 1969

Milton, G. W., and Lane Brown, M. M. The limited role of attenuated smallpox virus in the management of advanced malignant melanoma. Aust NZ J Surg *35*, 286–290, 1966

Milton, G. W., McGovern, V. J., and Lewis, M. G. Malignant Melanoma of the Skin and Mucous Membrane. London: Churchill Livingstone, 1977

Minden, P., McClatchy, J. K., Wainberg, M., and Weiss, D. W. Shared antigens between mycobacterium bovis (BCG) and neoplastic cells. J Natl Cancer Inst *53*, 1325–1331, 1974a

Minden, P., Sharpton, T. R., and McClatchy, J. K. Shared antigens between human malignant melanoma cells and mycobacterium bovis (BCG). J Immunol *116*, 1407–1414, 1976

Minden, P., Wainberg, M., and Weiss, D. W. Protection against guinea pig hepatomas by pretreatment with subcellular fractions of mycobacterium bovis (BCG). J Natl Cancer Inst *52*, 1643–1645, 1974b

Minor, P. D., and Smith, J. A. Explanation of degree of correlation of sibling generation times in animal cells. Nature *248*, 241–243, 1974

Minton, J. P., Rossio, J. L., Dixon, B., and Dodd, M. C. The effect of Corynebacterium parvum on the humoral and cellular immune system in patients with breast cancer. Clin Exp Immunol *24*, 441–447, 1976

Mintz, B., and Illmensee, K. Normal genetically mosaic mice produced from malignant teratocarcinoma cells. Proc Natl Acad Sci USA *72*, 3585–3589, 1975

Misdorp, W., and den Herder, B. A. Bone metastasis in mammary cancer. A report of 10 cases in the female dog and some comparison with human cases. Br J Cancer *20*, 496–503, 1966

Mitchell, D. N., Rees, R. J. W., and Salsbury, A. J. Human myeloma marrow cells in immunologically deficient mice. Br J Cancer *30*, 33–41, 1974

Mitchell, M. S., Mokyr, M. B., and Kahane, I. Stimulation of the lymphoid cells by components of BCG. J Natl Cancer Inst *55*, 1337–1342, 1975

Mitcheson, H. D., and Castro, J. E. Clinical studies with Corynebacterium parvum. Dev Biol Stand *38*, 509–514, 1978

Mitchison, J. M. The Biology of the Cell Cycle. London: Cambridge University Press, 1971

Mitchison, N. A. Passive transfer of transplantation immunity. Proc R Soc Lond B *142*, 72–87, 1954

Mitchison, N. A. Studies on the immunological response to foreign tumor transplants in the mouse. I. The role of lymph node cells in conferring immunity by adoptive transfer. J. Exp Med *102*, 157–177, 1955

Mitchison, N. A., and Dube, O. L. Studies on the immunological response to foreign tumor transplants in the mouse. II. The relation between hemagglutinating antibody and graft resistance in the normal mouse and mice pretreated with tissue preparations. J Exp Med *102*, 179–197, 1955

Miyabo, S., Fujimura, A., Matsuda, T., and Murakami, M. Gastric cancer containing insulin and associated with hypoglycemia. Diabetes *17*, 286–289, 1968

Miyaji, T. Multiple primary malignant tumors among autopsy cases in Japan during the thirteen years 1958–1970, p 3, In Severi, L. (Ed): Fifth Perugia International Conference on Cancer, 1973. Perugia Univ, 1974

Mizejewski, G. J., and Allen, R. P. Immunotherapeutic suppression in transplantable solid tumours with anti AFP serum. Nature 250, 50–52, 1974

Mizuno, D., Yoshioka, O., Akamatsu, M., and Kataoka, T. Antitumor effect of intracutaneous injection of bacterial lipopolysaccharide. Cancer Res 28, 1531–1537, 1968

Mobbs, B. G. The uptake of tritiated oestradiol by dimethylbenzanthracene-induced mammary tumours of the rat. J Endocrinol 36, 409–414, 1966

Moertel, C. G. Multiple primary malignant neoplasms. Recent Results Cancer Res 7, 1–108, 1966

Moertel, C. G. In discussion, Mavligit, G. M., p 604, In Terry, W. D., and Windhorst, D. (Eds): Immunotherapy of Cancer: Present Status of Trials in Man. New York: Raven Press, 1978

Moertel, C. G., O'Connell, M. J., Ritts, R. E., Schutt, A. J., Reitemeier, R. J., Hahn, R. G., Frytak, S. K., and Rubin, J. A controlled evaluation of combined immunotherapy (MER-BCG) and chemotherapy for advanced colorectal cancer, pp 573–584, In Terry, W. D., and Windhorst, D. (Eds): Immunotherapy of Cancer: Present Status of Trials in Man. New York: Raven Press, 1978

Moertel, C. G., Ritts, R. E., Schutt, A. J., and Hahn, R. G. Clinical studies of methanol extraction residue fraction of bacillus Calmette-Guérin as an immunostimulant in patients with advanced cancer. Cancer Res 35, 3075–3083, 1975

Mohos, S. C., and Kidd, J. G. Effects of various immune rabbit serums on the cells of several transplanted mouse lymphomas in vitro and in vivo. J Exp Med 105, 233–263, 1957

Mohr, U., Althoff, J., Kinzel, V., Suss, R., and Volm, M. Melanoma regression induced by chalone: A new tumour inhibiting principle acting in vivo. Nature 220, 138–139, 1968

Mohr, U., Boldingh, H. W., and Althoff, J. Identification of contaminating clostridium spores as the oncolytic agent in some chalone preparations. Cancer Res 32, 1117–1121, 1972a

Mohr, U., Boldingh, W. H., Emminger, A., and Behagel, H. A. Oncolysis by a new strain of clostridium. Cancer Res 32, 1122–1128, 1972b

Mokyr, M. B., Braun, D. P., Usher, D., Reiter, H., and Dray, S. The development of in vitro and in vivo antitumor cytotoxicity in noncy-
totoxic, MOPC-315-tumor-bearer, spleen cells "educated" in vitro with MOPC-315 tumor cells. Cancer Immunol Immunother 4, 143–150, 1978

Mokyr, M. B., and Mitchell, M. S. Activation of lymphoid cells by BCG in vitro. Cell Immunol 15, 264–273, 1975

Mole, R. H. The development of leukaemia in irradiated animals. Br Med Bull 14, 174–177, 1958

Möller, E. Contact-induced cytotoxicity by lymphoid cells containing foreign isoantigens. Science 147, 873–879, 1965

Möller, E., Lapp, W., and Lindholm, L. Allogeneic inhibition in tolerant animals. Transplant Proc 1, 543–547, 1969

Möller, E., and Möller, G. Quantitative studies of the sensitivity of normal and neoplastic mouse cells to the cytotoxic action of isoantibodies. J Exp Med 115, 527–553, 1962

Möller, G. Effect on tumour growth in syngeneic recipients of antibodies against tumour-specific antigens in methylcholanthrene-induced mouse sarcomas. Nature 204, 846–847, 1964

Möller, G., and Möller, E. Foreword: The Concept of Immunological Surveillance Against Neoplasia. Transplant Rev 28, 3–15, 1976

Moloney, J. B. The murine leukemias. Fed Proc 21, 19–31, 1962

Mondovi, B. Biochemical and ultrastructural lesions, pp 3–15, In Wizenberg, M. J., and Robinson, J. E. (Eds): Proc Intern Symp Cancer Therapy by Hyperthermia and Radiation. Baltimore: Am Coll Radiol Press, 1976

Mondovi, B., Strom, R., Rotilio, G., Agro, A. F., Cavaliere, R., and Rossi-Fanelli, A. The biochemical mechanism of selective heat sensitivity of cancer cells I. Studies on cellular respiration. Eur J Cancer 5, 129–136, 1969

Monis, B., and Weinberg, T. Cytochemical study of esterase activity of human neoplasms and stromal macrophages. Cancer 14, 369–377, 1961

Moon, H. D., Simpson, M. E., and Evans, H. M. Inhibition of methylcholanthrene carcinogenesis by hypophysectomy. Science 116, 331, 1952

Moore, A. E. Destruction of sarcoma 180 by Russian encephalitis virus with host survival. Proc Am Assoc Cancer Res 1, 39, 1953

Moore, D. H. Charney, J., Kramarsky, B., Lasfargues, E. Y., Sarkar, N. H., Brennan, M. J., Burrows, J. H., Sirsat, S. M., Paymaster, J. C., and Vaidya, A. B. Search for a human breast cancer virus. Nature 229, 611–615, 1971

Moore, D. H., Sarkar, N. H., Kelly, C. E., Pillsbury, N., and Charney, J. Type B particles in human milk. Tex Rep Biol Med 27, 1027–1039, 1969

Moore, G. E., and Gerner, R. E. Cancer immunity—Hypothesis and clinical trial of lymphocytotherapy for malignant diseases. Ann Surg 172, 733–739, 1970

Moore, G. E., Gerner, R. E., and Franklin, H. A. Culture of normal human leukocytes. JAMA 199, 519–524, 1967

Moore, G. E., and Moore, M. B. Autoinoculation of cultured human lymphocytes in malignant melanoma. NY State Med 69, 460–462, 1969

Moore, G. E., Sandberg, A., and Amos, D. B. Experimental and clinical adventures with large doses of gamma and other globulins as anti-cancer agents. Surgery 41, 972–983, 1957a

Moore, G. E., Sandberg, A., and Schubarg, J. R. Clinical and experimental observations of occurrence and fate of tumor cells in blood stream. Ann Surg 146, 580–587, 593–595, 1957b

Moore, M., Lawrence, N., and Nisbet, N. W. Tumour inhibition mediated by BCG in immunosuppressed rats. Int J Cancer 15, 897–911, 1975

Moore, M., Lawrence, N., and Nisbet, N. W. Inhibition of transplanted sarcomas mediated by BCG in rats with a defined immunological deficit. Biomedicine 24, 26–31, 1976

Moore, M., Lawrence, N., and Witherow, P. J. Suppression of transplanted rat sarcomata mediated by bacillus Calmette-Guérin (BCG). Eur J Cancer 10, 673–682, 1974

Moore, M., and Robinson, N. Cell-mediated cytotoxicity in carcinoma of the human urinary bladder. Cancer Immunol Immunother 2, 233–243, 1977

Moore, T. L., Kubchik, H. Z., Marcon, N., and Zamchek, N. Carcinoembryonic antigen assay in cancer of the colon and pancreas and other digestive tract disorders. Am J Digest Dis 16, 1–7, 1971

Morahan, P. S., and Kaplan, A. M. Macrophage activation and anti-tumor activity of biologic and synthetic agents. Int J Cancer 17, 82–89, 1976

Morales, A., Eidinger, D., and Bruce, A. W. Intracavitary BCG in the treatment of superficial bladder cancer. J Urol 116, 180–183, 1976

Morales, A., Eidinger, D., and Bruce, A. W. Adjuvant BCG immunotherapy in recurrent superficial bladder cancer, pp 225–231, In Terry, W. D., and Windhorst, D. (Eds): Immunotherapy of Cancer: Present Status of Trials in Man. New York: Raven Press, 1978

More, D. G., and Nelson, D. S. Antigen induced mitosis in liver macrophages of immunized mice. Experientia 28, 566–567, 1972

More, D. G., Penrose, J. M., Kearney, R., and Nelson, D. S. Immunological induction of DNA synthesis in mouse peritoneal macrophages. An expression of cell-mediated-immunity. Int Arch Allergy 44, 611–630, 1973

Moreschi, C. Ueber Antigene und pyrogene Wirkung des Typhusbacillus bei leukämischen Kranken. Z Immuno-Forsch 21, 410–421, 1914

Morgan, A. G., and Soothill, J. F. Measurement of the clearance function of macrophages with ^{125}I-labelled polyvinyl pyrrolidone. Clin Exp Immunol 20, 489–497, 1975

Morgan, C. N., and Lloyd-Davies, O. V. The comparative results and treatment for cancer of the rectum. Postgrad Med J 26, 135–141, 1959

Mori, R., Nomoto, K., and Takeya, K. Tumor formation by polyoma virus in neonatally thymectomized mice. Proc Jpn Acad 40, 445–447, 1964

Mori, W., Masuda, M., and Miyanaga, T. Hepatic artery ligation and tumor necrosis in the liver. Surgery 59, 359–363, 1966

Moroni, C., and Shumann, G. Are endogenous C-type viruses involved in the immune system? Nature 269, 600–601, 1977

Moroson, H., and Schechter, M. Treatment of rat fibrosarcoma by radiotherapy plus immune adjuvant. Biomedicine 25, 97–100, 1976

Morrison, A. S., Black, M. M., Lowe, C. R., MacMahon, B., and Yuasa, S. Some international differences in histology and survival in breast cancer. Int J Cancer 11, 261–267, 1973

Morton, D. L. Successful isoimmunization against a spontaneous mammary tumor on C3H/HEN mice. Proc Am Assoc Cancer Res 3, 346, 1962

Morton, D. L., Eilber, F. R., Holmes, E. C., Hunt, J. S., Ketcham, A. S., Silverstein, M. J., and Sparks, F. C. BCG immunotherapy of malignant melanoma: Summary of a seven-year experience. Ann Surg 180, 635–643, 1974

Morton, D. L., Eilber, F. R., Holmes, E. C., Sparks, F. C., and Ramming, K. P. Present status of BCG immunotherapy of malignant melanoma. Cancer Immunol Immunother 1, 93–98, 1976

Morton, D. L., Eilber, F. R., and Malmgren, R. A. Immune factors in human cancer: Malignant melanomas, skeletal and soft tissue sarcomas. Proc Exp Tumor Res 14, 25–42, 1971a

Morton, D. L., Eilber F. R., Malmgren, R. A., and Wood, W. Immunological factors which influence response to immunotherapy in malignant melanoma. Surgery 68, 158–164, 1970

Morton, D. L., Goldman, L., and Wood, D. A. Acquired immunological tolerance and carcinogenesis by the mammary tumor virus. II. Immune responses influencing growth of spontaneous mammary adenocarcinomas. J Natl Cancer Inst 42, 321–329, 1969a

Morton, D. L., Hall, W. T., and Malmgren, R. A. Human liposarcomas: Tissue culture containing foci of transformed cells with viral particles. Science 165, 813–816, 1969b

Morton, D. L., Holmes, E. C., Eilber, F. R., Sparks, F. C., and Ramming, K. P. Adjuvant immunotherapy of malignant melanoma: Preliminary results of a randomized trial in patients with lymph node metastases, pp 57–64, In Terry, W. D., and Windhorst, D. (Eds): Immunotherapy of Cancer: Present Status of Trials in Man. New York: Raven Press, 1978

Morton, D. L., Holmes, E. C., Eilber, F. R., and Wood, W. C. Immunological aspects of neoplasia. A rational basis for immunotherapy. Ann Intern Med 74, 587–604, 1971b

Morton, D. L., Joseph, W. L., Ketcham, A. S., Gleehoed, G. W., and Adkins, P. C. Surgical resection and adjunctive immunotherapy for selected patients with multiple pulmonary metastases. Ann Surg 178, 360–366, 1973

Morton, D. L., and Malmgren, R. A. Human osteosarcomas: Immunologic evidence suggesting an associated infectious agent. Science 162, 1279–1281, 1968

Morton, D. L., Malmgren, R. A., Hall, W. T., and Schidlovsky, B. S. Immunologic and virus studies with human sarcomas. Surgery 66, 152–161, 1969c

Morton, D. L., Malmgren, R. A., Holmes, E. C., and Ketcham, A. S. Demonstration of antibodies against human malignant melanoma by immunofluorescence. Surgery 64, 233–240, 1968

Morton, D. L., Miller, G. F., and Wood, D. A. Demonstration of tumor-specific immunity against antigens unrelated to the mammary tumor virus in spontaneous mammary adenocarcinomas. J Natl Cancer Inst 42, 289–301, 1969d

Möse, J. R., and Möse, G. Onkolyseversuche mit apathogen anaeroben Sporenbildnern am Ehrlich-tumor der Maus. Z Krebsforsch 63, 63–74, 1959

Möse, J. R., Möse, G., Probst, A., and Heppner, F. Onkolyse maligner Tumoren durch den Clostridienstamm M 55. Med Klin 62, 189–193, 220–225, 1967

Mosedale, B., and Smith, M. A. Corynebacterium parvum and anaesthetics. Lancet 1, 168, 1975

Motta, R. The passive immunotherapy of murine leukemia. I. The production of antisera against leukaemic antigens. Rev Eur Etudes Clin Biol 15, 161–167, 1970

Motta, R. Passive immunotherapy of leukemia and other cancer. Adv Cancer Res 14, 161–179, 1971

Mozes, E., Shearer, G. M., Sela, M., and Braun, W. Conversion with polynucleotides of a genetically controlled low immune response to a high response in mice immunized with a synthetic polypeptide antigen, pp 197–213, In Beers, E. F., and Braun, W. (Eds): Biological Effects of Polynucleotides. New York: Springer-Verlag, 1971

Müftüoğlu, A. Ü., and Balkur, S. Passive transfer of tuberculin sensitivity to patients with Hodgkin's disease. N Engl J Med 277, 126–129, 1967

Muggia, F. M. Immunotherapy of cancer. A short review and commentary on current trials. Cancer Immunol Immunother 3, 5–9, 1977

Muggleton, P. W., Prince, G. H., and Hilton, M. L. Effect of intravenous BCG in guineapigs and pertinence to cancer immunotherapy in man. Lancet 1, 1353–1355, 1975

Muhm, J. R., Brown, L. R., and Crowe, J. K. Use of computed tomography in the detection of pulmonary nodules. Mayo Clin Proc 52, 345–348, 1977

Mulvihill, J. J., Miller, R. W., and Fraumeni, J. F. (Eds): Genetics of Human Cancer. New York: Raven Press, 1977

Muna, N. M., Marcus, S., and Smart, C. Detection by immunofluorescence of antibodies specific for human malignant melanoma cells. Cancer 23, 88–93, 1969

Murphy, J. B. The lymphocyte in resistance to tissue grafting, malignant disease and tuberculosis infection. Monogr Rockefeller Inst Med Res No. 21, 1926

Murray, G. Experiments in immunity in cancer. Can Med Assoc J 79, 249–259, 1958

Murray, G. Experiments in host resistance to cancer (in human subjects). Am J Surg 109, 763–764, 1965

Murray, J. G. Cancer Research Campaign breast study. Br J Surg 61, 772–774, 1974

Murray, J. G., et al. Management of early cancer of the breast. Report on an international multicentre trial supported by the Cancer Research Campaign. Br Med J 1, 1035–1038, 1976

Murray-Lyon, I. M., Dawson, J. L., Parsons, V. A., Rake, M. O., Blendis, L. M., Laws, J. W., and Williams, R. Treatment of secondary hepatic tumours by ligation of hepatic artery and infusion of cytotoxic drugs. Lancet 2, 172–175, 1970

N

Nachtigal, D., Eshel-Zussman, R., and Feldman, M. Restoration of the specific immunological reactivity of tolerant rabbits by conjugated antigens. Immunology 9, 543–551, 1965

Nachtigal, D., and Feldman, M. The immune response to azo-protein conjugates in rabbits unresponsive to the protein carriers. Immunology 7, 616–625, 1964

Nachtigal, D., Zan-Bar, I., and Feldman, M. The role of specific suppressor T cells in immune tolerance. Transplant Rev 26, 87–105, 1975

Nadler, S. H., and Moore, G. E. Clinical immunologic study of malignant disease. Response to tumour transplants and transfer of lymphocytes. Ann Surg 164, 482–490, 1966

Nadler, S. H., and Moore, G. E. Immunotherapy of malignant disease. Arch Surg 99, 376–381, 1969

Nadler, S. H., and Moore, G. E. Response to injection of cultured human tumor cells. Arch Surg 100, 244–248, 1970

Nagasawa, H., and Yanai, R. Effects of prolactin or growth hormone on growth of carcinogen-induced mammary tumors of adreno-ovariectomized rats. Int J Cancer 6, 488–495, 1970

Naha, P. M., and Ashworth, M. On the theory of clonal selection in carcinogenic transformation. Br J Cancer 30, 448–458, 1974

Nahmias, A. J., Josey, W. E., Naib, Z. M., Luce, C., and Guest, B. Antibodies to herpesvirus hominis types 1 and 2 in humans. II. Women with cervical cancer. Am J Epidemiol 91, 547–561, 1970

Naib, Z. M., Nahmias, A. J., Josey, W. E., and Kramer, J. H. Genital herpetic infection: Association with cervical dysplasia and carcinoma. Cancer 23, 940–945, 1969

Nairn, R. C., Fothergill, J. E., McEntegart, M. G., and Richmond, H. G. Loss of gastro-intestinal-specific antigen in neoplasia. Br Med J 1, 1791–1793, 1962

Nairn, R. C., Nind, A. P. P., Guli, E. P. G., Davies, D. J., Little, J. H., Davis, N. C., and Whitehead, R. H. Anti-tumour immunoreactivity in patients with malignant melanoma. Med J Aust 1, 397–403, 1972

Nairn, R. C., Nind, A. P. P., Guli, E. P. G., Muller, H. K., Rolland, J. M., and Minty, C. C. J. Specific immune response in human skin carcinoma. Br Med J 4, 701–705, 1971a

Nairn, R. C., Nind, A. P. P., Guli, E. P. G., Davies, D. J., Rolland, J. M., McGiven, A. R., and Hughes, E. S. R. Immunological reactivity in patients with carcinoma of colon. Br Med J 4, 706–709, 1971b

Nairn, R. C., Philip, J., Ghose, T., Porteous, I. B., and Fothergill, J. E. Production of a precipitin against renal cancer. Br Med J 1, 1702–1704, 1963

Nairn, R. C., Richmond, H. G., McEntegart, M. G., and Fothergill, J. E. Immunological differences between normal and malignant cells. Br Med J 2, 1335–1340, 1960

Nakahara, W., and Fukuoka, F. The newer concept of cancer toxin. Adv Cancer Res 5, 157–177, 1958

Nakano, M., and Braun, W. Cell-released non-specific stimulators of antibody-forming cell populations. J Immunol 99, 570–575, 1967

Nandi, S. The histocompatibility-2 locus and susceptibility to Bittner virus borne by red blood cells in mice. Proc Natl Acad Sci USA 58, 485–492, 1967

Nathan, C. F., and Terry, W. D. Decreased phagocytosis by peritoneal macrophages from BCG-treated mice. Induction of the phagocytic defect in normal macrophages with BCG in vitro. Cell Immunol 29, 295–311, 1977

Nathanson, L. Regression of intradermal malignant melanoma after intralesional injection of Mycobacterium bovis strain BCG. Cancer Chemother Rep 56, 659–665, 1972

Nathanson, L. Immunology and immunotherapy of human breast cancer. Cancer Immunol Immunother 2, 209–224, 1977

National Cancer Institute Radiation Oncology Committee. Radiation therapy and immunotherapy. The value of immunotherapy in the control of local and regional cancer. Cancer 37, 2108–2119, 1976

Nauts, H. C. The apparently beneficial effects of bacterial infections on host resistance to cancer: End results in 435 cases. Monograph No. 8. New York: Cancer Research Institute, 1969

Nauts, H. C. Enhancement of natural resistance to renal cancer: Beneficial effects of concurrent infections and immunotherapy with bacterial vaccines. Monograph No. 12 New York: Cancer Research Institute, 1973

Nauts, H. C. Ewing's sarcoma of bone: End results following immunotherapy (bacterial toxins) combined with surgery and/or radiation. Monograph No. 14. New York: Cancer Research Institute, 1974

Nauts, H. C. Multiple myeloma: Beneficial effects of acute infections or immunotherapy (bacterial vaccines). Monograph No. 3. New York: Cancer Research Institute, 1975a

Nauts, H. C. Osteogenic sarcoma: End results following immunotherapy (bacterial vaccines) 165 cases, or concurrent infections, inflammation or fever, 41 cases. Monograph No. 15. New York: Cancer Research Institute, 1975b

Nauts, H. C. Beneficial effects of immunotherapy (bacterial toxins) on sarcoma of the soft tissues, other than lymphosarcoma: End results in 186 determinate cases with microscopic confirmation of diagnosis 49 operable, 137 inoperable. Monograph No. 16. New York: Cancer Research Institute, 1975c

Nauts, H. C. Giant cell tumor of bone: End results following immunotherapy (Coley toxins) alone or combined with surgery and/or radiation—66 cases—and concurrent infection—4 cases. Monograph No. 4. New York: Cancer Research Institute, 1976a

Nauts, H. C. Immunotherapy of Cancer by bacterial vaccines, In 3rd Int Symp Detection and Prevention of Cancer, New York, 1976b

Nauts, H. C. Immunological factors affecting incidence, prognosis and survival in breast cancer. Part I. The immunopotentiating effects of concurrent infections, inflammation or fever. Part II. Immunotherapy, effects of bacterial vaccines. Monograph No. 17. New York: Cancer Research Institute, 1977

Nauts, H. C. Bacterial vaccine therapy of cancer. Dev Biol Stand 38, 487–494, 1978

Nauts, H. C., and Fowler, G. A. End results in lymphosarcoma treated by toxin therapy alone or combined with surgery and/or radiation. Monograph No. 6. New York: Cancer Research Institute, 1969

Nauts, H. C., Swift, W. Z., and Coley, B. L. The treatment of tumors by bacterial toxins as developed by the late William B. Coley, M.D., reviewed in the light of modern research. Cancer Res 6, 205–216, 1946

Neff, J. R., and Enneking, W. F. Adoptive immunotherapy in primary osteosarcoma: An interim report. J Bone Joint Surg 57, 145–148, 1975

Negroni, G., and Hunter, E. Rejection of polyoma virus-induced neoplasms in mice inoculated with complement and antiserum. J Natl Cancer Inst 51, 265–268, 1973

Neidhart, J. A., and LoBuglio, A. E. Transfer-factor therapy of malignancy. Semin Oncol 1, 379–385, 1974

Nelson, D. S. Antigens of nasopharyngeal carcinoma. Clin Exp Immunol 8, 863–869, 1971

Nelson, D. S. Production by stimulated macrophages of factors depressing lymphocyte transformation. Nature 246, 306–307, 1973

Nelson, D. S. Antigens of carcinoma of the cervix uteri. A study by means of immunofluorescence. Clin Exp Immunol 16, 53–62, 1974

Nelson, D. S. (Ed); Immunobiology of the Macrophage. New York: Academic Press, 1976

Nelson, D. S. Autoantibodies in cancer patients. Pathology 9, 155–160, 1977

Nelson, D. S., and Nelson, M. Immunological and related aspects of nasopharyngeal carcinoma. Australas Radiol 15, 227–232, 1971

Nelson, H. S. Delayed hypersensitivity in cancer patients: Cutaneous and in vitro lymphocyte response to specific antigens. J Natl Cancer Inst 42, 765–770, 1969

Nelson, M., and Nelson, D. Macrophages and resistance to tumours. I. Inhibition of delayed-type hypersensitivity reactions by tumour cells and by soluble products affecting macrophages. Immunology 34, 277–290, 1978

Nemoto, T., Han, T., Minowada, J., Angkur, V., Chamberlain, A., and Dao, T. L. Cell-mediated immune status of breast cancer patients: Evaluation by skin tests, lymphocyte stimulation, and counts of rosette-forming cells. J Natl Cancer Inst 53, 641–645, 1974

Neveu, P. J. The effects of BCG on both cellular and humoral immunity during the early response to a hapten carrier complex. Clin Exp Immunol 26, 169–172, 1976

Neveu, T., Branellec, A., and Biozzi, G. Adjuvant effect of Corynebacterium parvum on antibody production and on induction of delayed hypersensitivity to conjugated proteins. Ann Inst Pasteur 106, 771–777, 1964

Newlands, E. S., Oon, C. J., Roberts, J. T., Elliott, P., Mould, R. F., Topham, C., Madden, F. J. F., Newton, K. A., and Westbury, G. Clinical trial of combination chemotherapy and specific active immunotherapy in disseminated melanoma. Br J Cancer 34, 174–179, 1976

Newman, C. E., Ford, C. H. J., Davies, D. A. L., and O'Neill, G. J. Antibody-drug synergism: An assessment of specific passive immunotherapy in bronchial carcinoma. Lancet 2, 163–166, 1977

Newman, W., and Southam, C. M. Virus treatment in advanced cancer. Cancer 7, 106–118, 1954

Newstead, G. L., Griffiths, J. D., and Salsbury, A. J. Fibrinolytic activity of carcinoma of the colorectum. Surg Gynecol Obstet 143, 61–64, 1976

Newton, K. A., Humble, J. G., Wilson, C. W., Pegg, D. E., and Skinner, M. E. G. Total thoracic supervoltage irradiation followed by the intravenous infusion of stored autogenous marrow. Br Med J 1, 531–535, 1959

Ngu, V. A. Host defenses to Burkitt tumor. Br Med J 1, 345–347, 1967

Nicholls, M. F., and Siddons, A. H. M. Spontaneous disappearance of lung metastases from hypernephroma. Br J Surg 47, 531–533, 1960

Nicolson, G. L. Difference in topology of normal and tumour cell membranes shown by different surface distribution of ferritin conjugated concanavalin A. Nature 233, 244–246, 1971

Nicolson, G. L., and Winkelhake, J. L. Organ specificity of blood-borne tumour metastasis determined by cell adhesion? Nature 255, 230–232, 1975

Niederhuber, J. E. The role of I region gene products in macrophage-T lymphocyte interaction. Immunol Rev 40, 28–52, 1978

Niederman, J. C., McCollum, R. W., Henle, G., and Henle, W. Infectious mononucleosis: Clinical manifestations in relation to EB virus antibodies. JAMA 203, 205–209, 1968

Nikoskelainen, J., Ablashi, D. V., Isenberg, R. A., Neel, E. U., Miller, R. G., and Stevens, D. A. Cellular immunity in infectious mononucleosis. II. Specific reactivity to Epstein-Barr virus antigens and correlation with clinical and hematological parameters. J Immunol 121, 1239–1244, 1978

Nilsson, A., Revesz, L., and Stjernsward, J. Suppression of strontium-90-induced development of bone tumors by infection with bacillus Calmette-Guérin (BCG). Radiat Res 26, 378–382, 1965

Nilsson, U. R., and Müller-Eberhard, H. J. Deficiency of the fifth component of complement in mice with an inherited complement defect. J Exp Med 125, 1–16, 1967

Nimberg, R. B., Glasgow, A. H., Menzoian, J. O., Constantian, M. B., Cooperband, S. R., Mannick, J. A., and Schmid, K. Isolation of an immunosuppressive peptide fraction from the serum of cancer patients. Cancer Res 35, 1489–1494, 1975

Nishioka, K., Tachibana, T., Klein, G., and Clifford, P. Complementological studies on tumor immunity. Measurement of C1 bound to tumor cells and immune adherence with Burkitt lymphoma cells. Gann Monogr No. 7, p 49, 1968

Nishioka, M., Ibata, T., Okita, K., Harada, T., and Fujita, T. Localization of α-fetoprotein in hepatoma tissues by immunofluorescence. Cancer Res 32, 162–166, 1972

Nkrumah, F. K., and Perkins, I. V. Burkitt's lymphoma in Ghana: Clinical features and response to chemotherapy. Int J Cancer 11, 19–29, 1973

Nkrumah, F. K., Perkins, A. B., and Biggar, R. J. Combination chemotherapy in abdominal Burkitt's lymphoma. Cancer 40, 1410–1416, 1977

Nomoto, K., and Takeya, K. Immunologic properties of methylcholanthrene-induced sarcomas of neonatally thymectomized mice. J Natl Cancer Inst 42, 445–453, 1969

Noonan, C. D., Margulis, A. R., and Wright, R. Bronchial arterial patterns in pulmonary metastases. Radiology 84, 1033–1042, 1965

Noonan, F. P., Gardner, M.A.H., Clunie, G. J. A., Isbister, W. H., and Halliday, W. J. Control of tumor growth in mice by thoracic duct drainage: Relationship to blocking factor in lymph. Int J Cancer 13, 640–649, 1974

Nordlund, J. J., Wolff, S. M., and Levy, H. B. Inhibition of biologic activity of poly I:poly C by human plasma. Proc Soc Exp Biol Med 133, 439–444, 1970

Norman, R. L. Vaccinia treatment of melanoma. Lancet 2, 867, 1975

Normann, S. J., and Sorkin, E. Cell-specific defect in monocyte function during tumor growth. J Natl Cancer Inst 57, 135–140, 1976

Normann, S. J. and Sorkin, E. Anti-inflammatory effects of tumour bearing, pp 303–313, In Willoughby, D. A., Giroud, J. P., and Velo, G. P. (Eds): Perspectives in Inflammation. Future Trends and Developments. Lancaster: MTP Press, 1977a

Normann, S. J., and Sorkin, E. Inhibition of macrophage chemotaxis by neoplastic and other rapidly proliferating cells in vitro. Cancer Res 37, 705–711, 1977b

North, R. J., Kirstein, D. P., and Tuttle, R. L. Subversion of host defense mechanisms by murine tumors. I. A circulating factor that suppresses macrophage-mediated resistance to infection. J Exp Med 143, 559–573, 1976a

North, R. J., Kirstein, D. P., and Tuttle, R. L. Subversion of host defense mechanisms by murine tumors. II. Counter-influence of concomitant antitumor immunity. J Exp Med 143, 574–584, 1976b

Norton, L., Simon, R., Brereton, H. D., and Bogden, A. E. Predicting the course of Gompertzian growth. Nature 264, 542–555, 1976

Nouza, K. The theory, practice and treatment of graft-versus-host reactions. Rev Fr Etudes Clin Biol 13, 747–762, 1968

Novinsky, M. Zur Frage über Impfung der krebsigen Geschwülste. Zentralb Med (Wissench) 14, 790–791, 1876

Nowell, P. C., and Cole, L. J. Hepatomas in mice: Incidence increased after gamma irradiation at low dose rates. Science 148, 96–97, 1965

Noyes, W. F. Studies on the human wart virus. II. Changes in primary human cell cultures. Virology 25, 358–363, 1965

Nungester, W., Bierwaltes, E., and Knorpp, C. [Cited by Vial and Callahan (1957) as personal communication], 1952

Nunn, M., Djeu, J., Glaser, M., Lavrin, B., and Herberman, R. B. Natural cytotoxic reactivity of rat lymphocytes against syngeneic Gross virus-induced lymphoma. J Natl Cancer Inst 56, 393–399, 1976

Nussenzweig, R. S. Increased nonspecific resistance to malaria produced by administration of killed Corynebacterium parvum. Exp Parasitol 21, 224–231, 1967

O

Ochoa, M., Wanebo, H. J., and Lewis, J. L. C. parvum and combination chemotherapy in advanced ovary cancer. Proc Am Assoc Cancer Res 17, 170, 1976

O'Conor, G. T. Malignant lymphoma in African children: II. A pathological entity. Cancer 14, 270–283, 1961

Oehler, J. R., Lindsay, L. R., Nunn, M. E., and Herberman, R. B. Natural cell-mediated cytotoxicity in rats. I. Tissue and strain distribution, and demonstration of a membrane receptor for the Fc portion of IgG. Int J Cancer 21, 204–209, 1978a

Oehler, J. R., Lindsay, L. R., Nunn, M. E., Holden, H. T., and Herberman, R. B. Natural cell-mediated cytotoxicity in rats. II. In vivo augmentation of NK-cell activity. Int J Cancer 21, 210–220, 1978b

Oettgen, H. F., Old, L. J., Farrow, J., and Lawrence, H. S. Effects of transfer factor in cancer patients. J Clin Invest 50, 71a, 1971

Oettgen, H. F., Old, L. J., Farrow, J. H., Valentine, F. T., Lawrence, H. S., and Thomas, L. Effect of dialyzable transfer factor in patients with breast cancer. Proc Natl Acad Sci USA 71, 2319–2323, 1974

Octtgen, H. F., Old, L. J., McLean, E. P., and Carswell, E. A. Delayed hypersensitivity and transplantation immunity elicited by soluble antigens of chemically induced tumours in inbred guinea pigs. Nature 220, 295–297, 1968

Oettgen, H. F., Pinsky, C. M., and Delmonte, L. Treatment of cancer with immunomodulators. Med Clin North Am 60, 511–537, 1976

Ojo, E., Haller, O., Kimura, A., and Wigzell, H. An analysis of conditions allowing Corynebacterium parvum to cause either augmentation or inhibition of natural killer cell activity against tumor cells in mice. Int J Cancer 21, 444–452, 1978a

Ojo, E., Haller, O., and Wigzell, H. Corynebacterium parvum-induced peritoneal exudate cells with rapid cytolytic activity against tumor cells are non-phagocytic cells with characteristics of natural killer cells. Scand J Immunol 8, 215–222, 1978b

Ojo, E., and Wigzell, H. Natural killer cells may be the only cells in normal mouse lymphoid cell populations endowed with cytolytic ability for antibody-coated tumor target cells. Scand J Immunol 7, 297–306, 1978

Olcott, C. T. A transplantable nephroblastoma (Wilms' tumor) and other spontaneous tumors in a colony of rats. Cancer Res 10, 625–628, 1950

Old, L. J. Cancer immunology. Sci Am 236, 62–79, 1977

Old, L. J., Benecerraf, B., Clarke, D. A., and Carswell, E. A. The role of the reticuloendothelial system in the host reaction to neoplasia. Cancer Res 21, 1281–1300, 1961

Old, L. J., and Boyse, E. A. Immunology of experimental tumors. Annu Rev Med 15, 167–186, 1964

Old, L. J., and Boyse, E. A. Specific antigens of tumors and leukemias of experimental animals. Med Clin North Am 50, 901–912, 1966

Old, L. J., Boyse, E. A., Clarke, D. A., and Carswell, E. A. Antigenic properties of chemically induced tumors. Ann NY Acad Sci 101, 80–106, 1962

Old, L. J., Boyse, E. A., and Lilly, F. Formation of cytotoxic antibody against leukemias induced by Friend virus. Cancer Res 23, 1063–1068, 1963

Old, L. J., Boyse, E. A., Oettgen, H. F., de Harven, E., Geering, G., Williamson, B., and Clifford, P. Precipitating antibody in human serum to an antigen present in cultured Burkitt's lymphoma cells. Proc Natl Acad Sci USA 56, 1699–1704, 1966

Old, L. J., Boyse, E. A., and Stockert, E. Mouse leukaemias. Typing of mouse leukaemias by serological methods. Nature 201, 777–779, 1964

Old, L. J., Clarke, D. A., and Banacerraf, B. Effect of bacillus Calmette-Guérin infection on transplanted tumours in the mouse. Nature 184, 291–292, 1959

Old, L. J., Stockert, E., Boyse, E. A., and Geering, G. A study of passive immunization against a transplanted G+ leukemia with specific antiserum. Proc Soc Exp Biol Med 124, 63–68, 1967

Old, L. J., Stockert, E., Boyse, E. A., and Kim, J. H. Antigenic modulation. Loss of TL antigen from cells exposed to TL antibody. Study of the phenomenon in vitro. J Exp Med 127, 523–539, 1968

Oldham, R. K., Ortaldo, J. R., and Herberman, R. B. Natural cytotoxic reactivity of rat lymphocytes against Gross virus-induced tumor cell lines as measured by ^{125}Iododeoxyuridine and tritiated proline microtoxicity assays. Cancer Res 37, 4467–4474, 1977

Oldham, R. K., Siwarski, D., McCoy, J. L., Plata, E. J., and Herberman, R. B. Evaluation of a cell-mediated cytotoxicity assay utilizing [125]Iododeoxyuridine-labelled tissue-culture target cells. Natl Cancer Inst Monogr 37, 49–58, 1973

Oliver, R. T. D. Active specific and non specific immunotherapy for patients with acute myelogenous leukaemia. Prog Immunol 3, 572–578, 1977

Oliver, R. T. D., and Pillai, A. Reactivity of antisera to oncorna virus proteins with human leukaemia cells. Proc R Soc Med 70, 556–559, 1977

Olivotto, M., and Bomford, R. In vitro inhibition of tumour cells growth and DNA synthesis by peritoneal and lung macrophages from mice injected with C. parvum. Int J Cancer 13, 478–488, 1974

Olsnes, S., and Pihl, A. Clinical significance of estrogen receptors in human breast cancer. Biomedicine 20, 377–383, 1974

Olurin, E. O., Sofowora, E. O., Afonja, A. O., Kolawole, T. M., and Junaid, T. A. Cushing's syndrome and bronchial carcinoid tumor. Cancer 31, 1514–1519, 1973

O'Meara, R. A. Q. Coagulative properties of cancer. Ir J Med Sci 394, 474–479, 1958

Omenn, G. S. Pathobiology of ectopic hormone production by neoplasms in man. Pathobiol Annu 3, 177–216, 1973

O'Neill, G. J., Henderson, D. C., and White, R. G. The role of anaerobic Coryneforms on specific and non-specific immunological reactions. I. Effect on particle clearance and humoral and cell-mediated immunological responses. Immunology 24, 977–995, 1973

Oon, C. J., Apsey, M., Buckleton, H., Cooke, K. B., Hanham, I., Hazarika, P., Hobbs, J. B., and McLeod, B. Human immune γ-globulin treated with chlorambucil for cancer therapy. Behring Inst Mitt 56, 228–235, 1974

Oppenheimer, B. S., Oppenheimer, E. T., Danishefsky, T., Stout, A. P., and Eirich, F. R. Further studies of polymers as carcinogenic agents in animals. Cancer Res 15, 333–340, 1955

Oppenheimer, B. S., Oppenheimer, E. T., and Stout, A. P. Sarcomas induced in rats by implanting cellophane. Proc Soc Exp Biol Med 67, 33–34, 1948

Order, S. E., Chism, S. E., and Hellman, S. Studies of antigens associated with Hodgkin's disease. Blood 40, 621–633, 1972

Order, S. E., Donahue, V., and Knapp, R. Immunotherapy of ovarian carcinoma. Cancer 32, 573–579, 1973

Order, S. E., and Hellman, S. Tumor associated antigens. A new perspective of Hodgkin's disease. JAMA 223, 174–175, 1973

Order, S. E., Kirkman, R., and Knapp, R. Serologic immunotherapy: Results and probable mechanism of action. Cancer 34, 175–183, 1974

Oren, M. E., and Herberman, R. B. Delayed cutaneous hypersensitivity reactions to membrane extracts of human tumor cells. Clin Exp Immunol 9, 45–56, 1971

O'Riordan, M. L., Robinson, J. A., Buckton, K. E., and Evans, H. J. Distinguishing between the chromosomes involved in Down's syndrome (trisomy 21) and chronic myeloid leukemia (Ph[1]) by fluorescence. Nature 230, 167–168, 1971

Orth, D. N., Nicholson, W. E., Mitchell, W. M., Island, D. P., and Liddle, G. W. Biologic and immunologic characterization and physical separation of ACTH and ACTH fragments in the ectopic ACTH syndrome. J Clin Invest 52, 1756–1769, 1973

Osborn, D. E., and Castro, J. E. Immunological response in patients receiving Corynebacterium parvum therapy. Clin Oncol 3, 155–164, 1977

Ossorio, R. C., Fahey, J. L., Wilson, W., Plotkin, D., Brossman, S., and Skinner, D. Toxicity of intravenous Corynebacterium parvum. Lancet 2, 1090–1091, 1975

Osunkoya, B. O. Evidence for anti-Burkitt tumour globulins in Burkitt tumour patients and healthy individuals. Br J Cancer 21, 302–311, 1967

Oth. D. Current questions on the tumour-associated antigens of chemically-induced tumours. I. In search of their characterization. Biomedicine 22, 350–357, 1975

Oth, D., and Barra, Y. Séparation de deux spécificités antigéniques tumorales différentes, chez deux variants isoantigéniques obtenus á partir d'une tumeur induite chimiquement dans des hybrides F1(A.CA×A.BY). CR Acad Sci D 278, 177–180, 1974

Oth, D., Berebbi, M., and Meyer, G. Tumor-associated antigens in isoantigenic variants of a 3-methylcholanthrene-induced sarcoma. J Natl Cancer Inst 55, 903–908, 1975

Oth, D., and Burg, C. Strength of the tumour specific antigens and of the hybrid effect of three chemically induced sarcomas of the same inbred strain origin. Folia Biol (Praha) 16, 374–380, 1970a

Oth, D., and Burg, C. Comparison of the neutralising effect of nonimmunized syngeneic and semi-syngeneic splenic cells towards parental tumour-cells. Eur J Clin Biol Res 15, 433–437, 1970b

Oth, D., and Liegey, A. Effect of multiple injections of allogeneic spleen cells on methylcholanthrene carcinogenesis in the mouse. Biomedicine 23, 17–19, 1975

O'Toole, C. Standardization of microcytotoxicity

assay for cell-mediated immunity. Natl Cancer Inst Monogr *37*, 19–24, 1973

O'Toole, C., Stejskal, V., Perlmann, P., and Karlsson, M. Lymphoid cells mediating tumor-specific cytotoxicity to carcinoma of the urinary bladder. Separation of the effector population using a surface marker. J Exp Med *139*, 457–466, 1974

Outzen, H. C., Custer, R. P., Eaton, G. J., and Prehn, R. T. Spontaneous and induced tumor incidence in germ-free "nude" mice. J Reticuloendothel Soc *17*, 1–9, 1975

Owen, J. J. T., and Seeger, R. C. Immunity to tumors of the murine leukaemia-sarcoma virus complex. Br J Cancer *28*, (Suppl I), 26–34, 1973

Owen, L. N. The treatment of malignant tumours of bone in the dog by intra-arterial injection or perfusion of epodyl (triethyleneglycol diglycidyl ether). Br J Cancer *18*, 407–418, 1964

Owen, L. N. Osteosarcoma in the dog. Proc R Soc Med *69*, 546–547, 1976

Owen, L. N. Lymphosarcoma in the dog. Proc R Soc Med *70*, 563–566, 1977

Ozer, H. L., and Jha, K. K. Malignancy and transformation: Expression in somatic cell hybrids and variants. Adv Cancer Res *25*, 53–93, 1977

P

Pack, G. T. Note on experimental use of rabies vaccine for melanomatosis. Arch Dermatol Syphilol *62*, 694–695, 1950

Pack, G. T. Tumors of Soft Somatic Tissues. New York: Hueber, 1958

Pack, G. T., Scharnagel, I., and Morfit, M. The principle of excision and dissection in continuity for primary and metastatic melanoma of the skin. Surgery *17*, 849–866, 1945

Palmer, A. M., and Symes, M. O. An investigation into the influence of a graft-versus-host reaction, induced by parent line cells, on the growth of lymphoma transplant in F1 hybrid mice. Folia Biol (Praha) *20*, 26–35, 1974

Palmer, B. V., Walsh, G., Smedley, P., McIntosh, I. H., and Greening, W. P. A survey of patients' reactions to intravenous Corynebacterium parvum therapy. Dev Biol Stand *38*, 529–533, 1978

Pantelouris, E. M. Absence of thymus in a mouse mutant. Nature *217*, 370–371, 1968

Papaioannou, V. E., McBurney, M. W., Gardner, R. L., and Evans, M. J. Fate of teratocarcinoma cells injected into early mouse embryos. Nature *258*, 70–73, 1975

Papamichail, M., Holborow, E. J., Keith, H. I., and Currey, H. L. F. Subpopulations of human peripheral blood lymphocytes distinguished by combined rosette formation and membrane immunofluorescence. Lancet *2*, 64–66, 1972

Papanicolaou, G. N. Atlas of Exfoliative Cytology. Cambridge, Mass.: Harvard Univ Press, 1954

Papatestas, A. E., and Kark, A. E. Peripheral lymphocyte counts in breast carcinoma. An index of immune competence. Cancer *34*, 2014–2017, 1974

Park, I. J., and Jones, H. W. Glucose-6-phosphate dehydrogenase and the histogenesis of epidermoid carcinoma of the cervix. Am J Obstet Gynecol *102*, 106–109, 1968

Parke, D. V. Research moves on, In 9th Annu Sympo Marie Curie Memorial Foundation—The Changing Face of Cancer, London, 1977a

Parke, D. V. The activation and induction of byphenyl hydroxylation and chemical carcinogenesis, In Estabrook, R. W., and Ullrich, V. (Eds): Microsomes and Drug Oxidations. Oxford: Pergamon Press, 1977b

Parke, D. V. Biochemistry of cancer, pp 113–156, In Raven, R. (Ed): Principles of Surgical Oncology. New York: Plenum Press, 1977c

Parker, R. C., Plummer, H. C., Siebenmann, C. O., and Chapman, M. G. Effects of histolyticus infection and toxin on transplantable mouse tumors. Proc Soc Exp Biol Med *66*, 461–467, 1947

Parker, R. G., Berry, H. C., Caderao, J. B., Gerdes, A. J., Hussey, D. H., Ornitz, R., and Rogers, C. C. Preliminary clinical results from US fast neutron teletherapy studies. Cancer *40*, 1434–1443, 1977

Parks, L. C., Smith, W. J., Beebe, B., Winn, L., Rafajho, R., Rolley, R., and Williams, G. M. Effects of heterologous anti-melanoma sera (Melogam) in melanoma patients. Proc Am Assoc Cancer Res *16*, 134, 1975

Parmiani, G., Carbone, G., and Prehn, R. T. In vitro "spontaneous" neoplastic transformation of mouse fibroblasts in diffusion chambers. J Natl Cancer Inst *46*, 261–267, 1971

Parmiani, G., and Invernizzi, G. Alien histocompatibility determinants on the cell surface of sarcomas induced by methylcholanthrene. I. In vivo studies. Int J Cancer *16*, 756–767, 1975

Parr, I. Wheeler, E., and Alexander, P. Similarities of the anti-tumour actions of endotoxin, lipid A and double-stranded RNA. Br J Cancer *27*, 370–389, 1973

Parr, I. B., Wheeler, E., and Alexander, P. Selective mobilization of specifically cytotoxic T-lymphocytes at sites of inflammation in relation to BCG-induced resistance to implants of syngeneic sarcoma in mice. J Natl Cancer Inst *59*, 1659–1666, 1977

Paslin, D., Dimitrov, N. V., and Heaton, C. Regression of a transplantable hamster melanoma by intralesional injections of Corynebacterium granulosum. J Natl Cancer Inst 52, 571–573, 1974

Pass, E., and Yashphe, D. J. Stimulation of antibody synthesis to soluble bovine γ-globulin by a methanol-extraction residue of BCG. Isr J. Med Sci 7, 609–610, 1971

Pasternak, G. Serologic studies on cells of Graffi virus-induced myeloid leukemia in mice. J Natl Cancer Inst 34, 71–84, 1965

Pasternak, G., and Graffi, A. Induction of resistance against isotransplantation of virus-induced myeloid leukaemias. Br J Cancer 17, 532–539, 1963

Pasternak, G., Hoffman, F., and Graffi, A. Growth of diethylnitrosamine-induced lung tumours in syngeneic mice specifically pretreated with x-ray killed tumour tissue. Folia Biol (Praha) 12, 299–304, 1966

Pasternak, G., Horn, K.-H., and Graffi, A. Immunologische Crossversuche mit Methylcholanthrentumoren eines Mäuseinzuchtstammes. Acta Biol Med Germ 9, 306–308, 1962

Paterson, R., and Russell, M. H. Clinical trials in malignant disease. Part III. Breast cancer: Evaluation of post-operative radiotherapy. J Fac Radiol 10, 175–180, 1959

Patey, D. H., and Dyson, W. H. The prognosis of carcinoma of the breast in relation to the type of operation performed. Br J Cancer 2, 7–13, 1948

Patt, H. M., and Blackford, M. E. Quantitative studies of the growth response of the Krebs ascites tumor. Cancer Res 14, 391–396, 1954

Patterson, W. B., Patterson, H. R., and Chute, R. N. Transplantable human tumors. Cancer 10, 1281–1292, 1957

Paukovits, W. R. Control of granulocyte production: Separation and chemical identification for specific inhibitor (chalone). Cell Tissue Kinet 4, 539–547, 1971

Paul, J. Cell and Tissue Culture (ed 5). London: Churchill Livingstone, 1975

Payne, L. N. Viral lymphomagenesis in the domestic fowl: A review. Proc R Soc Med 70, 559–563, 1977

Pazmino, N. H., Yuhas, J. M., and Milas, L. [Cited as unpublished result by Milas and Scott (1977)], 1977

Peacocke, I., Amos, B., and Lazlo, J. The detection of iso-antigens in leukemic cells during the cytotoxicity test. Blood 28, 665–673, 1966

Pearl, R. Cancer and tuberculosis. Am J Hyg 9, 97–159, 1929

Pearse, A. G. E. The cytochemistry and ultrastructure of polypeptide hormone-producing cells of the APUD series and the embryologic, physiologic and pathologic implications of the concept. J Histchem Cytochem 17, 303–313, 1969

Pearse, A. G. E., and Polak, J. M. Neural crest origin of the polypeptide (APUD) cells of the gastrointestinal tract and pancreas. Gut 12, 783–788, 1971

Pearson, G., Klein, G., Henle, G., Henle, W., and Clifford, P. Relation between Epstein-Barr viral and cell membrane immunofluorescence in Burkitt tumor cells. IV. Differentiation between antibodies responsible for membrane and viral immunofluorescence. J Exp Med 129, 707–718, 1969

Pearson, G. R., Redmon, L. W., and Bass, L. R. Protective effect of immune sera against transplantable Moloney virus-induced sarcoma and lymphoma. Cancer Res 33, 171–178, 1973a

Pearson, G. R., Redmon, L. W., and Pearson, J. W. Serochemotherapy against a Moloney virus-induced leukemia. Cancer Res 33, 1854–1857, 1973b

Pearson, J. W., Chaparas, S. D., and Chirigos, M. A. Effect of dose and route of bacillus Calmette Guérin in chemoimmunostimulation therapy of a murine leukemia. Cancer Res 33, 1845–1848, 1973

Pearson, J. W., Chirigos, M. A., Chaparas, S. D., and Sher, N. A. Combined drug and immunostimulation therapy against a syngeneic murine leukemia. J Natl Cancer Inst 52, 463–468, 1974

Pearson, J. W., Pearson, G. R., Gibson, W. T., Chermann, J. C., and Chirigos, M. A. Combined chemoimmunostimulation therapy against murine leukemia. Cancer Res 32, 904–907, 1972

Pearson, J. W., Perk, K., Chirigos, M. A., Pryor, J. W., and Fuhrman, F. S. Histological and combined chemoimmunostimulation therapy studies against a murine leukemia. Int J Cancer 16, 142–152, 1975

Pearson, M. N., and Raffel, S. Macrophage digested antigen as inducer of delayed hypersensitivity. J Exp Med 133, 494–505, 1971

Pearson, O. H., Llerna, O., Llerna, L., Molina, A., and Butler, T. Prolactin dependent rat mammary cancer: A model for man? Trans Assoc Am Physicians 82, 225–238, 1969

Peckham, M. J., Ford, H. T., McElwain, T. J., Harmer, C. L., Atkinson, K., and Austin, D. E. The results of radiotherapy for Hodgkin's disease. Br J Cancer 32, 391–400, 1975

Pees, H. W., and Seidel, B. Cell-mediated immune response of patients with meningiomas defined in vitro by a (³H)proline microcytotoxicity test. Clin Exp Immunol 24, 310–316, 1976

Pelfrene, A. F. Prevention of cancer. A luxury or an indispensability? Biomedicine 24, 2–3, 1976

Pellegrino, M. A., Ferrone, S., Dierlich, M. P.,

and Reisfeld, R. A. Variation in susceptibility of a human lymphoid cell line to immune lysis during the cell cycle. Lack of correlation with antigen density and complement binding. J Exp Med *140*, 578–590, 1974

Pellis, N. R., Tom, B. H., and Kahan, B. D. Tumor-specific and allospecific immunogenicity of soluble extracts from chemically induced murine sarcomas. J Immunol *113*, 708–711, 1974

Pels, E., and Den Otter, W. A cytophilic factor from challenged immune peritoneal lymphocytes renders macrophages specifically cytotoxic. J Int Res Commun *1*, 28, 1973

Pels, E., and Den Otter, W. The role of a cytophilic factor from challenged immune peritoneal lymphocytes in specific macrophage cytotoxicity. Cancer Res *34*, 3089–3094, 1974

Penn, I. Malignant tumors in organ transplant recipients, In Recent Results Cancer Research No. 35. New York: Springer-Verlag, 1970

Penn, I. Chemical immunosuppression and human cancer. Cancer *34*, 1474–1480, 1974

Penn, I. Malignancies associated with immunosuppressive or cytotoxic therapy. Surgery *83*, 492–502, 1978

Penn, I., Halgrimson, C. G., and Starzl, T. E. De novo malignant tumors in organ transplant recipients. Transplant Proc *3*, 773–778, 1971

Penn, I., Hammond, W., Brettschneider, L., and Starzl, T. E. Malignant lymphomas in transplantation patients. Transplant Proc *1*, 106–112, 1969

Penn, I., and Starzl, T. E. Malignant tumors arising de novo in immunosuppressed organ transplant recipients. Transplantation *14*, 407–417, 1972

Perlmann, P., and Holm, G. Cytotoxic effects of lymphoid cells in vitro. Adv Immunol *11*, 117–193, 1969

Perlmann, P., and Perlmann, H. Contactual lysis of antibody-coated chicken erythrocytes by purified lymphocytes. Cell Immunol *1*, 300–315, 1970

Perper, R. J., Oronsky, A. L., and Sanda, M. The effect of BCG on extravascular mononuclear cell accumulation in vivo. Int J Cancer *17*, 670–677, 1976

Persellin, R. H., and Ziff, M. The effect of gold salt on lysosomal enzymes of the peritoneal macrophage. Arthritis Rheum *9*, 57–65, 1966

Peter, H. H., Diehl, V., Kalden, J. R., Seeland, P., and Eckert, G. Humoral and cellular cytotoxicity in vitro against allogeneic and autologous human melanoma cells. Behring Inst Mitt, *56*, 167–177, 1975a

Peter, H. H., Kalden, J. R., Seeland, P., Diehl, V., and Eckert, G. Humoral and cellular immune reactions in vitro against allogeneic and autologous human melanoma cells. Clin Exp Immunol *20*, 193–207, 1975b

Peter, H. H., Pavie-Fischer, J., Fridman, W. H., Aubert, C., Cesarini, J., Roubin, R., and Kourilsky, F. M. Cell-mediated cytotoxicity in vitro of human lymphocytes against a tissue culture melanoma cell line (IGR3). J Immunol *115*, 539–548, 1975c

Peters, L. C., Hanna, M. G., Gutterman, J. U., Mavligit, G. M., and Hersh, E. M. Modulation of the immune response of guinea pigs by repeated BCG scarification. Proc Soc Exp Biol Med *147*, 344–349, 1974

Peters, L. J., and Hewitt, H. B. The influence of fibrin formation on the transplant ability of murine tumour cells: Implications for the mechanism of the Révész effect. Br J Cancer *29*, 279–291, 1974

Peters, L. J., McBride, W. H., Mason, K. A., and Milas, E. A Role for T lymphocytes in tumor inhibition and enhancement caused by systemic administration of Corynebacterium parvum. J Reticuloendothel Soc *24*, 9–18, 1978

Peters, V. Cutting the Gordian knot in early breast cancer. Ann R Coll Physicians Surg Can *8*, 186–192, 1975

Petitou, M., Rosenfeld, C., and Sinay, P. A new assay for cell-bound neuraminidase. Cancer Immunol Immunother *2*, 135–137, 1977

Peto, R. Guidelines on the analysis of tumour rates and death rates in experimental animals. Br J Cancer *29*, 101–105, 1974

Peto, R. Immunotherapy of acute myeloid leukemia, pp 341–346, In Terry, W. D., and Windhorst, D. (Eds): Immunotherapy of Cancer: Present Status of Trials in Man. New York: Raven Press, 1978a

Peto, R. [*In Discussion Mathé, Schwarzenberg et al. (1978)*], p 469, In Terry, W. D., and Windhorst, D. (Eds): Immunotherapy of Cancer: Present Status of Trials in Man. New York: Raven Press, 1978b

Peto, R. [*Discussion of Immunotherapy for melanoma*], p 147, In Terry, W. D., and Windhorst, D. (Eds): Immunotherapy of Cancer: Present Status of Trials in Man. New York: Raven Press, 1978c

Peto, R., and Galton, D. A. G. Chemoimmunotherapy of adult acute leukemia. Lancet *1*, 454, 1975

Peto, R., Pike, M. C., Armitage, P., Breslow, N. E., Cox, D. R., Howard, S. V., Mantel, N., McPherson, K., Peto, J., and Smith, P. G. Design and analysis of randomized clinical trials requiring prolonged observation of each patient. I. Introduction and design. Br J Cancer *34*, 585–612, 1976

Peto, R., Pike, M. C., Armitage, P., Breslow, N. E., Cox, D. R., Howard, S. V., Mantel, N., McPherson, K., Peto, J., and Smith, P. G. Design and analysis of randomized clinical trials requiring prolonged observation of each patient. II. Analysis and examples. Br J Cancer 35, 1–39, 1977

Peto, R., Roe, F. J. C., Lee, P. N., Levy, L., and Clack, J. Cancer and ageing in mice and men. Br J Cancer 32, 411–426, 1975

Petranyi, G. G., Benczur, M., Onody, C. E., Hollan, S. R., and Ivanyl, P. HL-A 3, 7 and lymphocyte cytotoxic activity. Lancet, 2, 736, 1974

Pettigrew, R. T., Galt, J. M., Ludgate, C. M., Horn, D. B., and Smith, A. N. Circulatory and biochemical effects of whole body hyperthermia. Br J Surg 61, 727–730, 1974a

Pettigrew, R. T., Galt, J. M., Ludgate, C. M., and Smith, A. N. Clinical effects of whole-body hyperthermia in advanced malignancy. Br Med J 4, 679–682, 1974b

Pfizenmaier, K., Trostmann, H., Röllinghoff, M., and Wagner, H. Temporary presence of self-reactive cytotoxic T lymphocytes during murine lymphocytic choriomeningitis. Nature 258, 238–240, 1975

Phillips, B., and Gazet, J. C. Transplantation of primary explants of human tumor to mice treated with ALS. Br J Cancer 24, 92–96, 1970

Pieroni, R. E., Bundeally, A. E., and Levine, L. The effect of actinomycin D on the lethality of poly I:C. J Immunol 106, 1128–1129, 1971

Pierpaoli, W., Haran-Ghera, N., and Kopp, H. G. Role of host endocrine status in murine leukaemogenesis. Br J Cancer 35, 621–629, 1977

Pierres, M., Germain, R. N., Dorf, M. E., and Benacerraf, B. Potentiation of a primary in vivo antibody response by alloantisera against gene products of the I region of the H2 complex. Proc Natl Acad Sci USA 74, 3975–3979, 1977

Piessens, W. F., Churchill, W. H., and David, J. R. Macrophages activated in vitro with lymphocyte mediators kill neoplastic but not normal cells. J Immunol 114, 293–299, 1975

Piessens, W. F., Heimann, R., Legros, N., and Heuson, J.-C. Effects of bacillus Calmette-Guérin (BCG) infection on residual disease of the rat mammary tumor after ovariectomy. Eur J Cancer 7, 377–380, 1971

Piessens, W. F., Lachapelle, F. L., Legros, N., and Heuson, J.-C. Facilitation of rat mammary tumour growth by BCG. Nature 228, 1210–1211, 1970

Pihl, E., Hughes, E. S. R., Nind, A. P. P., and Nairn, R. C. Colonic carcinoma: Clinicopath-ological correlation with immunoreactivity. Br Med J 3, 742–743, 1975

Pike, M. C., and Snyderman, R. Depression of macrophage function by a factor produced by neoplasms: A mechanism for abrogation of immune surveillance. J immunol 117, 1243–1249, 1976a

Pike, M. C., and Snyderman, R. Augmentation of human monocyte chemotactic response by levamisole. Nature 261, 136–137, 1976b

Pilch, D. J. F., and Planterose, D. N. Effect on Friend disease of double-stranded RNA of fungal origin. J Gen Virol 10, 155–166, 1971

Pilch, Y. H., deKernion, J. B., Skinner, D. G., Ramming, K. P., Schick, P. M., Fritze, D., Brower, P., and Kern, D. H. Immunotherapy of cancer with "immune" RNA: A preliminary report. Am J Surg 132, 631–637, 1976a

Pilch, Y. H., Fritze, D., deKernion, J. B., Ramming, K. P., and Kern, D. H. Immunotherapy of cancer with immune RNA in animal models and cancer patients. Ann NY Acad Sci 277, 592–608, 1976b

Pilch, Y. H., Fritze, D., Ramming, K. P., deKernion, J. B., and Kern, D. H. The mediation of immune responses by I-RNA to animal and human tumor antigens, pp 149–175, In Fink, M. A. (Ed): Immune RNA in Neoplasia. New York: Academic Press, 1976c

Pilch, Y. H., and Ramming, K. P. Transfer of tumor immunity with ribonucleic acid. Cancer 26, 630–636, 1970

Pilch, Y. H., and Ramming, K. P. Immunological enhancement of murine tumor isografts mediated by RNA from lymphoid organs of xenogeneic immunized animals. Transplantation 11, 10–19, 1971

Pilch, Y. H., Ramming, K. P., and deKernion, J. B. Clinical trials of immune RNA in the immunotherapy of cancer, pp 539–555, In Terry, W. D., and Windhorst, D. (Eds): Immunotherapy of Cancer: Present Status of Trials in Man. New York: Raven Press, 1978

Pilch, Y. H., Veltman, L. L., and Kern, D. H. Immune cytolysis of human tumour cells mediated by xenogeneic "immune" RNA: Implications for immunotherapy. Surgery 76, 23–34, 1974

Pilet, C., and Sabolovic, D. Brucella abortus et immunothérapie active non spécifique de la tumeur d'Ehrlich. Bull Assoc Fr Vet Microbiol Immunol 7, 43–57, 1970

Pimm, M. V. Intrapleural BCG treatment of experimental lung tumours. Lancet 2, 95–96, 1976

Pimm, M. V., and Baldwin, R. W. BCG immunotherapy of rat tumours in athymic nude mice. Nature 254, 77–78, 1975a

Pimm, M. V., and Baldwin, R. W. BCG therapy of pleural and peritoneal growth of transplanted rat tumours. Int J Cancer 15, 260–269, 1975b

Pimm, M. V., and Baldwin, R. W. Influence of whole body irradiation on BCG contact suppression of a rat sarcoma and tumour-specific immunity. Br J Cancer 34, 199–202, 1976a

Pimm, M. V., and Baldwin, R. W. C. parvum suppression of rat tumours in athymic nude mice. Br J Cancer 34, 453–455, 1976b

Pimm, M. V., and Baldwin, R. W. BCG treatment of malignant pleural effusions: Experimental development and clinical applications. Clin Oncol 2, 300–301, 1976c

Pimm, M. V., and Baldwin, R. W. Treatment of transplanted rat tumours with double-stranded RNA (BRL 5907). II. Treatment of pleural and peritoneal growths. Br J Cancer 33, 166–171, 1976d

Pimm, M. V., and Baldwin, R. W. Antigenic differences between primary methylcholanthrene-induced rat sarcomas and postsurgical recurrences. Int J Cancer 20, 37–43, 1977a

Pimm, M. V., and Baldwin, R. W. C. parvum immunotherapy of transplanted rat tumours. Int J Cancer 20, 923–932, 1977b

Pimm, M. V., Cook, A. J., and Baldwin, R. W. Failure of neuraminidase treatment to influence tumorigenicity or immunogenicity of syngeneically transplanted rat tumor cells. Eur J Cancer 14, 869–878, 1978

Pimm, M. V., Embleton, M. J., and Baldwin, R. W. Treatment of transplanted rat tumours with double-stranded RNA (BRL 5907). I. Influence of systemic and local administration. Br J Cancer 33, 154–165, 1976

Pimm, M. V., Hopper, D. G., and Baldwin, R. W. BCG treatment of malignant pleural effusions in the rat. Br J Cancer 34, 368–373, 1976

Pimm, M. V., Hopper, D. G., and Baldwin, R. W. Host responses in adjuvant contact suppression of experimental rat tumours. Dev Biol Stand 38, 349–354, 1978

Pinckard, R. N., Weir, D. M., and McBride, W. H. Factors influencing the immune response. III. The blocking effect of Corynebacterium parvum upon the induction of acquired immunological unresponsiveness to bovine serum albumin in the adult rabbit. Clin Exp Immunol 3, 413–421, 1968

Pines, A. A 5-year controlled study of BCG and radiotherapy for inoperable lung cancer. Lancet 1, 380–381, 1976

Pinkerton, H. Effects of adjuvants on benzpyrene tumorigenesis in hamsters. Proc Soc Exp Biol Med 141, 1089–1091, 1972

Pinsky, C. M., DeJager, R. L., Wittes, R. E., and Wong, P. P. Corynebacterium parvum as adjuvant to combination chemotherapy in patients with advanced breast cancer: Preliminary results of a prospective randomized trial, pp 647–653, In Terry, W. D., and Windhorst, D. (Eds): Immunotherapy of Cancer: Present Status of Trials in Man. New York: Raven Press, 1978a

Pinsky, C. M., Hirshaut, Y., and Oettgen, H. F. Treatment of malignant melanoma by intralesional injection of BCG. Natl Cancer Inst Monogr 39, 225–228, 1973

Pinsky, C. M., Hirshaut, Y., Wanebo, H. J., and Hilal, E. Y. Surgical adjuvant immunotherapy with BCG in patients with malignant melanoma: Results of a prospective, randomized trial, pp 27–33, In Terry, W. D., and Windhorst, D. (Eds): Immunotherapy of Cancer: Present Status of Trials in Man. New York: Raven Press, 1978b

Pinsky, C. M., Oettgen, H. F., El Domieri, A., Old, L. J., Beattie, E. J., and Buchenal, J. H. Delayed hypersensitivity reactions in patients with cancer. Proc Am Assoc Cancer Res 12, 100, 1971

Piper, C. E., and McIvor, K. L. Alloimmune peritoneal macrophages as specific effector cells: Characterization of specific macrophage cytotoxin. Cell Immunol 17, 423–430, 1975

Plata, F., Gomard, E., LeClerc, J. C., and Levy, J. P. Comparative in vitro studies of effector cell diversity in the cellular immune response to murine sarcoma virus (MSV)-induced tumors in mice. J Immunol 112, 1477–1487, 1974

Playfair, J. H. L. Cell cooperation in the immune response. Clin Exp Immunol 8, 839–856, 1971

Plescia, O. J., Smith, A. H., and Grinwick, K. Subversion of immune system by tumor cells and role of prostaglandins. Proc Natl Acad Sci USA, 72, 1848–1851, 1975

Pocock, S. J. Randomised clinical trials. Br Med J 1, 1661, 1977

Pollack, S. B. Effector cells for antibody-dependent cell mediated cytotoxicity. I. Increased cytotoxicity after priming with BCG-SS. Cell Immunol 29, 373–381, 1977

Pollack, S., Heppner, G., Brawn, R. J., and Nelson, K. Specific killing of tumor cells in vitro in the presence of normal lymphoid cells and sera from hosts immune to tumor antigens. Int J Cancer 9, 316–323, 1972

Pool, E. H., and Dunlop, G. R. Cancer cells in blood stream. Am J Cancer 21, 99–102, 1934

Poplack, D. G., Leventhal, B. G., Simon, R., Pomeroy, T., Graw, R. G., and Henderson, E. S. Treatment of acute lymphatic leukemia with chemotherapy alone or chemotherapy plus immunotherapy, pp 497–501, In Terry, W. D., and Windhorst, D. (Eds): Immunotherapy of Cancer: Present Status of Trials in Man. New York: Raven Press, 1978

Poplack, D. G., Sher, N. A., Chaparas, S. D., and Blaese, R. M. The effect of Mycobacterium bovis (bacillus Calmette-Guérin) on macrophage random migration, chemotaxis and pinocytosis. Cancer Res 36, 1233–1237, 1976

Porter, K. A. Pathology of the orthotopic homograft and heterograft, pp 422–471, In Starzl, T. E. (Ed): Experience in Hepatic Transplantation. Philadelphia: W. B. Saunders, 1969

Portman, B., Schindler, A.-M., Murray-Lyon, I. M., and Williams, R. Histological sexing of a reticulum cell sarcoma arising after liver transplantation. Gastroenterology 70, 82–84, 1976

Post, J., and Hoffman, J. A G2 population of cells in autogenous rodent sarcoma. Exp Cell Res 57, 111–113, 1969

Potmesil, M., Ludwig, D., and Goldfeder, A. Cell kinetics of irradiated experimental tumors: Relationship between the proliferating and the nonproliferating pool. Cell Tissue Kinet 8, 369–386, 1975

Pott, P. Chirurgical observations relative to the cancer of the scrotum [London 1775]. [Reprinted in Natl Cancer Inst Monogr No. 10, pp 7–13], 1963

Potter, C. W., Carr, L., Jennings, R., Rees, R. C., McGinty, F., and Richardson, V. M. Levamisole inactive in treatment of four animal tumours. Nature 249, 567–569, 1974

Potter, J. S., Taylor, M. J., and MacDowell, E. C. Transfer of acquired resistance to transplantable leukemia in mice. Proc Soc Exp Biol 37, 655–656, 1938

Potter, M. Immunoglobulin-producing tumours and myeloma proteins of mice. Physiol Rev 52, 631–719, 1972

Potter, M. R., and Balfour, B. M. Stimulation of syngeneic and allogeneic lymphoid cells by tumour cells in vitro. Br J Cancer 32, 5–15, 1975

Pouillart, P., Palangie, T., Schwarzenberg, L., Brugerie, H., Lheritier, J., and Mathé, G. Effect of BCG on haemopoietic stem cells. Biomedicine 23, 469–471, 1975

Povlsen, C. O., Fialkow, P. J., Klein, E., Rygaard, J., and Wiener, F. Growth and antigenic properties of a biopsy-derived Burkitt's lymphoma in thymus-less (nude) mice. Int J Cancer 11, 30–39, 1973

Powles, R. L. Immunotherapy for acute myelogenous leukemia using irradiated and unirradiated leukemia cells. Cancer 34, 1558–1562, 1974

Powles, R. L. Pitfalls in analysis of survival in clinical trials. Biomedicine 24, 327–328, 1976

Powles, R. L., Balchin, L. A., Fairley, G. H., and Alexander, P. Recognition of leukemia cells as foreign before and after autoimmunization. Br Med J 1, 486–489, 1971

Powles, R. L., Balchin, L. A., Smith, C., and Grant, C. K. Some properties of cryopreserved acute leukaemia cells. Cryobiology 10, 282–289, 1973a

Powles, R. L., Crowther, D., Bateman, C. J. T., Beard, M. E. J., McElwain, T. J., Russell, J., Lister, T. A., Whitehouse, J. M. A., Wrigley, P. F. M., Pike, M., Alexander, P., and Hamilton Fairley, G. Immunotherapy for acute myelogenous leukaemia. Br J Cancer 28, 365–376, 1973b

Powles, R. L., Lister, T. A., Oliver, R. T. D., Russell, J., Smith, C., Kay, H. E. M., McElwain, T. J., and Fairley, G. H. Safe methods of collecting leukaemia cells from patients with acute leukaemia for use as immunotherapy. Br Med J 4, 375–379, 1974

Powles, R. L., Russell, J., Lister, T. A., Oliver, T., Whitehouse, J. M. A., Malpas, J., Chapuis, B., Crowther, D., and Alexander, P. Immunotherapy for acute myelogenous leukaemia: A controlled clinical study 2½ years after entry of the last patient. Br J Cancer 35, 265–272, 1977 [Reprinted in Terry, W. D., and Windhorst, D. (Eds): Immunotherapy of Cancer: Present Status of Trials in Man, pp 315–326. New York: Raven Press, 1978]

Prager, M. D. Immunological stimulation with modified cancer cells. Biomedicine 18, 261–263, 1973

Prehn, R. T. Tumor-specific immunity to transplanted dibenz[ah]anthracene-induced sarcomas. Cancer Res 20, 1614–1617, 1960

Prehn, R. T. Failure of immunization against tumorigenesis. J Natl Cancer Inst 26, 223–227, 1961

Prehn, R. T. Specific isoantigenicities among chemically induced tumors. Ann NY Acad Sci 101, 107–113, 1962

Prehn, R. T. The role of immune mechanisms in the biology of chemically and physically induced tumors, pp 475–485, In Conceptual Advances in Immunology and Oncology. M. D. Anderson Hosp 16th Ann Symp—Fundamental Cancer Research. New York: Harper & Row, 1963a

Prehn, R. T. Tumor specific immunity to nonviral tumors. Can Cancer Conf 5, 387–395, 1963b

Prehn, R. T. The significance of tumor-distinctive histocompatibility antigens, pp 105–114, In Trentin, J. J. (Ed): Cross-reacting Antigens and Neo-antigens. Baltimore: Williams & Wilkins, 1967

Prehn, R. T. Analysis of antigenic heterogeneity within individual 3-methylcholanthrene-induced mouse sarcomas. J Natl Cancer Inst 45, 1039–1045, 1970

Prehn, R. T. Perspectives on oncogenesis: Does immunity stimulate or inhibit neoplasia? J Reticuloendothel Soc 10, 1–16, 1971

Prehn, R. T. The immune reaction as a stimulator of tumor growth. Science 176, 170–171, 1972

Prehn, R. T. Relationship of tumor immunogenicity to concentration of the oncogen. J Natl Cancer Inst 55, 189–190, 1975

Prehn, R. T. Tumor progression and homeostasis. Adv Cancer Res 23, 203–236, 1976a

Prehn, R. T. Do tumors grow because of the immune response of the host? Transplant Rev 28, 34–42, 1976b

Prehn, R. T. Immunostimulation of the lymphodependent phase of neoplastic growth. J Natl Cancer Inst 59, 1043–1049, 1977

Prehn, R. T., and Lappé, M. A. An immunostimulation theory of tumor development. Transplant Rev 7, 26–54, 1971

Prehn, R. T., and Main, J. M. Immunity to methylcholanthrene-induced sarcomas. J Natl Cancer Inst 18, 769–778, 1957

Presant, C. A., Bartolucci, A. A., Smalley, R. V., and Vogler, W. R. Effect of Corynebacterium parvum on combination chemotherapy of disseminated malignant melanoma, pp 113–121, In Terry, W. D., and Windhorst, D. (Eds): Immunotherapy of Cancer: Present Status of Trials in Man. New York: Raven Press, 1978

Preud'Homme, J. L., Klein, M., Verroust, P., and Seligman, M. Immunoglobulines monoclonales de membrane dans les leucémies lymphoides chroniques. Rev Eur Etudes Clin Biol 16, 1025–1031, 1971

Preussman, R. Chemical carcinogens in the human environment. Problems and quantitative aspects. Oncology 33, 51–57, 1976

Price, F. B., Hewlett, J. S., Deodhar, S. D., and Barna, B. The therapy of malignant melanoma with transfer factor. Cleve Clin Q 41, 1–4, 1974

Price, M. R., and Baldwin, R. W. Immunogeneic properties of rat hepatoma subcellular fractions. Br J Cancer 30, 394–400, 1974

Price, M. R., and Baldwin, R. W. Shedding of tumor cell-surface antigens. Cell Surf Rev 3, 423–471, 1977

Priester W. A. Esophogeal cancer in North China: High rate in human and poultry population in the same areas. Avian Dis 19, 213–215, 1975

Prinzmetal, M., Ornitz, E. M., Simkin, B., and Bergman, H. C. Arterio-venous anastomoses in liver, spleen and lungs. Am J Physiol 152, 48–52, 1948

Priori, E. S., Wilbur, J. R., and Dmochowski, L. Immunofluorescence tests of sera of patients with osteogenic sarcoma. J Natl Cancer Inst 46, 1299–1308, 1971

Pritchard, D. J., Reilly, C. A., and Finkel, M. P. Evidence for a human osteosarcoma virus. Nature New Biol 234, 126–127, 1971

Pritchard, H., and Micklem, H. S. Haemopoietic stem cells and progenitors of functional T-lymphocytes in the bone marrow of nude mice. Clin Exp Immunol 14, 597–607, 1973

Prochnownik, E. V., and Kirsten, W. H. Inhibition of reverse transcriptases of primate type C viruses by 7S immunoglobulin from patients with leukaemia. Nature 260, 64–67, 1976

Proctor, J., Rudenstam, C. M., and Alexander, P. Increased incidence of lung metastases following treatment of rats bearing hepatomas with irradiated tumour cells, and the beneficial effect of Corynebacterium parvum in this system. Biomedicine 19, 248–252, 1973a

Proctor, J. W., Rudenstam, C. M., and Alexander, P. A factor preventing the development of lung metastases in rats with sarcomas. Nature 242, 29–31, 1973b

Pross, H. F., and Jondal, M. Cytotoxic lymphocytes from normal donors. A functional marker of human non-T lymphocytes. Clin Exp Immunol 21, 226–235, 1975

Pruitt, J. C., Hilberg, A. W., and Kaiser, R. F. Malignant cells in peripheral blood. N Engl J Med 259, 1161–1164, 1958

Pruitt, J. C., Hilberg, A. W., Morehead, R. P., and Mengoli, H. F. Quantitative study of malignant cells in local and peripheral circulating blood. Surg Gynecol Obstet 114, 179–188, 1962

Purchase, H. G., Okazaki, W., and Burmester, B. R. Field trials with the herpes virus of turkeys (HVT) strain FC126 as a vaccine against Marek's disease. Poult Sci 50, 775–779, 1971

Purtilo, D. T., Cassel, C. K., Yang, J. P. S., Harper, R., Stephenson, S. R., Landing, B. H., and Vawter, G. F. X-linked recessive progressive combined variable immunodeficiency (Duncan's disease). Lancet 1, 935–941, 1975

Purves, H. D., and Griesbach, W. E. Studies on experimental goitre: Thyroid tumours in rats treated with thiourea. Br J Exp Pathol 28, 46–53, 1947

Purves, L. R., Bersohn, I., and Geddes, E. W. Serum alpha-feto-protein and primary cancer of the liver in man. Cancer 25, 1261–1270, 1970

Puvion, F., Fray, A., and Halpern, B. A cytochemical study of the in vitro interaction between normal and activated mouse peritoneal macrophages and tumor cells. J Ultrastruct Res 54, 95–108, 1976

Q

Quaglino, D., and Cowling, D. C. Cytochemical studies on cells from chronic lymphatic leukaemia and lymphosarcoma cultured with phytohaemagglutinin. Br J Haematol 10, 358–364, 1964

R

Rabbatt, A. G., and Jeejeebhoy, H. F. Heterologous antilymphocyte serum (ALS) hastens the appearance of methylcholanthrene-induced tumors in mice. Transplantation 9, 164–166, 1970

Rabotti, G. F., Grove, A. S., Sellers, R. L., and Anderson, W. R. Induction of multiple brain tumours (gliomata and leptomeningeal sarcomata) in dogs by Rous sarcoma virus. Nature 209, 884–886, 1966

Raff, M. C. Θ-Bearing lymphocytes in nude mice. Nature 246, 350–351, 1973

Raff, M. C. Immunological networks. Nature 265, 205–207, 1977

Raff, M. C., and Wortis, H. H. Thymus dependence of θ-bearing cells in the peripheral lymphoid tissues of mice. Immunology 18, 931–942, 1970

Rajewsky, M. F., and Gruneisen, A. Cell proliferation in transplanted rat tumors: influence of the host immune system. Eur J Immunol 2, 445–447, 1972

Ramming, K. P., and Pilch, Y. H. Mediation of immunity to tumor isografts in mice by heterologous ribonucleic acid. Science 168, 492–493, 1970

Ramming, K. P., and Pilch, Y. H. Transfer of tumor-specific immunity with RNA: Inhibition of growth of murine tumor isografts. J Natl Cancer Inst 46, 735–750, 1971

Ran, M., and Witz, I. P. Tumour-associated immunoglobulins. The elution of IgG2 from mouse tumors. Int J Cancer 6, 361–372, 1970

Rao, V. S., and Bonavida, B. Detection of soluble tumor-associated antigens in serum of tumor-bearing rats and their immunological role in vivo. Cancer Res 37, 3385–3389, 1977

Rapaport, F. T. Cross-reactive antigens, cancer and transplantation. Transplant Proc 6, 39–44, 1974

Rapaport, F. T. A possible role for cross-reacting antigens in conditioning immunological surveillance mechanisms in cancer and transplantation, pp 272–281, In Neter, E., and Milgrom, F. (Eds): The Immune System and Infectious Diseases, 4th Int Convoc—Immunology (Buffalo, N. Y., 1974). Basel: S. Karger, 1975

Rapaport, F. T., Dausset, J., Converse, J. M., and Lawrence, H. S. Biological and ultrastructural studies of leucocyte fractions as transplantation antigens in man. Transplantation 3, 490–500, 1965

Rapin, A. M. C., and Burger, M. M. Tumor cell surfaces: General alterations detected by agglutinins. Adv Cancer Res 20, 1–91, 1974

Rapp, F. Herpesviruses and cancer. Adv Cancer Res 19, 265–302, 1974

Ratner, A. C., Waldorf, D. S., and Van Scott, E. J. Alterations of lesions of mycosis fungoides lymphoma by direct imposition of delayed hypersensitivity reaction. Cancer 21, 83–88, 1968

Rauchwerger, J. M., Gallagher, M. T., Monie, H. J., and Trentin, J. J. "Xenogeneic resistance" to rat marrow transplantation: Maturation, split-dose irradiation, thymectomy, and Corynebacterium parvum (CP) studies. Fed Proc 32, 971, 1973

Ravdin, R. G., Lewison, E. F., Slack, N. H., Gardner, B., State, D., and Fisher, B. Results of a clinical trial concerning the worth of prophylactic oophorectomy for breast carcinoma. Surg Gynecol Obstet 131, 1055–1064, 1971

Rawls, W. E., Tomkins, W., and Melnick, J. L. The association of herpesvirus type 2 and carcinoma of the cervix. Am J Epidemiol 89, 547–554, 1969

Ray, P. K., Poduval, T. B., and Sundaram, K. Antitumor immunity. V. BCG-induced growth inhibition of murine tumors. Effect of hydrocortisone, antiserum against theta antigen, and gamma-irradiated BCG. J Natl Cancer Inst 58, 763–767, 1977

Rebuck, J. W., and Crowley, J. H. Method of studying leukocytic functions in vivo. Ann NY Acad Sci 59, 757–794, 1955

Reed, R. C. Increased regression of liver and lung

metastases of disseminated melanoma by the addition of Corynebacterium parvum to the imidazolecarboxamide, nitrosourea, and BCG regimen. Proc Am Assoc Cancer Res *17*, 214, 1976

Reed, R. C., Gutterman, J. U., Mavligit, G. M., Burgess, A. A., and Hersh, E. M. Corynebacterium parvum. Preliminary report of a phase I clinical and immunological study in cancer patients, pp 349–366, In Halpern, B. (Ed): Corynebacterium Parvum: Applications in Experimental and Clinical Oncology. New York: Plenum Press, 1975

Rees, J. A., and Symes, M. O. Observations on the increasing malignancy of tumours on prolonged growth: The influence of immunological changes in the host. Br J Cancer *15*, 121–129, 1971

Rees, J. A., and Symes, M. O. An in vivo test for the immunocompetence of human lymphocytes. Transplantation *16*, 565–569, 1973

Rees, L. H. The biosynthesis of hormones by nonendocrine tumours: A review. J Endocrinol *67*, 143–175, 1975

Rees, R. C., Price, M. R., Shan, L. P., and Baldwin, R. W. Detection of hepatoma-associated embryonic antigen in tumour-bearer serum. Transplantation *19*, 424–429, 1975

Refsum, S. B., and Berdall, P. Cell loss in malignant tumours in man. Eur J Cancer *3*, 235–236, 1967

Reif, A. E., and Kim, C.-A. H. Therapy of transplantable mouse leukaemias with antileukaemia sera. Nature *223*, 1377–1379, 1969

Reif, A. E., and Kim, C.-A. H. Leukemia L1210 therapy trials with antileukemia serum and bacillus Calmette-Guérin. Cancer Res *31*, 1606–1612, 1971

Reiner, J. Influence of multiple injections of normal syngeneic cells on tumor induction in mice. Cancer Res *30*, 2087–2088, 1970

Reiner, J., and Southam, C. M. Evidence of common antigenic properties in chemically induced sarcomas of mice. Cancer Res *27*, 1243–1247, 1967

Reiner, J., and Southam, C. M. Further evidence of common antigenic properties in chemically induced sarcomas of mice. Cancer Res *29*, 1814–1820, 1969

Reizenstein, P., Brenning, G., Engstedt, L., and Franzen, S. Effect of immunotherapy on survival and remission duration in acute non-lymphatic leukemia, pp 329–339, In Terry, W. D., and Windhorst, D. (Eds): Immunotherapy of Cancer: Present Status of Trials in Man. New York: Raven Press, 1978

Remington, J. S., and Merigan, T. C. Synthetic

polyanions protect mice against intracellular bacterial infection. Nature *226*, 361–363, 1970

Rénaud, M. La cutiréaction à la tuberculine chez les cancéreux. Bull Soc Med Paris *50*, 1441–1442, 1926

Renoux, G., and Renoux, M. Restauration par le phenylimidothiazole de la réponse immunologique des souris âgées. CR Acad Sci D Paris *274*, 3034–3035, 1972a

Renoux, G., and Renoux, M. Action du phenylimidothiazole (tétramisole) sur la réaction du greffon contre l'hôte. Rôle des macrophages. CR Acad Sci D Paris *274*, 3320–3323, 1972b

Renoux, G., and Renoux, M. Levamisole inhibits and cures a solid malignant tumour and its pulmonary metastases in mice. Nature New Biol *240*, 217–218, 1972c

Renoux, G., Renoux,M., and Branche, R. Stimulation of antibacterial vaccination in mice by polyadenylic acid:polyuridylic acid complex. Infect Immun *6*, 699–702, 1972

Renoux, G., Renoux, M., and Palat, A. Influences of levamisole on T-cell reactivity and on survival of untractable cancer patients. Fogarty Int Center Proc No. 28. Washington, D.C.: U.S. Govt Printing Office, 1975 [*Cited by Amery (1976)*]

Renoux, G., Renoux, M., Teller, M. N., McMahon, S., and Guillaumin, J. M. Potentiation of T-cell mediated immunity by levamisole. Clin Exp Immunol *25*, 288–296, 1976

Retik, A. B., Arons, M. S., Ketcham, A. S., and Mantel, N. The effect of heparin on primary tumors and metastases. J Surg Res *2*, 49–53, 1962

Revesz, L. Detection of antigenic differences in isologous host-tumor systems by pretreatment with heavily irradiated tumor cells. Cancer Res *20*, 443–451, 1960

Reynoso, G., Chu, M. T., Guinan, P., and Murphy, G. P. Carcinoembryonic antigen in patients with tumors of the urogenital tract. Cancer *30*, 1–4, 1972a

Reynoso, G., Chu, M. T., Holyoke, D., Cohen, E., Nemoto, T., Wang, J. J., Chuang, J., Guinan, P., and Murphy, G. P. Carcinoembryonic antigen in patients with different cancers. JAMA *220*, 361–365, 1972b

Ribacchi, R., and Giraldo, G. Leukemia virus release in chemically or physically induced lymphomas in BALB/c mice. Natl Cancer Inst Monogr *22*, 701–711, 1966

Ribi, E. E., Granger, D. L., Milner, K. C., and Strain, M. S. Tumor regression caused by endotoxins and mycobacterial fractions. J Natl Cancer Inst *55*, 1253–1257, 1975

Riccardi, C., Fioretti, M. C., Giampietri, A., Puccetti, P., Goldin, A., and Bonmassar, E. Growth inhibition of normal or drug-treated lymphoma cells in lethally irradiated mice. J Natl Cancer Inst 60, 1083–1090, 1978a

Riccardi, C., Puccetti, P., Santoni, A., and Herberman, R. B. [Cited by Herberman et al. (1979) as submitted for publication] 1978b

Rich, M. A., Geldner, A., and Meyers, P. Studies on murine leukemia. J Natl Cancer Inst 35, 523–536, 1965

Richards, V., and Klausner, C. The heterologous transplantation of human cancer in untreated Swiss-Webster mice. Surgery 44, 181–198, 1958

Richardson, R. L., Oldham, R. K., Pomeroy, T. C., Weese, J. L., McCoy, J. L., Cannon, G. B., Dean, J. H., and Herberman, R. B. Immunologic monitoring and immunotherapy in Ewing's sarcoma. Cancer Immunol Immunother 4, 87–94, 1978

Richie, E. R., Monie, H. J., Trentin, J. J., and Taub, R. N. Inhibition of the graft-versus-host reaction. III. Altered in vivo distribution of spleen cells pretreated with Fab fragments of antithymocyte globulin. Transplantation 19, 115–120, 1975

Richter, P. H. A network theory of the immune system. Eur J Immunol 5, 350–354, 1975

Richters, A., and Sherwin, R. P. The behaviour of lymphocytes in primary explants of human lung cancer in vitro. Lab Invest 13, 1520–1529, 1964

Riesco, A. Five year cancer cure: Relation to total amount of peripheral lymphocytes and neutrophils. Cancer 25, 135–140, 1970

Riesen, W., Noseda, G., Morell, A., Butler, R., Barandun, S., and Nydegger, U. E. Autoantibodies with antilipoprotein specificity and hypolipoproteinemia in patients with cancer. Cancer Res 35, 535–541, 1975

Rigby, P. G. Prolongation of survival of tumor-bearing animals by transfer of "immune" RNA with DEAE dextran. Nature 221, 968–969, 1969

Riggins, R. S., and Pilch, Y. H. Immunity to spontaneous and methylcholanthrene-induced tumors in inbred mice. Cancer Res 24, 1994–1996, 1964

Riggs, B. L., Arnaud, C. D., Reynolds, J. D., and Smith, L. H. Immunologic differentiation of primary hyperparathyroidism from hyperparathyroidism due to non parathyroid cancer. J Clin Invest 50, 2079–2083, 1971

Rios, A., and Simmons, R. L. Experimental cancer immunotherapy using a neuraminidase-treated non-viable frozen tumor vaccine. Surgery 75, 503–507, 1974a

Rios, A., and Simmons, R. L. Active specific immunotherapy of minimal residual tumor: Excision plus neuraminidase-treated tumor cells. Int J Cancer 13, 71–81, 1974b

Ritts, R. E., Pritchard, D. J., Gilchrist, G. S., Ivins, J. C., and Taylor, W. F. Transfer factor versus combination chemotherapy: An interim report of a randomized postsurgical adjuvant study in osteogenic sarcoma, pp 293–298, In Terry, W. D., and Windhorst, D. (Eds): Immunotherapy of Cancer: Present Status of Trials in Man. New York: Raven Press, 1978

Riveros-Moreno, V., Bomford, R., and Scott, M. T. Antitumor activity of purified cell walls from Corynebacterium parvum. J Natl Cancer Inst 60, 653–658, 1978

Robert, F., Oth, D., and Dumont, F. Cross-immunity between chemically-induced sarcomas, detected by transplantation in restricted genetic conditions. Eur J Cancer 9, 877–878, 1973

Roberts, M. M. Lymphocyte function in breast cancer. Eur Surg Res 6, 11–17, 1974

Roberts, M. M., Bass, E. M., Wallace, I. W. J., and Stevenson, A. Local immunoglobulin production in breast cancer. Br J Cancer 27, 269–275, 1973

Roberts, M. M., Bathgate, E. M., and Stevenson, A. Serum immunoglobulin levels in breast cancer. Cancer 36, 221–224, 1975

Roberts, M., and Jones-Williams, W. The delayed hypersensitivity reaction in breast cancer. Br J Surg 61, 549–552, 1974

Roberts, S., Jonasson, O., Long, L., McGrath, R., McGrew, E. A., and Cole, W. H. Clinical significance of cancer cells in the circulating blood: Two- to five-year survival. Ann Surg 154, 362–371, 1961

Roberts, S., Watne, A., McGrath, R., McGrew, E., and Cole, W. H. Technique and results of isolation of cancer cells from circulating blood. Arch Surg 76, 334–346, 1958

Robertson, H. T., and Black, P. H. Changes in surface antigens of SV40-virus transformed cells. Proc Soc Exp Biol Med 130, 363–370, 1969

Robins, R. A., and Baldwin, R. W. Immune markers on cancer cells. Cancer Immunol Immunother 2, 205–207, 1977

Robinson, E. Immunology and phytohaemagglutinin in cancer. Lancet 2, 753, 1966

Robinson, E., Ben-Hur, N., Shulman, J., Hochman, A., and Neuman, Z. Comparative study of skin homografts of normal donors and donors with malignant neoplasia in a host with malignant disease. A preliminary report. J Natl Cancer Inst 34, 185–190, 1965

Robinson, E., and Hochman, A. Comparative study of the lymphocyte transfer test with lymphocytes from normal donors and cancer patients. J Natl Cancer Inst 36, 819–824, 1966

Robinson, K. P., and Hoppe, E. The development of blood-borne metastases. Effect of local trauma and ischaemia. Arch Surg 85, 720–724, 1962

Robinson, R. A., DeVita, V. T., Levy, H. B., Baron, S., Husband, S. P., and Levine, A. S. A phase I–II trial of multiple-dose polyriboinosinic-polyribocytidylic acid in patients with leukemia or solid tumors. J Natl Cancer Inst 57, 599–602, 1976

Robson, M., and Moynihan, B. G. A. Diseases of the Stomach and Their Surgical Treatment (ed 2). London: Ballière, Tindall & Cox, 1904

Rocklin, R. E., Meyers, O. L., and David, J. R. An in vitro assay for cellular hypersensitivity in man. J Immunol 104, 95–102, 1970

Rodda, S. J., and White, L. O. Cytotoxic macrophages: A rapid nonspecific response to viral infection. J Immunol 117, 2067–2072, 1976

Roder, J. C., and Kiessling, R. Target-effector interaction in the natural killer cell system, I. Co-variance and genetic control of cytolytic and target-cell-binding subpopulations in the mouse. Scand J Immunol 8, 135–144, 1978

Roenigk, H., Deodhar, S., St. Jacques, R., and Burdick, K. Immunotherapy of malignant melanoma with vaccinia virus. Arch Dermatol 109, 668–673, 1974

Rohdenburg, G. L., and Prime, F. Effect of combined radiation and heat on neoplasms. Arch Surg 2, 116–129, 1921

Rojas, A. F., Feierstein, J. N., Glait, H. M., and Olivari, A. J. Levamisole action in breast cancer stage III, pp 635–645, In Terry, W. D., and Windhorst, D. (Eds): Immunotherapy of Cancer: Present Status of Trials in Man. New York: Raven Press, 1978

Rojas, A. F., Mickiewicz, E., Feierstein, J. N., Glait, H., and Olivari, A. J. Levamisole in advanced human breast cancer. Lancet 1, 211–215, 1976

Rollinghoff, M., Rouse, B. T., and Warner, N. L. Tumor immunity to murine plasma cell tumors. I. Tumor-associated transplantation antigens of NZB and Balb/c plasma cell tumors. J Natl Cancer Inst 50, 159–172, 1973

Rollinghoff, M., and Wagner, H. In vitro induction of tumor specific immunity II. The requirements for T lymphocytes and the protective potential against tumor growth in vivo. Eur J Immunol 3, 471–476, 1973a

Rollinghoff, M., and Wagner, H. In vivo protection against murine plasma cell tumor growth by in vitro activated syngeneic lymphocytes. J Natl Cancer Inst 51, 1317–1318, 1973b

Romsdahl, M. M. Influence of surgical procedures on development of spontaneous lung metastases. J Surg Res, 363–370, 1964

Rose, S. Augmentation of immune activity and its implications in cancer. J Surg Oncol 5, 137–166, 1973

Rosen, G., Wollner, N., and Wu, S. Prolonged disease-free survival in children with Ewing's sarcoma treated with radiation therapy and adjuvant 4-drug sequential chemotherapy. Cancer 33, 384–393, 1974

Rosenau, W., and Morton, D. L. Tumor-specific inhibition of growth of methylcholanthrene-induced sarcomas in vivo and in vitro by sensitized isologous lymphoid cells. J Natl Cancer Inst 36, 825–836, 1966

Rosenberg, E. B., Herberman, R. B., Levine, P. H., Halterman, R. H., McCoy, J. L., and Wunderlich, J. R. Lymphocyte cytotoxicity reactions to leukemia-associated antigens in identical twins. Int J Cancer 9, 648–658, 1972

Rosenberg, E. B., McCoy, J. L., Green, S. S., Donnelly, F. C., Siwarski, D. F., Levine, P. H., and Herberman, R. B. Destruction of human lymphoid tissue culture cell lines by human peripheral lymphocytes in ^{51}Cr release cellular cytotoxicity assays. J Natl Cancer Inst 52, 345–352, 1974

Rosenberg, S. A. Problems with the leukocyte migration inhibition technique in the study of human tumor immunity. Natl Cancer Inst Monogr 37, 139–140, 1973

Rosenberg, S. A., and David, J. R. Inhibition of leukocyte migration: An evaluation of this in vitro assay of delayed hypersensitivity in man to a soluble antigen. J Immunol 105, 1447–1452, 1970

Rosenberg, S. A., and Terry, W. D. Passive immunotherapy of cancer in animals and man. Adv Cancer Res 25, 323–388, 1977

Rosenstreich, D. L., Farrar, J. J., and Dougherty, S. Absolute macrophage dependency of T-lymphocyte activation by mitogens. J Immunol 116, 131–139, 1976

Rosenstreich, D. L., and Mizel, S. B. The participation of macrophages and macrophage cell lines in the activation of T lymphocytes by mitogens. Immunol Rev 40, 102–135, 1978

Rosenthal, A. S., Lipsky, P. E., and Shevach, E. M. Macrophage–lymphocyte interaction and antigen recognition. Fed Proc 34, 1743–1748, 1975

Ross, J. M. Carcinogenic action of radium in rabbit; Effect of prolonged irradiation with screened radium. J Pathol Bacteriol 43, 267–276, 1936

Roth, J. A., Silverstein, M. J., and Morton, D. L.

Metastatic potential of metastases. Surgery *79*, 669–673, 1976

Roubinian, J. R., Lane, M.-A., Slomich, M., and Blair, P. B. Stimulation of immune mechanisms against mammary tumors by incomplete T cell depletion. J Immunol *117*, 1767–1773, 1976

Roumiantzeff, M., Gamen, J., Musetescu, M., Mynard, M. C., Beranger, G., and Vincent-Falquet, J. C. Mouse tumour tests for quality control of C. parvum preparations. Dev Biol Stand *38*, 59–64, 1978

Roumiantzeff, M., Mynard, M. C., Coquet, B., Goldman, C., and Ayme, G. Acute and chronic toxicities in mammal and subhuman primates with inactivated corynebacterium suspension, pp 11–31, In Halpern, B. (Ed): Corynebacterium Parvum: Applications in Experimental and Clinical Oncology. New York: Plenum Press, 1975

Rous, P. An experimental comparison of transplanted tumour and a transplanted normal tissue capable of growth. J Exp Med *12*, 344–366, 1910a

Rous, P. A transmissible avian neoplasm (sarcoma of the common fowl). J Exp Med *12*, 696–705, 1910b

Rous, P. A sarcoma of the fowl transmissible by an agent separable from the tumor cells. J Exp Med *13*, 397–411, 1911

Rous, P., and Kidd, J. G. Conditional neoplasms and subthreshold neoplastic states. A study of the tar tumors of rabbits. J Exp Med *73*, 365–390, 1941

Rous, P., and Smith, W. E. Neoplastic potentialities of mouse embryo tissues. I and II. J Exp Med *81*, 597–620, 1945

Rousselot, L. M., Cole, D. R., Grossi, C. E., Conte, A. J., Gouzales, E. M., and Pasternack, B. S. Adjuvant chemotherapy with 5-fluorouracil in surgery for colorectal cancer. Dis Colon Rectum *15*, 169–174, 1972

Rowland, G. F., O'Neill, G. J., and Davies, D. A. L. Suppression of tumour growth in mice by a drug-antibody conjugate using a novel approach to linkage. Nature *255*, 487–488, 1975

Rowley, J. D. Do human tumors show a chromosome pattern specific for each etiologic agent? J Natl Cancer Inst *52*, 315–320, 1974

Rowntree, C. X-ray cancer. Br Med J *2*, 1111–1112, 1922

Rubens, R. D., and Dulbecco, R. Augmentation of cytotoxic drug action by antibodies directed at cell surface. Nature *248*, 81–82, 1974

Rubens, R. D., Vaughan-Smith, S., and Dulbecco, R. Augmentation of cytotoxic drug action and

x-irradiation by antibodies. Br J Cancer *32*, 352–354, 1975

Rubin, B. A. Analysis of a tolerance phenomenon evoked in adult mice by carcinogen hydrocarbons. Blood *20*, 113, 1962

Rubin, B. A. Alteration of the homograft response as a determinant of carcinogenicity. Prog Exp Tumor Res *14*, 138–195, 1971

Rubin, B. A., and Ida, N. Studies on the mechanisms of growth enhancement of transplanted mouse tumors by carcinogens. Proc Am Assoc Cancer Res *2*, 244, 1957

Ruckdeschel, J. C., Codish, S. D., Stranahan, A., and McKneally, M. F. Postoperative empyema improves survival in lung cancer: Documentation and analysis of a natural experiment. N Engl J Med *287*, 1013–1017, 1972

Rudenstam, C. M. Experimental studies on trauma and metastasis formation. Acta Chir Scand (Suppl) *391*, 12–18, 1968

Rudolph, R. H., Fefer, A., Thomas, E. D., Buckner, C. D., Clift, R. A., and Storb, R. Isogeneic marrow grafts for hematologic malignancy in man. Arch Intern Med *132*, 279–285, 1973

Ruhl, H., Vogt, W., Bochert, G., and Diamanstein, T. Stimulation of B cells by poly A:poly U and poly I:poly C in vitro. Immunology *26*, 937–941, 1974

Ruitenberg, E. J., and Steerenberg, P. A. Possible immunosuppressive effect of Corynebacterium parvum on infection with Trichinella spiralis. Nature New Biol *242*, 149–150, 1973

Ruitenberg, E. J., and van Noorle Jansen, L. M. [*Cited by Milas and Scott (1977).*] Zentralbl Bakteriol Parasitenkd Infektionskr Hyg Abt 1 Orig Reine A *231*, 197, 1975

Rumma, J., and Davies, D. J. Survival of F1 hybrid rats inoculated with a strain specific transplantable carcinoma following the induction of a systemic graft-versus-host reaction. Br J Cancer *32*, 134–138, 1975

Ruoslahti E., and Seppälä, M. Studies of carcino-fetal proteins. III. Development of a radioimmunoassay for α-fetoprotein. Demonstration of α-fetoprotein in serum of healthy human adults. Int J Cancer *8*, 374–383, 1971

Russell, B. R. G. The nature of resistance to the inoculation of cancer. ICRF Third Sci Rep *3*, 341–358, 1908

Russell, J. A., Chapuis, B., and Powles, R. L. Various uses of BCG and allogeneic acute leukemia cells to treat patients with acute myelogenous leukemia. Cancer Immunol Immunother *1*, 87–91, 1976

Russell, R. J., McInroy, R. J., Wilkinson, P. C., and White, R. G. A lipid chemotactic factor

from anaerobic coryneform bacteria including
Corynebacterium parvum with activity for
macrophages and monocytes. Immunology 30,
935–949, 1976

Russell, S. W., and Cochrane, C. G. The cellular
events associated with regression and progression of murine (Moloney) sarcoma. Int J Cancer 13, 54–64, 1974

Russell, S. W., Doe, W. F., and Cochrane, C. G.
Number of macrophages and distribution of
mitotic activity in regressing and progressing
Moloney sarcomas. J Immunol 116, 164–166,
1976

Russell, S. W., and McIntosh, A. T. Macrophages
isolated from regressing Moloney sarcomas are
more cytotoxic than those recovered from progressing sarcomas. Nature 268, 69–71, 1977

Ryan, J. J., Ketcham, A. S., and Wexler, H. Warfarin treatment of mice bearing autochthonous
tumors; Effect on spontaneous metastases. Science 162, 1493–1494, 1968a

Ryan, J. J., Ketcham, A. S., and Wexler, H. Reduced incidence of spontaneous metastases
with long term coumarin therapy. Ann Surg
168, 163–168, 1968b

Rygaard, J., and Povlsen, C. O. Heterotransplantation of a human malignant tumor to nude
mice. Acta Pathol Microbiol Scand 77, 758–
760, 1969

Rygaard, J., and Povlsen, C. O. Is immunological
surveillance not a cell-mediated immune function? Transplantation 17, 135–136, 1974a

Rygaard, J., and Povlsen, C. O. The mouse mutant
nude does not develop spontaneous tumours.
An argument against immunological surveillance. Acta Pathol Microbiol Scand 82, 99–
106, 1974b

Rygaard, J., and Povlsen, C. O. The nude mouse
vs the hypothesis of immunological surveillance. Transplant Rev 28, 43–61, 1976

Ryser, H. J. P. Chemical carcinogenesis. N Engl
J Med 285, 721–734, 1971

Rytömaa, T. The chalone concept. Int Rev Exp
Pathol 16, 156–205, 1976

Rytömaa, T., and Kiviniemi, K. Chloroma regression induced by the granulocytic chalone. Nature 222, 995–996, 1969

Rytömaa, T., and Kiviniemi, K. Regression of generalized leukaemia in rat induced by the granulocytic chalone. Eur J Cancer 6, 401–410,
1970

Rytömaa, T., Vilpo, J. A., Levanto, A., and Jones,
W. A. Effect of granulocyte chalone on acute
and chronic granulocytic leukaemia in man.
Report of seven cases. Scand J Haematol 27
(Suppl), 3–28, 1976

S

Saal, J. G., Rieber, E. P., Hadam, M., and Reith-
muller, G. Lymphocytes with T-cell markers
co-operate with IgG antibodies in the lysis of
human tumour cells. Nature 265, 158–160, 1977

Sachs, B. A., Becker, N., Bloomberg, A. E., and
Grunwald, R. P. "Cure" of ectopic ACTH
syndrome secondary to adenocarcinoma of the
lung. J Clin Endocrinol Metab 30, 590–597,
1970

Sadler, T. E., and Castro, J. E. Lack of immunological and anti-tumour effects of orally administered Corynebacterium parvum in mice.
Br J Cancer 31, 359–363, 1975

Sadler, T. E., and Castro, J. E. The effects of Corynebacterium parvum and surgery on the Lewis lung carcinoma and its metastases. Br J
Surg 63, 292–296, 1976a

Sadler, T. E., and Castro, J. E. Abrogation of the
anti-metastatic activity of C. parvum by antilymphocyte serum. Br J Cancer 34, 291–295,
1976b

Sadler, T. E., Cramp, W. A., and Castro, J. E.
Radiolabelling of Corynebacterium parvum
and its distribution in mice. Br J Cancer 35,
357–368, 1977

Sadler, T. E., Cramp, W. A., and Castro, J. E.
Distribution of ^{3}H-thymidine-labelled C. parvum in mice. Dev Biol Stand 38, 137–143,
1978

Sadowski, J. M., and Rapp, F. Inhibition by levamisole of metastases by cells transformed
by herpes simplex virus type 1. Proc Soc Exp
Biol Med 149, 219–222, 1975

Saksela, E., Timonen, T., Ranki, A., and Häyry,
P. Morphological and functional characterization of isolated effector cells responsible for
human natural killer activity to fetal fibroblasts
and to cultured cell line targets. Immunol Rev
44, 71–123, 1979

Sakurai, M. Studies on antigenicity of leukemia
and administration of antileukemic plasma to
the leukemic patients. Mie Med J 16, 79–92,
1966

Salama, F., Loke, R. G., and Hellebusch, A. A.
Carcinoma of the kidney producing multiple
hormones. J Urol 106, 820–822, 1971

Salaman, J. R., Millar, D., and Brown, P. Human
immunity to rat antigens. Transplantation 19,
505–510, 1975

Salaman, M. H. Immunodepression by mammalian
viruses and plasmodia. Proc R Soc Med 63,
11–15, 1970

Salaman, M. H., and Roe, F. J. C. Incomplete carcinogens: Ethyl carbamate (urethane) as an initiator of skin tumor formation in the mouse. Br J Cancer 7, 472–481, 1953

Salaman, M. H., and Wedderburn, N. The immunodepressive effect of Friend virus. Immunology 10, 445–458, 1966

Salaman, P. F. Double primaries. Proc R Soc Med 69, 704, 1976

Salih, H., Flax, H., Brander, W., and Hobbs, J. R. Prolactin dependence in human breast cancers. Lancet 2, 1103–1105, 1972

Salinas, F. A., and Hanna, M. G. Host response to tumor-associated fetal antigens. J Immunol 112, 1026–1034, 1974

Salinas, F. A., Smith, J. A., and Hanna, M. G. Immunological cross-reactivity of antigens common to tumor and fetal cells. Nature 240, 41–43, 1972

Salky, N. K., Di Luzio, N. R., Levin, A. G., and Goldsmith, H. S. Phagocytic activity of the reticuloendothelial system in neoplastic disease. J Lab Clin Med 70, 393–403, 1967

Salky, N. K., DiLuzio, N. R., P'Pool, D. B., and Sutherland, A. J. Evaluation of reticuloendothelial function in man. JAMA 187, 744–748, 1964

Salmon, S. E., and Jones, S. E. (Eds): Adjuvant Therapy of Cancer (Proc 1st Int Conference on the Adjuvant Therapy of Cancer, Tucson, Arizona, 1977). Amsterdam: Elsevier/North-Holland Biomedical Press, 1977

Salmon, S. E., and Seligman, M. Hypothesis: B-cell neoplasia in man. Lancet 2, 1230–1233, 1974

Salomon, J.-C., Galinha, A., Lascaux, V., Prin, J., Puvion, F., and Lynch, N. Intra-lesional injection of immunostimulants in bilateral rat tumors. Int J Cancer 18, 379–391, 1976

Salomon, J.-C., and Lynch, N. Intralesional injection of immunostimulants in rat and mouse tumors. Cancer Immunol Immunother 1, 145–151, 1976

Salsbury, A. J., White, C., Tsolakidis, P., McKinna, J. A., and Griffiths, J. D. Fibrinolysis and circulating malignant cells. Surg Gynecol Obstet 136, 733–736, 1973

Samellas, W. Spontaneous regression of pulmonary metastases from renal carcinoma. J Urol 85, 494–496, 1961

Sandberg, A. A., and Moore, G. F. Examination of blood for tumour cells. J Natl Cancer Inst 19, 1–12, 1957

Sander, S. The "in vitro" uptake of estrodiol in biopsies from 25 breast cancer patients. Acta Pathol Microbiol Scand 74, 301–302, 1968

Sanderson, C. J., and Frost, P. The induction of tumour immunity in mice using glutaraldehyde-treated tumour cells. Nature 248, 690–691, 1974

Sanderson, C. J., and Taylor, G. A. Antibody-dependent cell-mediated cytotoxicity in the rat. The role of macrophages. Immunology 30, 117–121, 1976

Sanford, B. H., An alteration in tumor histocompatibility induced by neuraminidase. Transplantation 5, 1273 1279, 1967

Sanford, B., and Codington, J. F. Further studies on the effect of neuraminidase on tumor cell transplantability. Tissue Antigens 1, 153–161, 1971

Sanford, B. H., Kohn, H. I., Daly, J. J., and Soo, S. F. Long-term spontaneous tumor incidence in neonatally thymectomized mice. J Immunol 110, 1437–1439, 1973

Sansing, W. A., Killion, J. J., and Kollmorgen, G. M. Evaluation of time and dose in treating mammary adenocarcinoma with immunostimulants. Cancer Immunol Immunother 2, 63–68, 1977

Santoli, D., and Koprowski, H. Mechanisms of activation of human natural killer cells against tumor and virus-infected cells. Immunol Rev 44, 125–163, 1979

Santos, G. W., Burke, P. J., Sensenbrenner, L. L., and Owens, A. H. Marrow transplantation and graft-versus-host disease in acute monocytic leukaemia. Exp Hematol 18, 20–25, 1969

Santos, G. W., Mullins, G. M., Bias, W. B., Anderson, P. N., Graziano, K. D., Klein, D. L., and Burke, P. J. Immunological studies in acute leukemia. Natl Cancer Inst Monogr 37, 69–75, 1973

Santos, G. W., Sensenbrenner, L. L., Anderson, P. N., Burke, P. J., Klein, D. L., Slavin, R. E., Schacter, B., and Borgaonkar, D. S. HL-A-identical marrow transplants in aplastic anemia, acute leukemia, and lymphosarcoma employing cyclophosphamide. Transplant Proc 8, 607–610, 1976

Santos, G. W., Sensenbrenner, L. L., Burke, P. J., Colvin, M., Owens, A. H., Bias, W. B., and Slavin, R. E. Marrow transplantation in man following cyclophosphamide. Transplant Proc 3, 400–404, 1971

Sarasin, A., and Meunier-Rotival, M. How chemicals may induce cancer. Biomedicine 24, 306–316, 1976

Sarkar, N. H., and Moore, D. H. On the possibility of a human breast cancer virus. Nature 236, 103–106, 1972

Sarma, D. S. R., Michael, R. O., Stewart, B. W.,

Cox, R., and Damjanov, I. Patterns of damage and repair of rat liver DNA induced by chemical carcinogenesis in vivo. Fed Proc *32*, 833, 1973

Sarma, K. P. The role of lymphoid reaction in bladder cancer. J Urol *104*, 843–849, 1970

Sarma, P. S., Shiu, G., Neubauer, R. H., Baron, S., and Huebner, R. J. Virus-induced sarcoma of mice: Inhibition by a synthetic polyribonucleotide complex. Proc Natl Acad Sci USA *62*, 1046–1051, 1969

Sarna, G. The resting cell: A chemotherapeutic problem. Parts I and II. Biomedicine *20*, 322–326, 384–389, 1974

Sato, H., Boyse, E. A., Aoki, T., Iritani, C., and Old, L. J. Leukemia-associated transplantation antigens related to murine leukemia virus. J Exp Med *138*, 593–606, 1973

Sauter, C., Cavalli, F., Lindenmann, J., Gmur, J. P., Berchtold, W., Alberto, P., Obrecht, P., and Senn, H. J. Viral oncolysis: Its application in maintenance treatment of acute myelogenous leukemia, pp 355–362, In Terry, W. D., and Windhorst, D. (Eds): Immunotherapy of Cancer: Present Status of Trials in Man. New York: Raven Press, 1978

Sauter, C., Gerber, A., Lindenmann, J., and Martz, G. Akute myeloische Leukämie: Behandlungsversuch mit einem an Myeloblasten adaptierten Myxovirus. Schweiz Med Wochenschr *102*, 285–290, 1972

Savary, C., and Lotzová, E. Suppression of natural killer cell cytotoxicity by splenocytes from Corynebacterium parvum-injected, bone marrow-tolerant, and infant mice. J Immunol *120*, 239–243, 1978

Savel, H. Effect of autologous tumor extracts on cultured human peripheral blood lymphocytes. Cancer *24*, 56–63, 1969

Scales, R. W., and Cruse, J. M. Abrogation of immunologic unresponsiveness by whole molecules and fragments of cross-reacting immunoglobulins. J Immunol *105*, 1072–1081, 1970

Scaletta, L. F., and Ephrussi, B. Hybridization of normal and neoplastic cells in vitro. Nature *205*, 1169–1171, 1965

Scanlon, E. F., Hawkins, R. A., Fox, W. W., and Smith, W. S. Fatal homotransplanted melanoma. A case report. Cancer *18*, 782–789, 1965

Schabel, F. M. In vivo leukemia cell kinetics and "curability" in experimental systems, pp 379–408, In The Proliferation and Spread of Neoplastic Cells. 21st Symp—Fundamental Cancer Research. University of Texas M. D. Anderson Hospital and Tumor Institute. Baltimore: Williams & Wilkins, 1968

Schabel, F. M. The use of tumor growth kinetics in planning "curative" chemotherapy of advanced solid tumors. Cancer Res *29*, 2384–2389, 1969

Schabel, F. M. Concepts for systemic treatment of micrometastases. Cancer *35*, 15–24, 1975

Schabel, F. M., Skipper, H. E., Laster, W. R., and Thompson, S. A. Experimental evaluation of potential anticancer agents. XX. Development of immunity to leukemia L1210 in BDF1 mice and effects of therapy. Cancer Chemother Rep *50*, 55–70, 1966

Shachat, D. A., Fefer, A., and Moloney, J. B. Effect of cortisone on oncogenesis by murine sarcoma virus (Moloney). Cancer Res *28*, 517–520, 1968

Schatten, W. E. An experimental study of postoperative tumor metastases. I. Growth of pulmonary metastases following total removal of primary leg tumor. Cancer *11*, 455–459, 1958

Schechter, B., Treves, A. J., and Feldman, M. Specific cytotoxicity in vitro of lymphocytes sensitized in culture against tumor cells. J Natl Cancer Inst *56*, 975–979, 1976

Scheid, M. P., Hoffmann, M. K., Komuro, K., Hammerling, U., Abbot, J., Boyse, E. A., Cohen, G. H., Hooper, J. A., Schulof, R. S., and Goldstein, A. L. Differentiation of T cells induced by preparations from thymus and by nonthymic agents. The determined state of the precursor cell. J Exp Med *138*, 1027–1032, 1973

Scheinberg, L. C., Suzuki, K., Davidoff, L. M., and Beilin, R. L. Immunization against intracerebral transplantation of a glioma in mice. Nature *193*, 1194–1195, 1962

Scheinberg, L. C., Suzuki, K., Edelman, F., and Davidoff, L. M. Studies in immunization against a transplantable cerebral mouse glioma. J Neurosurg *20*, 312–317, 1963

Schilling, J. A., Snell, A. C., and Favata, B. V. Heterologous ocular transplantation as a practical test for cancer. Cancer *2*, 480–490, 1949

Schilling, R. M., Phillips, R. A., and Miller, R. G. Requirement for non-T cells in the generation of cytotoxic T lymphocytes in vitro. I. Use of nude mice as source of non-T cells. J Exp Med *144*, 241–258, 1976

Schlager, S. I., and Dray, S. Tumor regression at an untreated site during immunotherapy of an identical distant tumor. Proc Natl Acad Sci USA *72*, 3680–3682, 1975

Schlager, S. I., Paque, R. E., and Dray, S. Complete and apparently specific local tumor regression using syngeneic or xenogeneic "tumor-immune" RNA extracts. Cancer Res *35*, 1907–1914, 1975

Schlom, J., Spiegelman, S., and Moore, D. RNA-dependent DNA polymerase activity in virus-like particles isolated from human milk. Nature 231, 97–100, 1971

Schlosser, J. V., and Benes, E. H. Immunotherapy of human cancer with phytohaemagglutinin stimulated lymphocytes. Proc Am Assoc Cancer Res 12, 82, 1971

Schmidtke, J. R., and Johnson, A. G. Regulation of the immune system by synthetic polynucleotides. I. Characteristics of adjuvant action on antibody synthesis. J Immunol 106, 1191–1200, 1971

Schoenberg, B. G., Fraumeni, J. F., Greenberg, R. A., and Christine, B. W. Multiple primary malignancies in Connecticut, 1935–1964. Clues to etiology, pp 3–12, In Severi, L. (Ed): Fifth Perugia Quadrennial International Conference on Cancer, 1973. Perugia Univ, 1974

Scholler, J., Bergs, V. V., and Groupe, V. Evidence for the cell-free transmission of chemically induced mammary carcinoma in the rat. Nature 209, 1037, 1966

Schöne, G. Untersuchungen über Karzinomimmunität bei Maüsen. München Med Wochenschr 53, 2517–2519, 1906

Schorlemmer, H. U., Davies, P., and Allison, A. C. Ability of activated complement components to induce lysosomal enzyme release from macrophages. Nature 261, 48–49, 1976

Schorlemmer, H. U., Hadding, U., Bitter-Suerman, D., and Allison, A. C. The role of complement cleavage products in killing of tumour cells by macrophages, pp 68–77, In James, K., McBride, B., and Stuart, A. (Eds): Proc EURES Symp—The Macrophage and Cancer. Edinburgh Univ Dept Surgery, 1977

Schrek, R. A quantitative study of the growth of the Walker rat tumor and the Flexner-Jobling rat carcinoma. Am J Cancer 24, 807–822, 1935

Schrek, R. A comparison of the growth curves of malignant and normal (embryonic and post-embryonic) tissues of the rat. Am J Pathol 12, 525–530, 1936a

Schrek, R. Further quantitative methods for the study of transplantable tumors. The growth of R39 sarcoma and Brown-Pearce carcinoma. Am J Cancer 28, 345–363, 1936b

Schulten, M. F., Heiskell, C. A., and Shields, T. W. The incidence of solitary pulmonary metastasis from carcinoma of the large intestine. Surg Gynecol Obstet 143, 727–729, 1976

Schulz, J. I., Florentin, I., Bourut, C., Bicker, U., and Mathé, G. Delayed-type hypersensitivity response and humoral antibody formation in mice treated with a new immunostimulant 2-[2-cyanaziridinyl-(1)]-2-[2-carbamoylaziridinyl-(1)-propane] (BM 12 531). IRCS Med Sci 6, 215, 1978

Schwartz, E. E., Upton, A. C., and Congdon, C. C. A fatal reaction caused by implantation of adult parental spleen tissue in irradiated F1 mice. Proc Soc Exp Biol Med 96, 797–800, 1957

Schwartz, R. H., David, C. S., Sachs, D. H., and Paul, W. E. T lymphocyte-enriched murine peritoneal exudate cells. III. Inhibition of antigen-induced T lymphocyte proliferation with anti-Ia antisera. J Immunol 117, 531–540, 1976

Schwartz, R. S. Immunoregulation, oncogenic viruses, and malignant lymphomas. Lancet 1, 1266–1268, 1972

Schwartz, R. S., and Beldotti, L. Malignant lymphomas following allogenic disease: Transition from an immunological to a neoplastic disorder. Science 149, 1511–1514, 1965

Schwartz, W. B., Curelop, S., Bennet, W., and Bartter, F. C. A syndrome of renal sodium loss and hyponatremia probably resulting from inappropriate secretion of antidiuretic hormone. Am J Med 23, 529–542, 1975

Schwarzenberg, L., Mathé, G., Schneider, M., Amiel, J. L., Cattan, A., and Schlumberger, J. R. Attempted adoptive immunotherapy of acute leukaemia by leucocyte transfusions. Lancet 2, 365–368, 1966

Schwarzenberg, L., Simmler, M. C., and Pico, J. L. Human toxicology of BCG applied in cancer immunotherapy. Cancer Immunol Immunother 1, 69–76, 1976

Scollard, D. Cellular cytotoxicity assays detect different effector cell types in vitro. Transplantation 19, 87–90, 1975

Scornik, J. C., and Cosenza, H. Antibody-dependent cell-mediated cytotoxicity. III. Two functionally different effector cells. J Immunol 113, 1527–1532, 1974

Scott, M. T. Biological effects of the adjuvant Corynebacterium parvum. I. Inhibition of PHA, mixed lymphocyte and G. V. H. reactivity. Cell Immunol 5, 459–468, 1972a

Scott, M. T. Biological effects of the adjucant Corynebacterium parvum. II. Evidence for macrophage-T-cell interaction. Cell Immunol 5, 469–479, 1972b

Scott, M. T. Corynebacterium parvum as a therapeutic antitumor agent in mice: I. Systemic effects from intravenous injection. J Natl Cancer Inst 53, 855–860, 1974a

Scott, M. T. Corynebacterium parvum as a therapeutic antitumor agent in mice. II. Local injection of C. parvum. J Natl Cancer Inst 53, 861–865, 1974b

Scott, M. T. Depression of delayed-type hypersensitivity by Corynebacterium parvum: Mandatory role of the spleen. Cell Immunol *13,* 251–263, 1974c

Scott, M. T. Corynebacterium parvum as an immunotherapeutic anticancer agent. Semin Oncol *1,* 367–378, 1974d

Scott, M. T. In vivo cortisone sensitivity of nonspecific antitumor activity of Corynebacterium parvum-activated mouse peritoneal macrophages. J Natl Cancer Inst *54,* 789–792, 1975a

Scott, M. T. Potentiation of the tumor-specific immune response by Corynebacterium parvum. J Natl Cancer Inst *55,* 65–72, 1975b

Scott, M. T. Failure of Corynebacterium parvum presensitization to modify the antitumor effects of systemic and local therapeutic injections of C. parvum in mice. J Natl Cancer Inst. *56,* 675–677, 1976

Scott, M. T. Studies using labelled C. parvum preparations in mice. Dev Biol Stand *38,* 123–127, 1978

Scott, M. T. Analysis of the principles underlying chemoimmunotherapy of mouse tumours. I. Treatment with cyclophosphamide followed by Corynebacterium parvum. Cancer Immunol Immunother *6,* 107–112, 1979a

Scott, M. T. Analysis of the principles underlying chemoimmunotherapy of mouse tumours. II. Treatment with Corynebacterium parvum followed by cyclophosphamide. Cancer Immunol Immunother *6,* 113–119, 1979b

Scott, M. T., and Decker, J. The distribution and effects of intrapleural Corynebacterium parvum in mice. A comparison with intravenous Corynebacterium parvum. Cancer Immunol Immunother *5,* 85–91, 1978

Scott, M. T., MacDonald, T. T., and Carter, P. B. C. parvum in germ-free mice. Cancer Immunol Immunother *4,* 135–137, 1978

Scott, M. T., and Milas, L. The distribution and persistence in vivo of Corynebacterium parvum in relation to its antitumor activity. Cancer Res *37,* 1673–1679, 1977

Scott, M. T., and Warner, S. L. The accumulated effects of repeated systemic or local injections of low doses of Corynebacterium parvum in mice. Cancer Res *36,* 1335–1338, 1976

Sealy, W. C. Non metastatic extrapulmonary manifestations of bronchogenic carcinoma. Surgery *68,* 906–913, 1970

Sedallian, J. P., and Triau, R. Principles d'une immunothérapie anti-cancéreuse à partir d'extraits embryonnaires. Lyon Med *29,* 1–24, 1968

Sedlacek, H. H., Bengelsdorff, H. J., Lemmer, A., and Seiler, F. R. Approaches to effective tumor immunotherapy with cells and the enzyme neuraminidase, p 363, In Proc Sixth International Conference on Lymphatic Tissues and Germinal Centers in Immune Reactions. New York: Plenum Press, 1979

Sedlacek, H. H., Meesmann, H., and Seiler, F. R. Regression of spontaneous mammary tumors in dogs after injection of neuraminidase-treated tumor cells. Int J Cancer *15,* 409–416, 1975

Sedlacek, H. H., and Seiler, F. R. Immunotherapy of neoplastic diseases with neuraminidase: Contradictions, new aspects, and revised concepts. Cancer Immunol Immunother *5,* 153–163, 1978

Seeger, R. C., and Owen, J. J. T. Anti-tumour cytotoxic effects mediated by minor and major cell populations of lymph nodes. Nature *252,* 420–421, 1974

Segall, A., Weiller, O., Genin, J., Lacour, J., and Lacour, F. In vitro study of cellular immunity against autochthonous human cancer. Int J Cancer *9,* 417–425, 1972

Segi, M. World incidence and distribution of skin cancer. Natl Cancer Inst Monogr *10,* 245–255, 1963

Seigler, H. F., Shingleton, W. W., Metzgar, R. S., Buckley, C. E., and Bergoc, P. M. Immunotherapy in patients with melanoma. Ann Surg *178,* 352–359, 1973

Seigler, H. F., Shingleton, W. W., Metzgar, R. S., Buckley, C. E., Bergoc, P. M., Miller, D. S., Fetter, B. F., and Phaup, M. B. Non-specific and specific immunotherapy in patients with melanoma. Surgery *72,* 162–174, 1972

Seiler, F. R., and Sedlacek, H. H. Chessboard vaccination—A pertinent approach to immunotherapy of cancer with neuraminidase and tumor cells? pp 479–488, In Proc Symp—Immunotherapy of Malignant Diseases. New York: Schattaner-Verlag, 1978

Sekla, B., Holečková, E., Janele, J., Lebansky, J., and Hněvkovsky, O. The effects of heterologous immune globulins upon human cancer in vivo. Neoplasma *14,* 641–647, 1967

Selawry, O. A., Carlson, J. C., and Moore, G. E. Tumor response to ionizing rays at elevated temperatures; Review and discussion. Am J Roentgenol *80,* 833–839, 1958

Selawry, O. S., Goldstein, M. N., and McCormick, T. Hyperthermia in tissue-cultured cells of malignant origin. Cancer Res *17,* 785–791, 1957

Sell, S. Radioimmunoassay of rat α-fetoprotein. Cancer Res *33,* 1010–1015, 1973

Sellers, E. A., Hill, J. M., and Lee, R. B. Effect of iodide and thyroid on production of tumours of thyroid and pituitary by propylthiouracil. Endocrinology *52,* 188–203, 1953

Sellwood, R. A., Kuper, S. W. A., Burn, J. L., and Wallace, E. N. Circulating cancer cells. Br Med J *1,* 1683–1686, 1964

Sendo, F., Aoki, T., Boyse, E. A., and Buofo, C. K. Natural occurrence of lymphocytes showing cytotoxic activity to Balb/C radiation-induced leukemia R101 cells. J Natl Cancer Inst 55, 603–609, 1975

Serrou, B., and Domas, J. Complications of BCG treatment in patients bearing solid tumors. Dev Biol Stand 38, 515–521, 1978

Serrou, B., Michel, H., Dubois, J. B., and Serre, A. Granulomatous hepatitis caused by BCG injection during immunotherapy of a malignant melanoma. Biomedicine 23, 236–240, 1975

Sethi, K. K., and Brandis, H. Neuraminidase-induced loss in the transplantability of murine leukemia L1210: Induction of immunoprotection and the transfer of induced immunity to normal DBA/2 mice by serum and peritoneal cells. Br J Cancer 27, 106–113, 1973

Sexauer, C. L., Nitschke, R., and Humphrey, G. B. Corynebacterium toxicity. Lancet 2, 199, 1976

Shah, L. P., Rees, R. C., and Baldwin, R. W. Tumour rejection in rats sensitized to embryonic tissue. I. Rejection of tumour cells implanted S.C. and detection of cytotoxic lymphoid cells. Br J Cancer 33, 577–583, 1976

Shand, F. L. Analysis of immunosuppression generated by the graft-versus-host reaction. I. A suppressor T-cell component studied in vivo. Immunology 29, 953–965, 1975

Shands, J. W., and Axelrod, B. J. Mouse peritoneal macrophages: Tritiated thymidine labeling and cell kinetics. J Reticuloendothel Soc 21, 69–76, 1977

Shapiro, D., and Fugmann, R. A role for chemotherapy as an adjunct to surgery. Cancer Res 17, 1098–1101, 1957

Sharma, B., and Terasaki, P. I. In vitro immunization to cultured human tumor cells. Cancer Res 34, 115–118, 1974

Sharpless, G. R., Davies, M. C., and Cox, H. R. Antagonistic action of certain neurotropic viruses toward a lymphoid tumor in chickens with resulting immunity. Proc Soc Exp Biol Med 73, 270–275, 1950

Shaw, R. K., Szwed, C., Boggs, D. R., Fahey, J. L., Frei, E., Morrison, E., and Utz, J. P. Infection and immunity in chronic lymphocytic leukemia. Arch Intern Med 106, 467–478, 1960

Sheard, C. E., Double, J. A., and Berenbaum, M. C. The sensitivity to chemotherapeutic agents of a rat tumour grown in immunosuppressed mice. Br J Cancer 25, 838–844, 1971

Shearer, G. M., Rehn, T. G., and Garbarino, C. A. Cell-mediated lympholysis of trinitrophenyl-modified autologous lymphocytes. Effector cell specificity to modified cell surface components controlled by the H-2K and H-2D serological regions of the murine major histocompatibility complex. J Exp Med 141, 1348–1364, 1975

Shearer, W. T. Stimulation of cells by antibody. Science 182, 1357–1359, 1973

Sheil, A. G. R. Cancer in renal allograft recipients in Australia and New Zealand. Transplant Proc 9, 1133–1136, 1977

Shellam, G. R. Gross-virus-induced lymphoma in the rat. V. Natural cytotoxic cells are non-T cells. Int J Cancer 19, 225–235, 1977

Shellam, G. R., and Hogg, N. Gross-virus-induced lymphoma in the rat. IV. Cytotoxic cells in normal rats. Int J Cancer 19, 212–214, 1977

Shellam, G. R., Knight, R. A., Mitchison, N. A., Gorczynski, R. M., and Maoz, A. The specificity of effector T cells activated by tumours induced by murine oncornaviruses. Transplant Rev 29, 249–276, 1976

Sherry, S., McAllister, W. H., Saltzstein, S. L., Kilburn, K. H., Levy, I., Harford, C. G., Kipnis, D., Packman, R. C., and Reiss, E. Cushing's syndrome associated with a parotid tumor: Clinocopathologic conference. Am J Med 34, 394–406, 1963

Sherwood, L. M., O'Riordan, J. L. H., Aurback, G. D. D., and Potts, J. T. Production of parathyroid hormone by non-parathyroid tumors. J Clin Endocrinol Metab 27, 140–146, 1967

Shields, R. New view of the cell cycle. Nature 260, 193–194, 1976

Shields, R. Gene derepression in tumours. Nature 269, 752–753, 1977

Shields, T. W., Robinette, C. D., and Keehn, R. J. Bronchial carcinoma treated by adjuvant cancer chemotherapy. Arch Surg 109, 329–333, 1974

Shigeno, N., Hammerling, U., Arpels, C., Boyse, E. A., and Old, L. J. Preparation of lymphocyte-specific antibody from anti-lymphocyte serum. Lancet 2, 320–323, 1968

Shin, H. S., Economou, J. S., Pasternack, G. R., Johnson, R. J., and Hayden, M. L. Antibody-mediated suppression of grafted lymphoma. J Exp Med 144, 1274–1283, 1976a

Shin, H. S., Pasternack, G. R., Economou, J. S., Johnson, R. J., and Hayden, M. L. Immunotherapy of cancer with antibody. Science 194, 327–328, 1976b

Shirakawa, S., Luce, J. K., Tannock, I., and Frei, E. Cell proliferation in human melanoma. J Clin Invest 49, 1188–1199, 1970

Shirato, E., Sinkovics, J. G., and Thornell, E. W. Passive immunization against murine lymphoma. Oncology 26, 80–86, 1972

Shivas, A. A., and Finlayson, N. D. C. The resistance of arteries to tumour invasion. Br J Cancer 19, 486–489, 1965

Shustik, C., Cohe, I. R., Schwartz, R. S., Latham-Griffin, E., and Waksal, S. D. T lymphocytes with promiscuous cytotoxicity. Nature 263, 699–701, 1976

Shyrock, H. S., and Siegel, J. S. The Methods and Materials of Demography. Washington, D.C.: U.S. Govt Printing Office, 1973

Sicevic, S. Generalized BCG tuberculosis with fatal course in two sisters. Acta Paediatr Scand 61, 178–184, 1972

Sieber, S. M., and Adamson, R. H. Toxicity of antineoplastic agents in man: Chromosomal aberrations, antifertility effects, congenital malformations and carcinogenic potential. Adv Cancer Res 22, 57–155, 1975

Siegel, B. V., and Morton, J. L. Depressed antibody response in the mouse infected with Rauscher leukaemia virus. Immunology 10, 559–562, 1966

Siegel, B. V., and Morton, J. L. Rauscher viral leukemogenesis in Balb/c mice treated with rabbit antimouse thymocyte serum. J Natl Cancer Inst 44, 573–579, 1970

Sikora, K., Stern, P., and Lennox, E. Immunoprotection by embryonal carcinoma cells for methylcholanthrene-induced murine sarcomas. Nature 269, 813–815, 1977

Silverman, N. A., Alexander, J. C., Potvin, C., and Chretien, P. B. In vitro lymphocyte reactivity and T cell levels in patients with melanoma: Correlations with clinical and pathological stage. Surgery 79, 332–339, 1976

Silvers, W. K., and Billingham, R. E. Studies on the immunotherapy of runt disease in rats. J Exp Med 129, 647–661, 1969

Simic, M. M., and Kanazir, D. T. Restoration of immunologic capacities in irradiated animals by nucleic acids and their derivatives, pp 386–403, In Plescia, O. J., and Braun, W. (Eds): Nucleic Acids in Immunology. New York: Springer-Verlag, 1968

Simmler, M. C., Schwarzenberg, L., and Mathé, G. Attempts at non-specific cell-mediated immunorestoration of immunodepressed cancer patients with BCG. Cancer Immunol Immunother 1, 157–161, 1976

Simmons, R. L., Aranha, G. V., Gunnarsson, A., Grage, T. B., and McKhann, C. F. Active specific immunotherapy for advanced melanoma utilizing neuraminidase-treated autochthonous tumor cells, pp 123–133, In Terry, W. D., and Windhorst, D. (Eds): Immunotherapy of Cancer: Present Status of Trials in Man. New York: Raven Press, 1978

Simmons, R. L., and Rios, A. Combined use of BCG and neuraminidase in experimental tumor immunotherapy. Surg Forum 22, 99–101, 1971a

Simmons, R. L., and Rios, A. Immunotherapy of cancer; Immuno-specific rejection of tumors in recipients of neuraminidase-treated tumor cells plus BCG. Science 174, 591–593, 1971b

Simmons, R. L., and Rios, A. Immunospecific regression of methylcholanthrene fibrosarcoma using neuraminidase. II. Intratumor injections of neuraminidase. Surgery 71, 556–564, 1972a

Simmons, R. L., and Rios, A. Immunospecific regression of methylcholanthrene fibrosarcoma using neuraminidase. III. Synergistic effect of BCG and neuraminidase-treated tumor cells. Ann Surg 176, 188–194, 1972b

Simmons, R. L., and Rios, A. Immunospecific regression of methylcholanthrene fibrosarcoma using neuraminidase. IV. Chemotherapeutic agents reverse the effects of tumor immunotherapy. Bull Bell Mus Pathobiol 3, 28–30, 1973a

Simmons, R. L., and Rios, A. Differential effect of neuraminidase on the immunogenicity of viral associated and private antigens of mammary carcinomas. J Immunol 111, 1820–1825, 1973b

Simmons, R. L., and Rios, A. Immunospecific regression of methylcholanthrene fibrosarcoma with the use of neuraminidase. V. Quantitative aspects of the experimental immunotherapeutic model. Isr J Med Sci 10, 925–938, 1974

Simmons, R. L., and Rios, A. Modified tumor cells in the immunotherapy of solid mammary tumors. Med Clin North Am 60, 551–565, 1976

Simmons, R. L., Rios, A., and Kersey, J. H. Regression of spontaneous mammary carcinomas using direct injections of neuraminidase and BCG. J Surg Res 12, 57–61, 1972

Simmons, R. L., Rios, A., Lundgren, G., Ray, P. K., McKhann, C. F., and Haywood, G. R. Immunospecific regression of methylcholanthrene fibrosarcoma with the use of neuraminidase. Surgery 70, 38–46, 1971a

Simmons, R. L., Rios, A., and Ray, P. K. Immunogenicity and antigenicity of lymphoid cells treated with neuraminidase. Nature New Biol 231, 179–181, 1971b

Simmons, R. L., Rios, A., Ray, P. K., and Lundgren, G. Effect of neuraminidase on the growth of methylcholanthrene fibrosarcoma in normal and immunosuppressed syngeneic mice. J Natl Cancer Inst 47, 1087–1094, 1971c

Simova, J., and Bubenik, J. Failure of bacillus Calmette-Guérin (BCG) infection to suppress the growth of transplanted mouse and rat sarcomas. Folia Biol (Praha) 19, 296–300, 1973

Simpson, E., and Nehlsen, S. L. Prolonged administration of antithymocyte serum in mice. II. Histopathological investigation. Clin Exp Immunol 9, 77–98, 1971

Simpson-Herren, L., Sanford, A. M., and Holmquist, J. P. Effects of surgery on the cell kinetics of residual tumor. Cancer Treat Rep (Suppl) 60, 1749–1760, 1976

Sims, P., and Grover, P. L. Epoxides in polycyclic aromatic hydrocarbon metabolism and carcinogenesis. Adv Cancer Res 20, 166–274, 1974

Singer, S. J., and Nicolson, G. L. The fluid mosaic model of the structure of cell membranes. Science 175, 720–731, 1972

Sjögren, H. O. Transplantation methods as a tool for detection of tumor-specific antigens. Prog Exp Tumor Res 6, 289–322, 1965

Sjögren, H. O. p 51, In Beers, R. F., Tilghman, R. C., and Bassett, E. G. (Eds): The Role of Immunological Factors in Viral and Oncogenic Processes. Baltimore: Johns Hopkins Univ Press, 1974

Sjögren, H. O., and Ankerst, J. Effect of BCG and allogeneic tumour cells on adenovirus type 12 tumorigenesis in mice. Nature 221, 863–864, 1969

Sjögren, H. O., Hellström, I., and Klein, G. Resistance of polyoma virus immunized mice to transplantation of established polyoma tumors. Exp Cell Res 23, 204–208, 1961a

Sjögren, H. O., Hellström, I., and Klein, G. Transplantation of polyoma virus-induced tumors in mice. Cancer Res 21, 329–337, 1961b

Sjögren, H. O., and Jonsson, N. Resistance against isotransplantation of mouse tumours induced by Rous sarcoma virus. Exp Cell Res 32, 618–621, 1963

Skipper, H. E., Schabel, F. M., and Wilcox, W. S. Experimental evaluation of potential anticancer agents. XIII. On the criteria and kinetics associated with "curability" of experimental leukemia. Cancer Chemother Rep 35, 3–9, 1964

Skipper, H. E., Schabel, F. M., and Wilcox, W. S. Experimental evaluation of potential anticancer agents. XIV. Further study of certain basic concepts underlying chemotherapy of leukemia. Cancer Chemother Rep 45, 5–29, 1965

Sklaroff, D. M., and Charkes, N. D. Bone metastases from breast cancer at the time of radical mastectomy. Surg Gynecol Obstet 127, 763–768, 1968

Skowron-Cendrzak, A., and Ptak, W. Suppression of local graft-versus-host reactions by mouse fetal and newborn spleen cells. Eur J Immunol 6, 451–452, 1976

Skurkovich, S. V., Kisljak, N. S., Machonova, L. A., and Begunenko, S. A. Active immunization of children suffering from acute leukaemia in acute phase with live allogeneic leukaemic cells. Nature 223, 509–511, 1969a

Skurkovich, S. V., Makhonova, L. A., and Reznichenko, F. M. Treatment of children with acute leukemia by passive cyclic immunization with autoplasma and autoleukocytes operated during the remission periods. Blood 33, 186–197, 1969b

Skurzak, H. M., Klein, E., Yoshida, T. O., and Lamon, E. W. Synergistic or antagonistic effect of different antibody concentrations on in vitro lymphocyte cytotoxicity in the Moloney sarcoma virus system. J Exp Med 135, 997 1002, 1972

Skurzak, H., Steiner, L., Klein, E., and Lamon, E. Cytotoxicity of human peripheral lymphocytes for glioma osteosarcoma and glia cell lines. Natl Cancer Inst Monogr 37, 93–102, 1973

Slack, N. H., Bross, J. D. J., Nemoto, T., and Fisher, B. Experience with bilateral primary carcinoma of the breast in a co-operative study. Surg Gynecol Obstet 136, 433–440, 1973

Slemmer, G. Interactions of separate types of cells during normal and neoplastic mammary gland growth. J Invest Dermatol 63, 27–47, 1974

Slettenmark, B., and Klein, E. Cytotoxic and neutralization tests with serum and lymph node cells of isologous mice with induced resistance against Gross lymphomas. Cancer Res. 22, 947–954, 1962

Šljivić, V. S., and Warr, G. W. Role of cellular proliferation in the stimulation of MPS phagocytic activity. Br J Exp Pathol 56, 314–321, 1975

Šljivić, V. S., and Watson, S. R. The adjuvant effect of C. Parvum: T-cell dependence of macrophage activation. J Exp Med 145, 45–57, 1977

Sloboda, A. E., and Landes, J. The comparative immunosuppressive effects of heterologous antisera to various C3H mouse tissues. J Immunol 104, 185–194, 1969

Small, M., and Trainin, N. Inhibition of syngeneic fibrosarcoma growth by lymphocytes sensitized on tumor-cell monolayers in the presence of the thymic humoral factor. Int J Cancer 15, 962–972, 1975

Small, M., and Trainin, N. Separation of populations of sensitized lymphoid cells into fractions inhibiting and fractions enhancing syngeneic tumor growth in vivo. J Immunol 117, 292–297, 1976

Smirnova, E. La greffe hétérogène des tumeurs malignes. Bull Biol Med Exp URSS, 4, 6–10, 1937

Smith G. V., Morse, P. A., Deraps, G. D., Raju, S., and Hardy, J. D. Immunotherapy of patients with cancer. Surgery 74, 59–68, 1973

Smith, H. G., Bast, R. C., Zbar, B., and Rapp, H. J. Eradication of microscopic lymph node metastases after injection of living BCG adjacent to the primary tumor. J Natl Cancer Inst *55*, 1345–1352, 1975

Smith, H. G., Harmel, M. G., Zwilling, B. S., Zbar, B., and Rapp, H. J. Regression of established intradermal tumors and lymph node metastases in guinea pigs after systemic transfer of immune lymphoid cells. J Natl Cancer Inst *58*, 1315–1322, 1977

Smith, J. A., and Martin, L. Do cells cycle? Proc Natl Acad Sci USA *70*, 1263–1267, 1973

Smith J. L., and Stehlin, J. S. Spontaneous regression of primary malignant melanomas with regional metastases. Cancer *18*, 1399–1415, 1965

Smith, L. H. Ectopic hormone production. Surg Gynecol Obstet *141*, 443–453, 1975

Smith, P. J., Robinson, C. M., and Reif, A. E. Specificity of antileukemia sera prepared by immunization with leukemia cells admixed with normal antigen-blocking sera. Cancer Res *34*, 169–175, 1974

Smith, R. The surgeon and the patient with cancer. J R Coll Surgeons Edinb *15*, 63–76, 1970

Smith, R. S., Huebner, R. J., Rowe, W. P., Schatten, W. E., and Thomas, L. B. Studies on the use of viruses in the treatment of carcinoma of the cervix. Cancer *9*, 1211–1218, 1956

Smith, R. T. Role of tumor Ag in tumor bearing, pp 3–14, In Smith, R. T., and Landy, M. (Eds): Immunobiology of the Tumor–Host Relationship. New York: Academic Press, 1975

Smith, R. T., and Konda, S. The stimulatory effect of bearing primary methylcholanthrene-induced tumors upon the murine lymphoreticular system. Int J Cancer *12*, 577–588, 1973

Smith, R. T., and Landy, M. (Eds): Immunological Surveillance. New York: Academic Press, 1970

Smith, S. E., and Scott, M. T. Biological effects of corynebacterium parvum. III. Amplification of resistance and impairment of active immunity to murine tumours. Br J Cancer *26*, 361–367, 1972

Smithers, D. W. A Clinical Prospect of the Cancer Problem. Edinburgh, London: Livingstone, 1960

Smithers, D. W. Cancer. An attack on cytologism. Lancet *1*, 493–499, 1962a

Smithers, D. W. Spontaneous regression of tumours. Clin Radiol *13*, 132–137, 1962b

Smithwick, E. M., and Berkovich, S. In vitro suspension of the lymphocyte response to tuberculin by live measles virus. Proc Soc Exp Biol Med *123*, 276–278, 1966

Snell, A. C. Heterotransplantation of tumors into various regions of the guinea-pig eye. Am J Ophthalmol *34*, 733–738, 1951

Snell, G. D. Methods for the study of histocompatibility genes. J Genet *49*, 87–103, 1948

Snell, G. D. The immunogenetics of tumor transplantation. Cancer Res *12*, 543–546, 1952

Snell, G. D., and Stevens, L. C. Histocompatibility genes of mice. III. H-1 and H-4, two histocompatibility loci in the first linkage group. Immunology *4*, 366–379, 1961

Snyder, H. W., Pincus, T., and Fleissner, E. Specificities of human immunoglobulins reactive with antigens in preparations of several mammalian type-C viruses. Virology *75*, 60–73, 1976

Snyderman, R., Dickson, J., Meadows, L., and Pike, M. Deficient monocyte chemotactic responsiveness in humans with cancer. Clin Res *22*, 430A, 1974

Snyderman, R., and Pike, M. C. An inhibitor of macrophage chemotaxis produced by neoplasms. Science *192*, 370–372, 1976

Snyderman, R., Pike, M. C., Blaylock, B. L., and Weinstein, P. Effects of neoplasms on inflammation: Depression of macrophage accumulation after tumour implantation. J Immunol *116*, 585–589, 1976

Snyderman, R., Pike, M. C., Meadows, L., Hemstreet, G., and Wells, S. Depression of monocyte chemotaxis by neoplasms. Clin Res *23*, 297A, 1975

Snyderman, R. K., Miller, D. G., and Lizardo, J. G. Prolonged skin homograft and heterograft survival in patients with neoplastic disease. Plast Reconstr Surg *26*, 373–377, 1960

Soderland, S. C., and Naum, Y. Growth of pulmonary alveolar macrophages in vitro. Nature *245*, 150–151, 1973

Sodomann, C. P., Malchow, H., and Schmidt, M. Die Wirkung von Polyinosin-Polycytidy-Saure (poly I: poly C) auf die Remissionszeit von Akuten Leukamien, pp 557–561, In Gross, R., and van de Loo, J. (Eds): Sonderdruck ans Leukamie. Berlin: Springer-Verlag, 1972

Sokal, J. E., Aungst, C. W., and Snyderman, M. Delay in progression of malignant lymphoma after BCG vaccination. N Engl J Med *291*, 1226–1230, 1974

Solowey, A. C., and Rapaport, F. T. Immunologic responses in cancer patients. Surg Gynecol Obstet *121*, 756–760, 1965

Solowey, A. C., Rapaport, F. T., and Lawrence, H. S. Cellular studies in neoplastic disease, pp 75–78, In Curton, E. S., et al (Eds): Histocompatibility Testing. Copenhagen: Munksgaard, 1967

Sophocles, A. M., and Nadler, S. H. Immunologic aspects of cancer. Surg Gynecol Obstet *133*, 321–331, 1971

Sorborg, M., and Bendixen, G. Human lymphocyte migration as a parameter of hypersensitivity. Acta Med Scand *181*, 247–256, 1967

Sordat, B., Fritsche, R., Mach, J. P., Carrel, S., Ozzello, L., and Cerrottini, J.-C. Morphological and functional evaluation of human solid tumors serially transplanted in nude mice, pp 269–278, In Rygaard, J., and Povlsen, C. O. (Eds): First Int Workshop on Nude Mice. Stuttgart: Gustav Fischer, 1974

Southam, C. M. Applications of immunology to clinical cancer. Past attempts and future possibilities. Cancer Res *21*, 1302–1316, 1961

Southam, C. M. The complex etiology of cancer. Cancer Res *23*, 1105–1115, 1963

Southam, C. M. Co-existence of allogeneic tumour growth and homograft immunity in man. Eur J Cancer *4*, 507–511, 1968

Southam, C. M., and Brunschwig, A. Quantitative studies of autotransplantation of human cancer; Preliminary report. Cancer *14*, 971–978, 1961

Southam, C. M., and Moore, A. E. Clinical studies of viruses as antineoplastic agents, with particular reference to Egypt 101 virus. Cancer *5*, 1025–1034, 1952

Southam, C. M., Moore, A. E., and Rhoads, C. R. Homotransplantation of human cell lines. Science *125*, 158–160, 1957

Southwick, H. W., Harridge, W. H., and Cole, W. H. Recurrence at the suture line following resection for carcinoma of the colon; Incidence following preventive measures. Am J Surg *103*, 86–89, 1962

Sparagana, M., Phillips, G., Hoffman, C., and Kucera, L. Ectopic growth hormone syndrome associated with lung cancer. Metabolism *20*, 730–736, 1971

Sparck, J. V., and Gross, K. The role of the host mesenchyme in the development of tumours after transplantation. Acta Pathol Microbiol Scand *77*, 24–38, 1969

Sparck, J. V., and Volkert, M. Effect of adoptive immunity on experimentally induced leukaemia in mice. Nature *206*, 578–579, 1965

Sparks, F. C., and Breeding, J. H. Tumor regression and enhancement resulting from immunotherapy with bacillus Calmette-Guérin and neuraminidase. Cancer Res *34*, 3262–3269, 1974

Sparks, F. C., O'Connell, T. X., Lee, Y.-T, N., and Breeding, J. H. BCG therapy given as an adjuvant to surgery: Prevention of death from metastases from mammary adenocarcinoma in rats. J Natl Cancer Inst *53*, 1825–1826, 1974

Spector, W. G. Macrophage turnover and traffic: A review, pp 15–18, In James, K., McBride, B., and Stuart, A. (Eds): Proc EURES Symp—The Macrophage and Cancer. Edinburgh Univ Dept Surgery, 1977

Spector, W. G., and Mariano, M. Macrophage behaviour in experimental granulomas, pp 927–938, In Van Furth, R. (Ed): Mononuclear Phagocytes in Immunity Infection and Pathology. Oxford: Blackwell, 1975

Spence, R. A., Swan, J. M., deBoer, W. G. R. M., Ghose, T. Nairn, R. C., Rolland, J. M., Ward, H. A., and Wright, S. H. B. A new immunoradioactive agent: ^{32}P-conjugated antibody. Clin Exp Immunol *3*, 865–872, 1968

Spence, R. J., Simon, R. M., and Baker, A. R. Failure of immunotherapy with neuraminidase-treated tumor cell vaccine in mice bearing established 3-methylcholanthrene-induced sarcomas. J Natl Cancer Inst *60*, 451–459, 1978

Spiegelman, S., Burney, A., Das, M. R., Keydar, J., Schlom, J., Travnicek, M., and Watson, K. Characterization of the products of RNA-directed DNA polymerases in oncogenic RNA viruses. Nature *227*, 563–567, 1970

Spitler, L. E., Sagebiel, R. W., Glogau, R. G., Wong, P. P., Malm, T. M., Chase, R. H., and Gonzales, R. L. A randomized double-blind trial of adjuvant therapy with levamisole versus placebo in patients with malignant melanoma, pp 73–79, In Terry, W. D., and Windhorst, D. (Eds): Immunotherapy of Cancer: Present Status of Trials in Man. New York: Raven Press, 1978

Spitler, L. E., Wybran, J., Fudenberg, H. H., Levin, A. S., Lewis, M. G. and Horn, L. Transfer factor therapy of malignant melanoma. Clin Res *21*, 654, 1973

Spivak, J. L. Phagocytic tumour cells. Scand J Haematol *11*, 253–256, 1973

Spratt, J. S. The rates of growth of skeletal sarcomas. Cancer *18*, 14–24, 1965

Spratt, J. S., and Spratt, T. L. Rates of growth of pulmonary metastases and host survival. Ann Surg *159*, 161–171, 1964

Sprent, J., and Miller, J. F. A. P. The interaction of thymus lymphocytes with histoincompatible cells. III. Immunological characteristics of antigen activated thymus-derived recirculating lymphocytes. Cell Immunol *3*, 213–230, 1972

Stanbridge, E. Suppression of malignancy in human cells. Nature *260*, 17–20, 1976

Stanley, E. R., Cifone, M., Heard, P. M., and Defendi, V. Factors regulating macrophage production and growth: Identity of colony-stimulating factor and macrophage growth factor. J Exp Med *143*, 631–647, 1976

Staquet, M. (Ed): The Design of Clinical Trials in Cancer Therapy. New York: Futura Publishing, 1973

Staquet, M., and Sylvester, R. A decision theory approach to phase II clinical trials. Biomedicine 26, 262–264, 1977

Starr, K. W. Hormonal imbalance and the sarcomata. Aust NZ J Surg 39, 142–150, 1969

Starr, S., and Berkovich, S. Effects of measles, gamma-globulin-modified measles and vaccine measles on the tuberculin test. N Engl J Med 270, 386–391, 1964

Starzl, T. Experience in Hepatic Transplantation. Philadelphia: W. B. Saunders, 1969

Starzl, T. E., Marchioro, T. L., Ridkind, D., Rowlands, D. T., and Waddell, W. R. Clinical experience with organ transplantation. South Med J 58, 131–147, 1965

Steel, C. M., and Ling, N. R. Immunopathology of infectious mononucleosis. Lancet 2, 861–862, 1973

Steel, G. G. Cell loss as a factor in the growth rate of human tumours. Eur J Cancer 3, 381–387, 1967

Steel, G. G. Growth Kinetics of Tumors. Oxford: Clarendon Press, 1977

Steel, G. G., Adams, K., and Barrett, J. C. Analysis of the cell population kinetics of transplanted tumours of widely-differing growth rate. Br J Cancer 20, 784–800, 1966

Steel, G. G., and Lamerton, L. F. The growth rate of human tumours. Br J Cancer 20, 74–86, 1966

Stehlin, J. S. Regional hyperthermia and chemotherapy by perfusion, pp 266–271, In Wizenberg, M. J., and Robinson, J. E. (Eds): Proc Int Symp—Cancer Therapy by Hyperthermia and Radiation. Baltimore: Am Coll Radiol Press, 1976

Stehlin, J. S., Giovanella, B. C., de Ipolyi, P. D., Muenz, L. R., and Anderson, R. F. Results of hyperthermic perfusion for melanoma of the extremities. Surg Gynecol Obstet 140, 339–348, 1975

Steinkuller, C. B., Krigbaum, L. G., and Weiss, D. W. Studies on the mode of action of the heterologous immunogenicity of a methanol-insoluble fraction of attenuated tubercle bacilli (BCG) Immunol 16, 255–275, 1969

Stephenson, H. E., Delmez, J. A., Renden, D. I., Kimpton, R. S., Todd, P. C., Charron, T. L., and Lindberg, D. A. B. Host immunity and spontaneous regression of cancer evaluated by computerized data reduction study. Surg Gynecol Obstet 133, 649–655, 1971

Stephenson, J. R., and Aaronson, S. A. Antigenic properties of murine sarcoma virus-transformed Balb/3T3 nonproducer cells. J Exp Med 135, 503–515, 1972

Stern, K. A new approach to tumour immunity. Nature 185, 787–788, 1960

Stern, K., Bartizal, C. A., and Divshony, S. Changes in reticuloendothelial phagocytosis in mice with spontaneous tumors. J Natl Cancer Inst 38, 469–480, 1967

Stevenson, G. T., Elliott, E. V., and Stevenson, F. K. Idiotypic determinants on the surface immunoglobulin of neoplastic lymphocytes: A therapeutic target. Fed Proc 36, 134, 1976

Stevenson, T. D., and von Haam, E. A study of factors affecting circulating tumor cells in experimental animals. Acta Cytol 10, 383–386, 1966

Steward, A. M., Nixon, D., Zamchek, N., and Aisenberg, A. Carcinoembryonic antigen in breast cancer patients: Serum levels and disease progress. Cancer 33, 1246–1252, 1974

Stewart, A. Low dose radiation cancers in man. Adv Cancer Res 14, 359–390, 1971

Stewart, B. W., Farber, E., and Mirvish, S. S. Induction by an hepatic carcinogen, 1-nitroso-5,6-dihydrouracil, of single and double strand breaks of liver DNA with rapid repair. Biochem Biophys Res Commun 53, 773–779, 1973

Stewart, S. E. The polyoma virus. Adv Virus Res 7, 61–90, 1960

Stewart, T. H. M. The presence of delayed hypersensitivity reactions in patients towards cellular extracts of their malignant tumours. Cancer 23, 1368–1379, 1969

Stewart, T. H. M., Hollinshead, A. C., Harris, J. E., Raman, S., Belanger, R., Crepeau, A., Crook, A. F., Hirte, W. E., Hooper, D., Klaassen, D. J., Rapp, E. F., and Sachs, H. J. Survival study of immuno-chemotherapy in lung cancer, pp 203–215, In Terry, W. D., and Windhorst, D. (Eds): Immunotherapy of Cancer: Present Status of Trials in Man. New York: Raven Press, 1978

Stewart, T. H. M., and Orizaga, M. The presence of delayed hypersensitivity reactions in patients towards cellular extracts of their malignant tumours. Cancer 28, 1472–1478, 1971

Stidolph, N. E. Malignant melanoma: Regression of metastases after excision of primary growth. Proc R. Soc Med 60, 1, 1967

Stiffel, C., Mouton, D., and Biozzi, G. Rôle des macrophages dans l'immunité non spécifique. Ann Inst Pasteur 120, 412–417, 1971

Stiffel, C., Mouton, D., Bouthillier, Y., Decreusefond, C., and Biozzi, G. Variabilité de la réponse de SRE à deux substances microbiennes selon l'espèce animale. J Reticuloendothel Soc 3, 439, 1966

Stjernsward, J. Effect of bacillus Calmette-Guérin and/or methylcholanthrene on the antibody-forming cells measured at the cellular level by a hemolytic plaque test. Cancer Res 26, 1591–1594, 1966

Stjernsward, J. Immune status of the primary host toward its own methylcholanthrene-induced sarcomas. J Natl Cancer Inst *40*, 13–22, 1968

Stjernsward, J. Immunosuppression by carcinogens. Antibiotica Chemother *15*, 213–233, 1969

Stjernsward, J., Almgard, L.-E., Franzen, S., von Schreeb, T., and Wadstrom. L. B. Tumour-distinctive cellular immunity to renal carcinoma. Clin Exp Immunol *6*, 965–970, 1970a

Stjernsward, J., Clifford, P., Singh, S., and Svedmyr, E. Indications of cellular immunological reactions against autochthonous tumour in cancer patients studied in vitro. East Afr Med J *45*, 1–14, 1968

Stjernsward, J., Clifford, P., and Svedmyr, E. General and tumour-distinctive cellular immunological reactions, pp 164–171, In Burkitt, D. P., and Wright, D. H. (Eds): General and Tumour-Distinctive Cellular Immunological Reactivity in Burkitt's Lymphoma. Edinburgh: E & S Livingstone, 1970b

Stjernsward, J., Johansson, B., Svedmyr, E., and Sundblad, R. Indication of tumour specific cell-bound immunological reactivity and depressed general reactivity in a pair of twins. Clin Exp Immunol *6*, 429–434, 1970c

Stjernsward, J., Jondal, M., Vanky, F., Wigzell, H., and Sealy, R. Lymphopenia and change in distribution of human B and T lymphocytes in peripheral blood induced by irradiation for mammary carcinoma. Lancet *1*, 1352–1356, 1972

Stjernsward, J., and Levin, A. Delayed hypersensitivity-induced regression of human neoplasms. Cancer *28*, 628–640, 1971

Stocks, P. A study of the age curve for cancer of the stomach in connection with a theory of the cancer producing mechanism. Br J Cancer *7*, 407–417, 1953

Stoker, M. Regulation of growth and orientation in hamster cells transformed by polyoma virus. Virology *24*, 165–174, 1964

Stoker, M. G. P. Abortive transformation by polyoma virus. Nature *218*, 234–238, 1968

Stoker, M. G. P. Tumour viruses and the sociology of fibroblasts. Proc R Soc Lond B *181*, 1–17, 1972

Stoker, M. G. P., and Rubin, H. Density dependent inhibition of cell growth in culture. Nature *215*, 171–172, 1967

Stoll, H. L., and Crissey, J. T. Epithelioma from single trauma. NY State Med *62*, 496–500, 1962

Storb, R., Bryant, J. I., Buckner, C. D., Clift, R. A., Fefer, A., Fialkow, P. J., Johnson, F. L., Neiman, P., and Thomas, E. D. Allogeneic marrow grafting for acute lymphoblastic leukemia: Leukemic relapse. Transplant Proc *5*, 923–926, 1973

Storb, R., Epstein, R. B., Graham, T. C., Kolb, H. J., Kolb, H., and Thomas, E. D. Rescue from canine graft-versus-host reaction by autologous or DL-A-compatible marrow. Transplantation *18*, 357–367, 1974

Stott, E. J., Probert, M., and Thomas, L. H. Cytotoxicity of alveolar macrophages for virus-infected cells. Nature *255*, 710–712, 1975

Stott, H., Stephens, R. J., Fox, W., and Roy, D. C. 5-Year follow-up of cytotoxic chemotherapy as an adjuvant to surgery in carcinoma of the bronchus. Br J Cancer *34*, 167–173, 1976

Stout, R. D., and Johnson, A. G. Regulation of the immune system by synthetic polynucleotides. V. Effect on cell-associated immunoglobulin receptors and immunological memory. J Exp Med *135*, 45–67, 1972

Straus, M. J., and Moran, R. E. Cell cycle parameters in human solid tumors. Cancer *40*, 1453–1461, 1977

Strauss, A. A. Immunologic Resistance to Carcinoma Produced by Electrocoagulation. Based on Fifty-Seven Years of Experimental and Clinical Results. Springfield, Ill.: Charles C. Thomas, 1969

Strauss, A. A., Appel, M., and Saphir, O. Electrocoagulation of malignant tumours. Am J Surg *104*, 37–45, 1962

Strauss, A. A., Appel, M., Saphir, O., and Rabinovitz, A. J. Immunologic resistance to carcinoma produced by electrocoagulation. Surg Gynecol Obstet *121*, 989–996, 1965

Strauss, A. A., Saphir, O., and Appel, M. The development of an absolute immunity in experimental animals and a relative immunity in human beings due to a necrosis of malignant tumors. Swiss Med J *86*, 606–608, 1956

Strickland, R. G., and Mackay, I. R. A reappraisal of the nature and significance of chronic atrophic gastritis. Am J Digest Dis *18*, 426–440, 1973

Strott, C. A., Nugent, C. A., and Tyler, F. H. Cushing's syndrome caused by bronchial adenomas. Am J Med *44*, 97–104, 1968

Strouk, V., Grundner, G., Fenyö, E. M., Lamon, E., Skurzak, H., and Klein, G. Lack of distinctive surface antigen on cells transformed by murine sarcoma virus. J Exp Med *136*, 344–352, 1972

Stuart, A. E. The heterogeneity of macrophages: A review, pp 1–14, In James, K., McBride, B., and Stuart, A. (Eds): Proc EURES Symp—The Macrophage and Cancer. Edinburgh Univ Dept Surgery, 1977

Study Group for Bronchogenic Carcinoma. Immunopotentiation with levamisole in resectable bronchogenic carcinoma: A double-blind controlled trial. Br Med J *3*, 461–464, 1975

Stutman, O. Tumour development after 3-methylcholanthrene in immunologically deficient athymic-nude mice. Science *183*, 534–536, 1974

Stutman, O. Tumor development after polyoma infection in athymic nude mice. J Immunol *114*, 1213–1217, 1975a

Stutman, O. Delayed tumour appearance and absence of regression in nude mice infected with murine sarcoma virus. Nature *253*, 142–144, 1975b

Stutman, O. Spontaneous, viral and chemically induced tumors in the nude mouse, pp 411–435, In Fogh, J., and Giovanella, B. C. (Eds): The Nude Mouse in Experimental and Clinical Research. New York: Academic Press, 1978

Stutman, O. Chemical carcinogenesis in nude mice: Comparison between nude mice from homozygous matings and heterozygous matings and the effect of age and carcinogen dose. J Natl Cancer Inst *62*, 353–358, 1979

Sugimura, T., Otaki, H., and Matsushima, T. Single strand scissions of DNA caused by a carcinogen, 4-Hydroxylaminoquinoline 1-oxide. Nature *218*, 392, 1968

Suit, H. D., Sedlacek, R., Silobrcic, V., and Lingood, R. M. Radiation therapy and Corynebacterium parvum in the treatment of murine tumors. Cancer *37*, 2573–2579, 1976a

Suit, H. D., Sedlacek, R., Wagner, M., and Orsi, L. Radiation response of C3H fibrosarcoma enhanced in mice stimulated by Corynebacterium parvum. Nature *255*, 493–494, 1975

Suit, H. D., Sedlacek, R., Wagner, M., Orsi, L., Silobrcic, V., and Rothman, J. Effect of Corynebacterium parvum on the response to irradiation of a C3H fibrosarcoma. Cancer Res *36*, 1305–1314, 1976b

Suit, H. D., and Silobrcic, V. Tumor-specific antigen(s) in a spontaneous mammary carcinoma of C3H mice. II. Active immunization of mammary-tumor-agent-free mice. J Natl Cancer Inst *39*, 1121–1128, 1967

Sullivan, P. W., and Salmon, S. E. Kinetics of tumor growth and regression in IgG myeloma. J Clin Invest *51*, 1697–1708, 1972

Summers, W. C. Dynamics of tumor growth: A mathematical model. Growth *30*, 333–338, 1966

Sumner, W. C., and Foraker, A. G. Spontaneous regression of human melanomas: Clinical and experimental studies. Cancer *13*, 79–81, 1960

Sutow, W. W., Sullivan, M. P., and Fernbach, D. J. Adjuvant chemotherapy in primary treatment of osteogenic sarcoma. Proc Am Assoc Cancer Res *15*, 20, 1974

Svec, J., Novotna, L., and Thurzo, V. Toward control of tumour and virus growth by helical RNA. I. Effect of poly I:C on tumour transplantation resistance in animals bearing tumours of viral and non viral origin. Neoplasma *19*, 447–452, 1972

Svet-Moldavsky, G. J., and Kadaghidze, Z. G. Anti-tumour effect of activated lymphocytes. Lancet *2*, 641–642, 1968

Svet-Moldavsky, G. J., Mkheidze, D. M., and Liozner, A. L. Rejection of skin grafts from tumour-bearing syngeneic donors. Nature *214*, 693–695, 1967

Swann, P. F., Magee, P. N., Mohr, U., Reznik, G., Green, U., and Kaufman, D. G. Possible repair of carcinogenic damage caused by dimethylnitrosamine in rat kidney. Nature *263*, 134–136, 1976

Swartzberg, J. E., Krahenbuhl, J. L., and Remington, J. S. Dichotomy between macrophage activation and degree of protection against Listeria monocytogenes and Toxoplasma gondii in mice stimulated with Corynebacterium parvum. Infect Immun *12*, 1037–1043, 1975

Swenberg, J. A., Koestner, A. Wechsler, W., Brunden, M. N., and Abe, H. Differential oncogenic effects of methylnitrosourea. J Natl Cancer Inst *54*, 89–96, 1975

Sykes, J., and Maddox, I. Prostaglandin production by experimental tumours and effects of anti-inflammatory compounds. Nature *237*, 59–61, 1972

Symes, M. O., Eckert, H., Feneley, R. C. L., Lai, T., Mitchell, J. P., Roberts, J. B. M., and Tribe, C. R. Adoptive immunotherapy and radiotherapy in the treatment of urinary bladder cancer. Br J Urol *50*, 328–331, 1978a

Symes, M. O., Eckert, H., Feneley, R. C. L., Lai, T., Mitchell, J. P., Roberts, J. B. M., and Tribe, C. R. The transfer of adoptive immunity by intraarterial injection of tumor-immune pig lymph node cells. Treatment of recurrent urinary bladder carcinoma after radical radiotherapy. Urology *12*, 398–401, 1978b

Symes, M. O., and Riddell, A. G. The use of immunized pig lymph node cells in the treatment of patients with advanced malignant disease. Br J Surg *60*, 176–180, 1973

Symes, M. O., Riddell, A. G., Feneley, R. C. L., and Tribe, C. R. The treatment of advanced bladder cancer with sensitized pig lymphocytes. Br J Cancer *28*, 276–284, 1973

Symes, M. O., Riddell, A. G., Immelman, E. J., and Terblanche, J. Immunologically competent cells in the treatment of malignant disease. Lancet *1*, 1054–1056, 1968

Symington, G. R., Mackay, I. R., and Lambert, R. P. Cancer and teratogenesis: Infrequent occurrence after medical use of immunosuppressive drugs. Aust NZ J Med *7*, 368–372, 1977

Szymaniec, S., and James, K. Studies on the Fc receptor bearing cells in a transplanted methycholanthrene-induced mouse fibrosarcoma. Br J Cancer *33,* 36–50, 1976

T

Tachibana, T., and Klein, E. Detection of cell-surface antigens on monolayer cells. Immunology *19,* 771–782, 1970

Tachibana, T., Worst, P., and Klein, E. Detection of cell surface antigens on monolayer cells. II. The application of mixed haemadsorption on a micro scale. Immunology *19,* 809–816, 1970

Tada, T., Taniguchi, M., and Takemori, T. Properties of primed suppressor T cells and their products. Transplant Rev *26,* 106–129, 1976

Takahashi, K. Squamous cell carcinoma of the esophagus: Stromal inflammatory cell infiltration as a prognostic factor. Cancer *14,* 921–933, 1961

Takasugi, M., Akira, D., Takasugi, J., and Mickey, M. R. Specificities in human cell-mediated cytotoxicity. J Natl Cancer Inst *59,* 69–82, 1977

Takasugi, M., and Hildemann, W. H. Lymphocyte-antibody interactions in immunological enhancement. Transplant Proc *1,* 530–534, 1969

Takasugi, M., and Klein, E. A microassay for cell-mediated immunity. Transplantation *9,* 219–227, 1970

Takasugi, M., and Klein, E. The methodology of micro-assay for cell-mediated immunity (MCI), pp 415–422, In Bloom, B. R., and Glade, P. R. (Eds): In Vitro Methods in Cell-mediated Immunity. New York: Academic Press, 1971

Takasugi, M., Mickey, M. R., and Tarasaki, P. I. Quantitation of the microassay for cell-mediated immunity through electronic image analysis. J Natl Cancer Inst Monogr *37,* 77–84, 1973a

Takasugi, M., Mickey, M. R., and Terasaki, P. I. Reactivity of lymphocytes from normal persons on cultured tumor cells. Cancer Res *33,* 2898–2902, 1973b

Takatsu, K., Hamaoka, T., Yamashita, U., and Kitagawa, M. Suppressed activity of thymus-derived cell in tumor-bearing host. Gann *63,* 273–275, 1972

Takeda, K., Aizawa, M., Kikuchi, Y., Yamawaki, S., and Nakamura, K. Autoimmunity against methylcholanthrene-induced sarcomas of the rat. Gann *57,* 221–240, 1966

Takita, H., and Brugarolas, A. Immunotherapy in bronchogenic carcinoma. Surg Forum *23,* 98–99, 1972

Takita, H., Takada, M., Minowada, J., Han, T., and Edgerton, F. Adjuvant immunotherapy of stage III cancer carcinoma, pp 217–223, In Terry, W. D., and Windhorst, D. (Eds): Immunotherapy of Cancer: Present Status of Trials in Man. New York: Raven Press, 1978

Takita, H., and Moayeri, H. Effects of Corynebacterium parvum and chemotherapy in lung carcinoma. Proc Am Soc Clin Oncol *17,* 292, 1976

Taliaferro, W. H., and Jaroslow, B. N. The restoration of hemolysin formation in x-rayed rabbits by nucleic acid derivatives and antagonists of nucleic acid synthesis. J Infect Dis *107* 341–350, 1960

Tan, Y. H. Chromosome 21 and the cell growth inhibitory effect of human interferon preparations. Nature *260,* 141–143, 1976

Tanaka, T., Cooper, E. H., and Anderson, C. K. Lymphocyte infiltration in bladder cancer. Rev Eur Etudes Clin Biol *15,* 1084–1089, 1970

Tanaka, T., Nakagawa, H., Kato, A., Yoshimura, M., Fujita, H., and Kumara, K. Effect of anti-thymocyte serum, anti-macrophage serum, and latex particles on the therapeutic efficacy of BCG or Corynebacterium liquefaciens (Propionibacterium acnes C7) in syngeneic mice. Gann *68,* 45–52, 1977

Tannock, I. F. The relation between cell proliferation and the vascular system in a transplanted mouse mammary tumor. Br J Cancer *22,* 258–273, 1968

Tannock, I. F. Population kinetics of carcinoma cells, capillary endothelial cells, and fibroblasts in a transplanted mouse mammary tumor. Cancer Res *30,* 2470–2476, 1970

Taranger, L. A., Chapman, W. H., Hellström, I., and Hellström, K. E. Immunological studies of urinary bladder tumors of rats and mice. Science *176,* 1337–1339, 1972

Tarin, D. (Ed): Tissue Interactions in Carcinogenesis. London, New York: Academic Press, 1972

Tashjian, A., Voelkel, E., Levine, L., and Goldhaber, P. Evidence that the bone resorption-stimulating factor produced by mouse fibrosarcoma cells is prostaglandin E_2. A new model for the hyper-calcemia of cancer. J Exp Med *136,* 1329–1343, 1972

Tatarinov, Y. S. Detection of embryospecific α-globulin in the blood serum of a patient with primary liver cancer. Vop Med Khim *10,* 90–91, 1964

Tatarinov, Y. S. Content of embryo-specific alpha-globulin in fetal and neonatal sera and sera from adult humans with primary carcinoma of the liver. Fed Proc (Transl Suppl) *25,* 344–346, 1966

Tattersall, M. H. N., and Tobias, J. S. How strong is the case for intensive cancer chemotherapy? Lancet *2,* 1071–1072, 1976

Taylor, G., and Odili, J. L. I. Histological evidence of tumor rejection after active immunotherapy in human malignant disease. Br Med J *2,* 183–188, 1972

Teasdale, C., Roux, L., Whitehead, R. H., Bolton, P. M., and Hughes, L. E. Analysis of PHA responsiveness of lymphocytes in cancer patients. Clin Oncol *2,* 306, 1976

Teimourian, B., and McCune, W. S. Surgical management of malignant melanoma. Am Surg *29,* 515–519, 1963

Temin, H. M. Mechanism of cell transformation by RNA tumor viruses. Annu Rev Microbiol *25,* 609–648, 1971a

Temin, H. M. The protovirus hypothesis: Speculations on the significance of RNA-directed DNA synthesis for normal development and for carcinogenesis. J Natl Cancer Inst *46*(2), iii–vii, 1971b

Temin, H. M. The cellular and molecular biology of RNA tumor viruses, especially avian leukosis-sarcoma viruses, and their relatives. Adv Cancer Res *19,* 47–104, 1974

Temin, H. M., and Baltimore, D. RNA-directed DNA synthesis and RNA tumor viruses. Adv Virus Res *17,* 129–186, 1972

Temple, A., Loewi, G., Davies, P., and Howard, A. Cytotoxicity of immune guinea-pig cells. II. The mechanism of macrophage cytotoxicity. Immunology *24,* 655–669, 1973

Terracini, B., and Stramignoni, A. Malignant lymphomas and renal changes in Swiss mice given nitrosomethylurea. Eur J Cancer *3,* 435–436, 1967

Terracini, B., and Testa, M. C. Carcinogenicity of a single administration of N-nitrosomethylurea: A comparison between newborn and five-week-old mice and rats. Br J Cancer 588–598, 1970

Terracini, B., Testa, M. C., Cabral, J. R., and Rossi, L. The roles of age at treatment and dose in carcinogenesis in C3Hf/Dp mice with a single administration of N-nitroso-N-methylurea. Br J. Cancer *33,* 427–439, 1976

Terranova, T., and Chiossone, F. Il fattore coagulazione nell'attechimento delle cellule neoplastiche immesse in circolo. Bull Soc Ital Biol Sper *28,* 1224–1225, 1952

Terry, W. D., and Windhorst, D. (Eds): Immunotherapy of Cancer: Present Status of Trials in Man. New York: Raven Press, 1978

Terz. J. J., Fu, Y. S., and King, E. R. Cell kinetics

of human tumors during radiation therapy. Proc Am Assoc Cancer Res *16,* 137, 1975

Terz, J. J., Lawrence, W., and Cox, B. Analysis of the cycling and non-cycling cell population of human solid tumors. Cancer *40,* 1462–1470, 1977

Thatcher, N., and Crowther, D. Effects of BCG and Corynebacterium parvum on immune reactivity in melanoma patients. Dev Biol Stand *38,* 449–453, 1978

Theilen, G., Hall, J. G., Pendry, A., Glover, D. J., and Reeves, B. R. Tumours induced in sheep by injecting cells transformed in vitro with feline sarcoma virus. Transplantation *17,* 152–155, 1974

Thiele, E., Arison, R. N., and Boxer, G. E. Oncolysis by clostridia. III. Effects of Clostridia and chemo-therapeutic agents on rodent tumors. Cancer Res *24,* 222–223, 1964

Thiry, L., Sprecher-Goldberger, S., Tack, L., Jacques, M., and Stienon, J. Comparison of the immunogenicity of hamster cells transformed by adenovirus and herpes simplex virus. Cancer Res *37,* 1301–1306, 1977

Thomas, E. D., Buckner, C. D., Clift, R. A., Fass, L., Fefer, A., Lerner, K. G., Neiman, P., Rowley, N., and Storb, R. Marrow grafting in patients with acute leukemia. Transplant Proc *5,* 917–922, 1973

Thomas E. D., Buckner, C. D., Fefer, A., Neiman, P. E., and Storb, R. Marrow transplantation in the treatment of acute leukemia. Adv Cancer Res *27,* 269–279, 1978

Thomas E. D., Buckner, C. D., Rudolph, R. H., Fefer, A., Storb, R., Neiman, P. E., Bryant, J. I., Chard, R. L., Clift, R. A., Epstein, R. B., Fialkow, P. J., Funk, D. D. Funk, E. R., Giblett, E. R., Lerner, K. C., Reynolds, F. A., and Slichter, S. Allogeneic marrow grafting for hematologic malignancy using HL-A matched donor–recipient pairs. Blood *38,* 267–287, 1971a

Thomas, E. D., Herman, E. C., Greenhough, W. B., Hager, E. B., Cannon, J. H., Sahler, O. D., and Ferrebee, J. W. Irradiation and marrow infusion in leukemia. Arch Intern Med *107,* 829–845, 1961

Thomas, E. D., Lochte, H. L., Cannon, J. H., Sahler, O. D., and Ferrebee, J. W. Supralethal whole body irradiation and isologous marrow transplantation in man. J Clin Invest *38,* 1709–1716, 1959

Thomas, E. D., Lochte, H. L., Lu, W. C., and Ferrebee, J. W. Intravenous infusion of bone marrow in patients receiving radiation and chemotherapy. N Engl J Med *257,* 491–496, 1957

Thomas, E. D., Rudolph, R. H., Fefer, A., Storb,

R., Slichter, S., and Buckner, C. D. Isogeneic marrow grafting in man. Exp Hematol 21, 16–18, 1971b

Thomas, E. D., Storb, R., Clift, R. A., Fefer, A., Johnson, F. L., Neiman, P. E., Lerner, K. G., Glucksberg, H., and Buckner, C. D. Bone-marrow transplantation. N Engl J Med 292, 832–843, 1975

Thomas, J. W. [Cited by Clements et al. (1976)] Conference on the Use of BCG in Therapy of Cancer, National Cancer Institute. 1972

Thomas, J. W., Plenderleith, I. H., Clements, D. V., and Landi, S. Observations in immunotherapy of lymphoma and melanoma patients. Clin Exp Immunol 21, 82–96, 1975

Thomas, J. W., Plenderleith, I. H., Landi, S., and Clements, D. V. BCG as maintenance therapy in non-Hodgkin's lymphoma, pp 297–302, In Proc Int Symp in Honour of Prof. Armand Frappier. New York: Grune & Stratton, 1976

Thomas, L. Discussion, pp 529–531, In Lawrence, H. S. (Ed): Cellular and Humoral Aspects of the Hypersensitivity States. London: Cassell, 1959

Thomas, P. R. M., George, R. J., Gazet, J. C., and Peckham, M. J. Immunotherapy for colorectal cancer. Lancet 1, 1349–1350, 1976

Thomas, W. R., Holt, P. G., Papadimitriou, J. M., and Keast, D. The growth of transplanted tumours in mice after chronic inhalation of fresh cigarette smoke. Br J Cancer 30, 459–462, 1974

Thomford, N. R., Woolner, L. B., and Clagett, O. T. The surgical treatment of metastatic tumors in the lungs. J Thorac Cardiovasc Surg 49, 357–363, 1965

Thomlinson, R. D., and Gray, L. H. The histological structure of some human lung cancers and the possible implications for radiotherapy. Br J Cancer 9, 539–549, 1955

Thompson, R. B. Lymphocyte transfer factor. Eur J Clin Biol Res 16, 201–204, 1971

Thompson, S. C. The colony forming efficiency of single cells and cell aggregates from a spontaneous mouse mammary tumour using the lung colony assay. Br J Cancer 30, 332–336, 1974

Thomson, D. M. P. Soluble tumour-specific antigen and its relationship to tumour growth. Int J Cancer 15, 1016–1029, 1975

Thomson, D. M. P., and Alexander, P. A cross-reacting embryonic antigen in the membrane of rat sarcoma cells which is immunogenic in the syngeneic host. Br J Cancer 27, 35–47, 1973

Thomson, D. M. P., Eccles, S., and Alexander, P. Antibodies and soluble tumor-specific antigens in blood and lymph of rats with chemi-

cally induced sarcomata. Br J Cancer 28, 6–15, 1973a

Thomson, D. N. P., Krupey, J., Freedman, S. O., and Gold, P. The radio-immunoassay of circulating carcinoembryonic antigen of the human digestive system. Proc Natl Acad Sci USA 64, 161–167, 1969

Thomson, D. M. P., Sellens, V., Eccles, S., and Alexander, P. Radioimmunoassay of tumour specific transplantation antigen of a chemically induced rat sarcoma: Circulating soluble tumour antigen in tumour bearers. Br J Cancer 28, 377–388, 1973b

Thomson, D. M. P., Steele, K., and Alexander, P. The presence of tumor-specific membrane antigen in the serum of rats with chemically induced sarcomata. Br J Cancer 27, 1–8, 1973c

Thor, D., Jureziz, R. E., Veach, S. R., Miller, E., and Dray, S. Cell migration inhibition factor released by antigen from human peripheral lymphocytes. Nature 219, 755–757, 1968

Thornes, R. D. Anticoagulant therapy in patients with cancer. J Ir Med Assoc 62, 426–429, 1969

Thornes, R. D. Warfarin as maintenance therapy for cancer. J Ir Coll Physicians Surg 2, 41–42, 1972a

Thornes, R. D. Fibrin and cancer. Br Med J 1, 110–111, 1972b

Thornes, R. D. Unblocking or activation of the cellular immune mechanism by induced proteolysis in patients with cancer. Lancet 2, 382–384, 1974

Thornes, R. D. Adjuvant therapy of cancer via the cellular immune mechanism or fibrin by induced fibrinolysis and oral anticoagulants. Cancer 35, 91–97, 1975

Thornes, R. D. Interpretation of management of levamisole-associated side effects, pp 157–164, In Chirigos, M. A. (Ed): Immune Modulation and Control of Neoplasia by Adjuvant Therapy. New York: Raven Press, 1978a

Thornes, R. D. Report on bowel tumour study data. Personal communication, 1978b

Thornes, R. D., Browne, D., D'Souza, D., and Holland, P. D. J. Activation or unblocking of T lymphocytes. Personal communication, 1978

Thornes, R. D., Smyth, H., Browne, O., O'Gorman, M., Reen, D. J., Farrell, D., and Holland, P. D. J. The effects of proteolysis on the human immune mechanism in cancer. J Med (Basel) 5, 92–97, 1974

Timmermans, A., Bentvelzen, P., Hageman, P. C., and Calafat, J. Activation of a mammary tumour virus in 020 strain mice by irradiation and urethane. J Gen Virol 4, 619–621, 1969

Ting, C.-C., and Herberman, R. B. Inverse relationship of polyoma tumour specific cell surface antigen to H-2 histocompatibility antigens. Nature 232, 118–120, 1971

Ting, C.-C., Lavrin, D. H., Shiu, G., and Herberman, R. B. Expression of fetal antigens in tumor cells. Proc Natl Acad Sci USA 69, 1664–1668, 1972

Ting, C.-C., Rodrigues, D., and Herberman, R. B. Expression of fetal antigens and tumor-specific antigens in SV40-transformed cells. II. Tumor transplantation studies. Int J Cancer 12, 519–523, 1973

Ting, R. C. Failure to induce transplantation resistance against polyoma tumour cells with syngeneic embryonic tissues. Nature 217, 858–859, 1968

Todaro, G. J. "Spontaneous" release of type C viruses from clonal lines of "spontaneously" transformed BALB/3T3 cells. Nature New Biol 240, 157–160, 1972

Todaro, G. J. RNA-tumour-virus genes and transforming genes: Patterns of transmission. Br J Cancer 37, 139–158, 1978

Todaro, G. J., and Gallo, R. C. Immunological relationship of DNA polymerase from human acute leukaemia cells and primate and mouse leukaemia virus reverse transcriptase. Nature 244, 206–209 [also Erratum Nature 245, 398] 1973

Todaro, G. J., and Martin, G. M. Increased susceptibility of Down's syndrome fibroblasts to transformation by SV40. Proc Soc Exp Biol Med 124, 1232–1236, 1967

Todd, D. W., Farrow, G. M., Winklemann, R. K., and Payne, W. S. Spontaneous regression of malignant melanoma. Mayo Clin Proc 41, 672–676, 1966

Tomatis, L., Mohr, U., and Davis, W. (Eds): Transplacental Carcinogenesis. IARC Sci Publ No. 4, 1973

Tønder, O., Morse, P. A., and Humphrey, L. J. Similarities of Fc receptors in human malignant tissue and normal lymphoid tissue. J Immunol 113,1162–1169, 1974

Toolan, H. W. Successful subcutaneous growth and transplantation of human tumors in x-irradiated laboratory animals. Proc Soc Exp Biol Med 77, 572–578, 1951

Toolan, H. W. Growth of human tumors in cortisone-treated laboratory animals: The possibility of obtaining permanently transplantable human tumors. Cancer Res 13, 389–394, 1953

Toolan, H. W. Transplantable human neoplasms maintained in cortisone-treated laboratory animals: H. S. No. 1; H. Ep., No. 1; H. Ep., No. 2; H. Ep., No. 3; and H. Emb. Rh., No. 1. Cancer Res 14, 660–666, 1954

Toolan, H. W. The transplantable human tumor. Ann NY Acad Sci 76, 733–741, 1958

Tooze, J. (Ed): The Molecular Biology of Tumor Viruses. New York: Cold Spring Harbor Lab, 1973

Tormey, D. C., Waalkes, T. P., Ahmann, D., Gehrke, C. W., Zumwatt, R. W., Snyder, J., and Hansen, H. Biological markers in breast carcinoma. I. Incidence of abnormalities of CEA, HCG, three polyamines, and three minor nucleosides. Cancer 35, 1095–1100, 1975

Toujas, L., Dazord, L., and Guelfi, J. Kinetics of proliferation of bone-marrow cell lines after injections of immunostimulant bacteria, pp 117–131, In Halpern, B. (Ed): Corynebacterium Parvum: Applications in Experimental and Clinical Oncology. New York: Plenum Press, 1975

Toujas, L., Sabolovic, D., Dazord, L., LeGarrec, Y., Toujas, J. P., Guelfi, J., and Pilet, C. The mechanism of immunostimulation induced by inactivated brucella abortus. Rev Eur Etude Clin Biol 17, 267–273, 1972

Trentin, J. J. Whole body x-ray and bone marrow therapy of leukemia in mice. Proc Am Assoc Cancer Res 2, 54, 1957

Treves, A. J., Carnaud, C., Trainin, N., Feldman, M., and Cohen, I. R. Enhancing T lymphocytes from tumor-bearing mice suppress host resistance to a syngeneic tumor. Eur J Immunol 4, 722–727, 1974

Treves, A. J., and Cohen, I. R. Recruitment of effector T lymphocytes against a tumor allograft by T lymphocytes sensitized in vitro. J Natl Cancer Inst 51, 1919–1925, 1973

Treves, A. J., Cohen, I. R., and Feldman, M. Immunotherapy of lethal metastases by lymphocytes sensitized against tumor cells in vitro. J Natl Cancer Inst 54, 777–780, 1975

Treves, A. J., Schechter, B., Cohen, I. R., and Feldman, M. Sensitization of T lymphocytes in vitro by syngeneic macrophages fed with tumor antigens. J Immunol 116,1059–1064,1976

Trinchieri, G., and Santoli, D. Antagonistic effects of interferon on natural killer and target cells, In Riethmüller, G., Wernet, P., and Cudkowicz, G. (Eds): Cytotoxic Cell Interaction and Immunostimulation. [Cited by Santoli and Koprowski (1979) as in press] New York: Academic Press, 1979

Tripodi, D., Parks, L. C., and Brugmans, J. Drug-induced restoration of cutaneous delayed hypersensitivity in anergic patients with cancer. N Engl J Med 289, 354–357, 1973

Trosko, J. E., and Chu, E. H. Y. The role of DNA repair and somatic mutation in carcinogenesis. Adv Cancer Res 21, 391–425, 1975

Truitt, R. L., and Pollard, M. Allogeneic bone marrow chimerism in germ-free mice. IV. Therapy of Hodgkin's-like reticulum cell sarcoma in SJL mice. Transplantation 21, 12–16, 1976

Tsakraklides, E., Smith, C., Kersey, J. H., and Good, R. A. Transplantation antigens (H-2) on virally and chemically transformed Balb/3T3 fibroblasts in culture. J Natl Cancer Inst 52, 1499–1504, 1974

Tsakraklides, F., Tsakraklides, V., Ashikari, H., Rosen, P. P., Siegal, F. P., Robbins, G. F., and Good, R. A. In vitro studies of axillary lymph node cells in patients with breast cancer. J Natl Cancer Inst 54, 549–556, 1975

Tsakraklides, V., Oslon, P., Kersey, J. H., and Good, R. A. Prognostic significance of the regional lymph node histology in cancer of the breast. Cancer 34, 1259–1267, 1974

Tsirimbas, A. D., Pichlmayr, R., Hornung, B., Pfisterer, H., Thierfelder, D., Brendel, W., und Stich, W. Therapeutische Wirkungen von heterologem Antihumanlymphocytenserum bei chronischer lymphatischer Leukämie. Klin Wochenschr 46, 583–586, 1968

Tsoi, M. S., and Weiser, R. S. Mechanisms of immunity to sarcoma 1 allografts in the C57BL/Ks mouse. I. Passive transfer studies with immune peritoneal macrophages in x-irradiated hosts. J Natl Cancer Inst 40, 23–30, 1968

Tubiana, M. The kinetics of tumor cell proliferation and radiotherapy. Br J Radiol 44, 325–347, 1971

Tubiana, M., and Malaise, E. P. Comparison of cell proliferation kinetics in human and experimental tumors: Response to irradiation. Cancer Treat Rep 60, 1887–1895, 1976

Tucker, D. F., Dennert, G., and Lennox, E. S. Thymus-derived lymphocytes as effectors of cell-mediated immunity to syngeneic and allogeneic transplants in the rat. J Immunol 113, 1302–1312, 1974

Tuffrey, M. A., and Batchelor, J. R. Tumour specific immunity against murine epitheliomas induced with 9,10-dimethyl-1,2-benzanthracene. Nature 204, 349–351, 1964

Turcotte, R., and Quevillon, M. Antitumor activity and other biological properties of two phenotypes isolated from BCG. Cancer Immunol Immunother 1, 25–30, 1976

Turk, J. L., and Willoughby, D. A. An analysis of the multiplicity of the effects of antilymphocyte serum. A comparison with the action of other immunosuppressive agents in the cell-mediated immune response and nonspecific inflammation. Antiobiot Chemother (Basel), 15, 267–294, 1969

Turkington, R. W. Prolactin receptors in mammary carcinoma cells. Cancer Res 34, 758–763, 1974

Turner, W., Chan, S. P., and Chirigos, M. A. Stimulation of humoral and cellular antibody formation in mice by poly IC. Proc Soc Exp Biol Med 133, 334–338, 1970

Tuttle, R. L., and North, R. J. Mechanisms of antitumor action of Corynebacterium parvum: Nonspecific tumor cell destruction at site of an immunologically mediated sensitivity reaction to C. parvum. J Natl Cancer Inst 55, 1403–1411, 1975

Twomey, P. L., Catalona, W. J., and Chretien, P. B. Cellular immunity in cured cancer patients. Cancer 33, 435–440, 1974

Tyler, A. A developmental immunogenetic analysis of cancer (Henry Ford Hosp Int Symp—Biological Interactions in Normal and Neoplastic Growth). Boston: Little, Brown, 1962

Tyzzer, E. E. Factors in the production and growth of tumor metastases. J Med Res 18, 309–333, 1912

Tyzzer, E. E. Tumor immunity. J Cancer Res 1, 125–155, 1916

U

Umezawa, H., Aoyagi, T., Suda, H., Hamada, M., and Takeuchi, T. Bestatin, a new amino-peptidase B inhibitor produced by actinomycetes. J Antibiot (Tokyo) 29, 97–99, 1976a

Umezawa, H., Ishisuka, M., Aoyagi, T., and Takeuchi, T. Enhancement of delayed-type hypersensitivity by bestatin, an inhibitor of amino-peptidase B and leucine aminopeptidase. J Antibiot (Tokyo) 29, 857–859, 1976b

Umiel, T., and Trainin, N. Immunological enhancement of tumor growth by syngeneic thymus-derived lymphocytes. Transplantation 18, 244–250, 1974

Unanue, E. R. The regulation of lymphocyte functions by the macrophage. Immunol Rev 40, 227–255, 1978

Ungar, B., Strickland, R. G., and Francis, C. M. The prevalence and significance of circulating antibodies to gastric intrinsic factor and parietal cells in gastric carcinoma. Gut 12, 903–905, 1971

Ungaro, P. C., Drake, W. P., Buchholz, D. H., and Mardiney, M. R. Alteration of the specificity of antitumor antisera by the use of passively administered antibody. Cancer Res 32, 1521–1525, 1972

Union Internationale Contre Le Cancer (UICC). Clinical Stage Classification and Presentation of Results: Malignant Tumours of the Breast. Geneva: UICC, 1960

Union Internationale Contre Le Cancer (UICC). Controlled Therapeutic Trials in Cancer. Geneva: UICC, 1974

Uphoff, D. E., and Law, L. W. Genetic factors influencing irradiation protection by bone marrow. II. The histocompatibility-2 (H-2) locus. J Natl Cancer Inst 20, 617–624, 1958

Upton, A. C., Kimball, A. W., Furth, J., Christenberry, K. W., and Benedict, W. H. Some delayed effects of atom-bomb radiations in mice. Cancer Res 20, 1–59, 1960

Upton, G. V., and Amatruda, T. T. Tumor peptides with CRF-like activity in the ectopic ACTH syndrome. N Engl J Med 285, 419–424, 1971

Urbach, F. (Ed): The Biological Effects of Ultraviolet Radiation (With Emphasis on the Skin). Oxford: Pergamon Press, 1969

Urban, J. A. Radical mastectomy with en bloc resection of internal mammary lymph node chain. Surg Clin North Am 36, 1065–1082, 1956

Urban, J. A. Bilaterality of cancer of the breast. Biopsy of the opposite breast. Cancer 20, 1867–1870, 1967

Urban, J. A. Biopsy of the "normal" breast in treating breast cancer. Surg Clin North Am 49, 291–301, 1969

Urban, J. A., and Baker, H. W. Radical mastectomy in continuity with en bloc resection of the internal mammary lymph node chain; A new procedure for primary operable cancer of the breast. Cancer 5, 992–1008, 1952

Urban, J. A., and Castro, E. B. Selecting variations in extent of surgical procedure for breast cancer. Cancer 28, 1615–1623, 1971

Usubuchi, I., Kudo, H., Sobajima, Y., Sato, T., Kakisaka, Y., and Nishimura, S. Inhibitory effect of cross-immunity on autotransplantation of methylcholanthrene-induced rat sarcomas. Tohoku J Exp Med 110, 155–160, 1973

Usubuchi, I., Sobajima, Y., Kudo, H., Hongo, T., and Sugawara, M. Cross-immunity among syngeneic tumors in mice. Tohoku J Exp Med 108, 79–84, 1972

V

Vaage, J. Non-cross-reacting resistance to virus induced mouse mammary tumours in virus infected C3H mice. Nature 218, 101–102, 1968a

Vaage, J. Non virus-associated antigens in virus-induced mouse mammary tumors. Cancer Res 28, 2477–2483, 1968b

Vaage, J. Concomitant immunity and specific depression of immunity by residual or re-injected syngeneic tumor tissue. Cancer Res 31, 1655–1662, 1971

Vadas, M. A., Miller, J. F. A. P., McKenzi, I. F. C., Chism, S. E., Shen, F. W., Boyse, E. A., Gamble, J. R., and Whitelaw, A. M. Ly and Ia antigen phenotypes of T cells involved in delayed-type hypersensitivity and in suppression. J Exp Med 144, 10–19, 1976

Vadlamudi, S., Padarathsingh, M., Bonmasser, E., and Goldin, A. Effect of combination treatment with cyclophosphamide and isogeneic or allogeneic spleen and bone marrow cells in leukemic (L1210) mice. Int J Cancer 7, 160–166, 1971

Vaheri, A., Ruoslahti, E., and Nordling, S. Neuraminidase stimulates division and sugar uptake in density-inhibited cell cultures. Nature New Biol 238, 211–212, 1972

Vaheri, A., Ruoslahti, E., Westermark, B., and Ponten, J. A common cell-type specific surface antigen in cultured human glial cells and fibroblasts: Loss in malignant cells. J Exp Med 143, 64–72, 1976

Vaitkevicius, V. K., Sugimoto, M., Reed, M. L., and Brennan, M. J. Effect of acute tissue injury on transplantability of autologous human cancer. Cancer 18, 665–670, 1965

Valdivieso, M., Hersh, E. M., Rodriguez, V., Gutterman, J. U., and Freireich, E. J. Chemoimmunotherapy of adenocarcinoma of the lung with Baker's antifol (BAF), FTOR-AFUR (FTOR) and Corynebacterium parvum (C.P.). Proc Am Assoc Cancer Res 17, 132, 1976

van Bekkum, D. W., and de Vries, M. J. The clinical application of bone marrow transplantation in the treatment of leukemia, pp 223–232, In Radiation Chimaeras. New York: Academic Press, 1967

van Bekkum, D. W., and Vos, O. Immunological aspects of homo- and heterologous bone marrow transplantation in irradiated animals. J Cell Comp Physiol 50 (Suppl), 139–156, 1957

Van Boxel, J. A., Paul, W. E., Frank, M. M., and Green, I. Antibody-dependent lymphoid cell-mediated cytotoxicity: Role of lymphocytes bearing a receptor for complement. J Immunol 110, 1027–1036, 1973

van den Brenk, H. A. S. Autoimmunization in human malignant melanoma. Br Med J 4, 171–172, 1969

van den Brenk, H. A. S., Burch, W. M., Kelly, H., and Orton, C. Venous diversion trapping and growth of blood-borne cancer cells en route to the lungs. Br J Cancer *31*, 46–61, 1975

van den Brenk, H. A. S., Stone, M., Kelly, H., Orton, C., and Sharpington, C. Promotion of growth of tumour cells in acutely inflamed tissues. Br J Cancer *30*, 246–260, 1974

van den Brenk, H. A. S., Stone, M., Kelly, H., Orton, C., and Sharpington, C. Lowering of innate resistance of the lungs to the growth of blood-borne cancer cells in states of topical and systemic stress. Br J Cancer *33*, 60–78, 1976

Vandeputte, M. The effect of heterologous anti-lymphocytic serum on the oncogenic activity of polyoma virus. Life Sci *7*, 855–865, 1968

Vandeputte, M., Datta, S. K., Billiau, A., and De Somer, P. Inhibition of polyoma-virus oncogenesis in rats by polyriboinosinic-ribocytidylic acid. Eur J Cancer *6*, 323–327, 1970

Vandeputte, M., Denys, P., Leyten, R., and De Somer, P. The oncogenic activity of the polyoma virus in thymectomized rats. Life Sci *2*, 475–478, 1963

Vandeputte, M., and De Somer, P. Influence of thymectomy on viral oncogenesis in rats. Nature *206*, 520–521, 1965

Van Duuren, E. L. Carcinogenic epoxides, lactones and haloethers and their mode of action. Ann NY Acad Sci USA *163*, 633–651, 1969

Vane, J. R. Inhibition of prostaglandin synthesis as a mechanism of action for aspirin-like drugs. Nature New Biol *231*, 232–235, 1971

Van Furth, R. The origin and turnover of promonocytes, monocytes and macrophages in normal mice, pp 151–165, In Van Furth, R. (Ed): Mononuclear Phagocytes. Oxford: Blackwell, 1970

Van Furth, R. Unsolved problems concerning the interaction between macrophages and tumour cells, pp 445–448, In James, K., McBride, B., and Stuart, A. (Eds): Proc EURES Symp—The Macrophage and Cancer. Edinburgh Univ Dept Surgery, 1977

Van Furth, R., and Cohn, Z. A. The origin and kinetics of mononuclear phagocytes. J Exp Med *128*, 415–433, 1968

Van Furth, R., and Diesselhoff-den Dulk, M. M. C. The kinetics of promonocytes and monocytes in the bone marrow. J Exp Med *132*, 813–828, 1970

Vanky, F., Klein, E., Stjernsward, J., and Nilsonne, U. Cellular immunity against tumor-associated antigens in humans: Lymphocyte stimulation and skin reaction. Int J Cancer *14*, 277–288, 1974

Vanky, F., Stjernsward, J., Klein, G., Steiner, L., and Lindberg, L. Tumour-associated specificity of serum-mediated inhibition of lymphocyte stimulation by autochthonous tumour cells. J Natl Cancer Inst *51*, 25–32, 1973

Vanky, F., Stjernsward, J., and Nilsonne, U. Cellular immunity against human sarcoma. J Natl Cancer Inst *46*, 1145–1151, 1971

Van Loveren, H., and Den Otter, W. In vitro activation of armed macrophages and the therapeutic application in mice. J Natl Cancer Inst *52*, 1917–1918, 1974

van Putten, L. M., Kram, L. K. J., van Dierdendonck, H. H. C., Smink, T., and Fuzy, M. Enhancement by drugs of metastatic lung nodule formation after intravenous tumour cell injection. Int J Cancer *15*, 588–595, 1975

Vanwijck, R. R., Godrick, E. A., Smith, H. G., Goldweitz, J., and Wilson, R. E. Stimulation or suppression of metastases with graded doses of tumor cells. Cancer Res *31*, 1559–1563, 1971

Vasarevic, B., Boranic, M., and Pavelic, Z. The effect of immunostimulation and chemotherapy on the growth of reticulosarcoma in mice. Biomedicine *21*, 462–464, 1974

Vaseduvin, D. M., Balakrishnan, K., and Talwar, G. P. Effect of neuraminidase on electrophoretic mobility and immune cytolysis of human uterine carcinoma cells. Int J Cancer *6*, 506–516, 1970

Vasiliev, J. M. The role of connective tissue proliferation in invasive growth of normal and malignant tissues: A review. Br J Cancer *12*, 524–536, 1958

Vaughan, J. W. Cancer vaccine and anticancer globulins as an aid in the surgical treatment of malignancy. JAMA *63*, 1258–1265, 1914

Veltri, R. W., Mengoli, H. F., Maxim, P. E., Westfall, S., Gopo, J. M., Huang, C.-W., and Sprinkle, P. M. Isolation and identification of human lung tumor associated antigen. Cancer Res *37*, 1313–1322, 1977

Verhaegen, H., de Cree, J., de Cock, W., and Verbruggen, F. Levamisole and the immune response. N Engl J Med *289*, 1148–1149, 1973

Verly, W. G., Deschamps, J., Pushpathadam, J., and Desrosiers, M. The hepatic chalone. I. Assay method for the hormone and purification of the rabbit liver chalone. Can J Biochem *49*, 1376–1383, 1971

Vesselinovitch, S. D., and Mihailovich, N. The inhibitory effect of griseofulvin on the 'promotion' of skin carcinogenesis. Cancer Res *28*, 2463–2465, 1968

Vetto, R. M., Burger, D. R., Nolte, J. E., Vandenbark, A. A., and Baker, H. W. Transfer factor immunotherapy. Cancer *37*, 90–97, 1976

Vial, A. B., and Callahan, W. The effect of some tagged antibodies on human melanoblastoma. Cancer *10*, 999–1003, 1957

Vidal, E. [*Cited by Southam (1961)*] La sérothérapie des tumeurs malignes, pp 293–342, In Travaux de la 2° Conférence Internationale pour l'étude du Cancer, Paris, 1910. 1911

Vilcek, J., Ng, M. H., Friedman-Kien, A. E., and Krawicw, T. Induction of interferon synthesis by synthetic double-stranded polynucleotides. J Virol 2, 648–650, 1968

Virchow, R. Ueber bewegliche thierische Zellen. Arch Pathol Anat Physiol Klin Med 28, 237–240, 1863

Visfeldt, J., Povlsen, C. O., and Rygaard, J. Chromosome analysis of human tumors following heterotransplantation to the mouse mutant nude. Acta Pathol Microbiol Scand 80, 169–176, 1972

Viza, D. Human leukemic and leukemoembryonic antigens, pp 369–378, In Anderson, N. G., and Coggin, J. H. (Eds): Embryonic and Fetal Antigens in Cancer. Springfield, Va.: U.S. Dept Commerce, 1971

Viza, D. C., Bernard-Degani, O., Bernard, C., and Harris, R. Leukaemia antigens. Lancet 2, 493–494, 1969

Viza, D., Davies, D. A. L., and Harris, R. Solubilization and partial purification of human leukaemic specific antigens. Nature 227, 1249–1251, 1970a

Viza, D., Davies, D. A. L., Todd, R., Bernard-Degani, O., Bernard, C., and Harris, R. Mise en évidence, isolement et purification partielle d'antigènes leucémique chez l'homme. Pr Med 78, 2259–2264, 1970b

Vogler, W. R., Bartolucci, A. A., Omura, A., Miller, D., Smalley, R. V., Knospe, W. H., and Goldsmith, A. S. A randomized clinical trial of BCG in myeloblastic leukemia conducted by the Southeastern Cancer Study Group, pp 365–373, In Terry, W. D., and Windhorst, D. (Eds): Immunotherapy of Cancer: Present Status of Trials in Man. New York: Raven Press, 1978

Vogler, W. R., and Chan, Y. K. Prolonging remission in myeloblastic leukaemia by Tice-strain bacillus Calmette-Guérin. Lancet 2, 128–131, 1974

Volkman, A. The origin and turnover of mononuclear cells in peritoneal exudates in rats. J Exp Med 124, 241–253, 1966

Volkman, A. Disparity in origin of mononuclear phagocyte populations. J Reticuloendothel Soc 19, 249–268, 1976

Von Ardenne, M. Theoretische und experimentelle Grundlagen der Krebs-Mehrschritt—Therapie (ed 2). Berlin: VEB Verlag Volk Gesundheit, 1971

von Leyden, E., and Blumenthal, F. Vorläufige Mitteilungen über einige Ergebnisse der Krebs-

forschung auf der I. Medizinischen Klinik. Dtsch Med Wochenschr 28, 637–638, 1902

Vose, B. M., Vanky, F., Argov, S., and Klein, E. Natural cytotoxicity in man: Activity of lymph node and tumor-infiltrating lymphocytes. Eur J Immunol 7, 753–757, 1977a

Vose, B. M., Vanky, F., and Klein, E. Lymphocyte cytotoxicity against autologous tumor biopsy cells in humans. Int J Cancer 20, 512–519, 1977b

Vose, B. M., Vanky, F., and Klein, E. Human tumor-lymphocyte interaction in vitro. V. Comparison of the reactivity of tumor-infiltrating blood and lymph-node lymphocytes with autologous tumor cells. Int J Cancer 20, 895–902, 1977c

Vredevoe, D. L., and Hays, E. F. Increased incidence of lymphoma in C3H/HeJ adult mice injected with Gross virus and antithymocytic serum. Infect Immun 2, 723–726, 1970

Vulchanov, V. H. On the antigenic reduction (loss of antigens) in human myeloid leukemia. Z Immun Allergieforsch 127, 436–444, 1964

W

Wade, H. An experimental investigation of infective sarcoma of the dog, with a consideration of its relationship to cancer. J Pathol Bacteriol 12, 384–425, 1908

Wagner, H., and Rollinghoff, M. In vitro induction of tumor specific immunity. I. Parameters of activation and cytotoxic reactivity of mouse lymphoid cells immunized in vitro against syngeneic and allogeneic plasma cell tumors. J Exp Med 138, 1–15, 1973

Wagner, H., and Rollinghoff, M. T cell-mediated cytotoxicity: Discrimination between antigen recognition, lethal hit and cytolysis phase. Eur J Immunol , 745–750, 1974

Wagner, J. L., and Haughton, G. Immunosuppression by antilymphocyte serum and its effect on tumors induced by 3-methylcholanthrene in mice. J Natl Cancer Inst 46, 1–10, 1971

Wagner, R. K., Gorlich, L., and Jungblut, P. W. Dehydrotestosterone receptor in human mammary cancer. Acta Endocrinol Suppl (Kbh) 173, 65, 1973

Wahl, D. V., Chapman, W. H., Hellström, I., and Hellström, K. E. Transplantation immunity to individually unique antigens of chemically induced bladder tumors in mice. Int J Cancer 14, 114–121, 1974

Wahl, S. M., and Rosenstreich, D. L. Role of B

lymphocytes in cell-mediated immunity I. Requirement for T cells or T-cell products for antigen-induced B-cell activation. J Exp Med 144, 1175–1187, 1976

Wahren, B. Cytotoxic assays and other immunologic studies of leukemias induced by Friend virus. J Natl Cancer Inst 31, 411–423, 1963

Wahren, B. Immunotherapy in Friend virus leukemia. II. Prevention of Friend leukemia by passive administration of immune serum and cells to young mice. J Natl Cancer Inst 41, 931–938, 1968

Wainberg, M. A., Deutsch, V., and Weiss, D. W. Stimulation of anti-tumour immunity in guinea-pigs by methanol extraction residue of BCG. Br J Cancer 34, 500–508, 1976

Wainberg, M. A., Margolese, R. G., and Weiss, D. W. Differential responsiveness of various substrains of inbred strain 2 guinea pigs to immunotherapy with the methanol extraction residue (MER) of BCG. Cancer Immunol Immunother 2, 101–108, 1977

Walford, R. L. Increased incidence of lymphoma after injections of mice with cells differing at weak histocompatibility loci. Science 152, 78–80, 1966

Walker, I. R., Strickland, R. G., Ungar, B., and Mackay, I. R. Simple atrophic gastritis and gastric carcinoma. Gut 12, 906–911, 1971

Walker, W. S. Functional heterogeneity of macrophages: Subclasses of peritoneal macrophages with different antigen-binding activities and immune complex receptors. Immunology, 26, 1025–1037, 1974

Wallace, A. C., and Hollenberg, N. K. The transplantability of tumours by intravenous and intralymphatic routes. Br J Cancer 19, 338–342, 1965

Wallis, V., Davies, A. J. S., and Koller, P. C. Inhibition of radiation-induced leukaemia by the injection of haematopoietic tissue; A study of chimaerism. Nature 210, 500–504, 1966

Wang, B. S., Onikul, S. R., and Mannick, J. A. Prevention of death from metastases by immune RNA therapy. Science 202, 59–60, 1978

Warnatz, H., and Scheiffarth, F. Cell-mediated immune response of in vitro sensitised lymphocytes to isogeneic methylcholanthrene-induced tumor cell lines. Transplantation 18, 273–279, 1974

Warner, N. L., Woodruff, M. F. A., and Burton, R. C. Inhibition of the growth of lymphoid tumours in syngeneic athymic (nude) mice. Int J Cancer 20, 146–155, 1977

Warner, T. F. C. S. Cell hybridisation in the genesis of ectopic hormone-secreting tumours. Lancet 1, 1259–1260, 1974

Warr, G. W., and James, K. Effect of C. parvum on the class and subclass of antibody produced in the response of different strains of mice to sheep erythrocytes. Immunology 28, 431–442, 1975

Warr, G. W., and Šljivić, V. S. Enhancement and depression of the antibody response in mice caused by Corynebacterium parvum. Clin Exp Immunol 17, 519–532, 1974

Warr, G. W., Willmott, N., and James, K. Effect of transplanted syngeneic myelomas on the antibody response of mice. Eur J Cancer 11, 351–357, 1975

Warren, B. A., and Shubik, P. The ultrastructure of capillary sprouts induced by melanoma transplants in the golden hamster. J R Microsc Soc 86, 177–187, 1966

Warren, S. The relation of "chronic mastitis" to carcinoma of the breast. Surg Gynecol Obstet 71, 257–273, 1940

Warren, S., and Gates, O. The fate of intravenously injected tumor cells. Am J Cancer 27, 485–492, 1936

Warren, S. L. Preliminary study of effect of artificial fever upon hopeless tumor cases. Am J Roentgenol 33, 75–87, 1935

Watkins, J. F., and Chen, L. Immunization of mice against Ehrlich ascites tumour using a hamster/Ehrlich tumour hybrid cell line. Nature 223, 1018–1022, 1969

Watne, A. C., Sandberg, A. A., and Moore, G. E. Prognostic implications of tumor cells in the blood. Proc Am Assoc Cancer Res 3, 160, 1960

Watson, R. D., Smith, A. G., and Levy, J. G. The use of immunoadsorbent columns for the isolation of antibodies specific for antigens associated with human bronchogenic carcinoma. Br J Cancer 29, 183–188, 1974

Watson, R. D., Smith, A. G., and Levy, J. G. The detection by immuno-diffusion of tumour associated antigenic components in extracts of human bronchogenic carcinoma. Br J Cancer 32, 300–309, 1975

Watson, S. R., and Šljivić, V. S. The role of macrophages in the adjuvant effect on antibody production of Corynebacterium parvum. Clin Exp Immunol 23, 149–153, 1976

Wattenberg, L. W. The role of the portal of entry in inhibition of tumorigenesis. Prog Exp Tumor Res 14, 89–104, 1971

Wattenberg, L. W., and Leong, J. L. Effects of phenothiazines on protective systems against polycyclic hydrocarbons. Cancer Res 25, 365–370, 1965

Webb, H. E., and Gordon Smith, C. E. Viruses in the treatment of cancer. Lancet 1, 1206–1209, 1970

Webb, H. E., Oaten, S. W., and Pike, C. P. Treatment of malignant ascitic and pleural effusions with Corynebacterium parvum. Br Med J *1*, 338–340, 1978

Webb, H. E., Wetherley-Mein, G., Gordon Smith, C. E., and McMahon, D. Leukaemia and neoplastic processes treated with Langat and Kyasanur Forest disease viruses: A clinical and laboratory study of 28 patients. Br Med J *1*, 258, 1966

Weber, F. P., Schwartz, E., and Hellenschmiel, R. Spontaneous inoculation of melanotic sarcoma from mother to foetus; Report of a case. Br Med J *1*, 537–539, 1930

Webster, D. J. T., Chare, M. J. B., and Baum, M. The effect of intravenous infusion of Corynebacterium parvum on an immune profile of women with breast cancer. Dev Biol Stand *38*, 467–470, 1978

Wedderburn, N. Effect of concurrent malarial infection on development of virus-induced lymphoma in Balb/c mice. Lancet *2*, 1114–1116, 1970

Weigle, W. O. Studies on the termination of acquired tolerance to serum protein antigens following injection of serologically related antigens. Immunology *7*, 239–247, 1964

Weigle, W. O. The immune response of rabbits tolerant to one protein conjugate following the injection of related protein conjugates. J Immunol *94*, 177–183, 1965

Weigle, W. O., Siekmann, D. G., Doyle, M. V., and Chiller, J. M. Possible roles of suppressor T cells in immunological tolerance. Transplant Rev *26*, 186–205, 1975

Weiler, E. Loss of specific cell antigen in relation to carcinogenesis, pp 165–167, In Wolstenholme, G. E., and O'Connor, M. (Eds): CIBA Fdn Symp—Carcinogenesis: Mechanisms of Action. London: Churchill, 1959

Weiner, R. S., Hubbard, J. D., and Mardiney, M. R. Production of tumor-specific antibody in the xenogeneic host: Use of blocking antibody. J Natl Cancer Inst *49*, 1063–1070, 1972

Weinhouse, S. Glycolysis, respiration, and anomalous gene expression in experimental hepatomas: G. H. A. Clowes Memorial Lecture. Cancer Res *32*, 2007–2016, 1972

Weiss, D. W. Nonspecific stimulation and modulation of the immune response and of states of resistance by the methanol-extraction residue fraction of tubercle bacilli. Natl Cancer Inst Monogr *35*, 157–171, 1972

Weiss, D. W. The questionable immunogenicity of certain neoplasms: What then the prospects for immunological intervention in malignant disease? Cancer Immunol Immunother *2*, 11–19, 1977

Weiss, D. W., Bonhag, R. S., and DeOme, K. B. Protective action of fractions of tubercle bacilli against isologous tumours in mice. Nature *190*, 889–891, 1961

Weiss, D. W., Bonhag, R. S., and Leslie, P. Studies on the heterologous immunogenicity of a methanol-insoluble fraction of attenuated tubercle bacilli (BCG). II. Protection against tumor isografts. J Exp Med *124*, 1039–1065, 1966

Weiss, D. W., Faulkin, L. J., and DeOme, K. B. Acquired resistance to spontaneous mammary carcinomas in autochthonous and isologous mice. Proc Am Assoc Cancer Res *4*, 71, 1963

Weiss, D. W., Faulkin, L. J., and DeOme, K. B. Acquisition of heightened resistance and susceptibility to spontaneous mouse mammary carcinomas in the original host. Cancer Res *24*, 732–741, 1964

Weiss, D. W., Stupp, Y., Many, N., and Izak, G. Treatment of acute myelocytic leukemia (AML) patients with the MER tubercle bacillus fraction: A preliminary report. Transplant Proc *7*, 545–552, 1975

Weiss, L. Neuraminidase, sialic acids, and cell interactions. J Natl Cancer Inst *50*, 3–19, 1973

Welin, S., Youker, J., and Spratt, J. S. The rates and patterns of growth of 375 tumors of the large intestine and rectum observed serially by double contrast. Am J Roentgenol *90*, 673–687, 1963

Wellings, S. R., Jensen, H. M., and Marcum, R. G. An atlas of subgross pathology of the human breast with special reference to possible precancerous lesions. J Natl Cancer Inst *55*, 231–273, 1975

Wells, S. A., Burdick, J. F., Christiansen, C., Ketcham, A. S., and Adkins, P. C. The demonstration of tumor associated delayed cutaneous hypersensitivity reactions in lung cancer patients and in patients with carcinoma of the cervix. Natl Cancer Inst Monogr *37*, 197–203, 1973a

Wells, S. A., Burdick, J. F., Joseph, W. L., Christiansen, C. L., Wolfe, W. G., and Adkins, P. C. Delayed cutaneous hypersensitivity reactions to tumor antigens and to non-specific antigens: Prognostic significance in patients with lung cancer. J Thorac Cardiovasc Surg *66*, 557–562, 1973b

Werner, G. H., Maral, R., Floch, F., Migliore-Samour, D., and Jolles, P. Adjuvant and immunostimulating activities of water-soluble substances extracted from Mycobacterium tuberculosis (var. hominis). Biomedicine *22*, 440–452, 1975

West, W. H., Cannon, G. B., Kay, H. D., Bonnard, G. D., and Herberman, R. B. Natural cytotoxic reactivity of human lymphocytes against a myeloid cell line: Characterization of effector cells. J Immunol *118*, 355–361, 1977

Westbury, G. Strategy in the management of melanoma. Proc R Soc Med *70*, 395–397, 1977

Westbury, G., Humble, J. G., Newton, K. A., Skinner, H. E. G., and Pegg, D. E. Disseminated malignant melanoma. Response to treatment by massive dosage of a cytotoxic agent combined with autogenous marrow replacement. Lancet *1*, 968–969, 1959

Westermark, N. The effect of heat upon rat tumours. Scand Arch Physiol *52*, 257–322, 1927

Whang-Peng, J., Canellos, G. P., Carbone, P. P., and Tjio, J. H. Clinical implications of cytogenetic variants in chronic myelocytic leukemia (CML). Blood *32*, 755–766, 1968

Wheatley, D. N., and Easty, G. C. The growth and infiltration of Ehrlich's ascites tumour in mice with reduced immunological responses. Br J Cancer *18*, 743–755, 1964

Whisnant, J. K. C. parvum clinical protocols: Prototypes and summary results in U.S. trials with Wellcome Coparvax. Dev Biol Stand *38*, 559–566, 1978

White, H., and Griffiths, J. D. Circulating malignant cells and fibrinolysis during resection of colorectal cancer. Proc R Soc Med *69*, 467–469, 1976

White, W. F. A biomathematical approach to the treatment of osteogenic sarcoma. Br J Surg *53*, 151, 1966

Whitehead, R. H., Thatcher, J., Teasdale, C., Roberts, G. P., and Hughes, L. E. T and B lymphocytes in breast cancer. Stage relationship and abrogation of T-lymphocyte depression by enzyme treatment in vitro. Lancet *1*, 330–333, 1976

Whitehouse, J. M. A. Circulating antibodies in human malignant disease. Br J Cancer *28* (Suppl), 170–174, 1973

Whitehouse, J. M. A., and Holborow, E. J. Smooth muscle antibody in malignant disease. Br Med J *4*, 511–513, 1971

Whitelaw, A. G. L., and Cohen, S. L. Ectopic production of calcitonin. Lancet *2*, 442, 1973

Whitney, R. B., Levy, J. G., and Smith, A. G. Influence of tumor size and surgical resection on cell-mediated immunity in mice. J Natl Cancer Inst *53*, 111–116, 1974

Whittaker, J. A., Bentley, P., Melville-Jones, G. R., and Slater, A. J. Granuloma formation in patients receiving BCG immunotherapy. J Clin Pathol *29*, 693–697, 1976

Whittaker, J. A., Lilleyman, J. S., Jacobs, A., and Balfour, I. Immunotherapy with intravenous BCG. Lancet *2*, 1454, 1973

Whittaker, J. A., and Slater, A. J. Immunotherapy of acute myelogenous leukemia using intravenous BCG, pp 393–404, In Terry, W. D., and Windhorst, D. (Eds): Immunotherapy of Cancer: Present Status of Trials in Man. New York: Raven Press, 1978

Whittaker, M. G., Rees, K., and Clark, C. G. Reduced lymphocyte transformation in breast cancer. Lancet *1*, 892–893, 1971

Wiener, E. The role of macrophages in the amplified in vitro response to sheep red blood cells by spleen cells from Corynebacterium parvum treated mice. Cell Immunol *19*, 1–7, 1975

Wiener, E., and Bandieri, A. Modifications in the handling in vitro of ^{125}I-labelled keyhole limpet haemocyanin by peritoneal macrophages from mice pretreated with the adjuvant. Immunology *29*, 265–274, 1975

Wiener, F., Fenyö, E. M., Klein, G., and Harris, H. Fusion of tumour cells with host cells. Nature New Biol *238*, 155–159, 1972

Wiener, F., Klein, G., and Harris, H. The analysis of malignancy by cell fusion. IV. Hybrid between tumor cells and a malignant L cell derivative. J Cell Sci *12*, 253–261, 1973

Wiener, F., Klein, G., and Harris, H. The analysis of malignancy by cell fusion V. Further evidence of the ability of normal diploid cells to suppress malignancy. J Cell Sci *15*, 177–183, 1974a

Wiener, F., Klein, G., and Harris, H. The analysis of malignancy by cell fusion. VI. Hybrids between different tumor cells. J Cell Sci *16*, 189–198, 1974b

Wigzell, H. Immunological depression of tumor growth in F1 hybrid/parental strain systems. Cancer Res *21*, 365–370, 1961

Wilkinson, P. C., O'Neill, G. J., McInroy, R. J., Cater, J. C., and Roberts, J. A. Chemotaxis of macrophages: The role of a macrophage-specific cytotaxin from anaerobic corynebacterium and its relation to immunopotentiation in vivo, pp 121–140, In Wolstenholme, G. E. W., and Knight, J. (Eds): Ciba Fdn Symp—Immunopotentiation. New Series 18. Amsterdam: ASP 1973a

Wilkinson, P. C., O'Neill, G. J., and Wapshaw, K. G. Role of anaerobic Coryneforms in specific and non-specific immunological reactions. II. Production of a chemotactic factor specific for macrophages. Immunology *24*, 997–1006, 1973b

Williams, D. E., Evans, D. M. D., and Blamey, R. W. The primary implantation of human tumours to the hamster cheek pouch. Br J Cancer *25*, 533–537, 1971

Williams, E. D. Tumours, hormones and cellular differentiation. Lancet 2, 1108–1109, 1969

Williams, E. D., Morales, A. M., and Horn, R. C. Thyroid carcinoma and Cushing's syndrome. J Clin Pathol 21, 129–135, 1968

Williams, R. C. Dermatomyositis and malignancy: A review of the literature. Ann Intern Med 50, 1174–1181, 1959

Williams, R. R., McIntire, K. R., Waldmann, T. A., Feinleib, M., Go, V. L. W., Kannel, W. B., Dawber, T. R., Castelli, W. P., and McNamara, P. N. Tumor-associated antigen levels (carcinoembryonic antigen, human chorionicgonadotropin, and alpha-fetoprotein) antedating the diagnosis of cancer in the Framingham Study. J Natl Cancer Inst 58, 1547–1551, 1977

Williams. W. H., and Krueger, R. G. Tumor-associated transplantation antigens of myelomas induced in Balb/c mice. J Natl Cancer Inst 49, 1613–1620, 1972

Willis, R. A. The spread of Tumours in the Human Body. London: Butterworth, 1952

Willis, R. A. Pathology of Tumours (ed 3). London: Butterworth, 1960

Willmer, E. N. (Ed): Cells and Tissues in Culture. Methods, Biology and Physiology. London, New York: Academic Press, 1965

Willoughby, D. A., and Wood, C. (Eds): The history and development of levamisole. R Soc Med Forum Immunother 1, 1–11, 1977

Wilson, R. H., Byers, E. H., Finney, W., Schrom, A., and Mallams, J. Studies in tumor autoimmunity. Clinical evaluation of induced host resistance to cancer. Acta Un Int Cancer 19, 84–88, 1963

Winchurch, R., and Braun, W. Antibody formation: Premature initiation by endotoxin or synthetic polynucleotides in newborn mice. Nature 223, 843–844, 1969

Winn, H. J. Immune mechanisms in homotransplantation. I. The role of serum antibody and complement in the neutralisation of lymphoma cells. J Immunol 84, 530–538, 1960a

Winn, H. J. The immune response and the homograft reaction. Natl Cancer Inst Monogr 2, 113–138, 1960b

Winn. H. J. Immune mechanisms in homotransplantation. II. Quantitative assay of the immunologic activity of lymphoid cells stimulated by tumor homografts. J Immunol 86, 228–239, 1961

Winn, H. J. The participation of complement in isoimmune reactions. Ann NY Acad Sci, 101, 23–44, 1962

Wintrobe, M. M., Lee, G. R., Boggs, D. R., Bithell,

T. C., Athens, J. W., and Forrester, J. Clinical Haematology (ed 7). Philadelphia: Lee & Febiger, 1974

Wise, L., Mason, A. Y., and Ackerman, L. V. Local excision and irradiation: An alternative method for the treatment of early mammary cancer. Ann Surg 174, 392–401, 1971

Wissler, R. W., Craft, K., Kesden, D., Polisky, B., and Dzoga, K. Inhibition of the growth of the Morris hepatoma (5123) in Buffalo rats using a mixture of pertussis vaccine and irradiated tumor, In Dausset, J., Hamburger, J., and Mathé, G. (Eds): Advances in Transplantation. Copenhagen: Munksgaard, 1968

Witebsky, E., Rose, N. R., and Shulman, S. Studies of normal and malignant tissue antigens. Cancer Res 16, 831–841, 1956

Witz, I. P. The biological significance of tumorbound immunoglobulins. Curr Topics Microbiol Immunol 61, 161–171, 1973

Witz, I. P. Tumor-bound immunoglobulin: In situ expressions of humoral immunity. Adv Cancer Res 25, 95–148, 1977

Witz, I., Klein, G., and Pressman, D. Moloney lymphoma antibodies from mice: Localization in spleens of Moloney lymphoma bearing mice. Proc Soc Exp Biol Med 130, 1102–1105, 1969

Witz, I., Yagi, Y., and Pressman, D. A normal component in rabbit IgG with affinity for mouse tissues. Immunology 15, 765–772, 1968a

Witz, I., Yagi, Y., and Pressman, D. Immunosuppressive activity of rabbit antisera directed against mouse lymphocytic leukemia L1210. Proc Soc Exp Biol Med 127, 562–565, 1968b

Woglom, W. H. Immunity to transplantable tumours. Cancer Rev 4, 129–214, 1929

Wolberg, W. H. Inhibition of migration of human autogenous and allogeneic leukocytes by extracts of patients' cancers. Cancer Res 31, 798–802, 1971

Wolf, A., Barfoot, R. K., and Johnson, R. A. Xenogeneic recognition of tumour specific plasma membrane antigens derived from mouse lymphoma cells. Immunology 22, 485–491, 1972

Wolfe, S. A., Tracey, D. E., and Henny, C. S. Induction of 'natural killer' cells by BCG. Nature 262, 584–586, 1976

Wolmark, N., and Fisher, B. The effect of a single and repeated administration of Corynebacterium parvum on bone marrow macrophage colony production in syngeneic tumor-bearing mice. Cancer Res 34, 2869–2872, 1974

Wolmark, N., Levine, M., and Fisher, B. The effect of a single and repeated administration of Corynebacterium parvum on bone marrow macrophage colony production in normal mice. J Reticuloendothel Soc *16*, 252–257, 1974

Wong-Staal, F., Gillespie, D., and Gallo, R. C. Proviral sequences of baboon endogenous type C RNA virus in DNA of human leukaemic tissues. Nature *262*, 190–195, 1976

Wood, A. W., Levin, W., Lu, A. Y. H., Yagi, H., Hernandez, O., Jerina, D. M., and Conney, A. H. Metabolism of benzo(a)pyrene and benzo(a)pyrene derivatives to metagenic products by highly purified hepatic microsomal enzymes. J Biol Chem *251*, 4882–4890, 1976

Wood, C. B., Gillis, C. R., and Blumgart, C. H. Use of historic controls in cancer studies. Lancet *2*, 251–252, 1976

Wood, G. W., and Gillespie, G. Y. Studies on the role of macrophages in regulation of growth and metastasis of murine chemically-induced fibrosarcomas. Int J Cancer *16*, 1022–1029, 1975

Wood, S. Pathogenesis of metastasis formation observed in vivo in the rabbit ear chamber. Arch Pathol *66*, 550–568, 1958

Wood, S., Holyoke, E. D., and Yardley, J. H. Mechanisms of metastasis production by bloodborne cancer cells, pp 167–223, In Proc 4th Can Cancer Conf. New York: Academic Press, 1961

Wood, W. C., and Morton, D. L. Microcytotoxicity tests: Detection of antibody in sarcoma patients cytotoxic to human sarcoma cells. Science *170*, 1318–1320, 1970

Wood, W. C., and Morton, D. L. Host immune response to a common cell-surface antigen in human sarcomas. Detection by cytotoxicity tests. N Engl J Med *284*, 569–572, 1971

Woodhall, B., Pickrill, K. L., Georgiade, N. G., Mahaley, M. S., and Dukes, H. T. Effect of hyperthermia upon cancer chemotherapy—Application to external cancer of head and face structures. Ann Surg *151*, 750–759, 1960

Woodruff, J. J., and Gesner, B. M. The effect of neuraminidase on the fate of transfused lymphocytes. J Exp Med *129*, 551–567, 1969

Woodruff, M. F. A. Evidence of adaptation in homografts of normal tissue, In Biological Problems of Grafting. Les Congrès et Colloques de L'Université de Liège *12*, 83–90, 1959

Woodruff, M. F. A. The Transplantation of Tissues and Organs. Springfield: C. C. Thomas, 1960

Woodruff, M. F. A. New approaches to the treatment of cancer. J R Coll Surg Edinb *6*, 75–92, 1961

Woodruff, M. F. A. Medical ethics and controlled trials. Br Med J *1*, 1339, 1963

Woodruff, M. F. A. Immunological aspects of cancer. Lancet *2*, 265–270, 1964

Woodruff, M. F. A. The One and the Many (London: R Soc Med). [*Reprinted in On Science and Surgery. Edinburgh University Press*] 1970

Woodruff, M. F. A. Residual cancer. Harvey Lect Series *66*, 161–176, 1972

Woodruff, M. F. A. Latent tumour metastases. Nature *258*, 776, 1975

Woodruff, M. F. A. Clinical research in oncology. Clin Oncol *2*, 289–291, 1976

Woodruff, M. F. A. Prospects for immunotherapy. Dev Biol Stand *38*, 573–580, 1977a

Woodruff, M. F. A. Prospects for immunotherapy of solid tumours. Prog Immunol *3*, 570–591, 1977b

Woodruff, M. F. A. Current state of clinical immunotherapy. Transplant Proc *11*, 1077–1081, 1979

Woodruff, M. F. A., and Boak, J. L. Inhibitory effect of pre-immunized CBA spleen cells on transplants of A-strain mouse mammary carcinoma in (CBA×A)F1 hybrid recipients. Br J Cancer *19*, 411–417, 1965

Woodruff, M. F. A., and Boak, J. L. Inhibitory effect of injection of Corynebacterium parvum on the growth of tumour transplants in isogeneic hosts. Br Cancer *20*, 345–355, 1966

Woodruff, M. F. A., Clunie, G. J. A., McBride, W. H., McCormack, R. J. M., Walbaum, P.R., and James, K. The effect of intravenous and intramuscular injection of Corynebacterium parvum. Allergie Immunol *6*, 201–202 1974a

Woodruff, M. F. A., Clunie, G. J. A., McBride, W. H., McCormack, R. J. M., Walbaum, P. R., and James, K. The effect of intravenous and intramuscular injection of Corynebacterium parvum, pp 383–388, In Halpern, B. (Ed): Corynebacterium Parvum: Applications in Experimental and Clinical Oncology. New York: Plenum Press, 1975

Woodruff, M. F. A., and Dunbar, N. The effect of Corynebacterium parvum and other reticuloendothelial stimulants on transplanted tumors in mice, pp 287–303, In Wolstenholme, G. E., and Knight, J. (Eds): Ciba Fdn Symp—Immunopotentiation. New Series 18. Amsterdam: ASP, 1973

Woodruff, M. F. A., and Dunbar, N. Effect of local injection of C. parvum on the growth of a murine fibrosarcoma. Br J. Cancer *32*, 34–41, 1975

Woodruff, M. F. A., Dunbar, N., and Ghaffar, A. The growth of tumours in T-cell deprived mice and their response to treatment with Corynebacterium parvum. Proc R Soc Lond B *184,* 97–102, 1973

Woodruff, M. F. A., Ghaffar, A., Dunbar, N., and Whitehead, V. L. Effect of C. parvum on immunization with irradiated tumour cells. Br J Cancer *33,* 491–495, 1976a

Woodruff, M. F. A., Ghaffar, A., and Whitehead, V. Modification of the effect of C. parvum on macrophage activity and tumour growth by x-irradiation. Int J Cancer *17,* 652–658, 1976b

Woodruff, M. F. A., Hitchcock, E., and Whitehead, V. L. Effect of C. parvum and active specific immunotherapy on intracerebral transplants of a murine fibrosarcoma. Br J Cancer *35,* 687–692, 1977

Woodruff, M. F. A., and Inchley, M. P. Cytolytic efficiency of rabbit-anti-mouse antilymphocytic globulin and its augmentation by antiglobulin. Clin Exp Immunol *9,* 839–851, 1971a

Woodruff, M. F. A., and Inchley, M. P. Synergistic inhibition of mammary carcinoma transplants in A-strain mice by antitumour globulin and C. parvum. Br J Cancer *25,* 584–593, 1971b

Woodruff, M. F. A., Inchley, M. P., and Dunbar, N. Further observations on the effect of C. parvum and anti-tumour globulin on syngeneically transplanted mouse tumours. Br J Cancer *26,* 67–76, 1972

Woodruff, M. F. A., McBride, W. H., and Dunbar, N. Tumour growth, phagocytic activity and antibody response in Corynebacterium parvum-treated mice. Clin Exp Immunol *17,* 509–518, 1974b

Woodruff, M. F. A., McCormack, R. J. M., and Walbaum, P. R. Unpublished, 1978a

Woodruff, M. F. A., and Nolan, B. Intravenous replacement of human splenic tissue. Lancet *2,* 689–690, 1961

Woodruff, M. F. A., and Nolan, B. Preliminary observations on treatment of advanced cancer by injection of allogeneic spleen cells. Lancet *2,* 426–429, 1963

Woodruff, M. F. A., Nolan, B., Anderton, J. L., Abouna, G. M., Morton, J. B., and Jenkins, A. McL. Long term survival after renal transplantation in man. Br J Surg *63,* 85–101, 1976c

Woodruff, M. F. A., Nolan, B., Robson, J. S., and MacDonald, M. K. Renal transplantation in man. Experience in 35 cases. Lancet *1,* 6–12, 1969

Woodruff, M. F. A., and Smith, L. H. Cytotoxic efficiency and effect on tumour growth of heterospecific antilymphocytic and antitumour sera. Nature *225,* 377–379, 1970

Woodruff, M. F. A., and Smith, L. H. Cytotoxic

efficiency and effect on tumour growth of heterospecific antilymphocytic and antitumour sera. In Le Sérum Antilymphocytaire. Colloques Int CNRS No. 190, 419–434, 1971

Woodruff, M. F. A., and Sparrow, M. Further observations on the induction of tolerance of skin homografts in rats. Transplant Bull *4,* 157–159, 1957

Woodruff, M. F. A., and Speedy, G. Inhibition of chemical carcinogenesis by C. parvum. Proc R Soc Lond B *201,* 209–215, 1978

Woodruff, M. F. A., and Symes, M. O. The significance of splenomegaly in tumour-bearing mice. Br J Cancer *16,* 120–130, 1962a

Woodruff, M. F. A., Symes, M. O., and Anderson, N. F. The effect of intraperitoneal injection of thoracic duct lymphocytes from normal and immunized rats in mice inoculated with the Landschutz ascites tumour. Br J Cancer *17,* 482–486, 1963a

Woodruff, M. F. A., and Symes, M. O. Evidence of loss of tumour-specific antigen on repeatedly transplanting a tumour in the strain of origin. Br J Cancer *16,* 484–488, 1962b

Woodruff, M. F. A., and Symes, M. O. The use of immunologically competent cells in the treatment of cancer: Experiments with a transplantable mouse tumour. Br J Cancer *16,* 707–715, 1962c

Woodruff, M. F. A., Symes, M. O., and Stuart, A. E. The effect of rat spleen cells on two transplanted mouse tumours. Br J Cancer *17,* 320–326, 1963b

Woodruff, M. F. A., and Warner, N. L. Effect of Corynebacterium parvum on tumor growth in normal and athymic (nude) mice. J Natl Cancer Inst *58,* 111–116, 1977

Woodruff, M., and Whitehead, V. L. Mechanism of inhibition of immunization with irradiated tumour cells by a large dose of Corynebacterium parvum. Proc R Soc Lond B *197,* 505–514, 1977

Woodruff, M. F. A., Whitehead, V. L., and Speedy, G. Studies with a spontaneous mouse tumour. I. Growth in normal mice and response to Corynebacterium parvum. Br J Cancer *37,* 345–355, 1978b

Woods, D. A. Influence of antilymphocyte serum on DMBA induction of oral carcinomas. Nature *224,* 276–277, 1969

World Health Organization. Immunotherapy of Cancer. Technical Rep Series 344. Geneva: WHO, 1966

World Health Organization. Immunodeficiency, pp 31–32. Technical Rep Series: 630. Geneva WHO, 1978

World Medical Association. International Code of Medical Ethics. Helsinki Declaration. Geneva, 1964

World Medical Association. Revised Helsinki Declaration. Geneva, 1975

Wrathmell, A. B. The growth patterns of two transplantable acute leukaemias of spontaneous origin in rats. Br J Cancer *33,* 172–180, 1976

Wrathmell, A. B., and Alexander, P. Immunogenicity of a rat leukaemia of spontaneous origin (SAL). Br J Cancer *33,* 181–186, 1976

Wright, P. W., Hellström, K. E., Hellström, I. E., and Bernstein, I. D. Serotherapy of malignant disease. Med Clin North Am *60,* 607–622, 1976

Wright, P.W., Hellström, K.E., Hellström, I.E., Warner, G., Prentice, R., and Jones, R.F., Serotherapy of malignant melanoma, pp 135–143, In Terry, W.D., and Windhorst, D. (Eds): Immunotherapy of Cancer: Present Status of Trials in Man. New York: Raven Press, 1978

Wybran, J., and Fudenberg, H. H. Thymus-derived rosette-forming cells in various human disease states: Cancer, lymphoma, bacterial and viral infections, and other diseases. J Clin Invest *52,* 1026–1032, 1973

Wybran, J., Spitler, L. E., Lieberman, R., and Fudenberg, H. H., "Active" T-cell rosettes and total T-rosettes in patients with melanoma following intratumoral inoculation of BCG: A clue to the mechanism of action of bacillus Calmette-Guérin? Cancer Immunol Immunother *1,* 153–156, 1976

Y

Yamagiwa, K., and Ichikawa, K. Experimentelle Studie uber die Pathogenese der Epithelialgeschwulste. Mitt Med Fak Tokio *15* 295–344, 1915

Yamagiwa, K., and Ichikawa, K. Experimental study of the pathogenesis of carcinoma. J Cancer Res *3,* 1–29, 1918

Yamamura, Y. Immunotherapy of Lung Cancer with oil-attached cell wall skeleton of BCG, pp 173–179, In Terry, W. D., and Windhorst, D. (Eds); Immunotherapy of Cancer: Present Status of Trials in Man. New York: Raven Press, 1978

Yamamura, Y., Azuma, I., Taniyama, T., Sugimura, K., Hirao, F., Tokuzen, R., Okabe, M.,

Nakahara, W., Yasumoto, K., and Ohta, M. Immunotherapy of cancer with cell wall skeleton of Mycobacterium bovis—bacillus Calmette-Guérin: Experimental and clinical results. Ann NY Acad Sci, *277,* 209–226, 1976a

Yamamura, Y., Ogura, T., Yoshimoto, T., Nishikawa, H., Sakatani, M., Itom, M., Masuno, T., Namba, M., Yazaki, H., Hirao, F., and Azuma, I. Successful treatment of the patients with malignant pleural effusion with BCG cell-wall skeleton. Gann *67,* 669–677, 1976h

Yamashita, U., and Kitagawa, M. Enhancing activity of synthetic polynucleotides on the induction of anti-hapten antibody response. Immunology *26,* 925–936, 1974

Yang, W. K. Isoaccepting transfer RNA's in mammalian differentiated cells and tumor tissues. Cancer Res *31,* 639–643, 1971

Yarkoni, E., and Bekierkunst, A. Nonspecific resistance against infection with Salmonella typhi and Salmonella typhimurium induced in mice by cord factor (trehalose-6,6'-dimycolate) and its analogues. Infect Immun *14,* 1125–1129, 1976

Yarkoni, E., Rapp, H. J., and Zbar, B. Immunotherapy of a guinea pig hepatoma with ultrasonically prepared mycobacterial vaccines. Cancer Immunol Immunother *2,* 143–146, 1977a

Yarkoni, E., Wang, L., and Bekierkunst, A. Stimulation of macrophages by cord factor and by heat-killed and living BCG. Infect Immun *16,* 1–8, 1977b

Yarkoni, E., Zbar, B., and Rapp, H. J. Host resistance to tumor growth in guinea pigs immunized with lyophilized tumor cells. Cancer Immunol Immunother *2,* 201–204, 1977c

Yashphe, D. J. Modulation of the immune response by a methanol insoluble fraction of attenuated tubercle bacilli (BCG). Clin Exp Immunol *12,* 497–506, 1972

Yashphe, D. J., and Weiss, D. W. Modulation of the immune response by a methanol insoluble fraction of attenuated tubercle bacilli. Primary and secondary responses to sheep red blood cells and T2 phage. Clin Exp Immunol *7,* 269–281, 1970

Yasumoto, K., Manabe, H., Veno, M., Ohta, M., Ueda, H., Iida, A., Nomoto, K., Azuma, I., and Yamamura, Y. Immunotherapy of human lung cancer with BCG cell-wall skeleton. Gann *67,* 787–795, 1976

Yefenof, E., and Klein, G. Antibody induced redistribution of normal and tumor associated surface antigens. Exp Cell Res *88,* 217–244, 1974

Yonemoto, R. H., Fujisawa, T., and Waldman, S. R. Selection of donors for transfer-factor immunotherapy. Proc Am Assoc Cancer Res *17*, 150, 1976

Yonemoto, R. H., and Terasaki, P. I. Cancer immunotherapy with HLA-compatible thoracic duct lymphocyte transplantation. Cancer *30*, 1438–1443, 1972

Yorkshire Breast Cancer Group. Observer variation in recording clinical data from women presenting with breast lesions. Br Med J *2*, 1196–1199, 1977

Yoshida, T. O., and Southam, C. M. Cell-associated immune reaction against autochthonous tumors in mice. Proc Am Assoc Cancer Res *4*, 74, 1963

Yoshikawa, S., Yamada, K., and Yoshida, T. O. Serum complement level in patients with leukemia. Int J Cancer *4*, 845–851, 1969

Youdim, S., and Sharman, M. Resistance to tumor growth mediated by Listeria monocytogenes: Collaborative and suppressive macrophage–lymphocyte interactions in vitro. J Immunol *117*, 1860–1865, 1976

Young, C. W. Interferon induction in cancer. Med Clin North Am *55*, 721–728, 1971

Young, L. S., Meyer, R. D., and Armstrong, D. Pseudomonas aeruginosa vaccine in cancer patients. Ann Intern Med *79*, 518–527, 1973

Young, S., and Cowan, D. M. Spontaneous regression of induced mammary tumours in rats. Br J Cancer *17*, 85–89, 1963

Young-Rodenchuk, J. M., and Gyenes, L. Differences in the sensitivity of tumor cells and normal lymphocytes towards lysis by alloantibodies and guinea pig or rabbit complement. Transplantation *20*, 20–25, 1975

Yuhas, J. M., Toya, R., and Wagner, E. Specific and non-specific stimulation of resistance to the growth and metastases of line 1 lung sarcoma. Cancer Res *35*, 242–244, 1975

Yuhas, J. M., and Ullrich, R. L. Responsiveness of senescent mice to the antitumor properties of Corynebacterium parvum. Cancer Res *36*, 161–166, 1976

Yunis, E. J., Martinez, C., Smith, J., Stutman, O., and Good, R. A. Spontaneous mammary adenocarcinoma in mice: Influence of thymectomy and reconstitution with thymus grafts or spleen cells. Cancer Res *29*, 174–178, 1969

Yutoku, M., Grossberg, A. L., and Pressman, D. Suppression of in vivo growth of mouse myelomas by purified rabbit antibodies against mouse myeloma cells. J Natl Cancer Inst *53*, 201–207, 1974

Z

Zacharski, L. R., and Linman, J. W. Lymphocytopenia: Its causes and significance. Mayo Clin Proc *46*, 168–173, 1971

Zagury, D., Bernard, J., Thierness, N., Feldman, M., and Berke, G. Isolation and characterization of individual functionally reactive cytotoxic T lymphocytes: Conjugation, killing and recycling at the single cell level. Eur J Immunol *5*, 818–822, 1975

Zamcheck, N., Moore, T. L., Dhar, P., and Kupchik, H. Immunologic diagnosis and prognosis of human digestive tract cancer. Carcinoembryonic antigens. N Engl J Med *286*, 83–86, 1972

Zankl, H., and Zang, H. D. Cytological and cytogenetic studies of brain tumors: Ph[1]-like chromosomes in human meningiomas. Humangenetik *12*, 42–49, 1971

Zankl, H., and Zang, H. D. Cytological and cytogenetic studies on brain tumors: Identification of the missing G chromosome in human meningiomas as No. 22 by fluorescence technique. Humangenetik *14*, 167–169, 1972

Zarling, J. M., Raich, P. C., McKeough, M., and Bach, F. H. Generation of cytotoxic lymphocytes in vitro against autologous human leukaemia cells. Nature *262*, 691–693, 1976

Zatz, M. M., White, A., and Goldstein, A. L. Alterations in lymphocyte populations in tumorigenesis. I. Lymphocyte trapping. J Immunol *111*, 706–742, 1973

Zbar, B., Bernstein, I. D., Bartlett, G. L., Hanna, M. G., and Rapp, H. J. Immunotherapy of cancer. Regression of intradermal tumors and prevention of growth of lymph node metastases after intralesional injection of living Mycobacterium bovis. J Natl Cancer Inst *49*, 119–128, 1972a

Zbar, B., Bernstein, I. D., and Rapp, H. J. Suppression of tumor growth at the site of infection with living bacillus Calmette-Guérin. J Natl Cancer Inst *46*, 831–839, 1971

Zbar, B., Rapp, H. J., and Ribi, E. E. Tumor suppression by cell walls of Mycobacterium bovis attached to oil droplets. J Natl Cancer Inst *48*, 831–835, 1972b

Zbar, B., Ribi, E. E., and Rapp, H. J. An experimental model for immunotherapy of cancer. Natl Cancer Inst Monogr *39*, 3–6, 1973

Zbar, B., and Tanaka, T. Immunotherapy of cancer: Regression of tumors after intralesional injection of living Mycobacterium bovis. Science 172, 271–273, 1971

Zeidman, I., and Buss, J. M. Transpulmonary passage of tumor cell emboli. Cancer Res 12, 731–733, 1952

Zeidman, I., McCutcheon, M., and Coman, D. R. Factors affecting the number of tumor metastases: Experiments with a transplantable mouse tumor. Cancer Res 10, 357–359, 1950

Zelerznick, L. D., and Bhuyan, B. K. Treatment of leukemic (L-1210) mice with double-stranded polyribonucleotides. Proc Soc Exp Biol Med 130, 126–128, 1969

Zembala, M., Ptak, W., and Hanczakowska, M. The role of macrophages in the cytotoxic killing of tumour cells in vitro. I. Primary immunisation of lymphocytes in vitro for target cell killing and the mechanism of lymphocyte–macrophage co-operation. Immunology 25, 631–644, 1973a

Zembala, M., Ptak, W., and Hanczakowska, M. Macrophage and lymphocyte co-operation in target cell destruction in vitro. Clin Exp Immunol 15, 461–466, 1973b

Ziegler, F. G., Lohmann-Matthes, M. L., and Fischer, H. Studies on the mechanism of macrophage-mediated cytotoxicity. Int Arch Allergy Appl Immunol 48, 182–191, 1975

Ziegler, L. Chemotherapy of Burkitt's lymphoma. Cancer 30, 1534–1540, 1972

Zighelboim, J., Bonavida, B., and Fahey, J. L. Evidence for several cell populations active in antibody dependent cellular cytotoxicity. J Immunol 111, 1737–1742, 1973

Zilber, L. A. Specific tumor antigens. Adv Cancer Res 5, 291–329, 1958

Zilber, L. A. Study of the tumor specificity of gastric cancer tissue. Ann NY Acad Sci 101, 264–270, 1962

Zilber, L. A., Krokova, I. N., Nartsikov, N. V., and Birvulina, T. I. O. [Cited by Levi and Schechtman (1963)] Serologicheskoi differenciacii ekstraktov sarkomi rousa i normalnoi tkani. Cop Onkol 4, 268–270, 1958

Zilber, L. A., and Ludogovskaya, L. A. Soluble antigens of gastric cancer. Folia Biol (Praha) 13, 331–334, 1967

Zilber, L. A., and Postnikova, Z. A. Induction of a leukemogenic agent by a chemical carcinogen in inbred mice. Natl Cancer Inst Monogr 22, 397–403, 1966

Zinkernagel, R. M., Althage, A., and Jensen, F. C. Cell-mediated immune response to lymphocytic choriomeningitis and vaccinia virus in rats. J Immunol 119, 1242–1247, 1977

Zinkernagel, R. M., Callahan, G. N., Althage, A., Cooper, S., Kelin, P. A., and Klein, J. On the thymus in the differentiation of "H-2 self-recognition" by T cells: Evidence for dual recognition? J Exp Med 147, 882–896, 1978a

Zinkernagel, R. M., Callahan, G. N., Althage, A., Cooper, S., Streilein, J. W., and Klein, J. The lymphoreticular system in triggering virus plus self-specific cytotoxic T cells: Evidence for T help. J Exp Med 147, 897–911, 1978b

Zinkernagel, R. M., and Doherty, P. C. H-2 compatibility requirement for T cell mediated lysis of target cells infected with lymphocytic choriomeningitis virus. Different cytotoxic T cell specificities are associated with structures coded for in H-2K or H-2D. J Exp Med 141, 1427–1436, 1975

Zoller, M., Price, M. R., and Baldwin, R. W. Inhibition of cell-mediated cytotoxicity to chemically induced rat tumours by soluble tumour and embryo cell extracts. Int J Cancer 17, 129–137, 1976

Zollinger, R. M., Timpkins, R. K., Amerson, T. R., Endahi, G. L., Kraft, A. R., and Moore, F. T. Identification of the diarrheogenic hormone associated with non-beta islet cell tumors of the pancreas. Ann Surg 168, 502–521, 1968

Zukoski, C. F., Killen, D. A., Ginn, E., Matter, B., Lucas, D. O., and Seigler, H. F. Transplanted carcinoma in an immunosuppressed patient. Transplantation 9, 71–74, 1970

Zur Hausen, H., Henle, W., Hummelor, K., Diehl, V., and Henle, G. Comparative study of cultured Burkitt tumor cells by immunofluorescence, autoradiography and electron microscopy. J Virol 1, 830–837, 1967

Zur Hausen, H., Schulte-Holthausen, H., Klein, G., Henle, W., Henle, G., Clifford, P., and Santesson, I. EBV DNA in biopsies of Burkitt tumours and anaplastic carcinomas of the nasopharynx. Nature 228, 1056–1058, 1970

Postscript

ADDENDUM TO SECTION 2.142

Hanto et al. have obtained evidence from serological and DNA hybridization studies that EB Virus is implicated in the development of lymphomas in immunosuppressed kidney transplant recipients. In two such lymphomas (one of which regressed completely while the other became disseminated and killed the patient), they observed a polyclonal population of cells showing histological features of malignancy that included cells lacking the usual surface markers of normal lymphocytes, cells showing chromosomal abnormalities, and cells in which the EBV genome was present. They suggest that the Ball proliferation evoked by EB Virus is limited in normal individuals by the action of T cells and NK cells, but that this homeostasis fails in immunosuppressed patients.

ADDENDUM TO SECTION 3.114

Evidence that metastases may develop from a minority population of cells in a tumor has been obtained in an experimental model by Katzav et al. They found that the cells of primary subcutaneous transplants of a tumor, which had been induced with melthylcholanthrene in a (C57 B1 $\times$ C3H) F1 hybrid mouse, expressed one parental haplotype (H-2^b) but not the other (H-2^k), whereas cells from pulmonary metastases expressed both parental haplotypes. Cloning studies showed that cells expressing both haplotypes constituted only a small portion of the original tumor cell population, and only clones of this kind were able to generate pulmonary metastases.

ADDENDUM TO SECTIONS 5.44 and 5.53

The cells in non-immunized animals, which are cytotoxic for tumor cells *in vitro,* appear to form a more heterogeneous population than was originally thought. Burton et al. have reported that fresh murine spleen cells include two kinds of NK cell: NK_L, which are active against lymphoma targets, and NK_S, which are active against non-lymphoid tumors. These categories can be distinguished by a variety of surface markers and by the fact that NK_A cells, but not NK_B cells, are deficient in mice homozygous for the beige mutation and also in mice treated with the bone-seeking radioactive isotype ^{89}Sr. A third category of cell (termed NK_C) was identified among spleen cells which had been cultured in vitro for 6 days. It was shown in other experiments (Hamilton; Burton and Winn) that NK_A also mediate ADCC against lymphoma targets.

Stutman et al. have identified a population of cells that they term natural cytotoxic (NC) cells in normal mouse spleens which kill murine fibrosarcoma cells labeled with ^{3}H-proline in 18–24 hour assays and which differ from NK cells as originally described in respect of cell suface antigens, radiosensitivity, and other properties. The cytotoxicity is blocked by the addition of mannose and other sugars, and Stutman et al. suggest that the targets recognized by NC cells may be simple sugars in the target cell membrane. The existence of a positive correlation between the TD_{50} (1-22) of different fibrosarcomas and the susceptibility of their cells to killing by NC cells in vitro suggests that NC cells may play a role in surveillance.

Rosse and Scuderi reported that the tumoricidal effect of immune sensitized mouse splenocytes, obtained by culturing spleen cells of tumor-immune mice with fibrosarcoma cells, in Winn assays was abolished if the recipient mice were previously given 900 $\hbar$ whole body irradiation. They showed that the recipient cells, which potentiate the effect of immune sensitized spleen cells in non-irradiated mice, were bone marrow derived and were present in nude mice, and were termed these recipient cells natural tumor growth regulatory cells.

The extent to which cell populations defined by different investigators coincide or overlap, and the function of these cells in vivo, remains to be seen, but it may well be that the NK_B cell of Burton et al. is the same as Stutman's NC cell.

REFERENCES

Hanto, D., Frizzera, K., Crajl-Peczalska, K., Purtilo, D. and Klein, G. EBV in the pathogenesis of polyclonal "post-transplant lymphoma." Transplant Proc, 1981 (in press)

Katzav, S., de Baetselier, P., Feldman, M. and Segal, S. Immunogenetic control of metastasis formation by a methylcholanthrene induced tumor (T-10) in mice. Transplant Proc, 1981 (in press)

Burton, R.C., Kumar, V., Bartlett, S.P. and Winn, H.J. Heterogeneity of natural killer cells in the mouse. Transplant Proc, 1981 (in press)

Hamilton, M.S., Burton, R.C., and Winn, H.J. Natural killing and antibody dependent cellular cytotoxicity of tumor targets are mediated by the same effector cell: a genetic and serological study. Transplant Proc, 1981 (in press)

Stutman, O., Figarella, E.F., Lattime, E., Cuttito, M., Wisun, R. and Pecoraro, G. In vitro and in vivo studies of natural cytotoxic (NC) cells against solid tumors in mice. Transplant Proc, 1981 (in press)

Rosse, C. and Scuderi, P. The role of bone marrow cells in the growth inhibition of transplanted methylcholanthrene-induced sarcoma (MCA) Transplant Proc, 1981 (in press)

AUTHOR INDEX

A

Aaronson, S. A. 93
Abbey Smith, R. 51
Abdou, N. I. 45
Abdou, N. L. 45
Abelev, G. I. 106
Abercrombie, M. 40
Ablashi, D. V. 25, 44
Achong, B. G. 13, 28
Ackerman, L. V. 83
Ackerman, N. R. 54
Adair, F. E. 76
Adams, G. E. 151
Adams, J. B. 77
Adams, K. 66, 67
Adamson, R. H. 21
Adamson, U. 284
Adlam, C. 200, 204, 212, 259
Adler, W. H. 82
Agostino, D. 56
Agwunobi, T. C. 84
Aherne, W. 48
Aherne, W. A. 66, 67
Aisenberg, A. C. 45, 81, 83
Aiuti, F. 100
Alam, I. 196
Albertini, R. J. 38
Albo, V. 237
Alexander, J. W. 10, 56
Alexander, P. 11, 24, 48, 49, 55, 59, 88, 91, 94, 95,
        105, 108, 117, 119, 123, 124, 126, 127, 135,
        147, 166, 176, 185, 186, 190, 191, 192, 208,
        213, 216, 217, 219, 223, 230, 232

Algire, G. H. 49
Allen, E. P. 52
Allen, R. P. 169, 170
Alley, C. D. 226
Allison, A. C. 24, 37, 120, 139, 140, 141, 144, 203,
        204
Allwood, G. G. 199
Alpert, E. 106
Al-Sarraf, M. 81, 82
Altemeier, W. A. 10
Althage, A. 121
Amaral, L. 85
Amatruda, T. T. 71
Ambrose, E. J. 40
Ambrus, J. L. 221
Ambus, U. 254
Amery, W. K. 267
Ames, B. N. 16
Amiel, J. L. 180, 192, 206, 208, 241, 242, 251,
        275, 276
Amino, N. 100
Amos, D. B. 43, 83, 137, 166, 237
Anastassiades, O. T. 96
Andersen, V. 102
Anderson, C. K. 48
Anderson, D. E. 8, 34
Anderson, E. E. 71
Anderson, J. M. 272
Anderson, N. F. 180
Anderson, N. G. 16, 106, 108, 109
Andreassen, M. 154
Andreini, P. 88
Andrews, G. A. 246
Andrien, J. M. 276
Ankherst, J. 41
Anthony, H. M. 82, 96, 257

Aoki, T. 25, 92, 93, 98, 111
Appel, M. 235
Appella, E. 92, 111
Aptekman, P. M. 224
Arcomano, J. P. 60
Ariel, I. M. 2
Armand, M.O. 2
Armitage, P. 17
Armstrong, B. 21
Armstrong, D. 98
Armstrong, M. Y. K. 33
Arnŏld, J. S. 22
Aschoff, K. A. L. 125
Ash, P. J. N. D. 27, 93
Asherson, G. L. 199
Ashikawa, K. 81, 85
Ashley, D. J. B. 17
Ashworth, M. 20
Ashworth, T. R. 54
Atkinson, J. B. 241
Attia, M. A. M. 93, 167
Aub, J. C. 40
Auclair, D. J. 189
Audibert, F. 196, 284
Auerbach, R. 49
Aungst, C. W. 252
Aurelian, L. 29
Auster, L. S. 23
Avis, F. 101
Avis, P. 107
Axel, R. 29, 30
Axelrad, A. A. 92
Axelrod, B. J. 125
Ayre, J. E. 274
Azuma, I. 196, 212
Azzarone, B. 79

B

Bach, F. H. 103
Bach, M. L. 103
Back, N. 221
Bagshawe, K. D. 87, 111, 149, 156, 207, 221, 224, 275
Baird, D. T. 77
Baird, L. G. 202
Bakemeier, R. F. 253, 256
Baker, A. R. 225
Baker, H. W. 153, 154
Baker, M. A. 50, 169
Baker, P. J. 137
Baker, W. H. 78
Balakrishnan, K. 101

Baldwin, R. W. 12, 43, 47, 75, 87, 90, 94, 108, 109, 110, 111, 112, 136, 149, 189, 192, 193, 194, 195, 206, 210, 218, 220, 221, 226, 229, 255
Balfour, B. M. 103
Balkur, S. 81
Ball, J. K. 35, 609
Balme, H. W. 78
Balner, H. 141, 190
Baltimore, D. 26
Band, P. R. 260, 262
Bandieri, A. 198
Bandlow, B. 126
Bang, O. 8
Bansal, S. C. 136, 167, 232
Bar, R. S. 29
Barfoot, R. K. 170
Barker, C. R. 43, 75, 90
Barker, H. R. 48
Barnes, D. W. H. 174, 175, 179
Barnes, J. W. 21
Baron, S. 218
Barr, M. 80
Barr, R. D. 46
Barr, Y. M. 28
Barra, Y. 111
Barrett, A. 77
Barrett, J. C. 66, 67
Barrett, M. K. 10, 11
Barski, G. 44
Bart, R. S. 219
Barth, R. F. 205
Bartlett, G. 94
Bartlett, G. L. 193, 194, 229
Barton, A. D. 64, 65
Bartsch, H. 16
Basham, C. 112, 125, 135, 202
Bashford, E. F. 10, 138
Basic, I. 124, 201, 202
Basombrio, M. A. 91
Bass, E. M. 48
Bast, R. C. 189
Basten, A. 91, 116, 173
Bataillon, G. 91, 100, 101
Batchelor, J. R. 89, 90, 137
Batson, O.V. 54
Bauer, F. W. 18
Bauer, H. 92, 108
Baum, H. 16, 36
Baum, M. 36, 83, 126, 151, 155, 161, 162, 201
Baumler, A. 43
Bayliss, W. M. 76
Bean, M. 101
Beardmore, G. L. 22
Beatson, G. T. 76
Beck, C. 71
Becker, N. 71
Becker, S. 129

Bedford, A. J. 69
Beech, M. 275
Begg, R. W. 79
Beilby, J. O. W. 29
Bekesi, J. G. 224, 225, 226, 273, 278
Bekierkunst, A. 35, 192, 196, 229
Beldotti, L. 32
Belisario, J. C. 264
Bell, J. W. 52
Bellone, C. J. 92
Belpomme, D. 276
Benacerraf, B. 114, 116, 118, 120, 121, 192
Bendich, A. 108
Bendixen, G. 102
Ben-Efraim, S. 191
Benes, E. H. 244
Ben-Ishay, Z. 124
Benjamin, S. A. 219, 220
Bennett, M. 122, 123
Ben-Sasson, Z. 112
Benson, R. C. 217, 218
Bentvelzen, P. 25, 27
Berardet, M. 192, 206, 208
Berczi, I. 225
Berdall, P. 67
Berebbi, M. 111
Berenbaum, M. C. 12, 13, 14, 157, 158, 228
Berenblum, I. 20, 24
Beretta, G. 253
Berg, J. W. 48, 96, 155
Bergenstal, D. M. 76
Bergheden, C. 122
Bergholtz, B. O. 121
Bergs, V. V. 27
Bergstrand, P. J. 65
Berkarda, F. B. 221
Berke, G. 116
Berkeley, W. N. 238, 239
Berkovich, S. 264
Berman, L. D. 37, 92, 140
Bernard, C. 82
Bernard, J. 172, 175, 179, 180, 181, 241
Berney, S. N. 182
Bernstein, A. 80
Bernstein, I. D. 184, 195
Berry, R. J. 158
Bersohn, I. 106
Berson, S. A. 71
Bertschmann, M. 111
Bessent, R. G. 60
Bevan, M. J. 20, 118
Bewley, D. K. 151
Bhan, R. D. 45
Bhuyan, B. K. 219
Bianco, A. R. 92
Bias, W. B. 99
Bichel, P. 68

Bicker, U. 283
Biddle, C. 138
Bielschowski, F. 31
Bierman, H. R. 54
Bierwaltes, E. 240
Biggar, R. J. 156
Biggs, P. M. 25
Bignall, J. R. 55
Bill, A. H. 30
Billingham, R. E. 87, 89, 136f, 179, 181
Binder, P. 226
Biniaminov, M. 268
Biozzi, G. 84, 180, 192, 197, 198, 199, 209
Biran, H. 263
Birbeck, M. S. C. 127
Birch, S. M. 98
Biskind, G. R. 31
Biskind, M. S. 31
Biskis, B. O. 22, 30, 65
Bittner, J. J. 10, 26
Björkland, B. 97
Björkland, V. 97
Black, M. M. 30, 48, 96, 102, 105
Black, P. H. 43
Blackford, M. E. 63
Blair, P. B. 26, 93
Blake, E. R. 11, 12, 53, 55, 56, 94, 144, 208, 234
Blake, J. 99
Blamey, R. W. 13, 88, 175
Blanden, R. V. 118, 191
Blaney, D. 150
Blaylock, B. L. 84
Bliznakov, E. G. 188
Block, K. J. 45
Bloom, H. J. G. 50, 78, 150
Blumenthal, F. 271
Blumgart, C. H. 5
Bluming, A. Z. 51, 104, 105, 253, 264
Boak, J. L. 84, 180, 181, 183, 197, 205, 210, 259, 261
Bodenham, D. C. 61, 156
Bodmer, W. F. 38
Boeryd, B. 221
Boetcher, D. A. 84
Bolhuis, R. L. H. 101
Bomford, R. 126, 198, 199, 201, 202, 203, 206, 209, 210, 211, 212, 222, 230
Bonadonna, G. 158
Bonavida, B. 100, 111, 136, 180
Bonhag, R. S. 192, 195
Bonmassar, E. 123
Bonnard, G. D. 85, 89
Boon, M. C. 31
Boone, C. W. 82, 111, 126, 214
Booth, S. N. 107
Boranic, M. 181, 182, 193
Borberg, H. 176

Borek, C. 40, 41
Borenfreund, E. 108
Borrie, J. 152
Borsos, T. 98, 171
Borst, P. 16
Bortin, M. M. 181, 182, 242
Bouck, N. 17
Bourali, C. 222
Bourali-Maury, C. 222
Bourque, R. A. 154
Bourut, C. 192
Bouvrain, A. 81, 82, 83
Bowen, J. G. 111, 112, 136
Boyd, W. 51
Boyer, P. J. J. 93
Boyle, M. D. P. 124
Boyse, E. A. 43, 87, 90, 92, 98, 111, 112, 117, 118,
    122
Braeman, J. 152
Branche, R. 217
Brandes, L. J. 247, 248
Brandis, H. 224, 240
Branellec, A. 198
Braun, W. 215, 216, 217, 218
Braunstein, H. 10
Brawn, R. J. 108
Breeding, J. H. 194, 226, 229
Breese, M. 201
Bremberg, S. 167
Brennan, M. J. 63
Brenner, H. J. 63, 65
Brent, L. 87, 136f, 179, 186
Bresnick, E. 20
Breur, K. 62
Breyere, E. J. 83
Brillantes, F. P. 31
Brinkley, D. M. 154
British Breast Group 4
British Medical Journal 6, 21, 60, 67, 77, 161, 275
Brittingham, T. E. 237
Britton, D. C. 67, 69
Briziarelli, G. 31, 76
Brncic, D. 174
Brooks, R. F. 66
Brooks, W. H. 81
Broom, B. C. 49
Broughton, E. S. 204
Brouty-Boyé, D. 222
Browdie, D. A. 201, 204
Brown, E. R. 239
Brown, G. 82
Brown, J. 29, 32, 34, 186
Brown, J. H. 152
Brown, J. M. 221
Brown, L. R. 2
Brown, M. B. 26, 27, 174
Brown, P. 83
Browning, H. C. 50

Brozovic, B. 200, 204
Bruce, A. W. 256
Bruce, W. R. 158
Bruchovsky, N. 77
Brugarolas, A. 274
Bruley-Rosset, M. 192
Brunner, K. T. 116
Brunner, K. W. 159
Brunschwig, A. 3, 51, 83
Bubbers, J. E. 116
Bubenik, J. 35, 92, 98, 101, 167, 176, 194
Buckley, C. E. 237
Buckner, C. D. 241
Buehler, H. G. 60
Buffet, R. F. 31
Bull, D. M. 102
Bullough, W. S. 74, 75
Bumpus, H. C. 60
Bundick, R. V. 13
Burch, P. R. J. 15, 17, 18, 21, 22, 74
Burchenal, J. H. 158, 160
Burdette, W. J. 34
Burdick, J. F. 80, 91, 264
Burg, C. 122
Burger, H. G. 71
Burger, M. M. 40, 41, 74
Burk, M. W. 100
Burki, K. 20
Burkitt, D. P. 28, 29, 51
Burmester, B. R. 25
Burn, J. I. 153, 154
Burnet, F. M. 15, 16, 18, 22, 38, 75, 80, 133, 134,
    144
Burney, A. 30
Burnham, T. K. 80
Burrows, D. 97
Burrows, M. T. 13
Burstein, N. A. 92
Burton, R. C. 89, 91, 93, 109, 132, 177
Busch, H. 68
Buss, J. M. 53
Bussey, H. J. R. 58
Buttle, G. A. H. 13
Byers, E. H. 272
Byers, L. A. 125
Byers, V. S. 30
Byfield, J. E. 99
Byrne, M. 101
Bystrin, J. -C. 112

C

Cahan, W. G. 152
Cairns, J. 17, 18, 38, 39

Calder, E. A. 115
Calderwood, S. K. 270
Caldwell, B. V. 12
Callahan, W. 240
Calne, R. Y. 143
Calmette, A. 189
Cameron, E. H. D. 77
Campanile, F. 132
Campbell, A. C. 152
Canellos, G. P. 45, 156
Cant, E. L. M. 32
Cantell, K. 284
Cantor, H. 118, 128, 129, 130, 132, 217
Carbone, G. 145
Cardenas, J. O. 254
Carey, R. W. 264
Carlson, J. C. 270
Carnaud, C. 177
Carnes, W. H. 26, 27
Carney, P. G. 24
Caro, R. A. 83
Carr, I. 49, 125, 194
Carr, T. E. F. 22, 27
Carrell, A. 13
Carrell, S. 112
Carruthers, C. 43
Carter, P. B. 199, 200
Carter, R. L. 127
Carter, S. B. 40
Carter, S. K. 159
Casale, G. P. 124, 127
Cascinelli, N. 255
Casey, M. J. 92
Caspary, E. A. 103, 135
Caspersson, T 42
Cassel, W. A. 214
Castermans-Elias, S. 269
Castro, E. B. 154
Castro, J. E. 13, 37, 108, 162, 199, 200, 205, 206,
      208, 209, 211, 212, 260, 262
Catalona, W. J. 81, 82
Cater, D. B. 186
Catterall, M. 151
Cavaliere, R. 270
Cavilli-Sforza, L. L. 38
Ceglowski, W. S. 38
Centanni, E. 188
Cerilli, G. J. 141, 144
Cerottini, J. -C. 116
Cerutti, I. 204
Chalkley, H. W. 49
Chamberlain, M. J. 218
Chambers, H. 271
Chambers, V. C. 125
Champion, H. R. 48
Chan, Y. K. 252
Chang, K. S. 92, 111
Chang, S. S. 140

Chang, Yu-Hui 84
Chaparas, S. D. 192
Chaplin, M. 237
Chapuis, B. 277
Char, D. H. 104
Chard, T. 171
Chare, M. J. B. 260
Charkes, N. D. 60
Charney, J. 29, 30, 98
Chase, M. W. 81
Chassoux, D. 194
Cheatle, G. L. 47
Checkik, B. E. 97
Chedid, L. 196, 284
Cheema, A. R. 244
Cheers, C. 216
Chen, L. 227
Cheng, V. S. T. 260, 262, 263
Chernyakhooskaya, I. Y. 178
Chesebro, B. 114, 116
Chess, L. 118
Chihara, G. 222
Chiossone, F. 221
Chirigos, M. A. 192, 221
Chism, S. E. 89, 97, 108, 109
Choay, J. 219
Choi, N. W. 32
Chretien, P. B. 81, 82, 99
Christie, G. H. 126, 198, 201, 202, 203
Chu, E. H. Y. 15, 101, 106
Chung, E. B. 193, 195
Churchill, W. H. 103
Chute, R. N. 13
Cifuentes, L. 202
Cinader, B. 275
Citrin, D. L. 2, 60
Clabaugh, W. A. 84
Clagett, O. T. 152
Clark, C. G. 82
Clark, I. A. 204
Clark, P. J. 76
Clarke, D. A. 190, 192
Clarkson, B. D. 67, 156, 263
Cleaver, J. E. 23, 66
Clements, D. V. 254
Clementson, K. J. 111
Cleveland, P. H. 100
Cleveland, R. P. 123, 191
Clifford, P. 29, 99, 101, 103, 237, 279
Cliffton, E. E. 56, 221
Clode-Hyde, M. 37
Cobb, L. M. 12, 13, 22
Coca, A. F. 271
Cochran, A. J. 51, 98, 99, 102, 257
Cochrane, C. G. 48, 49, 51, 127
Codington, J. F. 225
Coffin, J. M. 83
Coggin, J. H. 16, 106, 107, 108, 109

Cohen, A. 223
Cohen, A. M. 101, 136
Cohen, I. R. 177, 178
Cohen, R. B. 71
Cohen, S. A. 100
Cohen, Y. 83
Cohn, Z. A. 120, 125
Colby, C. 218
Cole, L. J. 22, 174
Cole, P. 29, 32, 34
Cole, W. H. 51, 52, 58, 60, 61, 239
Coley, W. B. 250, 251
Collavo, D. 140, 216
Collet A. J. 200, 201
Collins, F. M. 204
Collins, V. P. 63
Colnaghi, M. I. 91, 108, 110
Coman, D. R. 56
Comoglio, P. M. 167, 224
Comings, D. E. 16
Cone, L. 81
Cone, R. E. 216
Congdon, C. C. 174, 179
Connell, D. I. 166, 185
Constantini-Sourojon, M. 191
Cook, A. J. 226
Cook, J. W. 19
Cooke, R. 73
Cooper, E. H. 48, 68, 69
Cooper, M. 171
Cooperband, S. R. 217, 219
Cope, T. I. 275
Cornefert, F. 44
Cornell, C. J. 266
Corrin, B. 71
Corsigilia, V. F. 31
Cortes, E. P. 160
Cosenza, H. 100
Costanzi, J. J. 253
Cotchin, E. 8
Court Brown, W. M. 21
Cowan, D. M. 50
Cowling, D. C. 82
Cox, F. E. G. 204
Cox, H. R. 214
Cox, K. O. 204
Cox, M. L. 71
Cox, R. 20
Coyle, J. 201
Crain, R. C. 9
Cramp, W. A. 205
Creech, O. 152
Crepin, Y. 206
Crile, G. 78, 103, 104, 150, 154, 155, 270
Crile, G. W. 153
Crisler, C. 43
Criss, W. E. 16
Crissey, J. T. 23
Croce, C. M. 44

Crookston, J. H. 275
Crowe, J. K. 2
Crowley, J. H. 84
Crowther, D. 21, 257, 263
Crum, E. D. 247
Cruse, J. M. 227
Cudkowicz, G. 122, 123, 128, 130
Cullen, P. R. 99
Cullen, R. T. 201, 202, 203
Cummings, C. S. 197
Cunningham, T. J. 253, 274
Cunningham-Rundles, W. F. 261
Currey, H. L. F. 82
Currie, A. R. 69
Currie, G. A. 85, 99, 101, 112, 116, 119, 120, 125, 135, 202, 207, 224, 234, 238, 271, 272
Curtis, M. R. 9
Cushing, H. W. 51, 154
Custer, R. P. 141
Cutler, M. 47
Cuttner, J. 256
Czajkowski, N. P. 227, 274

D

Daams, J. H. 26
Da Fano, C. A. 47
Dahl-Iversen, E. 154
Dailey, J. E. 71
Dalton, A. 27
Damjanov, I. 20
Daniel, B. G. 16
Dao, T. L. 31
Dargeon, H. W. 54
Dausset, J. 110
David, C. S. 117
David, J. 51
David, J. R. 102
Davidson, J. A. 2
Davies, A. J. S. 48, 182
Davies, C. J. 60
Davies, D. A. L. 111, 112, 168, 173
Davies, D. J. 183
Davies, M. C. 214
Davies, P. 203
Davignon, L. 257, 258
Davis, H. H. 30
Davis, J. B. 30
Davis, N. C. 150
Davis, R. C. 141
Davis, S. 13
Davis, W. 19
Dawe, D. L. 216
Dawes, J. 198, 212
Day, D. 166

Day, E. D. 101
Dayan, A. D. 246
Dazord, L. 204
Dean, J. H. 216
De Bracco, M. M. de E. 100
de Carvalho, S. 238, 239
Decker, J. 205
Deckers, P. J. 186
De Clercq, E. 35, 218
De Cosse, J. 68, 166
Deeley, T. J. 152
Defendi, V. 44, 92
De Grast, G. C. 82
Degre, M. 35
Degroot, L. J. 100
De Jager, R. 259
De La Pava, S. 239
Della Porta, G. 91, 108
Delmez, J. A. 51
Delmonte, L. 268
de Long, R. P. 56
Delorme, E. J. 176, 184, 185
De Mars, R. 38
Denham, S. 117
den Herder, B. A. 9
Denlinger, R. H. 27
Dennert, G. 100, 227
Den Otter, W. 123, 124, 126, 127, 175, 178, 185
Dent, R. I. 264
Deodhar, S. D. 103, 104, 144
De Ome, K. B. 93, 192
De Pace, N. 264
Deringer, M. K. 11
Dersjant, H. 141
De Somer, P. 139
De Souza, I. 77
Dethlefsen, L. A. 62, 63, 67
Detre, S. I. 13
Deutsch, V. 195
De Vassal, F. 276
De Vita, V. 156, 265
De Vries, M. J. 175, 180, 241
Dhar, P. 107
Di Beradino, M. A. 17
Dickson, J. 84
Dickson, J. A. 270
Diehl, V. 51, 99, 101
Diesselhoff-den Dulk, M. M. C. 125
Di Luzio, N. R. 83, 123
Di Mayorca, G. 17
Dimitrov, N. V. 201, 210, 259
Dixon, W. J. 160
Dizon, Q. S. 84
Djerassi, I. 157
Djeu, J. Y. 130
Dmochowski, L. 26, 30
Doak, P. B. 142
Doak, S. M. 88, 174
Doe, W. F. 127

Doherty, P. C. 118
Doljansky, F. 112
Doll, R. 17, 21
Dolton, E. G. 159
Domas, J. 256
Dombernowsky, P. 68
Donahower, G. F. 71
Doniach, I. 32, 275
Dore, J. F. 98, 99, 225
Dorrance, G. M. 271
Dorsett, B. H. 95, 96
Double, J. A. 13, 14
Dougherty, S. 120
Douglas, H. C. 197
Douglass, H. O. 160, 244, 272
Doyle, F. H. 60
Drake, J. W. 38
Drake, W. P. 168, 171, 172
Drasher, M. L. 88
Dray, S. 214
Dresser, D. W. 173
Dreyfuss, Y. 26
Drogemuller, C. R. 187
d'Souza, J. P. 221
Dube, O. L. 136
Dubois, J. B. 192
Duclos, H. 81
Duffy, B. J. 22
Dukes, B. A. 77
Dukes, C. E. 34, 58, 78
Dulbecco, R. 25, 26, 28, 40, 166
Dullens, H. F. J. 123, 126, 185
Dumonde, D. C. 119
Dumont, F. 91
Dunbar, N. 197, 204, 206, 208, 209, 210, 211, 231
Dunkley, M. 116
Dunlop, G. R. 54
Dunning, W. F. 9
Dunphy, J. E. 51
Duplan, J. F. 181
Dupont, B. 247
Dupuy, J. M. 81
Dustin, P. 16
Dutton, R. W. 137
Dux, A. 33
Dwight, R. W. 160
Dykes, P. W. 261
Dyson, W. H. 154

E

Eady, R. P. 240
Eagle, H. 74
East, J. 140
Easton, J. M. 25

Easty, D. M. 40
Easty, G. C. 10, 40
Ebeling, A. H. 13
Eccles, S. A. 11, 48, 49, 59, 84, 85, 121, 126, 127, 147, 232
Eccleston, E. 217
Eckner, R. J. 92
Economides, F. 192
Eddington, G. M. 28
Eddy, B. E. 92
Edelstein, R. 259
Edlich, R. F. 152
Edwards, A. 100
Edwards, A. J. 88
Edwards, J. 100
Edwards, M. H. 61, 155
Edynak, E. M. 107
Egdahl, R. H. 186
Ehrke, M. J. 136
Ehrlich, P. 10, 87, 133, 138
Eichmann, K. 113, 233
Eidinger, D. 256
Eilber, F. R. 30, 81, 96, 98, 253, 279
Eisen, H. N. 93
Eisenberg, R. B. 56
Ekert, H. 252
El-Domeiri, A. A. 2, 60
Elgjo, K. 35
El Hassan, A. M. 84
Elias, E. G. 102
Elias, L. L. 102
Elkind, M. M. 38
Ellerman, V. 8
Elliott, E. V. 49, 170, 240
Ellis, H. 153
Ellis, H. A. 270
Ellison, M. L. 16
Ellman, L. 184
Elston, C. W. 156
Elves, M. W. 82
Embleton, M. J. 90, 94, 111, 191, 220, 229
Engelbart, K. 213
Engell, H. C. 54, 55
Engelsman, E. 77
Engeset, A. 53
Engstrom, P. F. 253
Enker, W. E. 226
Enneking, W. 245, 246
Ennis, R. S. 210
Eperon, J. 13
Ephrussi, B. 44
Epstein, M. A. 28
Erb, P. 119
Eshel-Zussman, R. 227
Eskeland, T. 45
Esselstyn, C. B. 103, 104
Essex, M. 26, 146
Eustace, J. C. 137, 171

Evans, C. A. 92, 223
Evans, C. R. 8
Evans, D. M. D. 13, 88
Evans, H. J
Evans, H. M. 31
Evans, R. 48, 100, 119, 123, 124, 126, 127, 176, 213, 216, 217
Everall, J. D. 264
Everson, T. C. 51, 58, 60, 61
Ewing, J. (i)
Ezdinli, E. Z. 42

F

Fadda, G. 35, 167
Fahey, J. L. 93, 99, 100, 171
Faiman, C. 71
Fairley, G. H. 80, 81, 101, 151, 272
Fakhri, O. 100
Falk, H. L. 34, 35
Falk, R. E. 234, 255
Faraci, R. P. 191, 224
Farber, E. 19, 20
Farber, S. 160
Farrar, J. J. 120
Farrell, C. 30
Farrow, J. H. 76
Fass, L. 104, 105, 175, 176, 237
Faulkin, L. J. 93
Fauve, R. M. 204, 216
Favata, B. V. 13
Fefer, A. 92, 114, 140, 165, 167, 168, 175, 176, 181, 241
Feigin, I. 49
Feigis, M. 191
Feinleib, M. 32
Fel, V. J. 43
Feldberg, W. 207, 283
Feldman, J. D. 136, 229
Feldman, M.(Mark) 119
Feldman, M.(Michael) 89, 90, 91, 137, 177, 215, 227
Feneley, R. C. L. 246
Fennely, J. J. 277
Fenyö, E. M. 45, 129
Feraci, R. P. 88
Ferluga, J. 191
Fett, J. W. 127
Fialkow, P. J. 13, 30, 45, 46, 242
Fidler, I. J. 126, 138, 175, 178
Field, A. K. 218
Field, E. J. 103, 135
Fingerhut, B. 12, 223
Finkel, M. P. 22, 30, 65

Finlayson, N. D. C. 54
Finley, T. N. 125
Finney, J. W. 272
Firshein, W. 215, 217, 218
Fischer, H. 119
Fisher, B. 47, 48, 53, 56, 59, 126, 152, 158, 161, 176, 191, 201, 208, 237, 260, 262
Fisher, E. R. 30, 47, 48, 53, 54, 56, 59, 152, 176
Fisher, H. E. 2
Fisher, J. C. 17, 94, 141, 206
Fisher, R. A. 262
Fishman, M. 185
Fitzgerald, P. J. 22
Flanagan, S. P. 139
Flax, H. 77
Fleissner, E. 30
Flickinger, J. T. 111
Floersheim. G. L. 175, 180
Florentin, I. 190, 191
Flynn, L. 246
Fogh, J. 139f
Foley, E. J. 88, 93
Folkman, J. 49, 50, 162
Foote, F. W. 30
Foraker, A. G. 51, 244
Forbes, I. J. 80, 126
Forbes, J. F. 5
Forbes, J. T. 91
Forbes, P. D. 38
Forni, G. 88, 90, 95, 167, 224
Forrest, A. P. M. 77, 153, 154
Forscher, B. K. 74
Foster, R. S. 201, 204
Fothergill, J. E. 75
Foulds, L. 50
Fox, W. 4, 7
Franchi, G. 221
Frank, G. L. 68
Franklin, H. A. 243
Franks, C. R. 13
Franks, L. M. 51, 54
Fraser, H. 9, 12
Fraser, J. 150
Fraumeni, J. F. 30, 34, 143
Fray, A. 202, 204
Fredette, V. 213
Freedman, H. H. 216, 218
Freedman, S. O. 106
Freeman, C. B. 277
Freeman, J. E. 151
Frei, E. 152
Frei, J. V. 27
Frenster, J. H. 244
Freund, H. 23
Friberg, S. 44
Fridman, W. H. 103
Friedell, G. H. 80
Friedewald, W. F. 20

Friedman, H. 38, 85
Friedman, J. M. 46
Frindel, E. 67
Friou, G. J. 216
Fritsche, R. 107
Fritze, D. 91, 186, 187
Froese, G. 225
Frøland, S. S. 100
Frost, M. J. 111
Frost, P. 200, 227
Fry, R. J. 66
Fu, Y. S. 68
Fuchs, W. A. 2
Fudenberg, H. H. 116
Fugman, R. 158
Fugman, R. A. 12
Fujimoto, S. 233
Fujisawa, T. 30
Fukuhara, S. 42
Fukunishi, R. 76
Fukuoka, F. 79
Fuller, P. C. 171
Fullerton, J. M. 51
Furnival, C. M. 60, 271
Furth, J. 11, 31, 86, 87
Furth, R. van. See van Furth, R.
Fusco, F. D. 71

G

Gabrilove, J. L. 71
Gaffney, P. R. 83
Gage, J. O. 112, 116, 119
Galasko, C. S. B. 2, 59, 60
Gale, R. T. 100
Gallagher, M. T. 123, 130
Gallily, R. 123, 124
Gallin, J. I. 247
Gallo, R. C. 27, 30
Galton, D. A. G. 248, 252
Gambacorta, J. P. 60
Garb, S. 89, 239
Garbarino, C. A. 118
Gardner, P. S. 180
Gardner, R. J. 83
Garland, H. 63
Garner, F. B. 255
Garrett, R. E. 214
Gartler, S. M. 46
Gasic, G. 174, 221
Gasic, T. 221
Gaston, M. R. 208
Gates, O. 55
Gates, S. L. 83

Gatti, R. A. 227
Gauci, C. L. L. 49
Gaudin, D. 17
Gautherie, M. 2
Gaylord, C. E. 100
Gazet, J. C. 13
Geddes, E. W. 106
Gee, T. S. 263
Geffard, M. 190
Gehan, E. A. 4, 160
Gelboin, H. V. 16, 19, 24, 34, 35
Geldner, A. 92
Gelfand, E. W. 97
Gelfant, S. 68
Gensler, W. T. 196
Gentile, J. M. 111
Gerber, P. 98
Gericke, D. 213
Gerner, R. E. 243, 244
Gershon, R. K. 137
Gesner, B. M. 182
Gewirtz, G. 71
Ghaffer, A. 115, 198, 201, 202, 203, 209
Ghose, T. 172, 173, 225, 240
Gianelli, F. 22
Gidlund, M. 129, 130
Gilden, R. V. 26
Gill, P. G. 262, 263
Gill, W. 150
Gillespie, A. V. 98
Gillespie, D. 30
Gillespie, G. Y. 127
Gillette, R. W. 82, 126
Gillis, C. R. 5
Gimbrone, M. A. 49
Giovanella, B. C. 13, 139f
Giraldo, G. 26
Girardi, A. J. 108
Girmann, G. 85
Glaser, M. 89, 199
Glaser, R. 29, 44
Glasgow, A. H. 85
Glaves, D. 108, 109, 111
Gleichmann, E. 33
Gleichmann, H. 33
Glenn, J. F. 71
Glick, J. L. 219
Gliedman, M. L. 152
Glincher, L. 118, 130
Globerson, A. 90, 91, 215
Glynn, J. P. 92, 140
Godrick, E. A. 225
Gold, P. 106
Goldberg, A. R. 219
Golde, D. W. 71, 125
Goldenberg, D. M. 13, 45
Goldenberg, G. H. 247

Goldin, A. 92
Golding, P. R. 275
Goldman, L. 135, 150
Goldman, R. 124
Goldsmith, H. S. 84
Goldstein, M. 269, 270
Goligher, J. C. 58
Golstein, P. 116
Golub, S. H. 82, 89
Gomard, E. 92, 93, 116
Gompertz, B. 64
Good, R. A. 81, 142
Goodwin, B. C. 16
Gorczynski, R. M. 82
Gordon, D. S. 260
Gordon, J. 90
Gordon, R. D. 118
Gordon, S. 120
Gordon Smith, C. E. 214
Gordon-Taylor, G. 51
Gorer, P. A. 10, 87, 89, 166
Gorodilova, V. V. 272
Gothoskar, B. P. 102
Gotohda, E. 176, 227, 231, 274
Gottlieb, J. A. 152
Goudie, R. B. 43
Gough, I. R. 271
Goulmy, E. 121
Gourley, R. D. 71
Grace, J. T. 3, 83, 97, 104
Grace, W. R. 206
Graff, R. J. 162
Graffi, A. 90, 91
Grage, T. 160
Graham, F. L. 25
Graham, J. B. 97, 98, 272
Graham, R. M. 97, 98, 272
Graham, S. 22
Graham-Pole, J. 30, 102
Grand, L. C. 31
Granda, J. L. 210
Granger, R. A. 124
Grant, G. A. 140, 141
Grant, J. P. 91, 108
Grant, R. M. 278
Grasso, P. 9
Graw, R. G. 241, 242, 243
Gray, G. R. 196
Gray, L. H. 69
Greaves, M. F. 82
Green, H. N. 20, 21, 75, 79
Greenberg, A. H. 100
Greene, H. S. N. 13, 50, 57, 61
Greene, M. I. 233
Gregg, R. S. 17
Gregorio, R. 47
Gresser, I. 222

Griesbach, W. E. 31
Griffin, A. C. 31
Griffith, A. H. 234
Griffiths, J. D. 55, 57
Griscelli, C. 247
Grob, P. J. 40, 41, 80
Gros, Ch. 2
Gross, K. 50
Gross, L. 25, 26, 31, 87, 88, 93
Grossberg, A. L. 168
Grosser, N. 103
Grossi, C. E. 56
Groupe, V. 27
Grover, P. L. 19
Gruneison, A. 88
Guegan, J. H. 25
Guelfi, J. 204
Guérin, C. 189
Guillou, P. J. 82
Gulati, S. C. 29, 30
Gunter, S. E. 197
Gunven, P. 28, 29, 115, 116
Gurdon, J. B. 17
Gurland, J. 62
Gurrioch, D. B. 82
Guthrie, D. 269
Gutterman, J. U. 104, 111, 234, 252, 253, 254, 273
Guyer, R. J. 263
Gyenes, L. 172
Gynning, I. 59
Gyure, L. 202

H

Haagensen, C. D. 154
Haaland, M. 10
Habel, K. 91, 92
Hackett E. 275
Haddow, A. 1, 24, 76, 223
Hadfield, G. 59
Hageman, P. C. 25
Hagmar, B. 221
Hakkinen, I. 107
Halbherr, T. 212
Halgrimson, C. G. 143
Hall, J. G. 135, 185
Hall, R. R. 270
Hall, S. J. 93
Hall, W. H. 31
Hall, W. T. 30
Hallahan, J. D. 60
Halle-Pannenko, O. 189, 192
Haller, O. 129, 132

Halliday, W. L. 103
Halpern, B. N. 190, 191, 192, 197, 200, 202, 204, 205, 206, 210, 211, 259, 262
Halsted, W. S. 153, 154
Halterman, R. H. 80, 97
Hamaoka, T. 216
Hamblin, T. J. 240
Hamburg, V. P. 91
Hamilton, D. N. H. 162
Hamilton, J. M. 8
Hamilton, M. S. 110
Hamilton, T. 154
Hamlin, I. M. E. 96
Hammond, C. B. 156
Hammond, V. 140
Hammond, W. G. 94
Han, T. 82, 104
Hanau, A. 10, 86
Hanczakowska, M. 124
Handler, A. H. 13
Handler, H. I. 16
Handley, R. S. 61, 154, 154f
Handley, W. S. 51, 52, 153
Hank, W. A. 264
Hanlon, J. T. 47
Hanna, M. G. 108, 192, 194, 228
Hansen, H. J. 106, 107
Hansen, W. H. 11
Haran, N. 20
Haran-Ghera, N. 32
Hard, G. C. 9
Harder, F. H. 91, 98
Harding, B. 100
Hardisty, R. N. 156
Hargreaves, R. 136
Harland, S. 149
Harnden, D. G. 16, 34, 45
Harridge, W. H. 58
Harries, E. J. 50, 150
Harris, H. 44, 45
Harris, J. R. 111
Harris, N. S. 232
Harris, R. 111
Harrison, R. G. 13
Hartley, J. W. 25
Hartman, J. T. 270
Hartmann, D. (Hartman, D.) 136
Hartmann, J. 237
Hartveit, F. 171, 186
Harvey, E. K. 57
Harvey, H. A. 260
Harvey, J. J. 140
Haskell, E. M. 260
Haskill, J. S. 48, 100, 127
Hattan, D. 141, 144
Hattler, B. G. 83
Hattori, T. 209, 242

Haughton, G. 92, 101, 122, 141
Hausman, M. S. 84
Hawkins, R. A. 4
Hay, D. 26
Hayat, M. 219
Haybittle, J. L. 150, 154
Hayes, E. F. 140
Hays, E. F. 26
Hayward, J. 154
Haywood, G. R. 43, 111
Healey, J. E. 54
Heaton, C. 210
Hedlöf, I. 97
Heidelberger, C. 20, 145
Heinonen, O. P. 21
Heiskell, C. A. 152
Hellman, S. 97, 168
Hellström, I. 30, 89, 90, 91, 92, 95, 100, 101, 109,
    116, 121, 122, 135, 136, 167, 232, 237
Hellström, K. E. 30, 90, 91, 101, 109, 116, 121,
    122, 135, 136, 167, 232, 237, 238
Helm, F. 269
Helpap, B. 68
Hems, G. 258
Henderson, B. E. 32
Henderson, D. C. 198
Henderson, M. A. 270
Hendrickx, A. C. 37
Henle, G. 98, 99
Henle, W. 98, 99
Henney, C. S. 116, 130, 191
Henon, P. 85
Hensle, T. W. 235
Heppner, F. 213
Herberman, R. B. 43, 80, 89, 93, 99, 100, 104,
    105, 108, 109, 127, 128, 129, 130, 131, 132,
    133, 191, 199, 201, 204, 217, 218
Herbst, A. L. 21
Héricourt, J. 238
Herman, E. C. 241
Herold, G. E. 80
Herrera, M. A. 107
Hersey, P. 100, 131, 168, 184, 280
Hersh, E. M. 80, 244, 252
Hershorn, K. 82
Heslop, B. F. 138
Heston, W. E. 34
Hevin, B. 204
Hewett, C. L. 19
Hewitt, H. B. 11, 12, 53, 55, 56, 94, 144, 208, 234
Hewlett, J. S. 252
Heyes, J. 219
Heyn, R. M. 252
Hibbs, J. B. 123, 124, 127, 191, 201, 202
Hieger, I. 19
Higgins, G. A. 159
Hilberg, A. W. 55

Hildemann, W. H. 171
Hiles, R. W. 156
Hilf, R. 85
Hilgard, P. 221
Hill, A. B. 5, 21
Hill, G. J. 160, 168
Hill, J. M. 31
Hill, L. E. 7
Hill M. 27
Hill, R. D. 51
Hilleman, M. R. 218, 265
Hillova, J. 27
Hines, J. R. 158
Hirano, M. 213
Hirayama, T. 32
Hirsch, H. M. 87, 93
Hirsch, M. S. 144
Hirsh, B. B. 27
Hirshaut, Y. 260, 263, 267
Hitchcock, E. 207, 210, 223, 230
Hiu, I. J. 196
Hoag, W. G. 9
Hobbs, J. R. 100
Hochberg, M. 50
Hochman, A. 83
Hochman, P. 128, 130
Hodges, C. V. 76
Hodgkinson, A. 71
Hodson, M. E. 80
Hoebeke, J. 221
Hoecker, G. 174
Hoerni, B. 253
Hofer, K. G. 67
Hoffken, K. 136, 229
Hoffman, F. 90
Hoffman, J. 68
Hoffmann, G. W. 113
Hogg, N. 124, 127, 131
Holborow, E. J. 80, 82
Holden, H. T. 48, 100, 127, 128, 129, 130, 131,
    132, 199, 201
Holden, W. D. 160
Holland, E. 54
Holland, J. F. 224, 225, 226, 273, 278
Hollenberg, N. K. 53
Hollinshead, A. 104, 111
Hollman, K. H. 29
Holloman, J. H. 17
Holm, G. 82, 99
Holmes, E. C. 93
Holtermann, O. A. 124, 127
Holyoke, E. D. 56
Hoover, H. C. 160, 268
Hoover, R. 143
Hoppe, E. 56
Hopper, D. G. 192, 194, 195, 221, 229
Horn, H. L. 237, 238

Horn, K. -H. 90, 91
Horn, L. 237
Horn, R. C. 71
Horning, E. S. 24
Horowitz, S. 152
Horsfall, F. L. 16
Hortobagyi, G. N. 254
Horwitz, K. B. 77
Houchens, D. P. 208
Houck, J. C. 74
Hough, D. W. 240
Howard, A. 99
Howard, J. G. 191, 198, 199, 204
Howard, J. M. 3
Howe, G. M. 21
Howell, K. M. 80
Hubbard, J. D. 171
Huber, B. 119
Hudson, C. N. 279
Huebner, R. J. 27, 220
Hueper, W. C. 22
Huggins, C. 31, 76
Hughes, L. E. 57, 81, 104, 273
Hughes, P. E. 19
Humble, J. G. 48
Humphrey, G. 260
Humphrey, L. J. 49, 161, 245, 273, 274
Humphries, R. E. 21
Hung, W. 71
Hunt, R. 37
Hunter-Craig, I. 264
Hustu, H. O. 160
Hutchin, P. 137
Hutter, R. V. P. 155
Huvos, A. G. 155
Hyman, R. 93

I

IARC 19, 21
Ichikawa, K. 19
Ida, N. 35
Ihle, J. N. 129
Iio, M. 83
Ikonopisov, R. L. 272
Ilfeld, D. 89, 177
Illmensee, K. 17
Im, H. M. 182
Inchley, M. P. 115, 171, 209, 231
Ingrand, J. 83
Inoue, M. 45
Invernizzi, G. 37, 111
Ioachim, H. L. 18, 48, 95, 96, 97

Iorio, A. 132
Irino, S. 26
Irvin, G. L. 137, 470
Irvine, W. J. 115
Irving, C. C. 20
Isa, A. M. 127
Isaacs, A. 221
Ishibashi, T. 190
Ishizuka, M. 216, 217, 218
Ishmael, D. R. 260
Island, D. 70
Israel, L. 81, 82, 83, 243, 259, 260, 261, 262, 263, 280
Israels, L. G. 172
Isselbacher, K. J. 106
Isturiz, M. A. 100
Ito, Y. 92
Itoh, T. 3
Ivanyi, J. 167
Iversen, O. H. 67, 68, 69
Ivins, J. C. 160, 248
Iwasaki, T. 55
Iwasutiak, R. 27
Izawa, T. 237

J

Jacob, F. 16
Jacobitz, J. L. 226
Jacobs, D. M. 195
Jacobs, J. B. 48
Jaffe, N. 160
Jagarlamoody, S. M. 89, 100, 244
Jakoubková, J. 275
James, K. 49, 81, 127, 198, 263
Jamieson, C. W. 225
Jandiski, J. 118
Jaroslow, B. N. 215
Jarrett, O. 26
Jarrett, W. 8, 26
Jayne, W. H. W. 48
Jeejeebhoy, H. F. 138, 141
Jehn, U. W. 102, 104, 112
Jenkins, G. D. 60
Jennette, J. C. 136, 229
Jensen, C. O. 10, 86, 223
Jensen, E. V. 77, 87, 161
Jensen, F. C. 121
Jensen, H. M. 30
Jerne, N. K. 113
Jerry, L. M. 136
Jesseph, J. E. 52
Jha, K. K. 44

Jick, H. 21
Johansson, B. 82, 83
Johnson, A. G. 215, 216, 217, 218, 284
Johnson, H. G. 216
Johnson, J. L. 197
Johnson, P. R. 184
Johnson, R. A. 170
Johnson, R. M. 152
Johnson, R. O. 62
Johnson, S. 141
Jolles, P. 212
Jonasson, O. 55
Jondal, M. 29, 82, 100, 115, 116, 132
Jones, B. M. 102
Jones, D. 219
Jones, H. E. H. 162
Jones, H. W. 46
Jones, J. E. 71
Jones, J. T. 200, 201, 204
Jones, P. D. E. 211
Jones, S. E. 160, 253
Jonsson, N. 92
Joo, P. 103
Joshi, V. V. 27
Jurin, M. 185
Jutila, J. W. 233

K

Kahan, B. D. 111
Kahane, I. 190
Kahn, M. C. 11
Kahn, M. F. 80
Kaiser, L. 70
Kaiser, R. F. 55
Kaliss, N. 10, 83
Kall, M. A. 89
Kallman, R. F. 50
Kamel, M. 188, 189, 206
Kamo, I. 85
Kampschmidt, R. F. 83
Kanazir, D. T. 215
Kandaloft, S. 154
Kaplan, A. M. 175, 201, 202, 210
Kaplan, E. L. 4
Kaplan, H. S. 26, 27, 31, 80, 174
Kappas, A. 162
Kark, A. E. 82
Karlson, A. G. 10
Kaschka-Dierich, C. 29
Katsuki, H. 159
Katz, D. H. 99, 107, 114, 118, 121, 184, 216
Katz, J. 99
Kausel, H. W. 255

Kay, H. E. M. 156, 252
Kearney, R. 91, 116, 273
Keast, D. 204
Kedar, E. 89, 177, 180
Keehn, R. J. 159
Keeler, C. E. 22
Keith, H. I. 82
Keller, A. R. 48
Keller, R. 123, 124, 126
Kellock, T. H. 271
Kelly J. F. 13
Kelly, M. T. 192
Kelly, P. A. 77
Kelly, W. D. 81
Kenis, Y. 160
Kennaway, E. L. 19, 21
Kennedy, C. T. C. 186
Kennedy, T. H. 31
Kenny, T. E. 69
Kerbel, R. S. 48, 49, 85, 188
Kerman, R. H. 257
Kern, D. H. 187, 249
Kerpe, S. 96
Kerr, J. F. R. 69, 70
Kersey, J. H. 142, 226, 230
Kessel, J. 60
Ketcham, A. S. 56, 81, 101, 136, 221, 224
Kiang, D. T. 71
Kidd, J. G. 20, 88, 167
Kieler, J. 94, 146
Kiessling, R. (Keissling, R.) 116, 127, 128, 129,
        130, 131, 132, 147
Kiger, N. 284
Kikuchi, K. 95
Kilburn, D. G. 82
Killion, J. J. 188, 225, 228
Kim, C. -A. H. 168, 169, 192
Kim, J. H. 112
Kim, J. S. 157
King, E. R. 68
King, T. J. 17
Kingma, F. J. 126
Kingston, A. 152
Kinlen, L. J. 22, 23, 34, 143, 144
Kirchner, H. 93, 199, 201
Kirkpatrick, C. H. 247
Kirsch, R. 757
Kirsten, W. H. 30
Kitabchi, A. E. 71
Kitagawa, M. 216, 217
Kiviniemi, K. 163
Klausner, C. 13
Kleenman, M. S. 106
Klein, E. 11, 45, 88, 91, 92, 94, 96, 97, 98, 99, 100,
        111, 112, 124, 127, 129, 137, 144, 146, 167, 269
Klein, G. 12, 13, 29, 44, 45, 46, 63, 87, 88, 91, 92,
        94, 95, 96, 97, 98, 99, 100, 101, 111, 112,
        113, 138, 144, 146, 169, 234

Klein, H. O. 157
Klein, J. 26
Klein, M. 45
Klein, P. A. 214, 224
Klemperer, M. R. 157
Knill-Jones, R. P. 71
Knorpp, C. 240
Knudson, A. G. 18, 34
Kobayashi, H. 214, 227, 274
Koch, M. A. 92
Kodama, T. 227, 274
Kohler, G. 283
Kohn, J. 106
Koldovsky, P. 87, 92, 98, 167, 170, 176, 177, 234
Koller, P. C. 88, 174
Kollmorgen, C. M. 188, 225, 228
Kölsch, E. 137
Komeda, T. 88
Komuro, K. 129
Konda, S. 82
Kondo, K. 3, 83, 104, 137
Kopf, A. W. 219
Kopp, H. G. 32
Koprowska, I. 214
Koprowski, H. 44, 132, 214
Korenman, S. G. 77
Kourilsky, F. M. 103
Kouznetzova, B. 36, 206, 212
Krahenbuhl, J. L. 124, 201
Krant, M. J. 81
Krebs, C. 26
Krebs, J. A. 51
Kreider, J. W. 219, 220
Krementz, E. T. 157, 245, 248, 255, 272
Krigbaum, L. G. 191
Kripke, M. L. 124, 195
Krivit, W. 237
Krueger, R. G. 93
Kruger, G. 88
Krupey, J. 107
Kufe, D. 30
Kumar, S. 80
Kung, J. T. 125, 202
Kuper, S. W. A. 55
Kuperman, O. 89, 191
Kurnick, N. B. 157, 241
Kurth, R. 30, 108

L

Lachmann, P. J. 230
Lacour, F. 220
Ladisch, S. 108
Lagrange, P. H. 189, 190, 224

Laing, C. A. 111
Laird, A. K. 62, 63, 64, 65
Laird, H. 26
Laki, K. 57
Lala, P. K. 10, 66, 68, 69, 70
Lamb, D. 81
Lambert, L. H. 124, 201, 202
Lambert, R. P. 143
Lamensans, A. 206
Lamerton, L. F. 66, 67
Lamon, E. W. 100, 114, 115, 116, 117
Lampson, G. P. 218
Lance, E. M. 200
Lancet, The 7, 8, 14, 51, 77
Landes, J. 168
Landi, S. 189
Landy, M. 90, 133
Lane, M. -A. 26
Lane Brown, M. M. 264
Langlands, A. O. 34, 154
Lankester, A. 40
Lapeyraque, F. 192, 213, 231
Lapp, W. 122
Lappé, M. A. 138, 147, 162
Laroye, G. J. 135
Larsen, V. 57
Larson, D. L. 80
Laszlo, J. 237
Lauder, I. 48
Lawrence, E. B. 74
Lavrin, D. H. 35, 93, 108, 127, 129, 130
Law, L. W. 24, 31, 87, 92, 111, 139, 140, 141, 179, 219, 220
Lawrence, H. S. 175, 247
Lawrence, N. 193, 195
Lawrence, W. 160
Lazlo, J. 43
Lebredo, M. G. 271
Leclerc, C. 196
Le Clerc, J. C. 25, 92, 93, 113, 116
Lederer, E. 35
Leditschke, J. F. 152
Lee, A, K. Y. 81
Lee, R. B. 31
Lee, J. A. H. 22
Lee, J. C. 129
Le Fever, A. V. 225
Le Garrec, Y. 35
Le Gendre, S. 171
Lehmann, A. R. 23
Lehoczky, A. 97
Leiberman, M. 26
Leighton, R. S. 52
Leis, H. P. 48, 105
Lejeune, F. 101, 272
Le Mevel, B. P. 108
Lemonde, P. 37
Lengerova, A. 176

Lennox, E. 37, 108
Lennox, E. S. 100
Leoffler, R. K. 63
Leonard, B. J. 217, 218
Leonard, E. J. 84
Leong, J. L. 34
Leskowicz, S. 81
Leslie, P. 195
Lespinats, G. 93
Levan, G. 42
Le Veen, H. H. 270
Leventhal, B. G. 97, 101, 103, 277
Levey, R. H. 116, 140
Levi, E. 89, 170, 239
Levi, E. L. 68
Levij, I. S. 34
Levin, A. 269
Levin, A. G. 3, 81
Levin, A. S. 248
Levin, W. 19
Levine, E. M. 40, 74
Levine, M. 201
Levine, P. H. 101
Levine, R. J. 72
Levinthal, J. D. 31
Levis, A. G. 158
Levy, H. B. 35, 219, 220, 266
Levy, I. S. 35
Levy, J. G. 91, 95, 111
Levy, J. P. 25, 92, 93, 113, 116
Levy, M. H. 124, 127
Levy, N. L. 101
Lewis, F. J. 152
Lewis, M. G. 99, 107, 136, 257
Lewis, M. R. 13, 224
Lewis, W. H. 13
Libansky, J. 81
Liddle, G. W. 70
Lieberman, M. W. 38
Lieberman, R. 257
Liegey, A. 37
Likhite, V. V. 206, 207, 210, 211, 230
Lilly, F. 33, 92
Lindahl, T. 13
Lindenmann, J. 214, 215, 221, 224, 265
Linder, D. 46
Linder, O. E. A. 83
Lindholm, L. 122
Lindsey, A. J. 22
Lindskog, G. E. 152
Lindstrom, G. A. 239
Linford, J. H. 172
Ling, N. R. 29, 134
Links, J. 25
Linman, J. W. 81
Linn, J. E. 71
Linscott, W. D. 172

Liozner, A. L. 83
Lipscomb, H. S. 71
Lipsky, P. E. 121
Lisafield, B. A. 124
Little, C. C. 10, 87
Little, V. A. 138
Littlejohn, K. 168
Littlewood, G. 79
Litwin, J. 206
Livnat, S. 178
Lizardo, J. G. 83
Lloyd-Davies, O. V. 58
Lo Buglio, A. E. 247, 248
Loc, T. B. 172
Lochte, H. L. 241
Loeb, L. 10
Loewi, G. 99
Logan, J. 81
Lo Gerfo, P. 107
Lohmann-Matthes, M. L. 119, 124
Loizner, A. L. 91
Lonai, P. 116
Londner, M. V. 186
London Hospital Clinical Trials Unit 5
Long, J. C. 45
Longmire, W. P. 160
Loor, F. 139
Lorenz, E. K. 174
Lotzová, E. 122, 123, 130
Loutit, J. F. 22, 27, 93, 174
Love, R. 214
Lozzio, B. B. 13
Lüben, G. 226
Luce, J. K. 152
Ludogovskaya, L. A. 97
Ludwig Lung Cancer Study Group 262
Luft, R. 76
Lund, P. K. 13
Lundak, R. L. 89
Lundblad, G. 97
Lundgren, G. 117, 178
Lynch, H. T. 34
Lynch, N. R. 188, 207
Lyons, M. J. 25
Lytton, B. 104

MC

McBean, M. A. 101
McBride, A. 277
McBride, W. H. 197, 198, 200, 201, 203, 204, 206, 210, 211, 212, 259, 272
McCallum, H. M. 43

McCarthy, R. E. 83
McClatchy, J. K. 191
McCloy, E. 99
McCollester, D. L. 111
McCormack, R. J. M. 261
McCormick, J. J. 23
McCormick, T. 270
McCorquodale, D. W. 76
McCoy, J. L. 92, 93, 102, 140
McCracken, A. 204
McCredie, J. A. 63, 239
McCune, W. S. 245
McCutcheon, M. 56
McDermott, M. V. 235
McDonald, H. R. 116, 270
McDonald, T. T. 199, 200
MacDowell, E. C. 174
McEndy, D. P. 31
McEwen, L. M. 97
McFarland, W. 241
McGinty, F. 194
MacGregor, A. B. 254
McGregor, D. D. 247
McGuigan, J. E. 71
McGuire, W. L. 77
McIllmurray, M. P. 279
McIntosh, A. T. 100, 127
McIntyre, R. O. 265, 266
McIvor, K. L. 124, 125
Mackaness, G. B. 189, 190, 224
McKay, E. N. 150
Mackay, I. R. 33, 81, 143
Mackay, W. D. 81, 88
McKearn, T. J. 181
McKhann, C. F. 43, 89, 91, 98, 100, 111, 244
Macklin, M. T. 34
McKneally, M. F. 255
McLaren, A. 17f
McLaughlin, J. F. 124
MacLean, N. 34
MacLennan, I. C. M. 99, 100
McLeod, G. R. 150
MacMahon, B. 29, 32, 34
McPeak, C. J. 245
MacPherson, B. R. 201, 204
McQuarrie, I. 1
McWhirter, R. 61, 65, 154

M

Mach, J. P. 107
Maciera-Coehlo, A. 40
Madden, J. L. 154

Maddox, I. 85
Madoc-Jones, H. 158
Maeda, Y. Y. 222
Magarey, C. J. 83, 155, 162
Magee, P. N. 21
Magrath, I. T. 160, 253
Maguire, H. 13
Mahaley, M. S. 101, 239
Mahé, E. 260
Maher, V. M. 23
Main, J. M. 88, 91, 94
Maini, M. M. 24
Makari, J. G. 97
Malaise, E. P. 67
Mallucci, L. 41
Malmgren, R. A. 24, 30, 96, 98, 213
Malpas, J. S. 160
Maluish, A. 103
Manes, C. 16
Mankiewicz, E. 257, 279
Mann, D. L. 97
Mann, F. C. 10
Mann, L. T. 60
Manni, J. A. 100
Mannick, J. A. 141, 186, 206, 208, 217, 219
Manning, D. D. 233
Mansell, P. W. A. 123, 245
Manson, L. A. 89
Marchalonis, J. J. 216
Marchant, J. 83
Marcove, R. C. 160, 272
Marcum, R. G. 30
Marcuse, R. A. 71
Mardiney, M. R. 168, 171, 172
Margolese, R. G. 195
Margulis, A. R. 54
Mariano, M. 126
Mark, J. 42
Marks, L. J. 71
Marmion, B. P. 206, 210, 211
Marquardt, H. 35
Marrone, J. A. 224
Marsh, B. 245, 246
Marshall, A. H. E. 49
Marshall, V. C. 23, 143
Martensson, L. 45
Marthaler, T. 159
Martin, D. S. 12
Martin, G. M. 34
Martin, L. 66
Martin, M. 192
Martin, M. S. 12
Martin, S. E. 147
Martin, W. J. 111, 147
Martinez, C. 140
Martinez, J. 283
Martland, H. S. 21

Martz, E. 116
Masina, M. H. 13
Mason, A. Y. 154
Mason, D. Y. 99
Mason, K. 208
Mastrangelo, M. J. 278
Masuda, M. 235
Mathé, G. 74, 172, 175, 179, 180, 181, 184, 185,
    188, 189, 192, 206, 213, 219, 223, 231, 234,
    241, 242, 243, 251, 255, 257, 275, 276, 277,
    279
Matsumoto, T. 88, 111
Matsushima, T. 20
Matthias, J. Q. 81
Maurer, A. M. 68
Maurer, W. 68
Maury, C. 222
Maver, C. 255
Mavligit, G. M. 104, 252, 253
Mawas, C. 81
Mayneord, W. V 63
Mayr, A. C. 259, 262
Mazurek, C. 209
Meador, C. K. 70
Meadows, L. 84
Medawar, P. B. 37, 87, 136f, 189
Medical Research Council 5, 6, 252
Medley, G. 100
Meerpohl, H. -G. 119
Meesmann, H. 226
Meier, H. 32, 220
Meier, P. 4
Mellors, R. C. 33
Mellstedt, H. 82, 284
Melnick, J. L. 29
Meltzer, M. S. 123, 124, 191
Mempel, W. 168
Menard, S. 108, 109
Mendelsohn, M. L. 62, 63, 66, 67
Menzies, D. N. 13
Meriadec de Byans, B. 107
Merigan, T. C. 35, 216, 218, 284
Merler, E. 49
Merrill, J. M. 22
Merrill, J. P. 281
Merritt, C. B. 182
Merritt, K. 215
Metcalf, D. 26, 32
Metcalf, W. 4
Metchnikoff, E. 125
Metchnikoff, O. 125
Metz, S. A. 72
Metzgar, R. S. 31
Meunier-Rotival, M. 19, 20, 38
Meyer, G. 111
Meyer, T. J. 196
Meyers, O. L. 102

Meyers, P. 92
Michaels, L. 56, 57, 268
Mickey, M. R. 100, 101, 127
Micklem, H. S 129
Mider, G. B. 79
Mihailovich, N. 34
Mihich, E. 100, 176
Miké, V. 160, 272
Mikulska, Z. B. 88, 91, 95, 126, 176
Milas, L. 36, 124, 197, 199, 200, 202, 204, 205,
    206, 207, 208, 210, 211, 259, 262
Miles, C. P. 42
Millar, D. 83
Miller, B. J. 54
Miller, D. G. 83, 167
Miller, E. C. 16, 19
Miller, G. F. 93
Miller, H. C. 60
Miller, J. A. 16, 19
Miller, J. F. A. P. 24, 25, 31, 116, 117, 120, 121,
    139, 140, 141, 176
Miller, J. H. 31
Miller, J. J. 83
Miller, O. J. 44
Miller, R. G. 116, 119
Miller, R. W. 30, 34
Miller, T. E. 190, 224
Miller, T. R. 250
Miller, W. R. 77
Millman, I. 212
Milne, I. 198
Milstein, C. 283
Milton, G. W. 51, 156, 264
Minden, P. 191, 195
Minor, P. D. 66
Minton, J. P. 260, 262, 263
Mintz, B. 16, 17
Mirvish, S. S. 20
Misdorp, W. 9
Mitchell, D. N. 13
Mitchell, M. S. 190
Mitcheson, H. D. 260
Mitchison, J. M. 66
Mitchison, N. A. 87, 88, 136, 174
Mitchley, B. C. V. 78
Mitelman, F. 42
Miyabo, S. 71
Miyaji, T. 19
Miyanaga, T. 235
Mizejewski, G. J. 169, 170
Mizel, S. B. 120
Mizuno, D. 213
Mkheidze, D. M. 83
Moayeri, H. 260
Mobbs, B. G. 77
Moertel, C. C. 18, 253, 256
Mohos, S. C. 167

Mohr, U. 19, 213
Mokyr, M. B. 177, 190
Mole, R. H. 27
Möller, E. 11, 115, 122, 134, 145, 147
Möller, G. 115, 117, 134, 145, 147, 166, 167, 178
Moloney, J. B. 25, 140
Mondovi, B. 270
Monga, J. N. 140
Monis, B 49
Monod, J. 16
Moon, H. D. 31
Moore, A. E. 3, 214, 264
Moore, D. H. 25, 29, 30, 99
Moore, G. E. 55, 243, 244, 245, 270, 273
Moore, G. F. 55
Moore, M. 101, 111, 193, 195
Moore, M. B. 244
Moore, T. L. 107
Morahan, P. S. 175, 201, 202, 210
Morales, A. 71, 256
Moran, R. E. 67
More, D. G. 126
Moreno, R. 222
Moreschi, C. 80
Morfit, M. 153
Morgan, A. G. 83
Morgan, C. N. 58
Mori, A. 209
Mori, R. 139
Mori, W. 235
Morii, S. 76
Moroni C. 136
Moroson, H. 208
Morrison, A. S. 48
Morrow, H. S. 83
Morse, P. A. 49, 248
Morton, D. L. 30, 38, 81, 89, 91, 93, 96, 98, 101, 135, 136, 152, 168, 176, 224, 253, 254, 279
Möse, G. 213
Möse, J. R. 213, 264
Mosedale, B. 204
Mosley, J. G. 84
Mosonov, I. 101
Motta, R. 172, 234
Mouton, D. 206
Moynihan, B. G. A. (Lord Moynihan) 153
Mozes, E. 216
Muckle, D. S. 270
Müftüoğlu, A. Ü. 81
Muggia, F. M. 269, 271
Muggleton, P. W. 195
Muhlbock, O. 33
Muhm, J. R. 2
Müller, W. 159
Müller-Eberhard, H. J. 171
Mulvihill, J. J. 34

Muna, N. M. 98
Murphy, J. B. 48, 87
Murray, G. 238
Murray, J. A. 10
Murray, J. G. 155
Murray-Lyon, I. M. 157
Myers, D. D. 220
Myers, W. L. 216

N

Nachtigal, D. 137, 215, 227
Nadkarni, J. S. 29, 45
Nadler, S. H. 87, 234, 245, 273
Nagasawa, H. 77
Naha, P. M. 20
Nahmias, A. J. 29
Naib, Z. M. 29
Nairn, R. G. 43, 75, 98, 99, 101
Nakahara, W. 79
Nakano, M. 215, 216, 218
Nakas, Y. 91
Nandi, S. 26
Nathan, C. F. 191
Nathanson, L. 96, 234, 255
National Cancer Institute 234
Natvig, J. B. 100
Nauts, H. C. 52, 235, 247, 250
Neff, J. R. 245, 246
Negroni, G. 172
Nehlsen, S. L. 141
Neidhart, J. A. 247, 248
Nelson, D. S. 29, 80, 82, 85, 91, 98, 116, 120, 126, 127, 200
Nelson, M. 29, 85, 92
Nemoto, T. 82
Neveu, P. J. 190
Neveu, T. 198
Newlands, E. S. 278
Newman, C. E. 239
Newman, W. 264
Newstead, G. L. 57
Newton, K. A. 241
Ngu, V. A. 237
Nicholls, M. F. 60
Nicholson, J. T. 250
Nicolson, G. L. 41, 57
Niederhuber, J. E. 120
Niederman, J. C. 29
Nigam, S. P. 172
Nikoskelainen, J. 29
Nilsonne, U. 103, 104
Nilsson, A. 35

Nilsson, U. R. 171
Nimberg, R. B. 85
Nisbet, N. W. 127
Nishioka, K. 96, 99
Nishioka, M. 106
Nkrumah, F. K. 156
Nolan, B. 242, 243
Nomoto, K. 139, 146
Noonan, C. D. 54
Noonan, F. P. 231
Noonan, K. D. 41
Nordin, A. A. 116
Nordling, S. 41
Nordlund, J. J. 266
Norman, R. L. 271
Normann, S. J. 84
North, R. J. 84, 85, 198, 200, 210, 212
Norton, L. 65
Nouza, K. 180
Novinsky, M. 10
Nowell, P. C. 22
Noyes, W. F. 28
Nungester, W. 240
Nunn, A. J. 7
Nunn, M. E. 127, 128, 129, 130, 131
Nussenzweig, R. S. 204

O

Ochoa, M. 259, 262
O'Connell, L. G. 277
O'Conor, G. T. 28
Odili, J. L. I. 272
Oehler, J. R. 131, 204
Oettgen, H. F. 87, 95, 111, 197, 234, 247, 267, 268
Ojo, E. 128, 130
Okazaki, W. 25
Olcott, C. T. 9
Old, J. L. 35, 43, 87, 88, 90, 91, 92, 98, 112, 117, 138, 168, 190, 192
Oldham, R. K. 101, 128, 131
Olivecrona, H. 76
Oliver, R. T. D. 31, 99, 278
Olivotto, M. 201, 202, 206, 209, 210
Olsnes, S. 77
Olsson, L. 251
Olurin, E. O. 71
O'Meara, R. A. Q. 57
Omenn, G. S. 72
O'Neill, G. J. 168, 173, 198, 201
Onikul, S. R. 208
Oon, C. J. 240, 246

Opler, S. R. 48, 96
Oppenheimer, B. S. 24
Oppenheimer, E. T. 24
Orbach-Arbouys, S. 190
Order, S. E. 97, 168, 169, 170
Oren, M. E. 104
O'Riordan, M. L. 42
Orizaga, M. 104
Ormerod, M. G. 124
Oronsky, A. L. 191
Ortaldo, J. R. 131
Orth, D. N. 71
Osborn, D. E. 260, 262
Osoba, D. 116
Ossorio, R. C. 260, 262
Osunkoya, B. O. 99
Otaki, H. 20
Oth, D. 37, 90, 91, 111, 122
O' Toole, C. 101, 115
Otsu, K. 88
Outzen, H. C. 141, 142
Owen, J. J. T. 116
Owen, L. N. 8, 9, 192
Ozer, H. L. 44

P

Pack, G. T. 23, 153, 264
Pacque, R. E. 186
Palat, A. 268
Palmer, A. M. 184
Palmer, B. V. 262
Palmer, J. C. 89
Paluch, E. 95, 96
Pantelouris, E. M. 139
Papaioannou, V. E. 17
Papamichail, M. 82
Papanicolaou, G. N. 55
Papatestas, A. E. 82
Park, I. J. 46
Parke, D. V. 16, 19
Parker, R. 37
Parker R. C. 213
Parker, R. G. 151
Parks, L. C. 239
Parmiani, G. 37, 111, 145
Parr, I. B. 190, 192, 213, 219, 220
Parsons, M. 96
Paslin, D. 210
Pass, E. 191
Pasternak, G. 90, 91, 92, 98
Paterson, R. 154
Patey, D. H. 154

Patt, H. M. 63
Patterson, H. R. 13
Patterson, W. B. 13
Paukovits, W. R. 74
Paul, J. 14
Paull, J. 174
Pavelic, Z. 193
Pavia, R. A. 45
Payne, L. N. 8, 25
Pazmino, N. H. 36
Peacocke, I. 43
Pearl, R. 188
Pearse, A. G. E. 71
Pearson, G. 29, 99
Pearson, G. R. 114, 136, 166, 167
Pearson, J. W. 166, 192, 208, 221
Pearson, M. N. 227
Pearson, O. H. 77
Peckham, M. J. 68, 156
Pees, H. W. 101
Pelfrene, A. F. 21
Pellegrino, M. A. 115
Pellis, N. R. 111
Pels, E. 124
Peltier, A. 263
Penn, I. 60, 143, 144
Pereira, H. G. 37
Perkins, I. V. 156
Perlmann, H. 99
Perlmann, P. 99
Perper, R. J. 191
Persellin, H. H. 210
Peter H. H. 102, 131
Peters, L. C. 190
Peters, L. J. 11, 207
Peters, V. 154
Petitou, M. 226
Peto, R. 4, 5, 9, 17, 21, 252, 276, 277, 281
Petranyi, G. G. 132
Pettigrew, R. T. 270
Pfizenmaier, K. 130
Phillips, B. 13
Phillips, R. A. 119
Phillips, T. M. 99
Pierce, G. E. 90, 91, 116
Pieroni, R. E. 217
Pierpaoli, W. 32
Pierrepoint, C. G. 8
Pierres, M. 233
Piessens, W. F. 35, 123, 193
Pihl, A. 77
Pihl, E. 101
Pike, M. C. 84, 85, 141, 268
Pilch, D. J. F. 35
Pilch, Y. H. 94, 186, 187, 249
Pilet, C. 213
Pillai, A. 31

Pimm, M. V. 47, 108, 110, 189, 192, 194, 195, 206, 210, 220, 221, 226, 229, 255
Pinckard, R. N. 198, 200
Pincus, T. 30, 33
Pines, A. 254
Pinkel, D. 160
Pinkerton, H. 35
Pinn, V. W. 106
Pinsky, C. M. 81, 253, 255, 259, 268
Piper, C. E. 124
Plante, C. 213
Planterose, D. N. 35
Plata, F. 116
Platt, R. D. 16
Playfair, J. H. L. 118
Plescia, O. J. 85
Pocock, S. J. 5
Polak, J. M. 71
Pollack, S. B. 115, 190
Pollard, M. 92, 181, 183
Polliack, A. 34
Pool, E. H. 54
Pope, J. H. 28
Poplack, D. G. 191, 276
Porter, K. A. 126
Portman, B. 126
Poskanzer, D. C. 21
Posner, A. S. 210
Post, J. 68
Postnikova, Z. A. 26
Potmesil, M. 68
Pott, P. 19
Potter, C. W. 221
Potter, J. S. 174
Potter, M. 45, 93
Potter, M. R. 103
Pouillart, P. 191, 192, 213, 231
Povlsen, C. E. 13, 141
Powles, R. L. 5, 273, 277
Prager, M. D. 227
Pratt, C. B. 160
Prehn, R. T. 46, 50, 88, 90, 91, 93, 94, 107, 137, 138, 140, 145, 146, 147, 175
Presant, C. A. 260
Prescott, R. J. 154
Pressman, D. 168, 169
Preston, F. W. 83
Preud'Homme, J. L. 45
Preussman, R. 22
Prewitt, J. M. S. 62
Price, F. B. 247, 248
Price, M. R. 111, 112
Priester, W. A. 8
Prime, F. 270
Prinzmetal, M. 54
Prioleau, W. H. 137
Priori, E. S. 30

Pritchard, D. J. 30
Pritchard, H. 129
Prochnownik, E. V. 30
Proctor, J. W. 147, 208, 230, 232
Pross, H. F. 49, 91, 100, 101, 132
Pruitt, J. C. 55
Pryce, D. M. 96
Pryor, J. 221
Ptak, W. 124, 181
Pulvertaft, R. J. V. 48
Purchase, H. G. 25
Purtilo, D. T. 29
Purves, H. D. 31
Purves, L. R. 106
Puvion, F. 201, 202

Q

Quaglino, D. 82
Quevillon, M. 189

R

Rabbatt, A. G. 141
Rabotti, G. F. 26
Rabson, A. S. 24, 219, 220
Rabourdin, A. 206
Radov, L. A. 48, 100, 127
Raff, M. C. 113, 139
Raffel, S. 227
Raidt, D. J. 89
Rajewski, K. 233
Rajewski, M. F. 88
Ralph, P. 93
Ramming, K. P. 186, 187
Ramot, B. 268
Ran, M. 96
Rao, V. S. 111, 136
Rapaport, F. T. Preface, 81, 146, 247
Rapin, A. M. C. 40, 41 74
Rapp, F. 28, 221
Rapp, H. J. 98, 191, 195, 196, 229
Rask-Nielsen, H. C. 26
Ratner, A. C. 269
Rauchwerger, J. M. 122
Ravdin, R. G. 161
Rawls, W. E. 29
Ray, P. K. 193, 195, 224
Rebuck, J. W. 84

Redmon, C. W. 114, 136, 166, 167
Reed, R. C. 260, 262, 263, 279
Rees, J. A. 50, 83
Rees, K. 82
Rees, L. H. 71
Rees, R. C. 108, 109
Rees, R. J. W. 13
Refsum, S. B. 67
Regamey, R. H. 234
Rehn, T. G. 118
Reid, D. E. 212, 259
Reif, A. E. 168, 169, 171, 192
Reilly, C. A. 30
Reiner, J. 37, 91
Reittie, J. R. 13
Reizenstein, P. 277
Remington, J. S. 124, 201, 202, 216
Réynaud, M. 81
Renoux, G. 216, 221, 268
Renoux, M. 216, 221, 268
Retik, A. B. 221
Revesz, L. 35, 63, 88
Reynoso, G. 106, 107
Rezzesi, F. 188
Rhoads, C. R. 3
Ribacchi, R. 26
Ribi, E. E. 196
Riccardi, C. 132, 133
Rich, M. A. 92
Richards, V. 13
Richardson, R. L. 257
Richardson, W. W. 50, 150
Richet, C. 238
Richie, E. R. 180
Richmond, H. G. 75
Richter, P. H. 113
Richters, A. 48
Riddell, A. G. 246
Riesco, A. 82
Riesen, W. 80
Rigby, P. G. 186
Riggi, S. J. 83
Riggins, R. S. 94
Riggs, B. L. 71
Rinfert, A. P. 31
Rios, A. 225, 226, 230, 231
Ritts, R. E. 248
Riveros-Moreno, V. 212
Robbins, S. L. 19
Robert, F. 91
Roberts, M. M. 48, 81, 96, 97, 98, 104, 105
Roberts, S. S. 55, 58
Robertson, H. T. 43
Robinette, C. D. 159
Robins, R. A. 87, 149
Robinson, C. M. 171
Robinson, E. 83

Robinson, K. P. 56
Robinson, N. 101
Robinson, R. A. 265, 266
Roboz, J. P. 225, 273, 278
Robson, M. 153
Rocklin, R. E. 102, 103
Rodda, S. J. 124
Roder, J. C. 128, 131
Rodrigues, D. 108
Rodriguez, V. 252
Roe, F. J. C. 17, 20, 140, 141
Roelants, G. E. 139
Roenigk, H. 265
Rogers, G. T. 111
Rogoway, W. M. 244
Rohdenburg, G. L. 270
Roitt, I. M. 162
Rojas, A. F. 267
Rolley, R. J. 94
Rollinghoff, M. 89, 93, 116, 117, 177
Romsdahl, M. M. 56
Rose, N. R. 271
Rose, S. 232
Rosen, G. 160
Rosen, S. N. 71
Rosenau, W. 91, 176
Rosenbaum, A. S. 54
Rosenberg, E. B. 101, 128
Rosenberg, E. D. 80
Rosenberg, S. A. 102, 165, 234, 238, 244, 246
Rosenfeld, C. 226
Rosenstreich, D. L. 119, 120
Rosenthal, A. S. 121
Ross, J. M. 22
Rossi, G. B. 123
Roth, J. A. 52
Roubinian, J. R. 116
Roumiantzeff, M. 206, 259
Rous, P. 8, 10, 19, 20
Rouse, B. T. 93
Rousselot, L. M. 160
Rowe, W. P. 25
Rowland, G. F. 173
Rowley, J. D. 42
Rowley, M. 81
Rowntree, C. 21
Rubens, R. D. 166
Rubin, B. A. 35
Rubin, H. 40
Ruckdeschel, J. C. 235
Ruddle, N. H. 124
Rudenstam, C. M. 56, 147, 208, 230, 232
Rudolph, R. H. 241
Ruhl, H. 216, 217
Ruitenberg, E. J. 204
Rumma, J. 183
Ruoslahti, E. 41, 106

Russ, S. 271
Russell, B. R. G. 47
Russell, J. A. 277
Russell, M. 239
Russell, M. H. 154
Russell, R. J. 212
Russell, S. W. 48, 49, 51, 100, 127
Russfield, A. B. 83
Ryan, J. J. 56, 221
Ryan, R. F. 157
Ryggard, J. 13, 141
Ryser, H. J. P. 20
Rytömaa, T. 74, 75, 162, 163

S

Saal, J. G. 100, 115
Sabin, A. B. 92
Sabolovic, D. 213
Sachs, B. A. 71
Sachs, L. 40
Sadler, T. E. 205, 206, 208, 209, 211, 212
Sadowski, J. M. 221
Saffer, E. 176
Sagebiel, R. W. 46
St. Arneault, G. 224, 225
Sakato, N. 93
Sakouhi, M. 219
Saksela, E. 131, 133
Sakurai, M. 237
Salama, F. 72
Salaman, J. R. 83
Salaman, M. H. 20, 38
Salaman, P. F. 19
Salih, H. 77
Salinas, F. A. 108
Salky, N. K. 83
Salmon, S. E. 33, 63, 160
Salomon, J. -C. 188, 194, 207, 229
Salsbury, A. J. 13, 55, 57
Samellas, W. 60
Sample, W. F. 82
Samuelson, L. E. 118
Sanda, M. 191
Sandberg, A. A. 55, 237
Sander, S. 77
Sanders, B. R. 127
Sanderson, C. J. 100, 227
Sanford, B. H. 141, 224, 225
Sansing, W. A. 188
Santoli, D. 131, 132
Santos, G. W. 99, 101, 241, 242
Saphir, O. 235

Sarasin, A. 19, 20, 38
Sarkar, N. H. 29
Sarkar, S. 93
Sarma, D. S. R. 20
Sarma, K. P. 48
Sarma, P. S. 35
Sarna, G. 166
Sato, H. 92, 93
Sauter, C. 265
Savary, C. 130
Savel, H. 104
Scales, R. W. 227
Scaletta, L. F. 44
Scanlon, E. F. 3
Schabel, F. M. 158, 167
Schachat, D. A. 140
Scharnagel, I. 153
Schatten, W. E. 11
Schechter, B. 89
Schechter, M. 208
Schechtman, A. 89, 170, 239
Scheid, M. P. 129
Scheiffarth, F. 89
Scheinberg, L. C. 90
Schidlowsky, B. S. 30
Schilling, J. A. 13
Schilling, R. M. 119
Schlager, S. I. 186
Schlom, J. 29, 30
Schlosser, J. V. 244
Schlossman, S. F. 118
Schmidt, D. 270
Schmidtke, J. R. 216
Schoenberg, B. G. 18
Scholler, J. 27
Schöne, G. 105
Schorlemmer, H. U. 125, 203
Schour, L. 88
Schrek, R. 63
Schrodt, T. 102
Schulten, M. F. 152
Schulz, J. I. 283
Schumann, G. 136
Schwartz, E. E. 179
Schwartz, R. H. 121
Schwartz, R. S. 33, 144
Schwartz, W. B. 71
Schwartzbach, M. 89
Schwarzenberg, L. 234, 241, 243, 251, 256, 257,
        276
Scollard, D. 116
Scornik, J. C. 100
Scott, E. J. Van See Van Scott, E. J.
Scott, M. T. 36, 124, 197, 198, 199, 200, 201, 202,
        204, 205, 206, 207, 208, 209, 210, 211, 212,
        230, 259, 262
Sealy, W. C. 71

Searle, J. 69
Sedallian, J. P. 170
Sedlacek, H. H. 226, 227
Seeger, R. C. 116
Segall, A. 102
Segi, M. 22
Segre, D. 216
Sehon, A. H. 225
Seidel, B. 101
Seigler, H. F. 89, 278
Seiler, F. R. 226
Sekla, B. 89, 239
Selawry, O. A. 270
Selawry, O. S. 270
Seligman, M. 33
Sell, S. 106
Sellars, A. H. 150
Sellers, E. A. 31
Sellwood, R. A. 55
Sendo, F. 129
Seppälä, M. 106
Serrou, B. 192, 256
Sethi, K. K. 224, 226
Sexauer, C. L. 262
Shah, L. P. 108
Shah, S. A. 270
Shand, F. L. 126, 137, 175
Shands, J. W. 125
Shane, S. B. 71
Shapiro, D. 158
Sharma, B. 89
Sharman, M. 213
Sharpless, G. R. 214
Sharpton, T. B. 191
Shaw, R. K. 80
Sheard, C. E. 12, 13, 14
Shearer, G. M. 118
Shearer, W. T. 138
Shcil, A. G. R. 23, 143
Shellam, G. R. 92, 127, 131
Shen, E. W. 130
Shen, L. 100
Sherry, S. 71
Sherwin, R. P. 48
Sherwood, L. M. 71
Shevach, E. M. 121
Shields, R. 66, 72
Shields, R. R. 221
Shields, T. W. 152, 159
Shigeno, N. 170
Shin, H. S. 169
Shingleton, W. W. 83
Shirakawa, S. 42, 67, 69
Shirato, E. 168
Shiu, G. 35
Shivas, A. A. 54, 153
Shroff, S. 2, 60

Shubik, P. 20, 49
Shulman, S. 271
Shustik, C. 117
Shyrock, H. S. 63
Sicevic, S. 257
Siddons, A. H. M. 60
Sieber, S. M. 21
Siegel, B. V. 38, 168
Siegel, J. S. 64
Sikora, K. 37, 108, 230
Silagi, S. 219
Siler, V. E. 150
Silissi, G. 50
Silobrcic, V. 93
Silverman, M. S. 137
Silverman, N. A. 82
Silvers, W. K. 89, 181
Sime, G. C. 99
Simic, M. M. 215
Simmler, M. C. 257
Simmons, R. L. 182, 224, 225, 226, 230, 231, 253, 278, 279
Simon, R. M. 225
Simons, M. 30
Simova, J. 194
Simpson, E. 118, 141
Simpson, M. E. 31
Simpson-Herren, L. 68
Sims, P. 19
Sinay, P. 226
Singer, S. J. 41
Singh, S. 237
Singla, O. 205
Sjögren, B. 76
Sjögren, H. O. 37, 87, 90, 91, 92, 93, 136, 137, 167, 232
Skegg, D. 21
Skidmore, B. J. 114
Skinner, P. E. 8
Skipper, H. E. 158
Sklaroff, D. M. 60
Skowron-Cendrzak, A. 181
Skurkovich, S. V. 244, 273
Skurzak, H. M. 101, 115
Slack, N. H. 47
Slater, A. J. 252, 256
Slavina, E. G. 178
Slemmer, G. 50
Slettermark, B. 88, 92, 98
Šljivić, V. S. 198, 200, 203, 204
Sloboda, A. E. 168
Small, M. 137, 175, 177
Smirnova, E. 13
Smith, A. G. 91, 95, 111
Smith, Abbey R. See Abbey Smith, R.
Smith, C. 88, 91, 95
Smith, C. E. Gordon See Gordon Smith, C. E.

Smith, E. T. 116
Smith, G. V. 248, 255
Smith, H. G. 176, 194
Smith, J. A. 66, 108
Smith, J. B. 82
Smith, J. L. 51
Smith, K. S. 103
Smith, L. H. 70
Smith, L. (Lyndsay) H. 115, 168, 169
Smith, M. A. 204
Smith, P. J. 171
Smith, R. (Sir Rodney Smith, Lord Smith) 148
Smith, R. S. 264
Smith, R. T. 82, 90, 91, 111, 133
Smith, S. E. 199, 206
Smith, W. E. 19
Smith, W. J. 239
Smith, W. S. 4
Smithers, D. W. 15, 51, 80
Smithwick, E. M. 264
Snell, A. C. 13
Snell, G. D. 10, 87, 121, 122, 162
Snell, M. E. 13
Snodgrass, M. J. 226
Snyder, H. W. 30
Snyderman, M. 252
Snyderman, R. 83, 84, 85, 268
Snyderman, R. K. 83
Soderland, S. C. 125
Sodomann, C. P. 265
Sokal, J. E. 252
Solowey, A. C. 81, 247
Sommers, S. C. 13
Soothill J. F. 83
Sophocles A. M. 87, 234
Sorborg, M. 102
Sordat, B. 13
Sorkin, E. 84
Southam, C. M. 3, 20, 21, 84, 88, 90, 91, 234, 264, 271
Southwick, H. W. 58
Sparagana, M. 71
Sparck, J. V. 50, 76
Sparks, F. C. 192, 194, 226, 229
Sparrow, M. 179
Spector, B. D. 142
Spector, W. G. 126
Speedy, G. 36, 94, 208, 211
Speer, F. D. 48, 96
Spence, R. A. 173
Spence, R. J. 225
Spiegelman, S. 29, 30
Spitler, L. E. 247, 248, 267
Spivak, J. L. 72
Spratt, J. S. 63
Spratt, T. L. 63
Sprent, J. 176

Spriggs, A. I. 55
Stanbridge, E. 44
Stanley, E. R. 187
Stanton, M. F. 92, 103
Staquet, M. 5
Starling, E. H. 76
Starr, K. W. 78
Starr, S. 264
Starzl, T. E. 143, 246
Steel, C. M. 29, 134
Steel, G. G. 66, 67, 69
Steerenberg, P. A. 204
Stefani, S. S. 257
Stehlin, J. S. 13, 51, 157, 270
Steinkuller, C. B. 191
Stephenson, H. E. 51
Stephenson, J. R. 93
Stern, K. 84, 91
Stern, P. 37, 108
Stevens, L. C. 121, 122
Stevens, N. 21
Stevens, R. A. 92
Stevens, R. E. 76
Stevenson, F. K. 240
Stevenson, G. T. 173, 240
Stevenson, T. D. 57
Steward, A. M. 107
Stewart, A. 22
Stewart, B. W. 20
Stewart, C. C. 221
Stewart, F. W. 30
Stewart, S. E. 24
Stewart, T. H. M. 104, 274
Stich, H. F. 24
Stidolph, N. E. 61
Stiffel, C. 200, 206
Stimpfling, J. H. 122
Stjernsward, J. 35, 51, 80, 82, 83, 91, 101, 103,
        104, 134, 152, 167, 190, 269
Stockert, E. 92, 112
Stocks, P. 17
Stoker, M. 25, 37, 40
Stolfi, R. L. 12
Stoll, H. L. 23
Stonehill, E. 108
Storb, R. 183, 234, 241
Stott, E. J. 124
Stott, H. 159
Stout, A. P. 24
Stout, R. D. 216
Stramignoni, A. 27
Straus, M. J. 67
Strauss, A. A. 235, 270
Strickland, R. G. 33
Strong, L. C. 10, 34
Strott, C. A. 71
Strouk, V. 93

Stuart, A. 258
Stuart, A. E. 84, 125, 180, 184, 185
Study Group for Bronchogenic Carcinoma 267
Stumpf, R. 137
Stutman, O. 139, 140, 141
Sugimura, T. 20
Suit, H. D. 93, 206, 207, 208, 210
Sullivan, P. W. 63
Summers, W. C. 65
Sumner, W. C. 51, 244
Sunderland, J. 31
Suter, R. B. 83
Sutherland, I. 151
Sutow, W. W. 160
Sutton, H. 31, 38, 76
Suvansri, U. 157
Suzanger, M. 270
Svec, J. 220
Svedmyr, E. 80
Svedmyr, E. A. J. 116
Svet-Moldavsky, G. J. 83, 91, 178
Svoboda, J. 91, 92, 170
Swann, P. F. 38
Swartzberg, J. E. 204
Swenberg, J. A. 27
Swift, W. Z. 52, 250
Sykes, J. 85
Sylvester, R. 5
Symes, M. O. 50, 83, 88, 113, 180, 181, 184, 185,
        243, 246
Symington, G. R. 143
Szymaniec, S. 49

T

Tachibana, T. 91, 98
Tada, T. 117
Takahashi, K. 48
Takahashi, M. 66
Takahashi, T. 111
Takasugi, M. 100, 101, 127, 132, 171
Takatsu, K. 82
Takeda, K. 91
Takemori, T. 117
Takeya, K. 139, 146
Takita, H. 82, 260, 274, 279
Taliaferro, W. H. 215
Talwar, G. P. 101
Tan, Y. H. 222
Tanaka, T. 48, 193, 194
Taniguchi, M. 117
Tannock, I. F. 50, 69
Taranger, L. A. 91